Apley and Solomon's

Concise System of Orthopaedics and Trauma

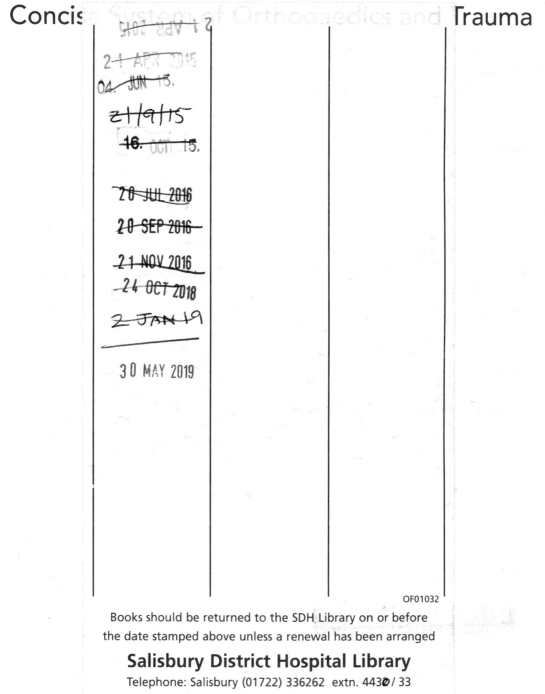

Apley and Solomon's Concise System of Orthopaedics and Trauma

FOURTH EDITION

Louis Solomon MB ChB MD FRCS FRCSEd
Emeritus Professor of Orthopaedic Surgery, University of Bristol, Bristol, UK

David Warwick MD FRCS FRCS(Orth) Eur Dip Hand Surg
Professor, University of Southampton and Consultant Hand Surgeon,
University Hospital Southampton, Southampton, UK

Selvadurai Nayagam BSc MCh(Orth) FRCS(Orth)
Consultant Orthopaedic Surgeon, Royal Liverpool Children's Hospital
and Royal Liverpool University Hospital, Liverpool, UK

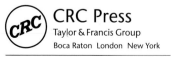

CRC Press
Taylor & Francis Group
Boca Raton London New York

CRC Press is an imprint of the
Taylor & Francis Group, an **informa** business

CRC Press
Taylor & Francis Group
6000 Broken Sound Parkway NW, Suite 300
Boca Raton, FL 33487-2742

© 2014 by Taylor & Francis Group, LLC
CRC Press is an imprint of Taylor & Francis Group, an Informa business

No claim to original U.S. Government works

Printed on acid-free paper
Version Date: 20140319

Printed and bound in India by Replika Press Pvt. Ltd.

International Standard Book Number-13: 978-1-4441-7431-1 (Paperback)
International Standard Book Number-13: 978-1-4822-6039-7 (International Students' Edition, restricted territorial availability)

Library of Congress Cataloging-in-Publication Data

Solomon, Louis, author.
  Apley's concise system of orthopaedics and fractures / Louis Solomon, David Warwick, Selvadurai Nayagam. -- Fourth edition.
     p. ; cm.
  Concise system of orthopaedics and fractures
  Based on (work): Apley's system of orthopaedics and fractures / Louis Solomon, David Warwick, Selvadurai Nayagam.
  Includes bibliographical references and index.
  ISBN 978-1-4441-7431-1 (pbk. : alk. paper)
  I. Warwick, David, 1962- author. II. Nayagam, Selvadurai, author. III. Solomon, Louis. Apley's system of orthopaedics and fractures. Digest of (work): IV. Title. V. Title: Concise system of orthopaedics and fractures.
  [DNLM: 1. Orthopedics--methods. 2. Fracture Fixation--methods. WE 168]

RD731
617.5--dc23   2014004724

Visit the Taylor & Francis Web site at
http://www.taylorandfrancis.com

and the CRC Press Web site at
http://www.crcpress.com

CONTENTS

PREFACE

Although the name of this new edition is slightly changed, we are confident that the Apley spirit has been kept alive. Yes, we are now able to perform tests and imaging studies that were unknown in years gone by, and true, there are now more shortcuts to diagnosis than before. Even so, the most useful and important tools to assist in an understanding of our patients and the management of their problems are our own hands and our clinical acumen. That has always been the focus of the book that arose out of Apley's teachings.

Why do we call it a System of orthopaedics and not simply a textbook? What Alan Apley had in mind when he set up his famous courses in orthopaedics almost 60 years ago was to imbue his listeners – the orthopaedic surgeons of the future – with not only the theory of this subject but also the clinical habits that would lead them to all the observations and connections from which they could construct a credible diagnosis and a reliable plan of treatment. *Look – Feel – Move* became not merely a mantra for those who had been at his classes but a constant reminder that diagnosis is more than inspired guesswork; it is the result of a systematic consideration of all the appearances and issues (the trivial as well as the obviously unusual) from which the alert mind will choose what is truly relevant. It is that approach that we have tried to preserve, however many clever instruments come into play during this repeatedly exciting enterprise.

As in previous editions, the book is divided into three parts: General Orthopaedics, comprises the main categories of clinical examination, special investigations and individual chapters on the most common groups of musculoskeletal disorders such as infection, arthritis, metabolic bone disease, developmental abnormalities, tumours, central neurological conditions and peripheral nerve disorders. This section ends with a chapter on the principles of operative orthopaedics and other methods commonly used in treating patients with musculoskeletal complaints.

The second part, Regional Orthopaedics, examines the specific manifestations and treatment of these conditions in each of the major bodily regions.

The third part, Fractures and Joint Injuries, covers the principles of trauma surgery. It begins with a chapter on the emergency management of the severely injured patient – a comprehensive review of the internationally accepted Advanced Trauma Life Support (ATLS) Program – followed by a chapter on the principles of fracture management, and then individual chapters on the management of fractures and dislocations in each anatomical region.

A hallmark of the book has been the liberal spread of 'on the spot' pictures and illustrations, culled from our clinical encounters during the last 50 years. The early authors were (and are) avid collectors of these real-life images, which together with their captions provide an instant summary of the accompanying text.

A question that crops up repeatedly is 'Which group of readers are we aiming at?' Most obviously medical students, trainees in orthopaedic surgery, and even their consultant teachers who want a concise review of subjects with which they are already familiar. Then many others as well: trainees in related surgical specialties; doctors and nurses working in accident and emergency units; experienced general practitioners; physiotherapists, occupational therapists and 'paramedics' who deal with physical abnormalities. Our hope is that they will enjoy these pages as much as we have enjoyed their preparation.

L.S.
D.W.
S.N.

PREFACE TO THE FIRST EDITION

For many years a course in orthopaedics and fractures, designed primarily for F.R.C.S. candidates, has been held at Pyrford. As the course grew and developed, so did the desire to cover the field as comprehensively as possible. Eventually, as a prophylactic against writer's cramp, lecture notes were issued. Re-written and amplified, these form the basis of the present book. The aim has been to prepare a text comprehensive enough for postgraduates, yet simple enough for undergraduates.

Many students, whether postgraduate or undergraduate, are not lacking in factual knowledge so much as in a methodical approach. The presentation used is designed to overcome this handicap and to inculcate method. Physical signs are described in a constant sequence throughout and, as far as possible, a standard system of headings is used both for orthopaedic disorders and for fractures.

In practice the same doctor usually deals with orthopaedics and with fractures; and rightly so, for they share many principles in common. Consequently a book dealing with both subjects may be appropriate and convenient. To this end brevity was important. I have tried to avoid wordiness and to present facts concisely. Illustrations have not been included; their value is not denied but, if the reader keeps the patient constantly in mind, and punctiliously follows the precept of 'LOOK, FEEL, MOVE', illustrations should not be indispensable. Their absence has been accepted as a challenge to provide unambiguous verbal descriptions instead.

The combination of method and compactness will, it is hoped, help the busy house surgeon, casualty officer, or the doctor who only occasionally practises orthopaedics, to find his way quickly in a large and complex subject.

In preparing this book I have leaned heavily on others. Many of their ideas have made such instant appeal that I have absorbed them and can no longer recall their source or adequately acknowledge my indebtedness. An immeasurable debt is, however, due to my teacher George Perkins, whose influence has, I hope, pervaded both my work and my teaching.

On many occasions I have sought the help of my colleague Mr. F. A. Simmonds, who has never failed to give sound advice. I am greatly indebted to Dr. I. Churchill-Davidson for his ungrudging and detailed help in writing the sections on radiotherapy. Mr. Gordon Hadfield read through the entire text and his many valuable suggestions are deeply appreciated. It is a pleasure to pay tribute to the diligence and skill of my secretary, Miss L. Freeland, and to acknowledge the constructive suggestions and friendly co-operation of the publishers.

A. Graham Apley
January 1959

CONTRIBUTORS

PRINCIPAL AUTHORS

Louis Solomon MB ChB MD FRCS FRCSEd
Emeritus Professor of Orthopaedic Surgery
University of Bristol
Bristol, UK

David Warwick MD FRCS FRCS(Orth) Eur
Dip Hand Surg
Professor, University of Southampton
Southampton, UK

Consultant Hand Surgeon
University Hospital Southampton
Southampton, UK

Selvadurai Nayagam BSc MCh(Orth)
FRCS(Orth)
Consultant Orthopaedic Surgeon
Royal Liverpool Children's Hospital and Royal
Liverpool University Hospital
Liverpool, UK

ADDITIONAL AUTHORS

Gavin W. Bowyer MChir FRCS(Orth)
Consultant Trauma and Orthopaedic Surgeon
University Hospital Southampton
Southampton, UK

Gorav Datta MD FRCS(Tr + Orth)
Consultant Trauma and Orthopaedic Surgeon
University Hospital Southampton
Southampton, UK

Nick Hancock MBChB FRCS(Tr + Orth)
Consultant Trauma and Orthopaedic Surgeon
University Hospital Southampton
Southampton, UK

Max Jonas MB BS FRCA
Consultant and Senior Lecturer in Critical Care
University Hospital Southampton
Southampton, UK

Amir Ali Qureshi FRCS(Tr + Orth) MRCS
MBBCh
Consultant Trauma and Orthopaedic Surgeon
University Hospital Southampton
Southampton, UK

David Sutton BM DA FRCA
Consultant Anaesthetist
University Hospital Southampton Major Trauma
Centre
Southampton, UK

Pre-Hospital Emergency Physician
South Central Ambulance Service

Clinical Governance Lead
Hampshire and Isle of Wight Air Ambulance

ACKNOWLEDGEMENTS

Advances in medical research and practice during the last two decades have led to ever greater specialization and the need for multi-authorship in modern textbooks. The Apley System was no exception: the 9th edition of the main textbook, published 2 years ago, sported three Principal Authors and 24 Contributing Authors. They were duly acknowledged in that edition and we express our gratitude to them again with the appearance of this new 4th edition of the concise version which is based on the more advanced publication.

In addition we have enlisted six new Contributing Authors whose remit has been an up-dating of specific chapters in the present *Concise System*; they are listed in the front pages and we extend to them our sincere thanks for filling the gaps in our earlier presentations. Although they would not have known Alan Apley and his inimitable teaching style, they have fitted into our authorial team splendidly.

No textbook would see the light of day without the help of their Publishing Editors and Copy Editors. We have had the good fortune to work with Dr Joanna Koster, Publisher at CRC Press (Taylor & Francis Group), and our eagle-eyed Copy Editors Kate Nardoni and Ruth Maxwell at Cactus Design. We pay them our sincere thanks. Thanks also to Dr Allen Zimbler, passionate collector of antiquarian books, for tracing a fine copy of the 1st Edition.

We never forget that writing a textbook is not a single-handed job. Behind the persons pounding the computer keys there are our partners and families: some take part in organizing the work, some offer helpful comments, others offer a ready ear to listen to the problems that beset every author, all of them endure the long periods of silence around us the writers. We can never thank them enough for the many ways in which they help us in our somewhat selfish endeavours.

Finally, we owe a huge debt of gratitude to the many patients who have allowed us to intrude upon their suffering and use their stories to populate our book.

L.S.
D.W.
S.N.

ABBREVIATIONS

1,25-DHCC	1,25-dihydroxycholecalciferol
25-HCC	25-hydroxycholecalciferol
^{99m}Tc-HDP	^{99m} technetium hydroxymethylene diphosphonate
ABG	arterial blood gas
ACL	anterior cruciate ligament
ACTH	adrenocorticotropic hormone
AIDS	acquired immunodeficiency syndrome
ALS	advanced life support
AP	anteroposterior
APC	anteroposterior compression
APPT	activated partial thromboplastin time
ARDS	acute respiratory distress syndrome
ATLS	Advanced Trauma Life Support
AVN	avascular necrosis
BCP	basic calcium phosphate
BMD	bone mineral density
BMP	bone morphogenetic protein
BSA	body surface area
BVM	bag–valve–mask
(anti-) CCP	(anti-)cyclic citrullinated peptide (antibody)
CE	centre–edge (angle)
CMC	carpometacarpal
CNS	central nervous system
CPPD	calcium pyrophosphate dihydrate
CRP	C-reactive protein
CSF	cerebrospinal fluid
CT	computed tomography
CVP	central venous pressure
DDH	developmental dysplasia of the hip
DEXA	dual-energy x-ray absorptiometry
DIP	distal interphalangeal
DISI	dorsal intercalated segment instability
DMARD	disease-modifying antirheumatic drug
DNA	deoxyribonucleic acid
DVT	deep vein thrombosis
ECG	electrocardiography
EDS	Ehlers–Danlos syndrome
EDF	elongation–derotation–flexion
EMG	electromyography

ESR	erythrocyte sedimentation rate
$EtCO_2$	end-tidal carbon dioxide
FAI	femoroacetabular impingement
FAST	Focussed Assessment Sonography for Trauma
FDP	flexor digitorum profundus
FDS	flexor digitorum superficialis
FPE	fatal pulmonary embolism
GAG	glycosaminoglycan
GCS	Glasgow Coma Score
HIV	human immunodeficiency virus
HLA	human leucocyte antigen
HMSN	hereditary motor and sensory neuropathy
HRT	hormone replacement therapy
ICP	intracerebral pressure
ICU	intensive care unit
Ig	immunoglobulin
IL	interleukin
INR	international normalized ratio
IO	intraosseous
IP	interphalangeal
IV	intravenous
JIA	juvenile idiopathic arthritis
LC	lateral compression
LCL	lateral collateral ligament
LMA	laryngeal mask airway
LMN	lower motor neuron
MBC	minimum bactericidal concentration
MCL	medial collateral ligament
MCP	metacarpophalangeal
MED	multiple epiphyseal dysplasia
MHC	major histocompatibility complex
MIC	minimum inhibitory concentration
MODS	multiple organ failure or dysfunction syndrome
MPFL	medial patellofemoral ligament
MPS	mucopolysaccharidoses
MRI	magnetic resonance imaging
MRSA	methicillin-resistant *Staphylococcus aureus*
MTP	metatarsophalangeal
NF	neurofibromatosis

NP	nasopharyngeal	RF	rheumatoid factor
NSAID	non-steroidal anti-inflammatory drug	RICE	rest, ice, compression and elevation
		RSI	rapid sequence intubation
OA	osteoarthritis	SED	spondyloepiphyseal dyplasia
OAF	osteoclast-activating factor	SIJ	sacroiliac joint
OI	osteogenesis imperfecta	SLAP	superior part of the glenoid
OP	oropharyngeal		labrum anteriorly and posteriorly
PA	posteroanterior	TB	tuberculosis
$PaCO_2$	arterial carbon dioxide tension	TFCC	tears of the triangular
PaO_2	arterial oxygen tension		fibrocartilage complex
PCL	posterior cruciate ligament	TNF	tumour necrosis factor
PE	pulmonary embolism	UMN	upper motor neuron
PEA	pulseless electrical activity	VISI	volar intercalated segment
PET	positron emission tomography		instability
PIP	proximal interphalangeal	VP	ventriculoperitoneal
PNS	peripheral nervous system	V/Q	ventilation–perfusion
PPE	personal protective equipment	VS	vertical shear
PTH	parathyroid hormone	VTE	venous thromboembolism
PVNS	pigmented villonodular synovitis	WBC	white blood cell
RA	rheumatoid arthritis	WHO	World Health Organization

PART 1

GENERAL ORTHOPAEDICS

DIAGNOSIS IN ORTHOPAEDICS

'Information consists of differences that make a difference'
Gregory Bateson

Diagnosis begins with the systematic gathering of information – from the patient's history, the physical examination, x-ray appearances and special investigations. It should, however, never be forgotten that every orthopaedic disorder is part of a larger whole – a patient who has a unique personality, a job and hobbies, a family and a home; all have a bearing upon, and are in turn affected by, the disorder and its treatment.

HISTORY

'Taking a history' is a misnomer. The patient tells a story; it is we the listeners who construct a history. The story may be maddeningly disorganized; the history has to be systematic. Carefully and patiently compiled, it can be every bit as informative as examination or laboratory tests.

As we record it, certain key words will inevitably stand out: *injury, pain, stiffness, swelling, deformity, instability, weakness, altered sensibility* and *loss of function*. Each symptom is pursued for more detail: we need to know when it began, whether suddenly or gradually, spontaneously or after some specific event; how it has changed or progressed; what makes it worse; what makes it better.

While listening, we consider if the story fits some pattern that we recognize, for we are already thinking of a diagnosis. Every piece of information should be thought of as part of a larger picture which gradually unfolds in our understanding. The surgeon-philosopher Wilfred Trotter (1870–1939) put it well: '*Disease reveals itself in casual parentheses*'.

SYMPTOMS

Pain

Pain is the most common symptom. Its precise location is important, so ask the patient to point to where it hurts. But don't assume that the site of pain is always the site of pathology; 'referred' pain and 'autonomic' pain can be very deceptive.

Referred pain

Pain arising in or near the skin is usually localized accurately. Pain arising in deep structures is more diffuse and is sometimes of unexpected distribution; thus, hip disease may manifest with pain in the knee (so might an obturator hernia!). This is not because sensory nerves connect the two sites; it is due to inability of the cerebral cortex to distinguish between sensory messages from embryologically related sites (see Fig 1.1).

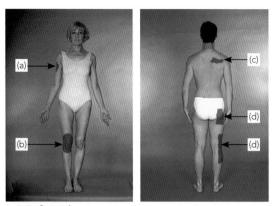

1.1 Referred pain Common sites of referred pain:
(a) from the shoulder; (b) from the hip; (c) from the neck;
(d) from the lumbar spine.

Autonomic pain

Pain that does not fit the usual pattern is often dismissed as 'inappropriate' (i.e. psychologically determined). But pain can also affect the autonomic nerves that accompany the peripheral blood vessels and this is much more vague, more widespread and often associated with vasomotor and trophic changes. It is poorly understood, often doubted, but nonetheless real.

Stiffness

Stiffness may be generalized (typically in rheumatoid arthritis and ankylosing spondylitis) or localized to a particular joint. Patients often have difficulty distinguishing stiffness from painful movement; limited movement should never be assumed until verified by examination.

Ask when it occurs: regular early morning stiffness of many joints is one of the cardinal features of rheumatoid arthritis, whereas transient stiffness of one or two joints after periods of inactivity is typical of osteoarthritis.

'*Locking*' is a term used to describe the sudden inability to complete a certain movement; it suggests a mechanical block, e.g. due to a loose body or a torn meniscus becoming trapped between the articular surfaces. Unfortunately, patients use the term for any painful limitation of movement; much more reliable is a history of 'unlocking' when the offending body suddenly moves out of the way.

Swelling

Swelling may be in the soft tissues, the joint or the bone; to the patient they are all the same. It is important to establish whether the swelling followed an injury, whether it appeared rapidly (probably a haematoma or a haemarthrosis) or slowly (soft-tissue inflammation or a joint effusion), whether it is painful (acute inflammation, infection – or a tumour!), whether it is constant or comes and goes and, most importantly, whether it is increasing in size.

Deformity

The common deformities are well described in terms such as round shoulders, spinal curvature, knock-knees, bow-legs, pigeon-toes and flat-feet. Some 'deformities' are merely variations of the normal (e.g. short stature or wide hips); others disappear spontaneously with growth (e.g. flat feet or bandy legs in an infant). However, if the deformity is progressive, or if it appears on only one side of the body, it may be serious.

Weakness

Generalized weakness is a feature of all chronic illness and any prolonged joint dysfunction will inevitably lead to weakness of the associated muscles. However, weakness affecting a single group of muscles suggests a more specific neurological disorder. Try to establish precisely which movements are affected; this may give an important clue to the site of the lesion.

Instability

The patient complains that the joint 'gives way' or 'jumps out'. If this happens repeatedly it suggests ligamentous deficiency, recurrent subluxation or some internal derangement such as a loose body.

Change in sensibility

Tingling or numbness signifies interference with nerve function: pressure from a neighbouring structure (e.g. a prolapsed intervertebral disc), local ischaemia (e.g. nerve entrapment in a fibro-osseous

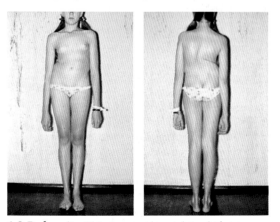

1.2 Deformity This young girl complained of a prominent right hip; the real deformity was scoliosis.

tunnel) or a peripheral neuropathy. It is important to establish its exact distribution; from this we can tell whether the fault lies in a peripheral nerve or in a nerve root.

Loss of function

Functional disability is more than the sum of individual symptoms and its expression depends upon the needs of the patient. The patient may say 'I can't sit for long' rather than 'I have backache', or 'I can't put my socks on' rather than 'my hip is stiff'. Moreover, what to one patient is merely inconvenient may, to another, be incapacitating. Thus a lawyer or a teacher may readily tolerate a stiff knee provided it is painless and does not impair walking; but to a plumber, the same disorder might spell economic disaster.

PREVIOUS DISORDERS

Patients should always be asked about previous accidents, illnesses, operations and drug therapy. They may give vital clues to the present disorder.

FAMILY HISTORY

Patients often wonder (and worry) about inheriting a disease or passing it on to their children. To the doctor, information about musculoskeletal disorders in the patient's family may help with both diagnosis and counselling.

SOCIAL BACKGROUND

No history is complete without enquiry about the patient's background: details about work, travel, recreation, home circumstances and the level of support from family and friends. These always impinge on the assessment of disability; occasionally a particular activity (at work, on the sports field or in the kitchen) is responsible for the entire condition.

EXAMINATION

In Conan Doyle's story 'A Case of Identity', Sherlock Holmes has the following conversation with Dr Watson:

Watson: You appeared to read a good deal upon [your client] which was quite invisible to me.
Holmes: Not invisible but unnoticed, Watson.

Some disorders can be diagnosed at a glance: who would mistake the facies of acromegaly or the hand deformities of rheumatoid arthritis for anything else? Nevertheless, even in these cases a systematic approach is rewarding; it provides information about the patient's particular disability, it keeps reinforcing good habits and the patient feels that he or she has been properly attended to.

The examination actually begins from the moment we set eyes on the patient. We observe his or her general appearance, posture and gait. Are they walking freely or do they use a stick? Are they in pain? Do their movements look natural? Can you spot any distinctive features immediately: a characteristic facial appearance; a spinal curvature; a short limb; any type of asymmetry? He or she may have a tell-tale gait suggesting a painful hip, an unstable knee or a foot-drop. The clues are endless and the game is played by everyone (qualified or lay) at each new encounter throughout life. In the clinical setting the assessment needs to be more focused.

When we proceed to the structured examination, the patient must be suitably undressed; no mere rolling up of a trouser leg is sufficient. If one limb is affected, both must be exposed so that they can be compared.

We examine first the good limb, then the bad. The student is often inclined to rush in with both hands – a temptation that must be resisted. Only by proceeding in a purposeful, orderly way can we avoid missing important signs. The system we normally use is simple but comprehensive: first we *look,* then we *feel* and then we *move*. Thereafter we may add *special manoeuvres* to assess neurological integrity or test for joint instability.

Obviously the sequence may sometimes have to be changed because a patient is in pain or severely disabled; you would not try to 'move' a limb with a suspected fracture when an x-ray can provide the answer. Furthermore, resuscitation will always take priority and in severely injured patients the detailed local examination may have to be curtailed or deferred.

- Look
  - First at the patient's general shape, posture and gait, noting any obvious deformity;
  - Then, with noteworthy areas suitably exposed, at the skin: are there any old scars?
  - Then at the local shape: is there swelling, wasting, a lump or some local deformity?
  - Then at the local posture: nerve lesions may cause characteristic changes in normal posture.

- Feel
  - The skin: is it warm or cold; moist or dry; and is sensation normal?
  - The soft tissues: is there a lump and where does it arise? Are the pulses normal?

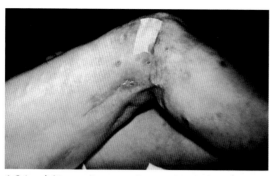

1.3 Look Scars often give clues to the previous history. The faded scar on this patient's thigh is an old operation wound – internal fixation of a femoral fracture. The other scars are due to postoperative infection; one of the sinuses is still draining.

- The bones and joints: are the outlines normal? Is there excessive fluid in the joint?
- Tenderness: if you know precisely *where* the trouble is, you're halfway to knowing *what* it is.

■ Move
- *Active movement*: ask the patient to move the joint and test for power.
- *Passive movement*: here it is the examiner who moves the joint in each anatomical plane. The range of movement should be expressed in degrees, starting from zero which is the neutral or anatomical position of the joint. Note whether movement is painful and whether it is associated with crepitus.
- *Abnormal movement*: is the joint unstable?

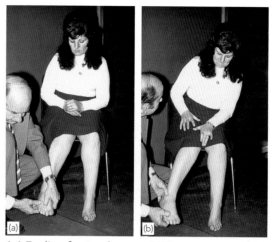

1.4 Feeling for tenderness (a) The wrong way – there is no need to look at your fingers, you should know where they are. (b) It is much more informative to look at the patient's face!

■ Special manoeuvres
- Special tests for conditions such as joint instability are described in the relevant chapters. One of the most telling clues to diagnosis is reproducing the patient's symptoms by applying a specific, *provocative movement*. Shoulder pain due to impingement of the subacromial structures may be 'provoked' by moving the joint in a way that is calculated to produce such impingement; the patient recognizes the similarity between this pain and his or her daily symptoms. Likewise, a patient who has

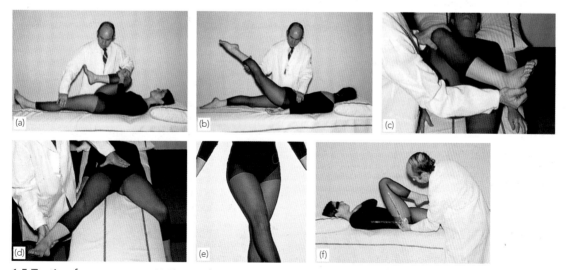

1.5 Testing for movement (a) Flexion; (b) extension; (c) rotation; (d) abduction; (e) adduction. The range of movement can be estimated by eye or measured accurately using a goniometer (f).

had a previous dislocation can be so vividly reminded of that event, by stressing the joint in a way that it again threatens to dislocate, that he or she goes rigid with anxiety at the anticipated result – this is aptly called the *apprehension test*.

TERMINOLOGY

Bodily surfaces, planes and positions are described in relation to the anatomical position: standing erect, facing the viewer, legs together with the knees pointing directly forwards and arms held by the sides with the palms facing forwards.

The principal planes of the body are named *sagittal*, *coronal* and *transverse*; they define the direction across which the body (or body part) is viewed in any description. Sagittal planes, parallel to each other, pass vertically through the body from front to back; the midsagittal or median plane divides the body into right and left halves. Coronal planes are also orientated vertically, corresponding to a frontal view, at right angles to the sagittal planes; transverse planes pass horizontally across the body.

Anterior (or *ventral*) signifies the frontal aspect and *posterior* (or *dorsal*) the rear aspect of the body or a body part. In the foot the upper surface is called the *dorsum* and the sole is called the *plantar* surface.

Medial means facing towards the midline of the body and *lateral* away from the midline. These terms are usually applied to a limb, the clavicle or one half of the pelvis. Thus the inner aspect of the thigh lies on the medial side of the limb and the outer part of the thigh lies on the lateral side. We could also say that the little finger lies on the medial or ulnar side of the hand and the thumb on the lateral or radial side of the hand.

Proximal and *distal* are used mainly for parts of the limbs, meaning respectively the upper end and the lower end as they appear in the anatomical position. Thus the knee joint is formed by the distal end of the femur and the proximal end of the tibia.

The longitudinal arrangements of adjacent limb segments are also named: the knees and elbows, for example, are normally angulated slightly outwards (*valgus*) while the opposite – 'bow-legs' – is more correctly described as *varus*. Tortile arrangements of segments of a long bone (or an entire limb) are named *lateral* (or *external*) rotation and *medial* (or *internal*) *rotation*. *Pronation* and *supination* are also rotatory movements, but the terms are applied only to movements of the forearm and the foot.

Flexion and *extension* are joint movements in the sagittal plane, most easily imagined in hinge joints like the knee, the elbow and the joints of the fingers and toes. Flexion means bending the joint and extension means straightening it. In the ankle flexion is also called *plantarflexion* (pointing the foot downwards) and extension is called *dorsiflexion* (drawing the foot upwards).

Abduction and *adduction* are movements in the coronal plane, away from or towards the midline. Not quite for the fingers and toes, though: here abduction and adduction mean away from and towards the longitudinal midline of the hand or foot!

Specialized movements, such as opposition of the thumb, lateral flexion and rotation of the spine and inversion or eversion of the foot, will be described in the relevant chapters.

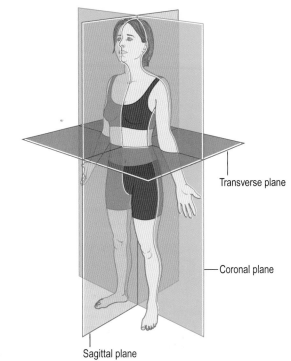

1.6 The principal planes of the body Diagram showing planes as viewed in the anatomical position: sagittal, coronal and transverse.

NEUROLOGICAL EXAMINATION

If the symptoms include weakness or inco-ordination or a change in sensibility, or if they point to any disorder of the neck or back, a complete neurological examination of the related part is mandatory.

Once again we follow a systematic routine, first looking at the general appearance, then assessing motor function (muscle tone, power and reflexes) and finally testing for sensory function (both skin sensibility and deep sensibility). See Chapter 10 for further details.

Appearance

Some neurological disorders result in postures that are so characteristic as to be almost diagnostic: e.g. the claw hand of an ulnar nerve lesion or a drop-wrist due to radial nerve palsy. Usually, however, it is when the patient moves that we can best appreciate the type and extent of motor disorder; e.g. the 'spastic' movement of cerebral palsy and the flaccid posture of a lower motor neuron lesion.

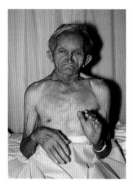

1.7 Posture Posture is often diagnostic. This patient's 'drop-wrist' – typical of a radial nerve palsy – is due to carcinomatous infiltration of the supraclavicular lymph nodes on the right.

Concentrating on the affected part, we look for trophic changes that signify loss of sensibility: the smooth, hairless skin that seems to be stretched too tight; atrophy of the fingertips and the nails; scars that tell of accidental burns; and ulcers that refuse to heal. Muscle wasting is rapidly assessed by comparing the two limbs.

Tone and power

Tone in individual muscle groups is tested by moving the nearby joint to stretch the muscle. Increased tone (spasticity) is characteristic of upper motor neuron disorders such as cerebral palsy and stroke. It must not be confused with rigidity (the 'lead-pipe' or 'cogwheel' effect) which is seen in Parkinson's disease. Decreased tone (flaccidity) is found in lower motor neuron lesions such as poliomyelitis. Muscle power is diminished in all three states; it is important to recognize that a 'spastic' muscle may still be weak.

Testing for power is not as easy as it sounds; the difficulty is making ourselves understood. The simplest way is to place the limb in the 'test' position, then ask the patient to hold it there as firmly as possible and resist any attempt by you,

the examiner, to change that position. The normal limb is examined first, then the affected limb and the two are compared. Finer muscle actions, such as those of the thumb and fingers, may be reproduced by first demonstrating the movement yourself, then testing it in the unaffected limb and then in the affected one. Muscle power is usually graded on the Medical Research Council scale.

We can also assess the patient's ability to perform complex movements by asking him or her to perform specific tasks, such as gripping a rod, holding a pen, doing up a button or picking up a pin.

Muscle power: Medical Research Council grading
■ Grade 0 No movement
■ Grade 1 Only a flicker of movement
■ Grade 2 Movement with gravity eliminated
■ Grade 3 Movement against gravity
■ Grade 4 Movement against resistance
■ Grade 5 Normal power

Tendon reflexes

A deep tendon reflex is elicited by rapidly stretching the tendon near its insertion. A sharp tap with the tendon hammer does this well; but all too often this is performed with a flourish and with such force that the finer gradations of response are missed. It is better to employ a series of taps, starting with the most forceful and reducing the force with each successive tap until there is no response. Comparing the two sides in this way, we can pick up fine differences showing that a reflex is 'diminished' rather than 'absent'. In the upper limb we test biceps, triceps and brachioradialis; and in the lower limb the patellar ligament and Achilles tendon.

The tendon reflexes are monosynaptic segmental reflexes; that is, the reflex pathway takes a 'short cut' through the spinal cord at the segmental level. Depression or absence of the reflex signifies interruption at some point along this pathway. It is a reliable pointer to the segmental level of dysfunction. An unusually brisk reflex, on the other hand, is characteristic of an upper motor neuron disorder (e.g. cerebral palsy, a stroke or injury to the spinal cord); the lower motor neuron is released from the normal central inhibition and there is an exaggerated response to tendon stimulation.

Superficial reflexes

The superficial reflexes are elicited by stroking the skin at various sites to produce a specific muscle contraction; the best known are the abdominal (T7–T12), cremasteric (L1, 2) and anal (S4, 5) reflexes. These are corticospinal (upper motor neuron) reflexes. Absence of the reflex indicates an upper motor neuron lesion (usually in the spinal cord) above that level.

The plantar reflex

Forceful stroking of the sole normally produces flexion of the toes (or no response at all). An extensor response (the big toe extends while the others remain in flexion) is characteristic of upper motor neuron disorders. This is the Babinski sign – a type of withdrawal reflex which is present in young infants and normally disappears after the age of 18 months.

Sensibility

Sensibility to touch and to pinprick may be increased (*hyperaesthesia*) or unpleasant (*dysaesthesia*) in certain irritative nerve lesions. More often, though, it is diminished (*hypoaesthesia*) or absent (*anaesthesia*), signifying pressure on or interruption of a peripheral nerve, a nerve root or the sensory pathways in the spinal cord. The area of sensory change can be mapped out on the skin and compared with the known segmental or dermatomal pattern of innervation (see Figure 10.4). If the abnormality is well defined it is an easy matter to establish the level of the lesion, even if the precise cause remains unknown.

Brisk percussion along the course of an injured nerve may elicit a tingling sensation in the distal distribution of the nerve (*Tinel's sign*). The point of hypersensitivity marks the site of abnormal nerve sprouting: if it progresses distally at successive visits this signifies regeneration; if it remains unchanged this suggests a local neuroma.

Tests for *temperature recognition* and *two-point discrimination* (the ability to recognize two touch-points a few millimetres apart) are sometimes used in the assessment of peripheral nerve disorders.

Deep sensibility can be examined in several ways. In the vibration test a sounded tuning-fork is placed over a peripheral bony point (e.g. the medial malleolus or the head of the ulna); the patient is asked if he or she can feel the vibrations and to say when they disappear. By comparing the two sides, differences can be noted. Position sense is tested by asking the patient to find certain points on the body with the eyes closed – for example, touching the tip of the nose with the forefinger. The sense of joint posture is tested by grasping the big toe and placing it in different positions of flexion and extension. The patient is asked to say whether it is 'up' or 'down'. Stereognosis, the ability to recognize shape and texture by feel alone, is tested by giving the patient (whose eyes are closed) a variety of familiar objects to hold and asking him or her to name each object.

The pathways for deep sensibility run in the posterior columns of the spinal cord. Disturbances are, therefore, found in peripheral neuropathies and in spinal cord lesions such as posterior column injuries or tabes dorsalis. The sense of balance is also carried in the posterior columns. This can be tested by asking the patient to stand upright with his or her eyes closed; excessive body sway is abnormal (*Romberg's sign*).

Cortical and cerebellar function

A staggering gait may imply drunkenness, an unstable knee or a disorder of the spinal cord or cerebellum. If there is no musculoskeletal abnormality to account for the sign, a full examination of the central nervous system will be necessary.

EXAMINING INFANTS AND CHILDREN

Paediatric practice requires special skills. You may have no first-hand account of the symptoms; a baby screaming with pain will tell you very little and over-anxious parents will probably tell you too much. When examining the child, you should be flexible. If he or she is moving a particular joint, take your opportunity to examine movement then and there. You will learn much more by adopting methods of play than by applying a rigid system of examination. And leave any test for tenderness until last!

Infants and small children

The baby should be undressed, in a warm room and placed on the examining couch. Look carefully for birthmarks, deformities and abnormal movements – or absence of movement. If there is no urgency or distress, take time to examine the head and neck, including facial features which may be characteristic of specific dysplastic syndromes. The back and limbs are then examined for abnormalities of position or shape. Examining for joint movement can be difficult. Active movements can often be stimulated by gently stroking the limb. When testing for passive mobility, be careful to avoid frightening or hurting the child.

In the neonate and throughout the first 2 years of life, examination of the hips is mandatory, even if the child appears to be normal. This is to avoid missing the subtle signs of developmental dysplasia of the hips (DDH) at the early stage when treatment is most effective.

It is also important to assess the child's general development by testing for the normal milestones which are expected to appear during the first 2 years of life.

Normal developmental milestones	
Newborn:	*Grasp reflex*: the infant will grasp the examiner's finger. *Morrow reflex*: slapping the couch causes the infant to reach arms out and move the legs about. *Tonic neck reflex*: if the baby's head is suddenly turned to one side, the elbow and knee on that side will be flexed and the opposite arm and leg extended.
4 months:	Newborn reflexes should disappear by 4 months.
6–12 months:	*Landau reflex*: when the child is held prone the head, back and lower limbs are involuntarily extended.
3–6 months:	Infant can hold the head up unsupported.
6–9 months:	Able to sit up.
9–12 months:	Crawling and standing up.
9–18 months:	Walking.
18–24 months:	Running.

Older children

Most children can be examined in the same way as adults, though with different emphasis on particular physical features. Posture and gait are very important; subtle deviations from the norm may herald the appearance of serious abnormalities such as scoliosis or neuromuscular disorders, while more obvious 'deformities' such as knock-knees and bow-legs may be no more than transient stages in normal development, similarly with mild degrees of 'flat-feet' and 'pigeon-toes'. More complex variations in posture and gait patterns, when the child sits and walks with the knees turned inwards (medially rotated) or outwards (laterally rotated),

are usually due to anteversion or retroversion of the femoral necks, sometimes associated with compensatory rotational 'deformities' of the femora and tibiae. Seldom need anything be done about this; the condition usually improves as the child approaches puberty and only if the gait is very awkward would one consider performing corrective osteotomies of the femora.

VARIATIONS AND DEFORMITIES

The word 'deformity' is derived from the Latin for 'misshapen', but the range of normality is so wide that variations should not automatically be designated as deformities and some undoubted 'deformities' are not necessarily pathological; for example, the generally accepted cut-off points for 'abnormal' shortness or tallness are arbitrary and people who in one population might be considered abnormally short or abnormally tall could, in other populations, be seen as quite ordinary. However, if one leg is short and the other long, noone would quibble with the use of the word 'deformity'! In any particular case, an assessment of 'deformity' will also depend on additional factors, such as the extent to which the appearance deviates from the norm, any symptoms to which it gives rise and the degree to which it interferes with function.

Postural deformity is something which the patient can, if properly instructed, correct voluntarily: e.g. a 'round back' due to slumped shoulders. However, a postural deformity may also be caused by temporary muscle spasm.

Structural deformity results from a permanent change in anatomical structure which cannot be voluntarily corrected.

'*Fixed deformity*' seems to mean that a joint is deformed and unable to move. Not so – it means that one particular movement cannot be completed. Thus the knee may be able to flex fully but not extend fully – at the limit of its extension it is still 'fixed' in a certain amount of flexion. This would be called a 'fixed flexion deformity'.

Varus and valgus

It may seem pedantic to replace 'bow-legs' and 'knock-knees' with '*genu varum*'and '*genu valgum*'. But comparable colloquialisms are not available for deformities of other joints and, besides, the formality is justified by the need for clarity and consistency. *Varus* means that the part distal to the apex of the deformity is displaced towards the midline, *valgus* away from the midline (see Fig 1.8).

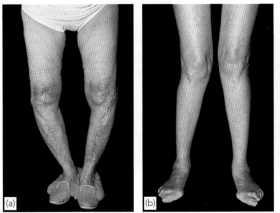
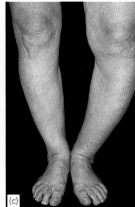

1.8 Varus and valgus (a) Varus knees due to osteoarthritis; (b) valgus deformity in rheumatoid arthritis; (c) another varus knee? No – the deformity here is in the tibia, due to Paget's disease.

Kyphosis and lordosis

Seen from the side, the normal spine has a series of curves – *convex* posteriorly in the dorsal region (*kyphosis*) and *concave* posteriorly in the cervical and lumbar regions (*lordosis*). Abnormally marked curvature constitutes a kyphotic or lordotic deformity (also sometimes referred to as *hyperkyphosis* and *hyperlordosis*).

Scoliosis

Seen from behind, the spine is straight. Any curvature in this (coronal) plane is called *scoliosis*. It is important to distinguish *postural scoliosis* from *structural* (*fixed*) *scoliosis*: the former is non-progressive and benign; the latter is usually progressive and may require treatment.

COMMON CAUSES OF DEFORMITY

In joints

- *Contracture of the overlying skin.* Typically with severe scarring across the flexor aspect of a joint.
- *Contracture of the subcutaneous fascia.* The classical example is Dupuytren's contracture in the palm of the hand.
- *Muscle contracture.* Fibrosis and contracture of muscles that cross a joint will cause a fixed deformity of the joint. This may be due to deep infection or fibrosis following ischaemic necrosis (Volkmann's ischaemic contracture).
- *Muscle imbalance.* Unbalanced muscle weakness or spasticity will result in joint deformity which, if not corrected, will eventually become fixed. This is seen typically in poliomyelitis and cerebral palsy.
- *Joint instability.* An unstable joint may look 'deformed' when force is applied.
- *Joint destruction.* Trauma, infection or arthritis may lead to severe deformity.

In bones

- *Genetic or developmental disorders.* Deformities can sometimes be diagnosed *in utero* (e.g. achondroplasia); some become apparent as the child grows (e.g. hereditary multiple exostosis) and some only in adulthood (e.g. multiple epiphyseal dysplasia).
- *Rickets* (in children) and *osteomalacia* (in adults) affect the entire skeleton.
- *Injuries involving the physis may result in asymmetrical growth*; the deformity emerges as the bone elongates.
- *Malunited fractures* can occur at any age.
- *Paget's disease* affects older people.
- *Postoperative iatrogenic deformity* should also be kept in mind.

BONY LUMPS

A bony lump may be due to faulty development, injury, inflammation or a tumour. Although x-ray examination is essential, the clinical features can be highly informative.

- *Size*: a lump attached to bone, or a lump which is getting bigger, is nearly always a tumour.
- *Site*: a lump at the metaphysis is most likely to be a tumour; a lump in the diaphysis may be fracture callus, inflammatory new bone or a tumour.
- *Shape*: a benign tumour has a well-defined margin; malignant tumours, inflammatory lumps and callus have an ill-defined edge.
- *Consistency*: benign tumours feel bony hard; a malignant tumour often feels spongy.
- *Tenderness*: marked tenderness suggests an inflammatory lesion, infection or perhaps even a malignant tumour.

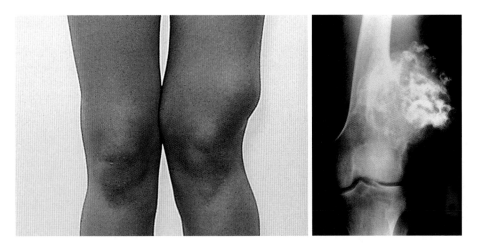

1.9 Bony lumps The lump above the left knee is hard, well defined and not increasing in size. The clinical diagnosis of cartilage-capped exostosis (osteochondroma) is confirmed by the x-rays.

- *Multiplicity*: multiple bony lumps are uncommon: they occur in hereditary multiple exostosis and in Ollier's disease.

STIFF JOINTS

It is convenient to distinguish three grades of joint stiffness:

- *All movements absent*: surgical fusion of a joint is called arthrodesis; pathological fusion is called ankylosis. Acute suppurative arthritis typically ends in bony ankylosis; tuberculous arthritis often heals by fibrosis and causes fibrous ankylosis.
- *All movements limited*: restriction of movement in all directions is characteristic of non-infective arthritis and is usually due to synovial swelling or capsular fibrosis.
- *One or two movements limited*: limitation of movement in some directions with full movement in others suggests a mechanical block or joint contracture.

LAX JOINTS

Generalized joint hypermobility occurs in about 5% of people and is familial. Hypermobile joints are not necessarily unstable – as witness the controlled performances of acrobats and gymnasts – but they do have a tendency to recurrent dislocation (e.g. of the shoulder or patella).

Severe joint laxity is a feature of certain rare connective tissue disorders such as Marfan's syndrome and osteogenesis imperfecta.

DIAGNOSTIC IMAGING

PLAIN FILM RADIOGRAPHY

Despite the remarkable technical advances of recent years, plain film x-ray examination remains the most useful method of diagnostic imaging. Whereas other methods may define some tissues and anatomical structures more accurately, the plain film provides information simultaneously on the size, shape, tissue 'density' and bone architecture – characteristics which, taken together, will usually suggest a diagnosis, or at least a range of possible diagnoses.

The radiographic image

Radiographic images are produced by the attenuation of x-rays as they pass through intervening tissues before striking an appropriately sensitized plate or film. The more dense and impenetrable the tissue, the greater the attenuation and therefore the more blank, or white, the image in the film. Thus, a metal implant appears intensely white, bone less so and soft tissues in varying shades of grey depending on their 'density'. Cartilage, which causes little attenuation, appears as a dark area between adjacent bone ends.

It is important to appreciate that these are two-dimensional images. Thus, if one image (say that of a bullet) is seen to be superimposed upon another (say that of a bone), it is impossible to tell whether the bullet is lying in front of the bone, behind the bone or inside the bone – unless you have another view of the area taken from a different angle. For this reason we always ask for at least two views projected at right angles to each other

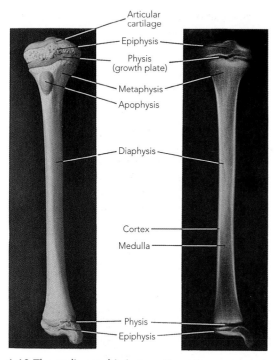

Articular cartilage
Epiphysis
Physis (growth plate)
Metaphysis
Apophysis
Diaphysis
Cortex
Medulla
Physis
Epiphysis

1.10 The radiographic image X-ray of an anatomical specimen to show the appearance of various parts of the bone in the x-ray image.

(anteroposterior and lateral), and sometimes special views to distinguish between bones overlapping each other.

How to read an x-ray

Although '*radiograph*' is more correct, the term 'x-ray' (or 'x-ray film') has become entrenched by usage. The process of 'reading an x-ray' should be as methodical as clinical examination. It is seductively easy to be led astray by some flagrant anomaly; systematic study is the only safeguard against missing important signs.

Start with a general orientation: identify the part, the particular view and, if possible, the type of patient. Then examine, in sequence, the soft tissues, the bones, the joints, the surrounding tissues.

- *The patient*: make sure that the name on the film is that of your patient; mistaken identity is a potent source of error. The clinical details are important; it is surprising how much more you can see on the x-ray when you know the background. For example, when considering a malignant bone lesion, simply knowing the patient's age may provide an important clue: under the age of 10 it is most likely to be a Ewing's sarcoma; between 10 and 20 years it is more likely to be an osteosarcoma; and over the age of 50 years it is likely to be a metastatic deposit.

- *Soft tissues*: unless examined early, these are liable to be forgotten. Look at the soft-tissue outlines to see if there is any swelling or wasting. Are there localized changes in tissue density (e.g. calcification)?

- *Bones*: take note of any generalized change in bone 'texture' (osteoporosis and abnormally thin cortices). Is there anything unusual about the shape of the bone? Look for deformity or local irregularities; examine the cortices for areas of destruction or new bone formation; then look for areas of reduced density (osteoporosis or destruction) or increased density (sclerosis). Remember that 'vacant' areas are not necessarily spaces or cysts; any tissue that is radiolucent may look 'cystic'.

- *Joints*: the radiographic 'joint' consists of the articulating bones and the 'space' between them. The 'joint space' is, of course, illusory; it is occupied by radiolucent articular cartilage. Look

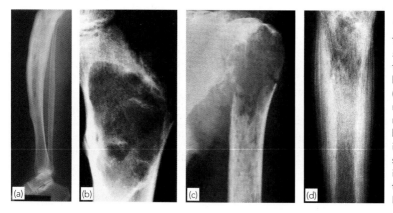

(a) (b) (c) (d)

1.11 X-rays – important features to look for (a) *General shape and appearance*: in this case the cortices are thickened and the bone is bent (Paget's disease). (b,c) *Interior density*: a vacant area may represent a true cyst (b) or radiolucent material infiltrating the bone, like the metastatic tumour in (c). *Periosteal reaction*: typically seen in healing fractures, bone infection and malignant bone tumours – as in this example of Ewing's sarcoma (d).

for narrowing of this 'space', which signifies loss of cartilage thickness, and examine the bone ends for flattening, erosion, cavitation or sclerosis – all features of arthritis. The joint margins may show osteophytes (typical of osteoarthritis) or erosions (typical of rheumatoid arthritis). Similarly, intervertebral disc 'spaces' are not gaps in the vertebral column; you must imagine the fibrous discs which occupy those 'spaces' and if a 'disc space' is abnormally flattened or narrowed it means that the intervertebral disc has collapsed.

OTHER X-RAY TECHNIQUES

Contrast radiography

Radio-opaque liquids may be used to outline cavities during x-ray examination (air or gas can be used in the same way). Common examples are sinography (outlining a sinus), arthrography (outlining a joint) and myelography (outlining the spinal theca).

Computed tomography (CT)

This method is capable of recording bone and soft-tissue outlines in cross-section. It is particularly useful for showing detailed fracture patterns, for displaying the shape of the spinal canal and for mapping the spread of tumours into the soft tissues. The computed data can also be reconstructed as a three-dimensional image. A disadvantage of CT is the relatively high radiation exposure. It should, therefore, be used with discretion.

Radionuclide scanning

A bone-seeking radio-isotope compound – usually ^{99m} technetium hydroxymethylene diphosphonate

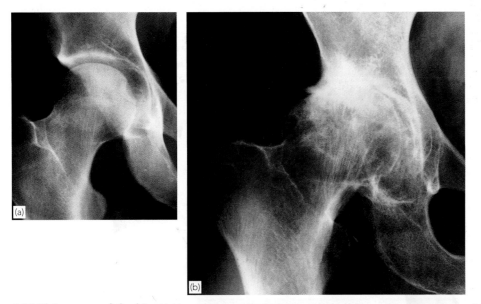

1.12 Plain x-rays of the hip (a) Normal hip: anatomical shape with joint 'space' (articular cartilage) fully preserved. (b) Advanced osteoarthritis: joint space markedly decreased; osteophytes at the joint margin.

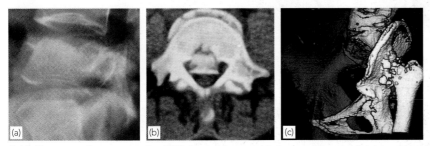

1.13 Computed tomography (CT) The plain x-ray (a) shows a fracture of the vertebral body but one cannot tell precisely how the bone fragments are displaced. The CT (b) shows clearly that they are dangerously close to the cauda equina. (c) Three-dimensional CT reconstruction of a congenital hip dislocation.

(^{99m}Tc-HDP) – is injected intravenously and its presence in the tissues is recorded with a gamma camera or rectilinear scanner. Increased uptake during the blood phase (immediately after injection) signifies hyperaemia; activity during the bone phase (about 3 hours later) suggests new bone formation. This information is valuable in the diagnosis of stress fractures (which often do not show on x-ray), bone infection and bone tumours.

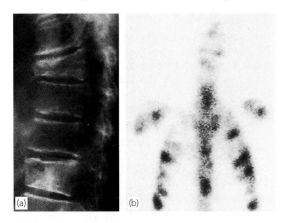

1.14 Radionuclide scanning (a) The plain x-ray showed a compression fracture, probably through a metastatic tumour. (b) The bone scan revealed generalized secondaries, here involving the spine and ribs.

MAGNETIC RESONANCE IMAGING (MRI)

Unlike x-ray imaging, MRI relies upon radio-frequency emissions from atoms and molecules in tissues exposed to a static magnetic field. It does not involve ionizing radiation. The images produced by these signals are similar to those of CT scans, but with even better contrast resolution and more refined differentiation of tissues.

Tissues containing abundant hydrogen (fat, cancellous bone and marrow) emit high-intensity signals and produce the brightest images; those containing little hydrogen (cortical bone, ligament, tendon and air) appear black; intermediate in the grey scale are cartilage, spinal canal and muscle. By adjusting various parameters, different tissues and organs can be displayed with extraordinary clarity. Bone tumours can be shown in their transverse and longitudinal extent and extraosseous spread can be accurately assessed. Moreover, there is the potential for characterizing the actual tissue, thus allowing a pathological as well as an anatomical diagnosis.

Other areas of usefulness are in the early diagnosis of bone ischaemia and necrosis, the investigation of backache and spinal disorders and the elucidation of cartilage and ligament injuries. In the knee, MRI is as accurate as arthroscopy in diagnosing meniscal tears and cruciate ligament injuries. It is also useful for diagnosing rotator cuff tears and labral injuries in the shoulder and ligament injuries around the ankle.

As MRI is so versatile and free of the risks of ionizing radiation, it is tempting to overindulge its use. It is well to remember that it is still only one diagnostic method among many.

DIAGNOSTIC ULTRASOUND

High-frequency sound waves, generated by a transducer, can penetrate several centimetres into the soft tissues; as they pass through the tissue interfaces some of these waves are reflected

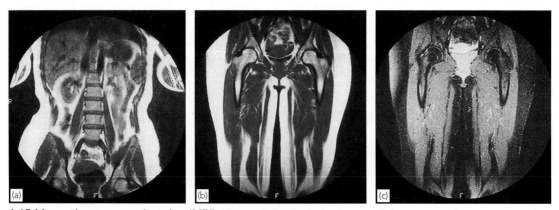

1.15 Magnetic resonance imaging (MRI) MRI can define both the shape and the structure of various tissues, thus revealing the presence and the extent of pathological change.

back (like echoes) to the transducer, where they are registered as electrical signals and displayed as images on a screen or plate. With modern equipment, tissues of varying density can be 'imaged' in gradations of grey that allow reasonable definition of the anatomy. Real-time display on a monitor gives a dynamic image, which is more useful than the usual static images on transparent plates. One major advantage of this technique is that the equipment is simple and portable and can be used almost anywhere. Another is that it produces no harmful side-effects.

As a result of the marked echogenic contrast between cystic and solid masses, ultrasonography is particularly useful for identifying hidden 'cystic' lesions such as haematomas, abscesses, popliteal cysts and arterial aneurysms. It is also capable of detecting intra-articular fluid.

One of the most useful applications is in screening newborn babies for developmental dysplasia of the hip, where the anatomical outlines can be identified even though they are entirely cartilaginous.

BONE BIOPSY

Bone biopsy is often the only means of establishing a diagnosis or distinguishing between local conditions that closely resemble one another, e.g. an area of bone destruction that could be due to a compression fracture, a bone tumour or infection. Even if it is obvious that the lesion is a tumour, we need to know what type of tumour, whether benign or malignant, primary or metastatic. Radical surgery should never be undertaken for a suspected neoplasm without first confirming the diagnosis histologically. In bone infection, the biopsy permits not only histological proof of acute inflammation but also bacteriological typing of the organism and tests for antibiotic sensitivity.

Open or closed?

Open biopsy is the most reliable way of obtaining a suitable sample of tissue, but it has several draw-backs: (1) it requires an operation, with the attendant risks of anaesthesia and infection; (2) tissue planes are opened up, predisposing to spread of infection or tumour; and (3) the incision may interfere with subsequent plans for tumour excision.

A carefully performed *closed biopsy*, using a needle or trephine, is the procedure of choice except when the lesion cannot be accurately localized or when the tissue consistency is such that a sufficient sample cannot be obtained.

Precautions

- The biopsy site and approach should be carefully planned with the aid of x-rays or other imaging techniques.
- If there is any possibility of the lesion being malignant, the approach should be sited so that the wound and biopsy track can be excised if later radical surgery proves to be necessary.
- The procedure should be carried out in an operating theatre, under anaesthesia (local or general) and with full aseptic technique.
- For deep-seated lesions, fluoroscopic control of the needle insertion is essential.
- The appropriate size of biopsy needle or cutting trephine should be selected.
- A knowledge of the local anatomy, and of the likely consistency of the lesion, is important. Large blood vessels and nerves must be avoided; potentially vascular tumours may bleed profusely and the means to control haemorrhage should be readily to hand. More than one surgeon has set out to aspirate an 'abscess' only to plunge a wide-bore needle into an aneurysm!
- Clear instructions should be given to ensure that the tissue obtained at the biopsy is suitably processed. If infection is suspected, the material should go into a culture tube and be sent to the laboratory as soon as possible. A smear may also be useful. Whole tissue is transferred to a jar containing formalin, without damaging the specimen or losing any material. Aspirated blood should be allowed to clot and can then be preserved in formalin for later paraffin embedding and sectioning. Tissue thought to contain crystals should not be placed in formalin as this may destroy the crystals; it should either be kept unaltered for immediate examination or stored in saline.
- No matter how careful the biopsy, there is always the risk that the tissue will be too scanty or too unrepresentative for accurate diagnosis. Close consultation with the radiologist and pathologist beforehand will minimize this possibility. In the best hands, needle biopsy has an accuracy rate of over 95%.

ELECTROPHYSIOLOGICAL STUDIES

Nerve and muscle function can be studied by electrical methods. Two types of investigation are employed: nerve conduction and electro-myography.

Nerve conduction

The time interval between stimulation of a motor nerve and muscle contraction can be measured accurately. If the test is repeated at two points a fixed distance apart along the nerve, the *conduction velocity* between these points can be determined. Normal values are about 40–60 m/s. Sensory nerve conduction can be measured in a similar way.

Conduction velocity is slowed in peripheral nerve damage or compression, and the site of the lesion can be established by taking measurements in different segments of the nerve.

If the nerve is divided, there is no response to stimulation of the nerve and an abnormal response to galvanic stimulation of the muscle – the '*reaction of degeneration*'. By plotting the voltage against the duration of stimulus necessary to produce contraction, a *strength/duration curve* can be obtained, which reflects the degree of muscle innervation after nerve injury. Serial examinations will show whether recovery is taking place.

Electromyography

Electromyography does not involve electrical stimulation. Instead, an electrode in the muscle is used to record motor unit activity at rest and during attempts to contract the muscle. Normally there is no electrical activity at rest, but on voluntary contraction characteristic oscilloscopic patterns appear. Changes in these patterns can identify certain neuropathic and myopathic disorders. After nerve injury there may be typical *denervation potentials*, and with recovery equally typical *re-innervation potentials*.

(See Chapter 10 for further details.)

CHAPTER 2

INFECTION

Micro-organisms may reach the bones and joints via the *blood stream* from a distant site, or by *direct invasion* from a skin puncture, operation or an open fracture. Depending on the type of organism, the site of infection and the host response, the result may be a *pyogenic osteomyelitis* or *arthritis*, a chronic *granulomatous reaction* (classically seen in tuberculosis) or an *indolent response to an unusual organism* (e.g. a fungal infection).

There is an important difference between bone infection and soft-tissue infection: since bone consists of a collection of rigid compartments, it is more susceptible than soft tissues to vascular damage and cell death from the build-up of pressure in acute inflammation. Unless it is rapidly suppressed, bone infection will inevitably lead to necrosis. The honeycomb of inaccessible spaces also makes it very difficult to eradicate infection once it is established.

The *host response* is crucial in determining the course of the disease. Susceptibility to infection is increased by: (a) *local factors* such as trauma, poor circulation, diminished sensibility, chronic bone or joint disease and the presence of foreign bodies; as well as (b) *systemic factors* such as malnutrition, general illness, diabetes, rheumatoid disease, corticosteroid administration and all forms of immunosuppression, either acquired or induced. Resistance is also diminished in the very young and the very old.

Bacterial colonization and resistance to antibiotics is also enhanced by the ability of certain microbes (including *Staphylococcus*) to adhere to avascular bone surfaces and foreign implants, protected from both host defences and antibiotics by a protein–polysaccharide slime (glycocalyx).

Acute pyogenic infection

Pyogenic infections are characterized by the formation of pus – a concentration of defunct leucocytes, dead and dying bacteria and tissue debris – which is often localized in an abscess. Pressure builds up within the abscess and infection may then extend directly along the tissue planes. It may also spread further afield via lymphatics (causing lymphangitis and lymphadenopathy) or via the blood stream (bacteraemia and septicaemia). The accompanying systemic reaction is due to the release of bacterial enzymes and endotoxins as well as cellular breakdown products from the host tissues.

Chronic infection

Chronic infection may follow on acute or, depending on the type of organism and the host reaction, it may be 'chronic' from the start. It usually involves the formation of granulation tissue (a combination of fibroblastic and vascular proliferation) leading to fibrosis. Some organisms provoke a non-pyogenic reaction involving the formation of cellular granulomas which consist largely of lymphocytes, modified macrophages and multi-nucleated giant cells; this is seen most typically in tuberculosis. Systemic effects are less acute but may ultimately be very debilitating, with lymphadenopathy, splenomegaly and tissue wasting.

Treatment

The principles of treatment are: (1) to provide analgesia and general supportive measures; (2) to rest the affected part; (3) to initiate antibiotic treatment or chemotherapy; (4) to evacuate pus and remove necrotic tissue; (5) to stabilize the bone if it has fractured; and (6) to maintain soft-tissue and skin cover.

ACUTE HAEMATOGENOUS OSTEOMYELITIS

Acute osteomyelitis almost invariably occurs in children; when adults are affected it may be because of lowered resistance or local trauma; damaged muscle is an ideal substrate for bacteria.

The causal organism is usually *Staphylococcus aureus*, less often *Streptococcus pyogenes* or *S. pneumoniae*. In young children *Haemophilus influenzae* used to be a fairly common pathogen for osteomyelitis and septic arthritis, but the introduction of *H. influenzae* type B vaccination has been followed by a much reduced incidence of this infection. Patients with sickle-cell anaemia are prone to infection by *Salmonella typhi*. Unusual organisms are also found in heroin addicts.

The blood stream is invaded, perhaps from a minor skin abrasion, a boil or – in the newborn – from an infected umbilical cord. In adults the source of infection may be a urethral catheter, an arterial line or a dirty needle and syringe.

In children the organisms usually settle in the vascular metaphysis of a long bone, most often at the proximal or distal end of the femur or the proximal end of the tibia. Predilection for this site has traditionally been attributed to the fact that the non-anastomosing terminal branches of the nutrient artery in that area twist back in hairpin loops before entering the venous network, causing the relative vascular stasis and consequent lowered oxygen tension that might favour bacterial colonization. This theory is still being argued over.

An important observation is that in infants, in whom there are still anastomoses between metaphyseal and epiphyseal blood vessels, infection can also reach the epiphysis.

Pathology

The classical changes are those seen in children: a progression through *inflammation – suppuration – necrosis – new bone formation –* to *resolution* or *intractable chronicity.*

Inflammation

The earliest change is an acute inflammatory reaction. The intraosseous pressure rises, causing intense pain and obstruction of blood flow.

Suppuration

By the second day pus appears in the medulla and forces its way along the Volkmann canals to the surface, where it forms a subperiosteal abscess. It then spreads along the shaft, to re-enter the bone at another level, or bursts out into the soft tissues. In infants, infection often extends into the epiphysis and thence into the joint. In older children the physis is a barrier to direct spread but where the metaphysis is partly intracapsular (e.g. at the hip, shoulder or elbow) pus may discharge through the periosteum into the joint. Vertebral infection may spread across the intervertebral disc to an adjacent vertebral body.

Necrosis

The rising intraosseous pressure, vascular stasis, infective thrombosis and periosteal stripping increasingly compromise the blood supply; by the end of 1 week there is usually evidence of necrosis. Pieces of bone may separate as sequestra which act as foreign-body irritants, causing persistent discharge through a sinus until they escape or are

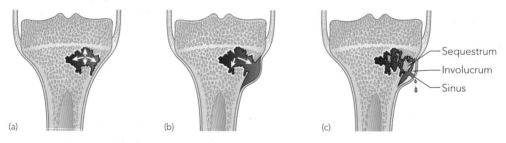

(a)   (b)   (c)

— Sequestrum
— Involucrum
— Sinus

2.1 Acute osteomyelitis – pathology (a) Infection in the metaphysis may spread towards the surface, to form a subperiosteal abscess. (b) Some of the bone may die, and is encased in periosteal new bone as a sequestrum. (c) The encasing involucrum is sometimes perforated by sinuses.

removed. However, the larger sequestra remain entombed in cavities of bone.

New bone formation

New bone forms from the deep layer of the periosteum. With time the new bone thickens to form a casing (or *involucrum*) enclosing the infected tissue and sequestra. If the infection persists, pus may discharge through perforations (*cloacae*) in the involucrum and track by sinuses to the skin surface; the condition is now established as a chronic osteomyelitis.

Resolution

If the infection is controlled and intraosseous pressure released at an early stage, this dire progress can be halted. The bone around the zone of infection becomes increasingly dense; this, together with the periosteal reaction, may result in overall thickening of the bone.

Clinical features

Children over the age of 4 years are most commonly affected. The patient presents with severe pain, malaise and a fever; in neglected cases toxaemia may be marked. Sometimes a history of a preceding skin lesion, an injury or a sore throat may be obtained.

The limb is held still and there is acute 'fingertip' tenderness near one of the larger joints. Even the gentlest manipulation is painful and joint movement is restricted (*pseudoparalysis*). Local redness, swelling, warmth and oedema are later signs and signify the presence of pus.

In infants, and especially in the *newborn*, the constitutional disturbance can be misleadingly mild; the baby simply fails to thrive and is drowsy but irritable. Suspicion should be aroused by a history of birth difficulties or umbilical artery catheterization. There may be metaphyseal tenderness and resistance to joint movement. Always look for other sites – multiple infection is not uncommon.

During the first year of life metaphyseal infection often spreads to the epiphysis and from there into the adjacent joint. Damage to the physis may eventually lead to retarded growth and deformity at that site.

In adults the commonest site of haematogenous infection is the spine. Suspicious features are backache and a mild fever, possibly following a urological procedure. It may take weeks for x-ray signs to appear, and even then the diagnosis may need to be confirmed by fine-needle aspiration and bacteriological culture.

Imaging

For the first 10 days *plain x-rays* show no abnormality. However, radio-isotope scans may show increased activity – a non-specific sign of acute inflammation. By the end of the second week there may be early radiographic signs of rarefaction of the metaphysis and periosteal new bone formation. Later still, if treatment is delayed or ineffectual, the bone may appear increasingly ragged. With healing there is sclerosis and thickening of the cortex. Sometimes sequestra are seen, separated from the surrounding bone.

Magnetic resonance imaging (MRI) shows pathological changes before x-rays and can help to distinguish between bone and soft-tissue infection. It is particularly useful in detecting a focus of infection in the axial skeleton.

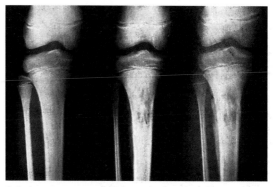

2.2 Acute osteomyelitis – x-rays During the first 2 weeks the x-ray looks normal; later the bone may look mottled and there are increasing signs of periosteal new bone formation.

Laboratory investigations

The white blood cell (WBC) count and erythrocyte sedimentation rate (ESR) are usually elevated and blood cultures may be positive. However, the most certain way to confirm the clinical diagnosis is to aspirate pus from the subperiosteal abscess or the adjacent joint. Even if no pus is found, a smear of the aspirate is examined immediately for cells and organisms. A sample is also sent for bacteriological examination and tests for sensitivity to antibiotics. Blood C-reactive protein (CRP) is a sensitive marker for monitoring progress during the course of treatment.

Differential diagnosis

- *Cellulitis*: this is often mistaken for osteomyelitis. There is widespread redness and lymphangitis. A source of skin infection may not be obvious and should be searched for (e.g. between the toes). If doubt remains about the diagnosis, MRI will help to distinguish between bone infection and soft-tissue infection.

- *Sickle-cell crisis*: patients with sickle-cell disease may present with features like those of acute osteomyelitis. Where *Salmonella* is endemic it would be wise to treat these patients with suitable antibiotics until infection is definitely excluded.

Treatment

Antibiotics

Blood and, if possible, aspiration samples are sent immediately for culture, *but the prompt administration of antibiotics is so vital that the result is not awaited before starting treatment*. Initially the choice of antibiotics is based on the findings from direct examination of the aspirate and a 'best guess' as to the most likely pathogen; a more appropriate drug can be substituted once the organism is identified and its antibiotic sensitivity is known. The following recommendations should be taken as a guide to empirical antibiotic therapy:

- *Neonates and infants up to 6 months of age*: initial antibiotic treatment should be effective against penicillin-resistant *S. aureus*, Group B streptococcus and Gram-negative organisms. Drugs of choice are flucloxacillin plus a third-generation cephalosporin like cefotaxime.
- *Children 6 months to 6 years of age*: empirical treatment in this age group should include cover against *H. influenzae*, unless it is known for certain that the child has had an antihaemophilus vaccination. This is best provided by a combination of intravenous flucloxacillin and cefotaxime or cefuroxime.
- *Older children and previously fit adults*: the vast majority in this group will have a staphylococcal infection and can be started on intravenous flucloxacillin and fusidic acid. Fusidic acid is preferred to benzylpenicillin partly because of the high prevalence of penicillin-resistant staphylococci and because it is particularly well concentrated in bone. However, for a known streptococcal infection benzylpenicillin is better. Patients who are allergic to penicillin should be treated with a second- or third-generation cephalosporin.
- *Elderly and previously unfit patients*: in these patients there is a greater than usual risk of Gram-negative infections, due to respiratory, gastrointestinal or urinary disorders. Here the choice would be a combination of flucloxacillin and a second- or third-generation cephalosporin.
- *Patients with sickle-cell disease*: these patients are prone to osteomyelitis, which may be caused by a staphylococcal infection but in many cases is due to *Salmonella* and/or other Gram-negative organisms. Chloramphenicol used to be the preferred antibiotic, though there were worries about the complication of aplastic anaemia. Now the antibiotic of choice is a third-generation cephalosporin or a fluoroquinolone like ciprofloxacin.
- *Heroin addicts and immunocompromised patients*: unusual infections (e.g. *Pseudomonas* or *Proteus*) are likely in these patients. Infants with human immunodeficiency virus (HIV) infection may also have picked up other sexually transmitted organisms during birth. These patients are best treated empirically with one of the third-generation cephalosporins or a fluoroquinolone preparation.
- *Patients at risk of methicillin-resistant S. aureus* (MRSA): those with acute haematogenous osteomyelitis who have a previous history of MRSA infection, or any patient with a bone infection admitted to a ward where MRSA is endemic, should be treated with intravenous vancomycin (or similar antibiotic) together with a third-generation cephalosporin.

The drugs should be administered intravenously (adjusting the choice of antibiotic once the results of antimicrobial sensitivity become available) until the patient's condition begins to improve and the CRP values return to normal levels – which usually takes 2–4 weeks depending on the virulence of the infection and the patient's general fitness. Thereafter, the antibiotic should still be administered orally for at least another 3–6 weeks; during that period it is important to track the serum antibiotic levels so as to ensure that the minimum inhibitory concentration (MIC) is maintained. CRP, ESR and WBC values are also checked at regular intervals and treatment is discontinued only when these are seen to remain normal.

Supportive treatment

Continuous bed rest is important. Osteomyelitis is extremely painful; the affected limb is splinted and adequate analgesics must be given.

Drainage

If antibiotics are given within the first 48 hours after the onset of symptoms, drainage may not be necessary. However, if the clinical features do not improve within 36 hours of starting treatment, or even earlier if there are signs of deep pus (swelling, oedema, fluctuation), and most certainly if pus is aspirated, the abscess should be drained by open operation under general anaesthesia.

If pus is found – and released – there is little to be gained by drilling into the medullary cavity. However, if there is no obvious abscess, it is reasonable to drill a few holes into the bone in various directions; if there is an intramedullary abscess, drainage can be best achieved by cutting a small window in the cortex. The wound is closed without a drain and the splint (or traction) is reapplied.

Once the signs of infection subside, movements are encouraged and the child is allowed to walk with the aid of crutches. Full weightbearing is usually possible after 3–4 weeks.

At present about one-third of patients with confirmed osteomyelitis are likely to need an operation; adults with vertebral infection seldom do.

Follow-up

Once the infection has subsided, movements are encouraged; however, the patient may have to use crutches for another few weeks. Outpatient follow-up is important, to ensure that there is no recurrence of infection.

Complications

- *Spread*: infection may spread to the joint (septic arthritis) or to other bones (metastatic osteomyelitis).
- *Pathological fracture*: occasionally the bone is so weakened that it fractures at the site of infection or operative perforation.
- *Growth disturbance*: if the physis is damaged there may later be shortening or deformity.

- *Persistent infection*: treatment must be prompt and effective. 'Too little too late' may result in chronic osteomyelitis.

SUBACUTE HAEMATOGENOUS OSTEOMYELITIS

Osteomyelitis may present in a relatively mild form, presumably because the organism is less virulent or the patient more resistant. The distal femur and the proximal and distal tibia are the favourite sites. The patient is usually a child or adolescent who has had pain near one of the large joints for several weeks. Laboratory investigations are often negative. The typical x-ray picture is of a small, oval cavity surrounded by sclerotic bone – the classic Brodie's abscess – but sometimes the lesion is more diffuse. A radio-isotope scan will show increased activity. If the condition is troublesome, the abscess is opened under antibiotic cover.

A small abscess is easily mistaken for an osteoid osteoma and the diagnosis may be made only when the lesion is explored. With a larger lesion there is the risk that it may be mistaken for a bone tumour. If the diagnosis is in doubt an open biopsy is called for.

Treatment

Treatment may be conservative if the diagnosis is not in doubt. Immobilization and antibiotics (flucloxacillin and fusidic acid) intravenously for 4 or 5 days and then orally for another 6 weeks often result in healing, though this may be slow. If the x-ray shows that there is no healing after conservative treatment, open curettage may be indicated; this is always followed by a further course of antibiotics.

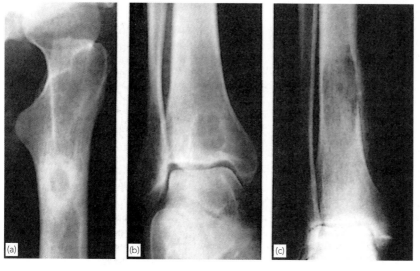

2.3 Subacute osteomyelitis (a,b) The classic Brodie's abscess looks like a small walled-off cavity in the bone with little or no periosteal reaction. (c) Sometimes rarefaction is more diffuse and there may be cortical erosion and periosteal reaction.

POST-TRAUMATIC OSTEOMYELITIS

Open fractures are always contaminated and are therefore prone to infection. The combination of tissue injury, vascular damage, oedema, haematoma, dead bone fragments and an open pathway to the atmosphere must invite bacterial invasion even if the wound is not contaminated with particulate dirt. This is the most common cause of osteomyelitis in adults.

S. aureus is the usual pathogen, but other organisms such as *Escherichia coli*, *Proteus mirabilis* and *Pseudomonas aeruginosa* are sometimes involved.

Clinical features

The patient becomes feverish and develops pain and swelling over the fracture site; the wound is inflamed and there may be a seropurulent discharge. Blood tests reveal increased CRP levels, leucocytosis and an elevated ESR; it should be remembered, though, that these inflammatory markers are non-specific and may be affected by tissue trauma.

X-ray appearances may be difficult to interpret because of bone fragmentation. MRI can be helpful in differentiating between bone and soft-tissue infection, but is less reliable in distinguishing between long-standing infection and bone destruction due to trauma.

A wound swab is obtained for microbiological examination and (if necessary) to test for antibiotic sensitivity.

Treatment

The management of open fractures is discussed on page 347. The essence of treatment is prophylaxis: thorough cleansing and debridement of dead and dying tissues, stabilization of the bone fragments, skin cover of the wound (either by suture or by skin grafting) if or when it is assuredly clean, and antibiotic administration.

In most cases a combination of flucloxacillin and benzylpenicillin (or sodium fusidate), given 6-hourly for 48 hours, will suffice. If the wound is contaminated, it is advisable also to give metronidazole for 4 or 5 days to control both aerobic and anaerobic organisms.

Pyogenic wound infection, once it has taken root, is difficult to eradicate. The presence of necrotic soft tissue and dead bone, together with a mixed bacterial flora, conspire against effective antibiotic control. Regular wound dressing and repeated excision of all dead and infected tissue

may be necessary. Further treatment is essentially the same as for chronic osteomyelitis.

CHRONIC OSTEOMYELITIS

This used to be a common sequel to acute haematogenous osteomyelitis; nowadays it more frequently follows an open fracture or operation.

An area of bone has been destroyed by the acute infection leaving sequestra surrounded by dense sclerosed bone. The imprisoned sequestra provoke a chronic seropurulent discharge which escapes through a sinus (or several sinuses) at the skin surface.

Bacteria can remain dormant for years, giving rise to recurrent acute flares and purulent discharges. The usual suspects are *S. aureus*, *E. coli*, *S. pyogenes*, *Proteus* and *Pseudomonas*; in the presence of surgical implants, *S. epidermidis* is the commonest pathogen.

Clinical features

Following acute bone infection, the patient returns with recurrent bouts of pain, redness and tenderness at the affected site. Classic signs are healed and discharging sinuses and x-ray features of bone rarefaction surrounded by dense sclerosis and cortical thickening; within that area there may be an obvious sequestrum. A *sinogram* can help to localize the focus of active infection, and *bone scans* are useful in revealing hidden foci of inflammatory activity.

CT and *MRI* are invaluable in planning operative treatment: together they will show the extent of bone destruction and reactive oedema, hidden abscesses and sequestra.

Organisms cultured from discharging sinuses should be tested repeatedly for antibiotic sensitivity; with time, they often change their characteristics. *Note, however, that a superficial swab sample may not reflect the really persistent infection; samples should be taken from deeper tissues.*

Treatment

Treatment depends on the frequency of relapsing flare-ups; if seldom, it can be conservative. A sinus may be painless and need a dressing simply to protect the clothing; a flare often settles with a few days' rest, although if an abscess presents it should be incised. Antibiotics are often used, though most fail to penetrate the barrier of fibrous tissue and bone sclerosis. Sequestrectomy should be performed only if a sequestrum is radiologically visible and surgically accessible.

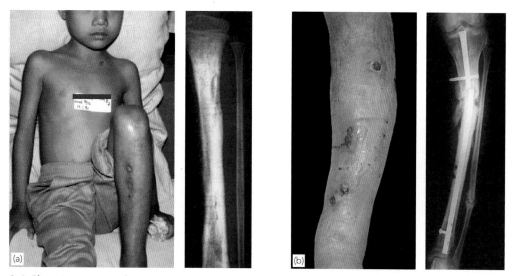

2.4 Chronic osteomyelitis Chronic osteomyelitis may follow on acute. This young boy in (a) presented with draining sinuses at the site of a previous acute infection. The x-ray shows densely sclerotic bone. (b) In adults, chronic osteomyelitis is usually a sequel to open trauma or operation.

In refractory or frequently recurring cases it may be possible to excise the infected and/or devitalized segment of bone and then close the gap by the *Ilizarov method* of 'transporting' a viable segment from the remaining diaphysis. This is especially useful if infection is associated with an ununited fracture (see page 155).

It is always wise to search for underlying systemic conditions (e.g. diabetes) that may have an adverse effect on the outcome.

Antibiotics

Chronic infection is seldom eradicated by antibiotics alone. Yet bactericidal drugs are important: (a) to suppress the infection and prevent its spread to healthy bone; and (b) to control acute flares. The choice of antibiotic depends on microbiological studies, but the drug must be capable of penetrating sclerotic bone and should be non-toxic with long-term use. Fusidic acid, clindamycin and the cephalosporins are good examples. Vancomycin and teicoplanin are effective in most cases of MRSA infection.

Antibiotics are administered for 4–6 weeks (starting from the beginning of treatment or the last debridement) before considering operative treatment. During this time serum antibiotic concentrations should be measured at regular intervals to ensure that they are kept above the *minimum bactericidal concentration* (MBC). Continuous collaboration with a specialist in microbiology is important.

Local treatment

A sinus may be painless and need dressing simply to protect the clothing. An acute abscess may need urgent incision and drainage.

Operation

A waiting policy, punctuated by spells of bed rest and antibiotics to control flares, may have to be endured until there is a clear indication for radical surgery: for chronic haematogenous infections this means intrusive symptoms, failure of adequate antibiotic treatment, and/or clear evidence of a sequestrum or dead bone; for post-traumatic infections, an intractable wound and/or an infected ununited fracture; for postoperative infection, similar criteria and evidence of bone erosion.

External fixation may need to be applied so that internal fixation devices can be removed. All infected and dead tissue must then be excised. After 3 or 4 days the wound is inspected and if there are renewed signs of tissue death the debridement is repeated – several times if necessary. Antibiotic cover is continued for at least 4 weeks after the last debridement.

There are several ways of dealing with the resulting 'dead space'. *Antibiotic-impregnated beads* can be laid in the cavity and left for 2 or 3 weeks and then replaced with cancellous bone grafts. *Bone grafts* have also been used on their own: in the *Papineau technique* the entire cavity is packed with small cancellous chips (preferably autogenous) mixed with an antibiotic and a fibrin sealant.

Where possible, the area is covered by adjacent muscle and the skin wound is sutured without tension.

Other methods involve the use of *muscle flaps with split-skin grafts* or a *free vascularized muscle flap transfer*.

A different approach is used in the *Lautenbach technique*. This involves radical excision of all avascular and infected tissue followed by closed irrigation and suction drainage of the bed using double-lumen tubes and an appropriate antibiotic solution in high concentration. The 'dead space' is gradually filled by vascular granulation tissue; the tubes are removed when cultures remain negative in three consecutive fluid samples and the cavity is obliterated.

In refractory cases it may be possible to excise the infected and/or devitalized segment of bone completely and then close the gap by the *Ilizarov method* of 'transporting' a viable segment from the remaining diaphysis. This is especially useful if infection is associated with an ununited fracture (see Chapter 12).

Whichever method is favoured, the bone must be covered with skin. For small defects split-thickness skin grafts may suffice; for larger wounds local musculocutaneous flaps, or free vascularized flaps, may be needed.

Aftercare

Success is difficult to measure; a minute focus of infection might escape the therapeutic onslaught, only to flare into full-blown osteomyelitis many years later. Prognosis should always be guarded; local trauma must be avoided and any recurrence of symptoms, however slight, should be taken seriously and investigated. The watchword is 'cautious optimism' – a 'probable cure' is better than no cure at all.

ACUTE SUPPURATIVE ARTHRITIS

Cause and pathology

The causal organism is usually *S. aureus*; in children between 1 and 4 years old, *H. influenzae* is an important pathogen unless they have been vaccinated against this organism.

The joint is invaded through a penetrating wound, by eruption of an adjacent bone abscess or by blood spread from a distant site. As infection spreads through the joint, articular cartilage is eroded; in infants the entire epiphysis (which is still cartilaginous) may be destroyed. If pus bursts out of the joint it will present as an abscess or a sinus. With healing, the raw articular surfaces may adhere, producing fibrous or bony ankylosis.

Clinical features

Typical features are acute pain and swelling in a single large joint – commonly the hip in children and the knee in adults. However, any joint can be affected. The patient becomes ill, with a rapid pulse and swinging fever. The WBC is raised and blood culture may be positive.

Many of the local signs can be elicited only in superficial joints. The skin looks red, the joint is held flexed and it is swollen. There is superficial warmth, diffuse tenderness and fluctuation. All movements are grossly restricted and often completely abolished by pain and spasm (pseudoparesis).

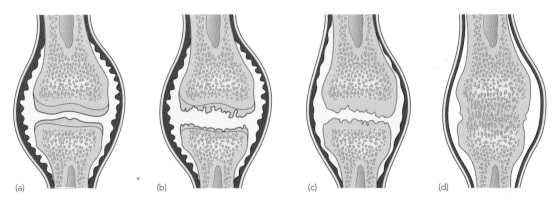

(a) (b) (c) (d)

2.5 Acute suppurative arthritis – pathology In the early stage (a), there is an acute synovitis with a purulent joint effusion. (b) Soon the articular cartilage is attacked by bacterial and cellular enzymes. If the infection is not arrested, the cartilage may be completely destroyed (c). Healing then leads to bony ankylosis (d).

In infants the emphasis is on septicaemia rather than joint pain. The baby is irritable and refuses to feed; there is a rapid pulse and sometimes a fever. Infection is usually suspected, but it could be anywhere! The joints should be carefully felt and moved to elicit the local signs of warmth, tenderness and resistance to movement. The umbilical cord should be examined for a source of infection. An inflamed intravenous infusion site should always excite suspicion.

Patients with rheumatoid arthritis, and especially those on corticosteroid treatment, may develop a 'silent' joint infection. Suspicion may be aroused by an unexplained deterioration in the patient's general condition; every joint should be carefully examined.

Imaging

X-rays may show soft-tissue swelling, widening of the joint space (due to the effusion) and periarticular osteoporosis during the first 2 weeks of bacterial arthritis. Later, when the articular cartilage is attacked, the 'joint space' is narrowed. In advanced cases there are signs of bone destruction.

Radionuclide imaging and *MRI* are helpful for detecting signs in difficult sites such as the sternoclavicular and sacroiliac joints.

Investigations

The diagnosis can usually be confirmed by joint aspiration and immediate microbiological investigation of the fluid. Blood cultures also may be positive, though only in about 50% of proven cases. Non-specific features of acute inflammation (leucocytosis, raised ESR and positive CRP) are suggestive but not diagnostic.

Diagnosis

Osteomyelitis near a joint may be indistinguishable from septic arthritis; the safest is to assume that both are present.

An *acute haemarthrosis*, either post-traumatic or due to a haemophilic bleed, can closely resemble infection. The history is helpful and joint aspiration will resolve any doubt.

Transient synovitis (*irritable joint*) in children causes symptoms and signs which are less acute, but there is always the fear that this is the beginning of an infection.

Gout and *pseudogout* in adults can be indistinguishable from joint infection and cellulitis. Aspirated fluid may look turbid but the presence of urate or pyrophosphate crystals will confirm the diagnosis.

Complications

- *Dislocation*: a tense effusion may cause dislocation.
- *Epiphyseal destruction*: in neglected infants the largely cartilaginous epiphysis may be destroyed, leaving an unstable pseudoarthrosis.
- *Growth disturbance*: physeal damage may result in shortening or deformity.
- *Ankylosis*: if articular cartilage is eroded, healing may lead to ankylosis.

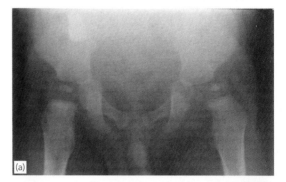
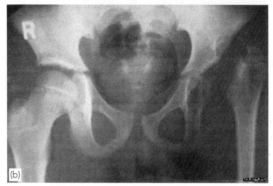

2.6 Suppurative arthritis – x-ray (a) In this child the left hip is subluxated and the soft tissues are swollen. (b) If the infection persists untreated, the cartilaginous epiphysis may be entirely destroyed leaving a permanent pseudarthrosis (Tom Smith's dislocation).

Treatment

The first priority is to aspirate the joint and examine the fluid. Treatment is then started without further delay and follows the same lines as for acute osteomyelitis.

Antibiotics

Intravenous antibiotics should be started as soon as joint fluid and blood samples have been taken for culture. If Gram-positive organisms are identified, flucloxacillin is suitable. If in doubt, a third-generation cephalosporin will cover both Gram-positive and Gram-negative organisms. Once the bacterial sensitivity is known the appropriate drug is substituted. Intravenous administration is continued for several weeks and is followed by oral antibiotics for a further 2 or 3 weeks.

Splintage

The joint must be rested either on a splint or in a widely split plaster. At the hip, the joint should be held abducted and 30 degrees flexed.

Drainage

Under anaesthesia, pus is drained and the joint washed out. This is best done by open operation, but in a superficial joint it can be achieved by repeated needle aspiration and irrigation or, in the case of the knee, by arthroscopy.

Once the patient's general condition is good and the joint is no longer inflamed, gentle and gradually increasing movements are encouraged. But if articular cartilage has been destroyed, the aim is to keep the joint immobile in the optimum position while ankylosis is awaited.

SEPTIC BURSITIS

Bursal infection is common, especially in the olecranon bursa at the back of the elbow and the prepatellar bursa, both of which are exposed to trauma in labourers and craftspeople who work on their knees. Olecranon bursitis is also seen in patients with rheumatoid arthritis or gout.

The condition usually starts as a non-septic bursitis which is then infected by an overlying skin abrasion or puncture. The common organism is *S. aureus*.

Pain, swelling and redness – sometimes extending well beyond the boundaries of the bursa itself – are typical features. The diagnosis is confirmed by aspirating the bursal fluid and submitting it for microscopic and bacteriological examination.

Treatment consists of local rest or splintage and intravenous administration of flucloxacillin (or a more appropriate antibiotic as dictated by sensitivity tests). If pus has formed, it must be released, preferably by open drainage. Intractable infection, or recurrent septic bursitis, may need prolonged antibiotic treatment and operative bursectomy.

TUBERCULOSIS

Tuberculosis is on the increase; bones or joints are affected in about 5% of patients. *Mycobacterium tuberculosis* has a predilection for the vertebral bodies and the large synovial joints.

Where pulmonary tuberculosis is endemic, skeletal tuberculosis is seen mainly in children and young adults. In non-endemic areas the disease usually appears in patients with chronic debilitating disorders or reduced immune defence mechanisms (e.g. acquired immunodeficiency syndrome [AIDS]).

Pathology

Infection reaches the skeleton by haematogenous seeding from the lung or intestine. There is a chronic inflammatory reaction, characteristically leading to granuloma formation and caseation. Spread into soft tissues leads to a subacute abscess (the so-called 'cold abscess') which may track along tissue planes and 'point' somewhere quite remote from the original site of bone infection. Infected material may discharge through the skin leaving a chronic sinus. Secondary pyogenic infection may follow.

Vertebral tuberculosis usually begins in the anterior part of the vertebral body near the intervertebral disc. After progressive bone destruction, the infection spreads across the disc into an adjacent vertebral body. The two vertebrae may collapse forwards, causing a sharp angulation, or gibbus, in the affected segment – usually in the lower thoracic or lumbar spine.

Joint tuberculosis may start either in the synovium or in a nearby metaphysis from where it spreads across the physis, through the articular surface into the synovial cavity. Either way, the presenting picture is of a chronic monarthritis affecting a large joint (usually the hip or knee, less often the shoulder or ankle). Secondary infection by pyogenic organisms is quite common. If the condition is not arrested, the articular surfaces will be destroyed. Healing is by fibrosis, resulting in a tight 'fibrous ankylosis' of the joint. Within this fibrocaseous tissue mycobacteria may lurk undiscovered, only to flare up again some years later.

Clinical features

The patient complains of pain and (in a superficial joint) swelling. Muscle wasting is characteristic and palpable synovial thickening is often striking. Movements are limited in all directions. As articular erosion progresses the joint becomes stiff and severely deformed; in late cases there may be a sinus.

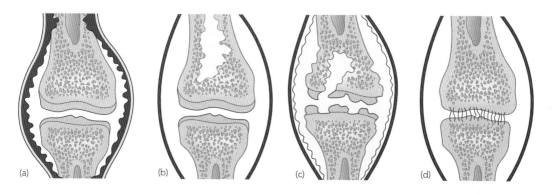

2.7 Tuberculous arthritis – pathology The disease may begin as synovitis (a) or osteomyelitis (b). From either it can extend to become a true arthritis (c); not all the cartilage is destroyed, and healing is usually by fibrous ankylosis (d).

In tuberculosis of the spine, pain may be deceptively slight. Consequently the patient may not present until there is a visible abscess or until collapse causes a localized kyphosis (gibbus). Spread along fascial planes may lead to a cold abscess pointing some distance away, e.g. in the loin or along the insertion of the psoas muscle in the groin.

Occasionally the presenting feature is weakness or loss of sensibility in the lower limbs. In areas where treatment is delayed or non-existent vertebral collapse may lead to paralysis (Pott's paraplegia); this is dealt with in Chapter 18.

X-rays

X-rays show soft tissue swelling and periarticular osteoporosis. In the early stages the joint space is retained but later there is narrowing and irregularity, with bone erosion on both sides of the joint. Cystic lesions may appear in the bone.

Tuberculous spondylitis may appear as localized bone erosion and collapse across an intervertebral disc space. Always look for soft-tissue traces of a paravertebral abscess.

Diagnosis

Except in regions where tuberculosis is common, diagnosis is often delayed simply because the disease is not suspected. In many respects it resembles rheumatoid arthritis in a single joint like the hip. Features suggesting tuberculosis, and calling for more active investigation, are a long history, involvement of only one joint, marked synovial thickening, marked muscle wasting and periarticular osteoporosis. The ESR is usually raised and the Mantoux test is positive. Synovial biopsy for histological examination and bacterial culture is often necessary.

In patients with spinal tuberculosis, metastatic bone disease, multiple myeloma, sarcoidosis and unusual infections such as brucellosis must be excluded.

Treatment

The mainstay of treatment is antituberculous chemotherapy, which should always include rifampicin and isoniazid, for 6 months or more. Resistance to isoniazid may call for the use of additional drugs (e.g. fluoroquinolones)

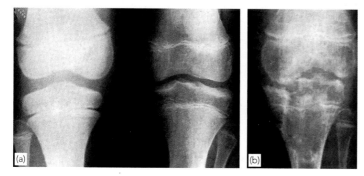

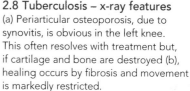

2.8 Tuberculosis – x-ray features
(a) Periarticular osteoporosis, due to synovitis, is obvious in the left knee. This often resolves with treatment but, if cartilage and bone are destroyed (b), healing occurs by fibrosis and movement is markedly restricted.

and follow-up treatment with a combination of drugs such as isoniazid, pyrazinamide and ethambutol for another 9 months. During the entire treatment period drugs and dosage should be adjusted and modified, depending on the individual patient's age, size, general health and drug reactions. If chemotherapy is started early, the joint may heal and function be completely restored.

Local measures include rest, traction and (occasionally) operation. Splintage should be continued for several months, by which time it is usually clear whether the joint has been saved. If the articular surfaces are destroyed, the joint is immobilized until all signs of disease activity have disappeared.

If the disease remains quiescent, arthrodesis – or even joint replacement – may be considered.

CHAPTER 3

INFLAMMATORY RHEUMATIC DISORDERS

The term 'inflammatory rheumatic disorders' covers a number of diseases that cause chronic pain, stiffness and swelling around joints and tendons. In addition, they are commonly associated with extra-articular features including skin rashes and inflammatory eye disease. Many – perhaps all – are due to a faulty immune reaction resulting from a combination of environmental exposures against a background of genetic predisposition.

RHEUMATOID ARTHRITIS

Rheumatoid arthritis (RA), the commonest cause of inflammatory joint disease, affects about 3% of the population, women three times more often than men. It usually appears in the fourth or fifth decade.

Cause

The cause is unknown, but it is believed that a foreign antigen – possibly a virus – sets off a chain of events culminating in a chronic inflammatory disorder in which abnormal immunological reactions are prominent. These include the production of antibodies (both immunoglobulin IgG and IgM) to the body's own IgG. Such 'autoantibodies' appear as serum rheumatoid factors (RFs) in 80% of patients with RA, and they can also be demonstrated in the synovium.

The abnormal immune response may be genetically predetermined, for patients with RA show increased frequencies of the human leucocyte antigen HLA-DR4.

Pathology

Although tissues throughout the body are affected, the brunt of the attack falls on synovium. The pathological changes, if unchecked, proceed in four stages:

- *Stage 1: preclinical*: well before RA becomes clinically apparent the immune pathology is already beginning. Raised erythrocyte sedimentation rate (ESR), C-reactive protein (CRP) and rheumatoid factor (RF) may be detectable years before the first diagnosis.
- *Stage 2: synovitis*: synovial membrane becomes inflamed and thickened, giving rise to a cell-rich effusion. Although painful and swollen, the joints and tendons are still intact and the disorder is potentially reversible.
- *Stage 3: destruction*: persistent inflammation causes joint and tendon destruction. Articular cartilage is eroded, partly by proteolytic enzymes, partly by vascular tissue in the folds of the synovial reflections, and partly due to direct invasion of the cartilage by a pannus of granulation tissue creeping over the articular surface. At the margins of the joint, bone is eroded by granulation tissue invasion and osteoclastic resorption. Similar changes occur in tendon sheaths, causing tenosynovitis and, eventually, partial or complete rupture of tendons. A synovial effusion, often containing

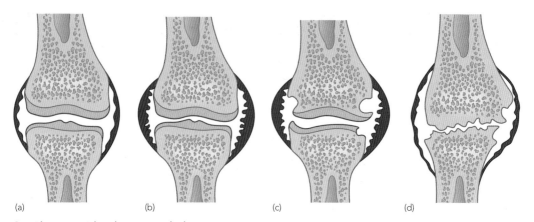

(a)   (b)   (c)   (d)

3.1 Rheumatoid arthritis – pathology (a) The normal joint. (b) Stage 1 – synovitis and joint swelling. (c) Stage 2 – early joint destruction with periarticular erosions. (d) Stage 3 – advanced joint destruction and deformity.

copious amounts of fibrinoid material, produces swelling of the joints, tendons and bursae.

- *Stage 4*: *deformity*: the combination of articular destruction, capsular stretching and tendon rupture leads to progressive instability and deformity.

Extra-articular features

The most characteristic extra-articular lesion is the *rheumatoid nodule*, a small granuloma occurring under the skin (especially over bony prominences), on tendons, in the sclera and in viscera. Other systemic features are *lymphadenopathy*, *vasculitis*, *muscle weakness* and *visceral disease* affecting the lungs, heart, kidneys, brain and gastrointestinal tract.

It used to be thought that the disease would eventually 'burn itself out', but this does not appear to be the case. Features of different stages can occur simultaneously in different joints and even when the arthritis is quiescent, systemic pathology may still be active.

Clinical features

The usual pattern is the insidious emergence of a symmetrical polyarthritis affecting mainly the hands and feet, together with early morning stiffness and a lack of well-being. Women are affected more often than men.

The *early stage* is marked by swelling, stiffness, increased warmth and tenderness of the proximal finger joints and the wrists, as well as of the tendon sheaths around these joints. X-ray examination may show soft-tissue swelling and periarticular osteoporosis. Gradually similar symptoms and signs appear in other joints: the elbows, shoulders, knees, ankles and feet. However, it is important to

remember that the condition occasionally begins in one of the larger joints and (at least for a while) can resemble an inflammatory monarthritis such as gonococcal or tuberculous synovitis.

As the *disease progresses* joint movements become increasingly restricted and isolated tendon ruptures appear at the wrists. Subcutaneous nodules may be felt over the olecranon process; although they occur in only 25% of patients, they are pathognomonic of RA.

In the *later stages* joint deformity becomes increasingly apparent and the acute pain of synovitis is replaced by the more constant ache of joint destruction. The combination of instability and tendon rupture produces the typical 'rheumatoid' deformities: ulnar deviation of the fingers, radial and volar displacement of the wrists, valgus knees, valgus feet and clawed toes. Joint movements are restricted and often very painful. About one-third of all patients develop pain and stiffness in the cervical spine. Function is increasingly disturbed and patients may need help with grooming, dressing and eating.

Extra-articular features such as muscle wasting, lymphadenopathy, nerve entrapment syndromes, skin atrophy or ulceration, scleritis, vasculitis and peripheral sensory neuropathy become increasingly apparent in patients with severe disease.

X-rays

Early on, x-rays show only the features of synovitis: soft-tissue swelling and periarticular osteoporosis. The later stages are marked by the appearance of marginal bony erosions and narrowing of the articular space, especially in the proximal joints of the hands and feet. In advanced disease, articular destruction and joint deformity are obvious.

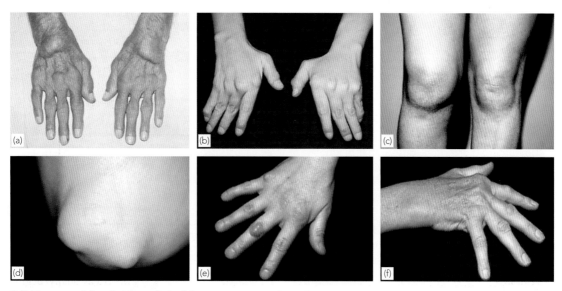

3.2 Rheumatoid arthritis – clinical features (a) Early features of swelling and stiffness of the proximal finger joints and the wrists. (b) The late hand deformities are so characteristic as to be almost pathognomonic. (c) Occasionally rheumatoid disease starts with synovitis of a single large joint (in this case the right knee). Extra-articular features include subcutaneous nodules (d,e) and tendon ruptures (f).

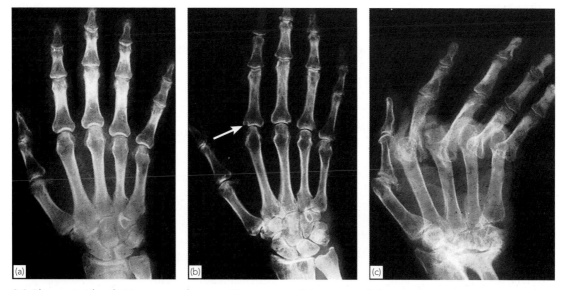

3.3 Rheumatoid arthritis – x-ray changes The progress of disease is well shown in this patient's x-rays. First there was only soft-tissue swelling and periarticular osteoporosis; later juxta-articular erosions appeared (arrow); ultimately the joints became unstable and deformed.

Blood investigations

Normocytic, hypochromic anaemia is common and is a reflection of abnormal erythropoiesis. It may be aggravated by chronic gastrointestinal blood loss caused by non-steroidal anti-inflammatory drugs (NSAIDS). In active phases the ESR and CRP concentration are usually raised.

Serological tests for RF are positive in about 80% of patients and antinuclear factors are present in 30%. Neither of these tests is specific and neither is required for a diagnosis of RA.

Diagnosis

The minimal criteria for diagnosing RA are: (1) bilateral, symmetrical polyarthritis, involving (2) the proximal joints of the hands or feet, present

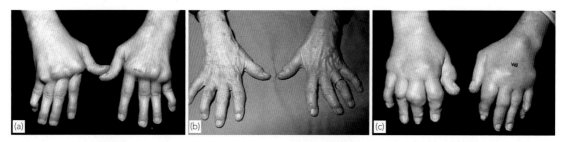

3.4 Rheumatoid arthritis – differential diagnosis All three patients presented with painful swollen fingers. In (a) mainly the proximal joints were affected (rheumatoid arthritis); in (b) the distal joints were the worst (Heberden's osteoarthritis); in (c) there were asymmetrical nodular swellings around the joints (gouty tophi).

for (3) at least 6 weeks. If, in addition, there are subcutaneous nodules or periarticular erosions on x-ray, the diagnosis is certain. *A positive test for RF in the absence of the above features is not sufficient to diagnose RA, nor does a negative test exclude the diagnosis if all the other features are present.* The chief value of the RF tests is in assessing prognosis; high titres herald more serious disease.

In the differential diagnosis of polyarthritis, several disorders must be considered:

- *Seronegative polyarthritis* is a feature of a number of conditions vaguely related to RA: psoriatic arthritis, juvenile chronic arthritis (Still's disease), systemic lupus erythematosus and other connective-tissue diseases.
- *Ankylosing spondylitis* may involve the peripheral joints, but it is primarily a disease of the sacroiliac and intervertebral joints, causing back pain and progressive stiffness.
- *Reiter's disease* affects the large joints and the lumbosacral spine. There is a history of urethritis or colitis and often also conjunctivitis.
- *Polyarticular gout* affects large and small joints, and tophi on fingers and toes may be mistaken for rheumatoid nodules.
- *Polyarticular osteoarthritis* affects the distal interphalangeal joints and causes nodular swellings with radiologically obvious osteophytes.
- *Polymyalgia rheumatica* occurs mostly in middle-aged or elderly women, causing marked stiffness and weakness after inactivity. Pain is most severe around the pectoral and pelvic girdles; tenderness is in muscles rather than joints. The ESR is almost always high. This is a form of giant-cell arteritis and carries the risk of temporal arteritis resulting in blindness. Corticosteroids provide rapid and dramatic relief of all symptoms.

> ⚠ **Swollen finger joints:**
> Proximal joints = inflammatory arthritis.
> Distal joints = osteoarthritis.

Complications

Infection

Patients with RA – and even more so those on corticosteroid therapy – are susceptible to infection. Sudden clinical deterioration, or increased pain in a single joint, should alert one to the possibility of septic arthritis and the need for joint aspiration.

Tendon rupture

Nodular infiltration may lead to tendon rupture. This is seen most often at the wrist, where it contributes significantly to the development of the characteristic rheumatoid deformities.

Joint rupture

Occasionally the joint lining ruptures and synovial contents spill into the soft tissues. Treatment is directed at the underlying synovitis – i.e. splintage and injection of the joint, with synovectomy as a second resort.

Secondary osteoarthritis

Articular cartilage erosion may leave the joint so damaged that, even if the rheumatoid disease subsides or is kept under control, the end stage will be very similar to advanced osteoarthritis.

Prognosis

Rheumatoid arthritis runs a variable course. When the patient is first seen it is difficult to predict the outcome, but high titres of RF, periarticular erosions, rheumatoid nodules, severe muscle wasting, joint contractures and evidence of vasculitis are bad prognostic signs. Women, on the whole, fare somewhat worse than men. Without

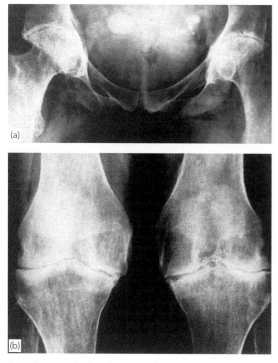

(a)

(b)

3.5 Rheumatoid arthritis – aftermath After the acute inflammatory phase has passed, the patient may be left with features of secondary osteoarthritis, especially in (a) the hips and (b) the knees.

effective treatment about 10% of patients improve steadily after the first attack of active synovitis; 60% have intermittent phases of disease activity and remission, but with a slow downhill course over many years; 20% have severe joint erosion, which is usually evident within the first 5 years; and 10% end up completely disabled. In addition, a reduction in life expectancy by 5–10 years is common and is often due to premature ischaemic heart disease. However, early aggressive medical treatment appears to reduce the morbidity and mortality.

Treatment

There is no cure for RA. A multi-disciplinary approach is needed from the beginning: ideally the therapeutic team should include a rheumatologist, orthopaedic surgeon, physiotherapist, occupational therapist, orthotist and social worker. Their deployment and priorities will vary according to the individual and the stage of the disease.

At the onset of the disease there will be uncertainty about its likely rate of progress. A poor prognosis is associated with female sex, multiple joint involvement, high ESR and CRP, positive RF and anticyclic citrullinated peptide antibody (CCP), younger age and the presence of erosions at diagnosis.

Principles of medical management

Treatment is aimed at controlling inflammation as rapidly as possible. *Corticosteroids* are used for their rapid action (initially an oral dose of 30 mg of prednisolone or 120 mg of methylprednisolone intramuscularly). The dose should be rapidly tapered off to prevent significant side-effects.

In addition, *disease-modifying antirheumatic drugs* (DMARDs) should be started at this time; the first choice is now methotrexate at doses of 10–25 mg/week. This may be used initially alone or in combination with sulfasalazine and hydroxychloroquine. Leflunomide can also be considered if methotrexate is not tolerated. Gold and penicillamine are now rarely used.

NSAIDs may be needed to control pain and stiffness. If there is no satisfactory response to DMARDs, it is wise to progress rapidly to *biological therapies* such as the tumour necrosis factor (TNF) inhibitors infliximab, etanercept and adalimumab.

Further measures include the *injection of long-acting corticosteroid preparations into inflamed joints and tendon sheaths*. It is sometimes feared that such injections may themselves cause damage to articular cartilage or tendons. However, there is little evidence that they are harmful, provided they are used sparingly and with full precautions against infection.

Physiotherapy and occupational therapy

Muscle tone and joint mobility are maintained by a balanced programme of exercise, and general advice on coping with the activities of daily living. Preventative splinting and orthotic devices may be helpful; however, it is important to encourage activity.

Surgical management

Operative treatment may be indicated at any stage of the disease if conservative measures alone are not effective. Early on this consists mainly of soft-tissue procedures (synovectomy, tendon repair or replacement and joint stabilization).

In late rheumatoid disease, severe joint destruction, fixed deformity and loss of function are clear indications for reconstructive surgery. Arthrodesis, osteotomy and arthroplasty all have their place and are considered in the appropriate chapters. However, it should be recognized that patients who are no longer suffering the pain of active synovitis and who are contented with a limited pattern of life may not want or need heroic surgery merely to improve their anatomy. Careful assessment for occupational therapy, the provision of mechanical aids and adjustments to their home environment may be much more useful.

It appears safe to continue methotrexate during elective orthopaedic surgery. However, doses of corticosteroids should be as low as possible and biological therapies such as the TNF inhibitors should be stopped prior to surgery where possible.

ANKYLOSING SPONDYLITIS

Like RA, this is a generalized chronic inflammatory disease but its effects are seen mainly in the spine and sacroiliac joints. It is characterized by pain and stiffness of the back, with variable involvement of the hips and shoulders and (more rarely) the peripheral joints. Its prevalence is about 0.2% in Western Europe, but is much lower in Japanese and African peoples. Males are affected more frequently than females (estimates vary from 2:1 to 10:1) and the usual age at onset is between 15 and 25 years.

Cause

The disease tends to run in families; close relatives may have either classic ankylosing spondylitis or one of the other 'spondarthritides' such as Reiter's disease, psoriatic arthritis or enteropathic arthritis. The fact that all these conditions are associated with a particular tissue type, the HLA-B27, suggests a genetic predisposition; the specific clinical syndrome is probably triggered by some recent event – often genitourinary or bowel infection.

Pathology

There are three characteristic lesions: (1) *synovitis* of diarthrodial joints; (2) *inflammation at the fibro-osseous junctions* of syndesmotic joints, tendons and ligaments (*enthesopathy*); and (3) *ossification* across the periphery of the intervertebral discs.

The disease starts as an inflammation of the sacroiliac and vertebral joints and ligaments. Sometimes the hips and shoulders also are affected, and very occasionally the peripheral joints.

Pathological changes follow a constant sequence: inflammation – granulation tissue formation – erosion of articular cartilage or bone – replacement by fibrous tissue – ossification of the fibrous tissue – ankylosis. If many vertebrae are involved, the spine may become absolutely rigid. If the costovertebral joints are involved, respiratory excursion is diminished.

Clinical features

Most patients are young men who complain of persistent backache and stiffness, often worse in the early morning or after inactivity. About 10% have pain in peripheral joints.

The most typical sign is stiffness of the spine. All movements are diminished, but loss of extension is both the earliest and the most severe. The 'wall test' is useful: if a healthy person stands with his or her back to a wall, their heels, buttocks, scapulae and occiput could all be made to touch the wall simultaneously, but if extension is seriously diminished, this is impossible. In advanced cases the entire spine may be rigid ('poker back') and chest expansion is decreased to well below the normal 7 cm.

If the hips are involved, they also may go on to complete ankylosis. Occasionally, peripheral joints are swollen and tender. Some patients complain of painful heels and have tenderness at the insertion of the tendo Achilles.

Extraskeletal manifestations include general fatigue and loss of weight, ocular inflammation, aortic valve disease, carditis and pulmonary fibrosis.

Imaging

The cardinal x-ray feature is fuzziness or frank erosion of the sacroiliac joints. Later these joints become sclerosed and, eventually, completely ankylosed. More subtle changes can be revealed by MRI.

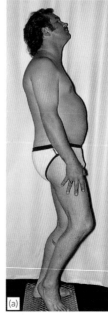
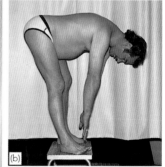

3.6 Ankylosing spondylitis – early The cardinal clinical feature is marked stiffness of the spine. (a) This patient manages to stand upright by keeping his knees slightly flexed. (b) It looks as if he can bend down to touch his toes, but his back is rigid and all the movement takes place at his hips.

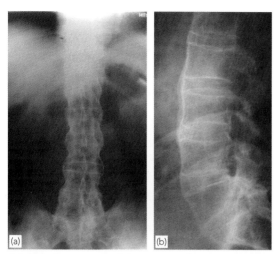

3.7 Ankylosing spondylitis – x-ray features Bony bridges (syndesmophytes) between the vertebral bodies convert the spine into a rigid column. Note that the sacroiliac joints have fused.

Ossification across the intervertebral discs produces bony bridges (syndesmophytes) spanning the gaps between adjacent vertebral bodies. Bridging at several levels gives the appearance of a 'bamboo spine'.

Peripheral joints may show erosive arthritis resembling that of RA.

Investigations

The ESR is usually elevated during active phases of the disease. HLA-B27 is present in 95% of Caucasian patients and one-half of their first-degree relatives.

Diagnosis

Diagnosis is easy in patients who present with chronic back pain and spinal rigidity. However, in over 10% of cases the disease starts in a peripheral joint and it may be several years before the true diagnosis reveals itself. Atypical onset is more common in women. A history of ankylosing spondylitis in a relative is strongly suggestive. There are three syndromes in particular which may cause confusion.

Other seronegative spondarthritides

These are a group of conditions which are related to ankylosing spondylitis and may, in fact, share a genetic and pathogenetic background. They are described in the next section of this chapter.

Diffuse idiopathic hyperostosis (Forestier's disease)

This is a radiological teaser. Clinical features are non-existent or mild, but x-rays (taken for other complaints) show widespread ossification of ligaments and tendon insertions. The inexperienced clinician may mistake these appearances for those of ankylosing spondylitis, but the absence of symptoms and signs of an inflammatory disorder should suggest the correct diagnosis.

Mechanical back pain

Low back pain in young adults is usually attributed to one of many 'mechanical' conditions, including muscle strain, facet joint dysfunction and discogenic disorders. Ankylosing spondylitis should be kept in mind, lest the diagnosis be missed merely for lack of thinking about it.

Treatment

The disease is not usually as crippling as RA and many patients continue to lead an active life. Treatment consists of: (1) general measures to maintain satisfactory posture and preserve movement; (2) anti-inflammatory drugs to counteract pain and stiffness; (3) the use of TNF inhibitors for severe disease; and (4) operations to correct deformity or restore mobility.

- *General measures*: patients are taught how to maintain satisfactory posture and encouraged to remain active and to perform spinal extension exercises every day.
- *NSAIDs*: these drugs may not retard the progress to ankylosis but they do control pain and counteract soft-tissue stiffness.
- *TNF inhibitors*: with the introduction of the TNF inhibitors it has become possible to treat the underlying inflammatory processes active in ankylosing spondylitis. This can result in significant improvement in disease activity including remission. TNF inhibitors are generally reserved for patients who cannot be helped by NSAIDs.
- *Operation*: significantly damaged hips can be treated by joint replacement, though this seldom provides more than moderate mobility. Moreover, the incidence of infection is higher than usual and patients may need prolonged rehabilitation. Deformity of the spine may be severe enough to warrant lumbar or cervical osteotomy. These are difficult and potentially hazardous procedures; fortunately they are seldom needed.

SERONEGATIVE SPONDARTHRITIS

A number of conditions usually associated with seronegative polyarthritis (i.e. without serum RFs) may show changes in the spine and sacroiliac joints indistinguishable from those of ankylosing spondylitis. The best defined of these conditions are *psoriatic arthritis*, *Reiter's disease* and the arthritis that sometimes accompanies *ulcerative colitis* or *Crohn's disease*; together with classic *ankylosing spondylitis* they are often grouped as the 'seronegative spondarthritides'.

The exact relationship between these disorders is unknown, but they share certain important features: (1) the characteristic spondylitis and sacroiliitis occur in all of them; (2) they are all associated with HLA-B27; (3) they show familial aggregation; and (4) there is considerable overlap within families, some members having one disorder and close relatives another.

PSORIATIC ARTHRITIS

About 4% of patients with chronic polyarthritis have psoriasis; not all, however, have psoriatic arthritis, which is a distinct entity and not simply 'RA plus psoriasis'. Unlike RA, psoriatic arthritis affects men and women equally and tends to run in families. The arthritis is not as clearly symmetrical as in RA and – in marked contrast to the latter – it occurs mainly in the interphalangeal joints of the fingers and toes. Bone destruction may be so severe that the digits are completely flail or badly deformed ('arthritis mutilans'). About one-quarter of the patients develop sacroiliac and vertebral changes like those of ankylosing spondylitis. HLA-B27 occurs in about 60% of those with overt sacroiliitis.

General treatment aims at controlling the skin disorder with topical preparations, and alleviating joint symptoms with NSAIDs. In resistant forms of arthritis, immunosuppressive agents have proved effective.

Local treatment consists of judicious splintage to prevent undue deformity, and surgery for unstable joints.

REITER'S DISEASE AND REACTIVE ARTHRITIS

'Classic' Reiter's disease is a clinical triad: polyarthritis, conjunctivitis and non-specific urethritis. However, the term is now used more loosely for a *reactive arthritis* associated with

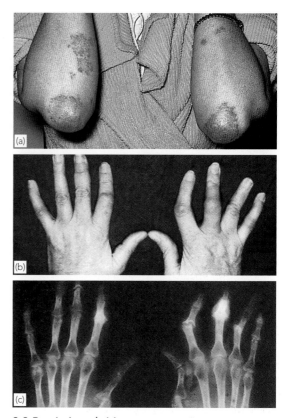

3.8 Psoriatic arthritis (a) Psoriasis of the elbows and forearms. (b) Typical finger deformities. (c) X-rays show distal joint involvement – clearly the disease is not simply rheumatoid arthritis in a patient with psoriasis.

non-specific urogenital or bowel infection. It is probably the most common type of large-joint polyarthritis in young men. Familial aggregation, overlap with other forms of seronegative spondarthritis in first-degree relatives, and an increased frequency of HLA-B27 in all these disorders point to a genetic predisposition. *Chlamydia trachomatis* has been implicated as the urogenital infective agent, but arthritis also occurs with bowel infection due to *Shigella*, *Salmonella* or *Yersinia enterocolitica*.

The joints themselves are not infected; the synovitis is the end stage of an abnormal immune response to infection elsewhere or to its products.

Clinical features

The *acute phase* of the disease is marked by an asymmetrical inflammatory arthritis of the lower limb joints – usually the knee and ankle but often the tarsal and toe joints as well. The joint may be acutely painful, hot and swollen with a tense effusion, suggesting gout or infection. Tendo

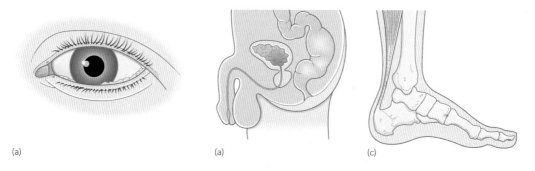

(a)   (a)   (c)

3.9 Reiter's syndrome The classic *'Reiter's triad'* consists of conjunctivitis, urethritis (sometimes colitis) and arthritis. Tenderness of the tendo Achilles and the plantar fascia is also common.

Achilles tenderness and plantar fasciitis (evidence of enthesopathy) are common, and the patient may complain of backache even in the early stage.

Typically there is a history of urethritis, prostatitis, cervicitis or diarrhoea. Ocular lesions include conjunctivitis, episcleritis and uveitis.

The acute disorder usually lasts for a few weeks or months and then subsides, but most patients have either recurrent attacks of arthritis or other features suggesting chronic disease.

The *chronic phase* is more characteristic of a spondarthropathy. Over one-half of the patients with Reiter's disease complain of mild, recurrent episodes of polyarthritis (including upper limb joints). About one-half of those again develop sacroiliitis and spondylitis, with features resembling those of ankylosing spondylitis.

Special investigations

Tests for HLA-B27 are positive in 75% of patients with sacroiliitis. The ESR may be high in the active phase. The causative organism can sometimes be isolated from urethral fluids or faeces, and tests for antibodies may be positive.

Diagnosis

If the condition affects only one or two joints it is usually mistaken for gout or infective arthritis. Examination of the synovial fluid for organisms and crystals will help to exclude these disorders.

Treatment

General treatment is indicated for active urogenital or bowel infection; a short course of antibiotics is usually sufficient, but for *Chlamydia* tetracycline daily for 6 months is recommended.

Symptomatic treatment includes the use of analgesia and NSAIDs. If the inflammatory response is aggressive then local injection of corticosteroids or even intramuscular methylprednisolone may be useful. If symptoms and signs do not resolve then DMARDs, as used in the treatment of RA, may be needed. Topical steroids may be used for uveitis.

JUVENILE IDIOPATHIC ARTHRITIS

Juvenile idiopathic arthritis (JIA) is the preferred term for non-infective inflammatory joint disease of more than 3 months' duration in children under 16 years. It embraces a group of disorders in all of which pain, swelling and stiffness of the joints are common features. The prevalence is about 1 per 1000 children, and boys and girls are affected with equal frequency.

The cause is probably similar to that of rheumatoid disease: an abnormal immune response to some antigen in children with a particular genetic predisposition. However, RF is usually absent.

The pathology, too, is like that of RA: a synovial inflammation leading to fibrosis and ankylosis; the joints tend to stiffen in whatever position they are allowed to assume (usually flexion) and growth is retarded.

Clinical features

JIA occurs in several characteristic forms: about 15% have a systemic illness and arthritis only develops somewhat later; the majority (60–70%) have a pauciarticular arthritis affecting a few of the larger joints; about 10% present with polyarticular arthritis, sometimes closely resembling RA; the remaining 5–10% develop a seronegative spondyloarthritis.

Systemic JIA

This, the classic Still's disease, is usually seen below the age of 3 years. It starts with intermittent fever, rashes and malaise; there may also be lymphadenopathy, splenomegaly and hepatomegaly. Joint swelling occurs some weeks or months after the onset; fortunately, it usually resolves when the systemic illness subsides but it may go on to a progressive seronegative polyarthritis with permanent deformity of the larger joints and fusion of the cervical apophyseal joints. By puberty there may also be stunting of growth, often abetted by the use of corticosteroids.

Pauciarticular JIA

This is by far the commonest form of JIA. It usually occurs below the age of 6 years and is more common in girls. Only a few joints are involved and there is no systemic illness. The child presents with pain and swelling of medium-sized joints (knees, ankles, elbows and wrists); RF tests are negative. A serious complication is chronic iridocyclitis, which occurs in about 50%. The arthritis often goes into remission after a few years but by then the child is left with asymmetrical deformities and growth defects that may be permanent.

Polyarticular seropositive JIA

This is usually seen in older children, mainly girls. The typical deformities of RA are uncommon and RF is usually absent. In some cases, however, the features can be indistinguishable from those of adult RA, with a positive RF test; these probably warrant the designation 'juvenile rheumatoid arthritis'.

Seronegative spondarthritis

In older children – usually boys – the condition may take the form of sacroiliitis and spondylitis; hips and knees are sometimes involved as well. Tests for HLA-B27 are often positive and this should probably be regarded as 'juvenile ankylosing spondylitis'.

Complications

- *Stiffness*: while most patients recover good function, some permanent loss of movement is common.
- *Growth defects*: there is general retardation of growth, sometimes aggravated by prolonged corticosteroid therapy.
- *Iridocyclitis*: this is most common in pauciarticular disease; untreated it may lead to blindness.
- *Amyloidosis*: in children with long-standing active disease there is a serious risk of amyloidosis, which may be fatal.

Treatment

General treatment is similar to that of RA. Corticosteroids should be used only for severe systemic disease and chronic iridocyclitis unresponsive to topical therapy.

Local treatment aims to prevent stiffness and deformity. Night splints are useful for the wrists, hands, knees and ankles; prone lying for some period each day may prevent flexion contracture of the hips. Between periods of splinting, active exercises are encouraged.

Fixed deformities may need correction by serial plasters; when progress is no longer being made, joint capsulotomy may help.

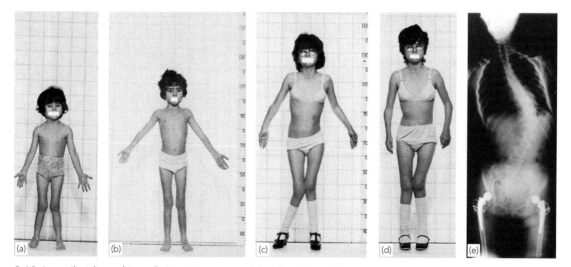

3.10 Juvenile idiopathic arthritis This young girl developed JIA when she was 5 years old. Here we see her at 6, 9 and 14 years of age (a,b,c). The arthritis became inactive, leaving her with a knee deformity which was treated by osteotomy (d). (e) X-ray of another girl who required hip replacements at the age of 14 years and, later, surgical correction of her scoliosis.

For painful, eroded joints operation is indicated. Useful procedures include custom-designed arthroplasties of the hip and knee (even in children), and arthrodesis of the wrist or ankle.

Outcome

Fortunately, most children with JIA recover from the arthritis and are left with only moderate deformity and limitation of function. However, 5–10% (and especially those with juvenile RA) are severely disabled and require treatment throughout life.

A significant number of children with JIA (about 3%) still die – usually as a result of renal failure due to amyloidosis, or following overwhelming infection.

SYSTEMIC CONNECTIVE-TISSUE DISEASES

'Systemic connective-tissue disease' is a collective term for a group of closely related conditions that have features which overlap with those of rheumatoid disease. Like RA, these are 'autoimmune disorders', probably triggered by viral infection in genetically predisposed individuals.

Systemic lupus erythematosus is the best known. It occurs mainly in young females and may be difficult to differentiate from RA. Although joint pain is usual, it is often overshadowed by systemic symptoms such as malaise, anorexia, weight loss and fever. Characteristic clinical features are skin rashes (especially a 'butterfly rash' on the face), Raynaud's phenomenon, peripheral vasculitis, splenomegaly, and disorders of the kidney, heart, lung, eyes and central nervous system. Anaemia, leucopenia and elevation of the ESR are common. Tests for antinuclear factor are always positive.

Corticosteroids are indicated for severe systemic disease and may have to be continued for life. Progressive joint deformity is unusual and the arthritis can almost always be controlled by anti-inflammatory drugs, physiotherapy and intermittent splintage.

A curious complication of systemic lupus is avascular necrosis (usually of the femoral head). This may be due in part to the corticosteroid treatment, but the disease itself seems to predispose to bone ischaemia.

FIBROMYALGIA

Fibromyalgia is not so much a diagnosis as a descriptive term for a condition in which patients complain of pain and tenderness in the muscles and other soft tissues around the back of the neck and shoulders and across the lower part of the back and the upper parts of the buttocks. What sets the condition apart from other 'rheumatic' diseases is the complete absence of demonstrable pathological changes in the affected tissues. Indeed, it is often difficult to give credence to the patient's complaints, an attitude which is encouraged by the fact that similar symptoms are encountered in some patients who have suffered trivial injuries in a variety of accidents; a significant number also develop psychological depression and anxiety.

The criteria for making the diagnosis were put forward by the American College of Rheumatology in 1990. These included symptoms of widespread pain in all four quadrants of the body, together with at least nine pairs of designated 'tender points' on physical examination. In practice, however, the diagnosis is often made in patients with much more localized symptoms and signs, and it is now quite common to attach this label to almost any condition associated with myofascial pain where no specific underlying disorder can be identified.

The cause of fibromyalgia remains unknown; no pathology has been found in the 'tender spots'. It has been suggested that this is an abnormality of 'sensory processing', which is perhaps another way of saying that the sufferers have a 'low pain threshold'; in fact they often do display increased sensitivity to pain in other parts of the body. There are also suggestions that the condition is related to stress responses which can be activated by sudden accidents or traumatic life events. This does not mean that such patients will necessarily show other features of psychological dysfunction and the condition cannot be excluded merely by psychological testing.

In mild cases, treatment can be limited to keeping up muscle tone and general fitness (hence the advice to have physiotherapy and then continue with daily exercises on their own), perhaps together with injections into the painful areas simply to reduce the level of discomfort. Patients with more persistent and more disturbing symptoms may benefit from various types of psychotherapy.

GOUT AND PSEUDOGOUT

Gout and its imitators form a group of conditions characterized by the presence of crystals in and around the joints, bursae and tendons. Three clinical disorders in particular are associated with this phenomenon:

- *Gout*: urate crystal deposition disorder.
- *Pseudogout*: calcium pyrophosphate dihydrate (CPPD) deposition disease.
- *Basic calcium phosphate* (BCP) *deposition disease.*

Characteristically, in each of these conditions, crystal deposition has three distinct consequences: (1) the deposit may be inert and asymptomatic; (2) it may induce an acute inflammatory reaction; or (3) it may result in slow destruction of the affected tissues.

GOUT

This is a disorder of purine metabolism characterized by hyperuricaemia, deposition of monosodium urate monohydrate crystals in joints and periarticular tissues and recurrent attacks of acute synovitis. Late changes include cartilage degeneration, renal dysfunction and uric acid kidney stones.

The clinical disorder was known to Hippocrates and its association with hyperuricaemia was recognized well over 100 years ago. The prevalence of symptomatic gout varies from 1 to over 10 per thousand, depending on the race, sex and age of the population studied. It is much commoner in Caucasian than in Black African peoples; it is more widespread in men than in women (the ratio may be as high as 20:1) and it is seldom seen before the menopause in females.

Although the risk of developing clinical features of gout increases with increasing levels of serum uric acid, only a fraction of those with hyperuricaemia develop symptoms. However, 'hyperuricaemia' and 'gout' are generally regarded as aspects of the same disorder.

Pathology

Hyperuricaemia

Nucleic acid and purine metabolism normally proceeds, through complex pathways, to the production of hypoxanthine and xanthine; the final breakdown to uric acid is catalysed by the enzyme xanthine oxidase. Monosodium urate appears in ionic form in all the body fluids; about 70% is derived from endogenous purine metabolism and 30% from purine-rich foods in the diet. It is excreted (as uric acid) mainly by the kidneys and partly in the gut.

Serum uric acid concentration varies considerably and some populations (for example New Zealand Maoris) have much higher levels than others. The term 'hyperuricaemia' is therefore generally reserved for individuals with a serum urate concentration which is significantly higher than that of the population to which they belong (more than two standard deviations above the mean); this is about 0.42 mmol/L for men and 0.35 mmol/L for women in Western Caucasian peoples. By this definition, about 5% of men and less than 1% of women have hyperuricaemia; the majority suffer no pathological consequences and they remain asymptomatic throughout life.

Clinical gout

Urate crystals are deposited in minute clumps in connective tissue, including articular cartilage; the commonest sites are the small joints of the hands and feet. For months, perhaps years, they remain inert. Then, possibly as a result of local trauma, the needle-like crystals are dispersed into the joint and the surrounding tissues where they excite an acute inflammatory reaction.

With the passage of time, urate deposits may build up in joints, periarticular tissues, tendons and bursae; common sites are around the metatarsophalangeal joints of the big toes, the Achilles tendons, the olecranon bursae and the pinnae of the ears. These clumps of chalky material, or tophi, vary in size from less than 1 millimetre to several centimetres in diameter. They may ulcerate through the skin or destroy cartilage and periarticular bone.

Urate calculi appear in the urine, and crystal deposition in the kidney parenchyma may cause renal failure.

Classification

Primary gout (95% of cases) occurs in the absence of any obvious cause and may be due to constitutional under-excretion (the vast majority) or over-production of urate. *Secondary gout* (5%) results from prolonged hyperuricaemia due to acquired disorders such as myeloproliferative diseases, administration of diuretics or renal failure.

This division is somewhat artificial; people with an initial tendency to 'primary' hyperuricaemia may develop gout only when secondary factors are introduced: for example obesity and alcohol abuse, or treatment with diuretics or salicylates which increase tubular reabsorption of uric acid.

Clinical features

Patients are usually men over the age of 30 years. Often there is a family history of gout.

The acute attack

The sudden onset of severe joint pain which lasts for 1–2 weeks is typical of acute gout. This is usually spontaneous but may be precipitated by minor trauma, operation, unaccustomed exercise or alcohol. The commonest sites are the metatarsophalangeal joint of the big toe, the ankle and finger joints and the olecranon bursa. The skin looks red and shiny and there is considerable swelling. The joint feels hot and extremely tender, suggesting a cellulitis or septic arthritis. Sometimes the only feature is acute pain and tenderness in the heel or the sole of the foot.

Hyperuricaemia is present at some stage, although not necessarily during an acute attack. The diagnosis can be established beyond doubt by finding the characteristic birefringent crystals in the synovial fluid.

Chronic gout

Recurrent acute attacks may eventually merge into polyarticular gout. Tophi may appear around joints, over the olecranon and in the pinna of the ear. A large tophus can ulcerate and discharge its chalky material. Joint erosion causes chronic pain, stiffness and deformity. Renal lesions include calculi and parenchymal disease.

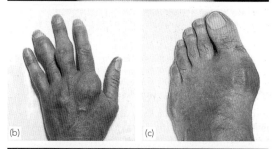

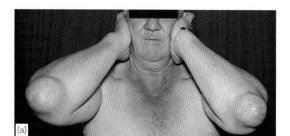

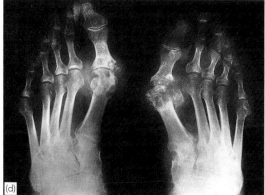

4.1 Gout (a) This is the typical 'gouty type', with his rubicund face, large olecranon bursae and small subcutaneous tophi over the elbows. (b,c) Tophaceous gout affecting the hands and feet; the swollen big toe joint is particularly characteristic. (d) X-rays show the typical periarticular excavations (tophi consisting of uric acid deposits) in the big toe metatarsophalangeal joints.

X-rays

During the acute attack x-rays show only soft-tissue swelling. Chronic gout may show asymmetrical, punched-out 'cysts' in the periarticular bone, joint space narrowing and secondary osteoarthritis.

Differential diagnosis

Pseudogout

Pyrophosphate crystal deposition may cause an acute arthritis indistinguishable from gout – except that it tends to affect large rather than small joints and is somewhat more common in women than in men. Articular calcification may show on x-ray. Demonstrating the crystals in synovial fluid establishes the diagnosis.

Infection

Cellulitis, septic bursitis, an infected bunion or septic arthritis must all be excluded, if necessary by immediate joint aspiration and examination of synovial fluid.

Rheumatoid arthritis

Polyarticular gout affecting the fingers may be mistaken for rheumatoid arthritis, and elbow tophi for rheumatoid nodules. In difficult cases, biopsy will establish the diagnosis.

Treatment

The acute attack

The acute attack should be treated by resting the joint, applying ice packs and giving full doses of a non-steroidal anti-inflammatory drug (NSAID). Colchicine, one of the oldest of medications, is also effective but may cause diarrhoea, nausea and vomiting. A tense effusion may require aspiration and intra-articular injection of corticosteroids. Oral corticosteroids are useful for patients in whom NSAIDs are contraindicated. The sooner treatment is started the more effective it is likely to be.

Interval therapy

Between attacks, attention should be given to simple measures such as losing weight, cutting out alcohol and eliminating diuretics. Urate-lowering drugs are indicated if acute attacks recur at frequent intervals, if there are tophi or if renal function is impaired. They should also be considered for asymptomatic hyperuricaemia if the plasma urate concentration is persistently above 6 mg/dL (0.36 mmol/L). However, one must remember that this starts a life-long commitment and many clinicians feel that people who have never had an attack of gout and are free of tophi or urinary calculi do not need treatment.

Uricosuric drugs (probenecid or sulfinpyrazone) can be used if renal function is normal. However, allopurinol, a xanthine oxidase inhibitor, is usually preferred, and for patients with renal complications or chronic tophaceous gout allopurinol is definitely the drug of choice.

Urate-lowering drugs should never be started before the acute attack has completely subsided, and they should always be covered by an anti-inflammatory preparation or colchicine, otherwise they may actually prolong or precipitate an acute attack. Patients who suffer an acute attack of gout while already on a constant dose of urate-lowering treatment should be advised to continue taking the drug at the usual dosage while the acute episode is being treated.

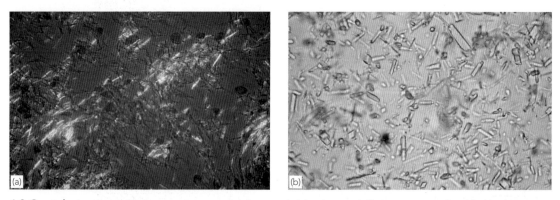

4.2 Crystals In polarized light, crystals appear bright on a dark background. If a compensator is added to the optical system, the background appears in shades of mauve and birefringent crystals as yellow or blue. In these two specimens (obtained from crystal deposits in two different joints) *urate crystals* (a) appear needle-like, 5–20 μm long and exhibiting strong negative birefringence, while the *pyrophosphate crystals* (b) are rhomboid-shaped, slightly smaller than urate crystals and showing weak positive birefringence. (Courtesy of Professor P. A. Dieppe.)

Surgery

With prolonged urate-lowering therapy, adjusted to maintain a normal serum uric acid level (less than 0.36 mmol/L), tophi may gradually dissolve. However, ulcerating tophi that fail to heal with conservative treatment can be evacuated by curettage; the wound is left open and dressings are applied until it heals.

CALCIUM PYROPHOSPHATE DIHYDRATE DEPOSITION

'CPPD deposition' encompasses three overlapping conditions: (1) *chondrocalcinosis* – the appearance of calcific material in articular cartilage and menisci; (2) *pseudogout* – a crystal-induced synovitis; and (3) *chronic pyrophosphate arthropathy* – a type of degenerative joint disease.

Pathology

Pyrophosphate is probably generated in abnormal cartilage by enzyme activity at chondrocyte surfaces; it combines with calcium ions in the matrix where crystal nucleation occurs on collagen fibres. The crystals grow into microscopic 'tophi' which appear in the cartilage matrix and in fibrocartilaginous structures such as the menisci of the knee and the intervertebral discs.

From time to time CPPD crystals are extruded into the joint where they excite an inflammatory reaction similar to gout.

Clinical features

The clinical disorder takes several forms, all of them appearing with increasing frequency in relation to age. Most of the patients are women over the age of 60 years.

Asymptomatic chondrocalcinosis

Calcification of the menisci is common in elderly people and is usually asymptomatic. When it is seen in association with osteoarthritis this does not necessarily imply cause and effect; both are common in elderly people and they are bound to be seen together in some patients. *X-rays* may reveal chondrocalcinosis in other asymptomatic joints. Chondrocalcinosis in patients under 50 years of age should suggest the possibility of an underlying metabolic disease or a familial disorder.

Acute synovitis (pseudogout)

The patient, typically a middle-aged woman, complains of acute pain and swelling in one of the larger joints – usually the knee. Sometimes the attack is precipitated by a minor illness or operation. The joint is tense and inflamed, though usually not as acutely as in gout. Untreated the condition lasts for a few weeks and then subsides spontaneously. *X-rays* may show signs of chondrocalcinosis, and the diagnosis can be confirmed by finding *positive birefringent crystals* in the synovial fluid.

Chronic pyrophosphate arthropathy

The patient, usually an elderly woman, presents with polyarticular 'osteoarthritis' affecting the larger joints, including joints such as the ankles, shoulders or elbows where 'primary' osteoarthritis is seldom seen. This is often diagnosed as 'generalized osteoarthritis' but the *x-ray features* are distinctive: (a) unusual calcification in articular cartilage and

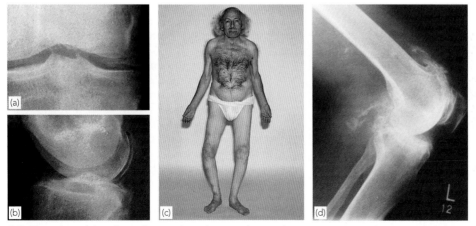

4.3 Chondrocalcinosis and pyrophosphate arthropathy (a,b) Chondrocalcinosis (calcification of articular cartilage and fibrous menisci) in the knee. (c) This middle-aged man presented with osteoarthritis in several large joints, including the elbow and ankle where osteoarthritis is uncommon. (d) A characteristic feature is patellofemoral arthritis associated with large, trailing osteophytes.

menisci as well as the periarticular soft tissues; together with (b) progressive degeneration of the articular surfaces.

Sometimes alternating bouts of acute synovitis and chronic arthritis may mimic rheumatoid disease. Occasionally joint destruction is so marked as to suggest neuropathic joint disease.

Diagnosis

Pseudogout must be distinguished from other acute inflammatory disorders such as gout and infection. Diagnosis rests on identifying the characteristic crystals in synovial fluid.

Chronic pyrophosphate arthropathy can resemble other types of polyarticular arthritis and will come into the differential diagnosis of rheumatoid arthritis and polyarticular osteoarthritis (see page 48).

Metabolic disorders such as hyperparathyroidism, haemochromatosis and alkaptonuria may be associated with calcification of articular cartilage and fibrocartilage as well as joint symptoms. It is important to exclude such generalized disorders before labelling a patient as 'just another case of chondrocalcinosis'.

Gout	Pseudogout
■ Smaller joints	■ Large joints
■ Pain intense	■ Pain moderate
■ Joint inflamed	■ Joint swollen
■ Hyperuricaemia	■ Chondrocalcinosis
■ Uric acid crystals	■ Calcium pyrophosphate crystals

Treatment

The treatment of pseudogout is similar to that of classic gout: rest, NSAIDs, joint aspiration and intra-articular injection of corticosteroid. Chronic pyrophosphate arthropathy is treated like osteoarthritis.

CALCIUM HYDROXYAPATITE DEPOSITION

BCP is a normal component of bone mineral, in the form of calcium hydroxyapatite crystals. It also occurs abnormally in dead or damaged tissue. Minute deposits in joints and periarticular tissues can give rise to either an acute reaction (synovitis or tendinitis) or a chronic, destructive arthropathy.

Prolonged hypercalcaemia or hyperphosphataemia, of whatever cause, may result in widespread metastatic calcification. However, by far the most common cause of BCP crystal deposition in and around joints is local tissue damage – strained or torn ligaments, tendon attrition and cartilage damage or degeneration.

Pathology

Minute BCP crystals are deposited in articular cartilage and in damaged tendons and ligaments – most notably around the shoulder and knee. The deposits grow by crystal accretion and may be detectable by x-ray.

In long-standing cases the calcific deposit has a chalky consistency. The mini-tophus may be completely inert, but in symptomatic cases it is surrounded by an acute vascular reaction and inflammation. Crystal shedding into joints may give rise to synovitis. More rarely this is complicated by the development of a rapidly destructive, erosive arthritis; bits of articular cartilage and bone or fragments of a meniscus may be found in the synovial cavity.

Clinical features

Two clinical syndromes are associated with BCP crystal deposition: (1) an acute or subacute periarthritis; and (2) a chronic rapidly destructive arthritis.

Acute or subacute periarthritis

This is by far the commonest form of BCP crystal deposition disorder. The patient, usually an adult between 30 and 50 years, complains of pain close to one of the larger joints – most commonly the shoulder or the knee. Symptoms may start suddenly, perhaps after minor trauma, and rise to a crescendo during which the soft tissues around the joint are swollen, warm and exquisitely tender. At other times the onset is more gradual and it is easier to localize the area of tenderness to one of the periarticular structures. Both forms of the condition are seen most commonly in rotator cuff lesions of the shoulder. Symptoms usually subside after a few weeks or months; sometimes they are aborted only when the calcific deposit is removed or the surrounding tissues are decompressed. In acute cases, operation may disclose a tense globule of creamy material oozing from between the frayed fibres of tendon or ligament.

Chronic destructive arthritis

BCP crystals are sometimes found in association with a chronic erosive arthritis; whether they cause

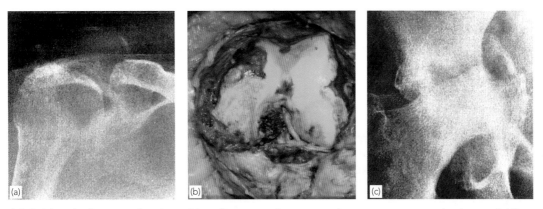

4.4 Calcium hydroxyapatite deposition disease Hydroxyapatite deposition is associated with several different clinical conditions: (a) painful supraspinatus calcium deposition; (b) severe articular destruction; and occasionally (c) a rapidly destructive arthropathy of the hip (or shoulder).

the arthritis or modify a pre-existing disorder remains uncertain.

A more dramatic type of rapidly destructive arthritis of the shoulder is occasionally seen in elderly patients with rotator cuff lesions. They have been attributed to BCP crystal (or mixed BCP and CPPD crystal) shedding into the joint. A similar rapidly destructive arthritis occasionally affects the hip.

X-rays

With periarthritis, calcification may be seen in tendons or ligaments close to the joint, most commonly in the rotator cuff around the shoulder.

Articular cartilage and fibrocartilaginous menisci and discs never show the type of calcification seen in CPPD deposition disease, but 'loose bodies' may be seen in synovial joints. Erosive arthritis causes loss of the articular space, with little or no sclerosis or osteophyte formation. The typical picture of rapidly destructive arthritis is one of severe erosion and destruction of subchondral bone. In advanced cases the joint may become unstable and, eventually, dislocated.

Treatment

Acute periarthritis should be treated by rest and NSAIDs. Resistant cases may respond to local injection of corticosteroids; this treatment should be used only to weather the acute storm – repeated injections for lesser pain may dampen the repair process in damaged tendons. Persistent pain and tenderness may call for operative removal of the calcific deposit or 'decompression' of the affected tendon or ligament.

Erosive arthritis is treated like osteoarthritis. However, rapidly progressive bone destruction calls for early operation: in the case of the shoulder, synovectomy and soft-tissue repair; for the hip, usually total joint replacement.

CHAPTER 5

OSTEOARTHRITIS AND RELATED DISORDERS

OSTEOARTHRITIS

Osteoarthritis (OA) is a chronic joint disorder in which there is progressive softening and disintegration of articular cartilage accompanied by new growth of cartilage and bone at the joint margins (osteophytes), and capsular fibrosis. It is defined as primary when no cause is obvious, and secondary when it follows a demonstrable abnormality.

Cause

The most obvious feature of OA is that it increases in frequency with age. This does not mean that it is an expression of senescence; it simply shows that OA takes many years to develop. To be sure, cartilage ageing does occur, resulting in splitting and flaking of the surface, but these changes are not progressive and they do not cause symptomatic arthritis.

OA results from a disparity between the stress applied to articular cartilage and the ability of the cartilage to withstand that stress. This could be due to one or a combination of two processes: (1) *weakening of the articular cartilage* (possibly due to genetic defects in type II collagen or to enzymatic activity in certain inflammatory disorders such as rheumatoid disease); and (2) *increased mechanical stress in some part of the articular surface*. Increased

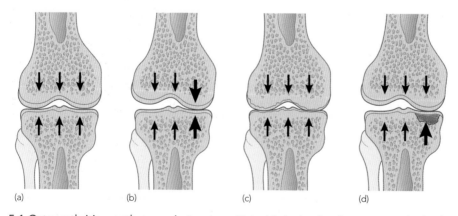

(a)   (b)   (c)   (d)

5.1 Osteoarthritis – pathogenesis In a normal joint (a), the loading forces are evenly distributed. Cartilage damage results from: (b) increased stress on some part of the articular surface; (c) a preceding inflammatory disorder which weakens the cartilage and renders it unable to bear even normal loads; or (d) abnormality of the subarticular bone which alters its ability to support the cartilage appropriately.

stress may be produced either by excessive impact loading or by reduction of the articular contact area in conditions causing joint incongruity. This would explain why an incongruent or an unstable joint almost inevitably develops OA. Theoretically, defects in the subchondral bone also may lead to stress concentration at particular sites.

The subsequent sequence of changes is still disputed, but at an early stage there appears to be damage to the cartilage collagen network and loss of proteoglycans from the matrix, giving rise to deformation and gradual structural disintegration.

Pathology

The cardinal features are: (1) progressive loss of articular cartilage thickness; (2) subarticular cyst formation and sclerosis; (3) re-modelling of the bone ends and osteophyte formation; (4) synovial irritation; and (5) capsular fibrosis.

The earliest morphological change is softening of the articular cartilage. The normally smooth and glistening surface becomes frayed or fibrillated, and eventually it is worn away to expose the underlying bone.

The subarticular bone reacts to these changes in several ways. In the area of greatest stress, cysts appear and the surrounding trabeculae become thickened or sclerotic. There is vascular congestion and the intraosseous pressure rises. Meanwhile, as the disease progresses, cartilage in peripheral, unstressed areas proliferates and ossifies, producing bony outgrowths (osteophytes). This re-modelling process restores a measure of congruity to the increasingly malopposed joint surfaces. It is clear,

therefore, that OA is not a purely degenerative disorder, and the term 'degenerative arthritis' – which is often used as a synonym for OA – is a misnomer. OA is a dynamic phenomenon, showing interacting features of both destruction and repair.

Although OA is not primarily an inflammatory disease, shedding of fragments from the fibrillated articular cartilage, as well as release of enzymes from damaged cells, may give rise to a low-grade synovitis. In the late stages, capsular fibrosis is common and may account for joint stiffness.

The cause of pain is problematic; articular cartilage and synovium have no nerve supply but the capsule is sensitive to stretching and the bone is sensitive to changes in pressure. Pain, therefore, may be due to both capsular fibrosis and vascular congestion of the subarticular bone.

Risk factors

- *Joint dysplasia*: disorders such as congenital acetabular dysplasia, Perthes' disease and slipped upper femoral epiphysis presage a greater than normal risk of OA in later life. Minor degrees of dysplasia are often asymptomatic and are spotted only later in life when OA starts to develop.
- *Trauma*: fractures involving the articular surface are obvious precursors of secondary OA; so too are lesser injuries which result in joint instability.
- *Occupation*: there is good evidence of an association between OA and certain occupations which cause repetitive stress, for example OA of the knees in workers engaged in continuous knee-bending activities.

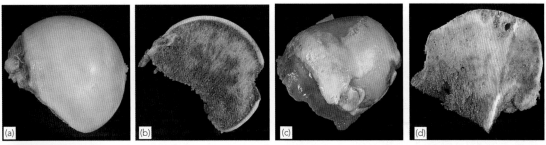

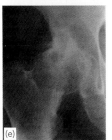

5.2 Osteoarthritis – pathology (a) Normal ageing causes slight degeneration of the articular surface, but the coronal section (b) shows that the cartilage thickness is well preserved. By contrast, in progressive osteoarthritis the weightbearing area suffers increasing damage. In the femoral head specimen (c), the superior surface is completely denuded of cartilage and there are large osteophytes around the periphery. In the coronal section (d), the subarticular cysts are clearly revealed; the x-ray (e) shows that the superolateral joint space (cartilage) has virtually disappeared and there are cysts in the underlying bone.

■ *Family history*: women whose mothers had generalized OA are more likely to develop the same condition. The particular trait responsible for this is not known.

Clinical features

Patients usually present after middle age, although it is likely that cartilage changes start 10 or even 20 years before that. Sometimes – especially in younger patients – there is a history of some preceding joint disorder or injury.

In some cases symptoms are confined to one or two large joints; in others (especially elderly women) multiple joints are affected, including the distal interphalangeal joints of the hand (polyarticular OA). Pain starts insidiously and increases slowly over months or years. It is aggravated by exertion and relieved by rest, although with time relief is less and less complete. Stiffness, characteristically, is worst after periods of rest. Typically symptoms follow an intermittent course, with periods of remission sometimes lasting for months. Swelling, deformity, tenderness, crepitus on movement, loss of mobility and muscle wasting are features of advanced disease. Ultimately the joint may become unstable.

In contrast to inflammatory joint disease, OA is unassociated with any systemic manifestations.

X-rays

The characteristic changes are: (1) narrowing of the joint 'space', due to cartilage depletion; (2) subarticular cyst formation and sclerosis; and (3) osteophyte formation. Initially the first two features are restricted to the major loadbearing part of the

joint, but in late cases the entire joint is affected. Evidence of previous disorders (congenital defects, old fractures, rheumatoid arthritis) may be present.

Clinical variants of OA

Although the features of OA in any particular joint are fairly consistent, the overall pattern of involvement shows variations which define a number of sub-groups.

Monarticular and pauciarticular OA

In its 'classic' form, OA presents with pain and dysfunction in one or two of the large weight-bearing joints. There may be an obvious underlying abnormality: acetabular dysplasia, old Perthes' disease or slipped epiphysis, long-standing joint deformity, a previous fracture or damage to ligaments or menisci. In many cases, however, the abnormality is so subtle that one may question whether the OA is 'primary' or 'secondary'.

Polyarticular (generalized) OA

This is far and away the most common form of OA, though most of the patients never consult an orthopaedic surgeon. The typical patient is a middle-aged woman who presents with pain, swelling and stiffness of the distal finger joints. The first carpometacarpal and the big toe metatarsophalangeal joints, or the knees and lumbar facet joints, may be affected as well.

The changes are most obvious in the hands. The interphalangeal joints become swollen and tender, and in the early stages they often appear to be inflamed. Over a period of years osteophytes and soft-tissue swelling produce a characteristic knobbly appearance of the distal interphalangeal joints (Heberden's nodes) and, less often, the proximal interphalangeal joints (Bouchard's nodes); pain may disappear but stiffness and deformity can be disturbing. Some patients present with painful knees or backache and the knobbly fingers are noticed only in passing.

OA in unusual sites

OA is uncommon in the shoulder, elbow, wrist and ankle. If any of these joints is affected one should suspect a previous abnormality – congenital or traumatic – or an associated generalized disease such as a crystal arthropathy.

Treatment

Early

There are three principles in the treatment of early OA: (1) relieve pain; (2) increase movement; (3) reduce load.

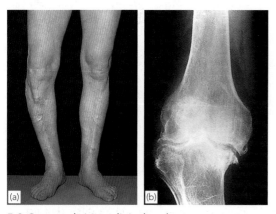

5.3 Osteoarthritis – clinical and x-ray (a) Varus deformity of the right knee due to osteoarthritis.
(b) The x-ray shows the classic features: disappearance of the joint 'space', subarticular sclerosis and osteophyte formation at the margins of the joint.

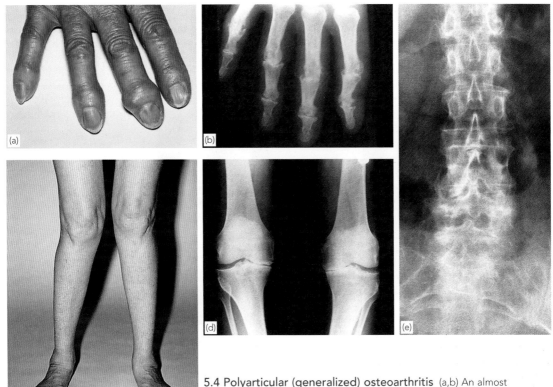

5.4 Polyarticular (generalized) osteoarthritis (a,b) An almost invariable feature of polyarticular osteoarthritis (OA) is involvement of the terminal finger joints – Heberden's nodes. There is a strong association with OA of the knees (c,d) and the lumbar facet joints (e).

Pain relief is achieved by analgesics and non-steroidal anti-inflammatory drugs (NSAIDs). Rest periods and modification of activities may also be necessary. NSAIDs are powerful prostaglandin inhibitors, which reduce the vascular congestion in the subchondral bone. Unfortunately they have a serious drawback: they cause gastrointestinal irritation and in some patients this leads to ulceration and bleeding. NSAIDs should be used only under medical supervision.

Joint mobility can often be improved by physiotherapy; even a small increase in range and power will reduce pain and improve function.

Load reduction can be achieved by using a walking stick, wearing soft-soled shoes, avoiding prolonged, stressful activity and by weight reduction. Physiotherapists and occupational therapists will give useful advice on how to modify daily activities and improve the work environment so as to reduce exposure to painful joint loading.

Intermediate

If symptoms increase despite conservative treatment, some form of operative treatment may be needed. This will usually be a 'holding' procedure, especially in younger patients who are not yet ready for a joint replacement. For OA of the knee, joint debridement (removal of interfering osteophytes, cartilage tags and loose bodies) can be performed arthroscopically. For both the hip and the knee, realignment osteotomy used to be popular, provided the joint was still stable and mobile; pain relief was often dramatic, probably because it provided vascular decompression of the subchondral bone as well as redistribution of loading forces towards less damaged parts. Nowadays this has been superseded by advances in joint replacement surgery.

Late

Joint replacement, in one form or another, is now the procedure of choice for OA in patients with severe symptoms, marked loss of function and significant restriction of daily activities. For OA of the hip and knee in middle-aged and older patients, total joint replacement by modern techniques promises improvement lasting for 15 years or longer, but techniques are improving year by year.

49

However, joint replacement operations are highly dependent on technical skills, implant design, appropriate instrumentation and postoperative care – requirements that cannot always be met, or may not be cost-effective, in all parts of the world.

Arthrodesis is sometimes indicated for joints in which permanent stiffness is not a drawback.

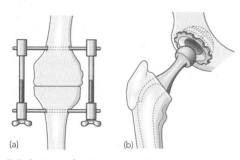

5.5 Osteoarthritis – operative treatment
(a) Compression arthrodesis of the knee. (b) Total joint replacement of the hip.

NEUROPATHIC ARTHRITIS (CHARCOT'S DISEASE)

Neuropathic arthritis is a rapidly progressive degeneration in a joint which lacks position sense and protective pain sensation. In the lower limb it is associated with tabes dorsalis, cauda equina lesions, peripheral neuropathies (especially diabetic) and congenital indifference to pain; in the upper limbs it is usually due to syringomyelia.

Pathology

The joint disorder is a rapidly progressive form of OA. There is marked destruction of articular cartilage and the underlying bone, and microscopic spicules of bone become embedded in the synovium. Ligaments and capsule are lax and at the joint periphery there is florid new bone formation.

Clinical features

The patient complains of instability, swelling and deformity; the symptoms may progress rapidly. The appearance of the joint suggests that movement would be agonising and yet it is often painless. The paradox is diagnostic.

Swelling and deformity are marked, yet there is no warmth or tenderness. Fluid is greatly increased and bits of bone can be felt everywhere. All movements are increased and the joint is unstable, yet painless.

The underlying neurological disorder should be sought.

X-rays

The joint may be subluxated or dislocated; gross bone destruction is obvious and there are irregular calcified masses in the capsule.

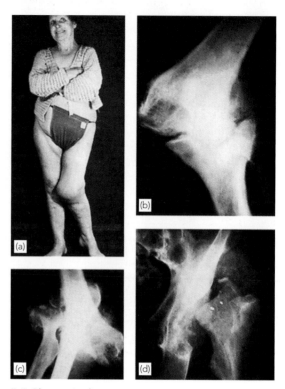

5.6 Charcot's disease (a,b) This patient with Charcot's disease developed neuropathic arthritis in her left knee. Her cheerful expression contrasts sharply with the gross joint destruction. (c,d) Other joints also can be affected by neuropathic disorders, as seen here in x-rays of the elbow and hip.

Treatment

The underlying condition may need treatment, but the affected joints cannot recover. They should, if possible, be stabilized by external splintage (e.g. a calliper). Operation is not advised.

HAEMOPHILIC ARTHROPATHY

Of the various bleeding disorders, two are associated with recurrent haemarthroses and progressive joint destruction: *classic haemophilia*, in which there is a deficiency of clotting factor VIII, and *Christmas disease*, due to deficiency of factor IX. These are rare X-linked recessive disorders manifesting in males but carried by females.

Plasma clotting factor levels above 40% of the

normal are compatible with normal control of haemorrhage. Patients with clotting factor levels above 5% ('*mild haemophilia*') may have prolonged bleeding after injury or operation; those with levels below 1% ('*severe haemophilia*') have frequent spontaneous joint and muscle haemorrhages.

Acute bleeding into a joint

With trivial injury a joint may rapidly fill with blood. Pain, warmth, boggy swelling, tenderness and limited movement are the outstanding features. The resemblance to inflammatory arthritis is striking but the history is diagnostic.

Treatment: the appropriate purified clotting factor must be given intravenously. If this is not available, cryoprecipitate or fresh-frozen plasma will do. Aspiration is avoided unless distension is severe or there is a strong suspicion of infection. A removable splint provides comfort, but once the acute episode has passed movement is encouraged.

Acute bleeding into muscles

A painful swelling appears in the arm or leg. There is a danger of a compartment syndrome and Volkmann's ischaemia, but decompression is unwise and ineffectual.

Treatment: treatment is by splintage and early factor replacement, followed by physiotherapy. Later, operation may be needed to correct any resulting joint deformity.

Joint degeneration

This, the sequel to repeated bleeding, usually begins before the age of 15 years. Chronic synovitis is followed by cartilage degeneration. An affected joint shows wasting and fixed deformity not unlike a tuberculous or rheumatoid joint. X-rays show

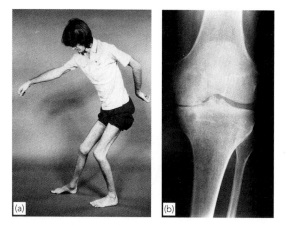

5.7 Haemophilic arthritis (a) This young man has developed contractures of the knees and ankles following repeated bleeds. (b) X-ray of the knee shows features of an erosive arthritis.

periarticular osteoporosis and progressive joint erosion.

Treatment: progressive degeneration is preventable by controlling bleeds, encouraging movement and counteracting joint deformity. Operative treatment is feasible but the clotting factor concentration should be raised to above 25% for factor VIII and above 15% for factor IX, and it should be kept at those levels throughout the postoperative period. Useful procedures are tendon lengthening (to correct contractures), osteotomy (for established deformity) and arthrodesis of the knee or ankle (for painful joint destruction). Synovectomy is sometimes performed but the benefits are dubious. Total hip replacement is technically feasible, but tissue dissection should be kept to a minimum and meticulous haemostasis is needed.

CHAPTER 6

OSTEONECROSIS (AVASCULAR NECROSIS)

OSTEONECROSIS

The prototypical example of avascular necrosis (AVN) is aseptic death of a large segment of the femoral head following fracture of the femoral neck and severance of the local blood supply. It is now recognized that aseptic osteonecrosis occurs at a number of other sites, due either to local injury or to non-traumatic conditions (including Perthes' disease, high-dosage corticosteroid administration and alcohol abuse) which result in ischaemia of a substantial segment of bone.

Table 6.1 Main conditions associated with non-traumatic osteonecrosis

Bone infections
Septic arthritis
Perthes' disease
Cortisone administration
Alcohol abuse
Sickle-cell disease
Gaucher's disease
Haemoglobinopathies
Caisson disease
Ionizing radiation

Sites most susceptible are the femoral head, femoral condyles, head of humerus and proximal poles of scaphoid and talus. What they have in common is that they lie at the outskirts of the bone's main vascular supply and they are largely enclosed by articular cartilage which is itself avascular and which restricts the area for entry of local blood vessels. Furthermore, at some of these sites the subarticular trabeculae are sustained largely by endarterioles with limited arterial connections.

Another factor which needs to be taken into account is that the vascular sinusoids which nourish the marrow and bone cells, unlike arterial capillaries, have no adventitial layer and their patency is determined by the volume and pressure of the surrounding marrow tissue, which itself is encased in unyielding bone. The system functions essentially as a closed compartment within which one element can expand only at the expense of the others. Local changes such as vascular stasis, haemorrhage or marrow swelling can, therefore, rapidly spiral to a vicious cycle of ischaemia, reactive oedema or inflammation, further marrow swelling, increased intraosseous pressure and further ischaemia.

The process described above can be initiated in at least four different ways: (1) severance of the local blood supply; (2) venous stasis and retrograde arteriolar stoppage; (3) intravascular thrombosis; and (4) compression of capillaries and sinusoids by marrow swelling. *Ischaemia, in the majority of cases, is due to a combination of several of these factors.*

Traumatic osteonecrosis

In fractures and dislocations of the hip the retinacular vessels supplying the femoral head are easily torn;

if, in addition, there is damage to or thrombosis of the ligamentum teres, osteonecrosis is inevitable. Other injuries which are prone to osteonecrosis are fractures of the scaphoid and talus; significantly, in these cases it is always the proximal fragment which suffers because the principal vessels enter the bones near their distal ends and course through the bone from distal to proximal.

Impact injuries and osteoarticular fractures at any of the convex articular surfaces behave in the same way and may cause localized ischaemic changes affecting a small segment of bone just below the articular surface. These small lesions are usually referred to as 'osteochondroses' and many of them have acquired eponyms which are now firmly embedded in orthopaedic history.

Non-traumatic osteonecrosis

The mechanisms here are more complex and may involve several pathways to intravascular stasis or thrombosis, as well as extravascular swelling and capillary compression. These changes, acting either independently or in combination, are believed to cause the critical bone ischaemia in osteonecrotic lesions associated with Perthes' disease, caisson disease, sickle-cell disease, Gaucher's disease, high-dosage corticosteroid medication and alcohol abuse

Pathology

Dead bone is structurally and radiographically indistinguishable from live bone. However, lacking a blood supply, it does not undergo renewal, and after a limited period of repetitive stress it collapses. The changes develop in four overlapping stages.

- *Stage 1: bone death without structural change*: within 48 hours after infarction there is marrow necrosis and cell death. However, for weeks or even months the bone may show no alteration in macroscopic appearance.
- *Stage 2: repair and early structural failure*: some days or weeks after infarction the surrounding, living bone shows a vascular reaction; new bone is laid down upon the dead trabeculae and the increase in bone mass shows on the x-ray as exaggerated density.
- *Stage 3: major structural failure*: small fractures begin to appear in the dead bone. The necrotic portion starts to crumble and the bone outline becomes distorted.
- *Stage 4: articular destruction*: cartilage, being nourished mainly by synovial fluid, is preserved even in advanced osteonecrosis. However, severe distortion of the surface eventually leads to cartilage breakdown and secondary osteoarthritis.

Clinical features

By the time the patient presents, the lesion is often well advanced. Pain is the usual complaint; it is felt near a joint and is accompanied by stiffness. Local tenderness may be present and the nearby joint may be swollen. Movements are usually restricted.

Imaging

- *X-rays*: the distinctive x-ray feature of AVN is a subarticular segment of increased bone density. This is not because dead bone is more radio-opaque than living bone; it is due to reactive

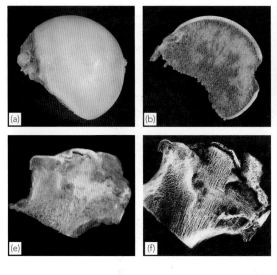

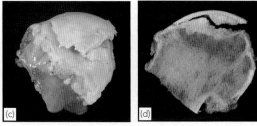

6.1 Osteonecrosis – pathology Three femoral head specimens showing different stages of pathology. (a,b) Normal femoral head with intact articular cartilage; the coronal section (b) shows the structurally perfect articular cartilage and vascularized subarticular bone. In the head with osteonecrosis (c) the articular cartilage is lifted off and the coronal section in (d) shows that this is due to a subarticular fracture through a necrotic segment in the dome of the femoral head. In the latest stage there is marked cartilage and bone destruction, shown here in the coronal section through the femoral head specimen (e) and a fine-detail x-ray (f).

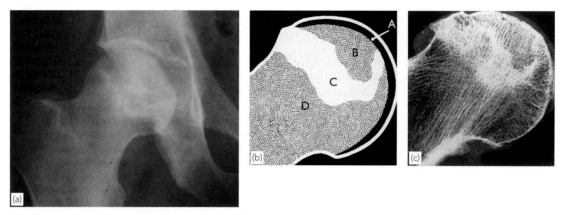

6.2 Osteonecrosis – x-ray (a) The cardinal x-ray feature is increased radiographic density in the weight-bearing part of the subarticular bone. The 'density' is due to new bone formation spreading into the necrotic segment. This is shown in the diagram (b) and the corresponding fine-detail x-ray of the femoral head specimen (c). (**A**, articular cartilage, **B**, dead bone, **C**, new bone formation, **D**, normal bone).

new bone formation in the surrounding living tissue which increases the total mass of calcified bone. Later changes are fracturing and collapse of the necrotic segment. A cardinal feature that distinguishes these progressive changes from those of osteoarthritis is that the radiographic 'joint space' retains its normal width because the articular cartilage is not destroyed until very late.

■ *Radioscintigraphy*: radionuclide scanning with ^{99m} technetium hydroxymethylene diphosphonate (^{99m} Tc-HDP) may reveal an avascular segment (a 'cold' area signifying diminished activity), e.g. after fracture of the femoral neck. More often, however, the picture is dominated by increased activity, reflecting hyperaemia and new bone formation in the area around the infarct.

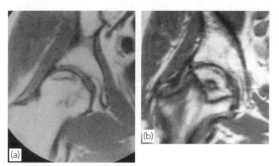

6.3 Osteonecrosis – MRI (a) Before any change is discernible on the plain x-ray, MRI will show a typical hypointense band in the T1-weighted image, outlining the ischaemic segment beneath the articular surface. (b) In this case the size of the ischaemic segment is much larger – and the likelihood of bone crumbling much greater.

■ *Magnetic resonance imaging* (*MRI*): the drawback in relying on x-ray examination is that changes appear only after several months. The only reliable method of picking up the early signs of osteonecrosis is by MRI.

Staging the lesion

It has long been recognized that the prognosis and planning of treatment for osteonecrosis depend largely on the stage at which the disorder is encountered. The most widely used system of staging is the one promoted by the International Association of Bone Circulation and Bone Necrosis (*Association Research Circulation Osseous – ARCO*) which applies mainly to femoral head necrosis.

Table 6.2 Modified ARCO staging of osteonecrosis

Stage 0	Patient asymptomatic and all clinical investigations 'normal' Biopsy shows osteonecrosis
Stage 1	X-rays normal MRI or radionuclide scan shows osteonecrosis
Stage 2	X-rays and/or MRI show early signs of osteonecrosis but no distortion of bone shape or subchondral intraosseous fracture ('crescent sign')
Stage 3	X-ray shows early abnormality but femoral head still spherical
Stage 4	Signs of flattening or collapse of femoral head
Stage 5	Changes as above plus loss of 'joint space'
Stage 6	Changes as above plus marked destruction of articular surfaces

Diagnosis of the underlying disorder

In many cases of osteonecrosis an underlying disorder will be obvious from the history: a known episode of trauma, an occupation such as deep-sea diving or working under compressed air, a family background of Gaucher's disease or sickle-cell disease, or a history of long-standing alcohol abuse.

There may be a record of high-dosage corticosteroid administration; for example, after organ transplantation where the drug is used for immunosuppression. However, smaller doses (e.g. as short-term treatment for asthma or as an adjunct in neurosurgical emergencies) can also be dangerous in patients with other risk factors. Combinations of drugs (e.g. corticosteroids and azathioprine, or corticosteroids after a period of alcohol abuse) also can be potent causes of osteonecrosis; occasionally corticosteroids have been given without the patient's knowledge.

Treatment

If possible, the cause should be eliminated. In ARCO stages 1 and 2, bone collapse can sometimes be prevented by a combination of weight-relief, splintage and (in some cases associated with venous stasis and marrow oedema) surgical decompression of the bone. Once bone collapse has occurred, and provided the area of involvement is less than 30% or in a non-loadbearing position (stages 3A and 3B), a realignment osteotomy, by transferring stress to an undamaged area, may relieve pain and prevent further bone distortion. In stages 4–6 the treatment is essentially the same as for osteoarthritis: (1) pain control and modification of daily activities; (2) arthrodesis of the joint if mobility is not a major issue, e.g. the ankle or wrist; or (3) partial or total joint replacement, the preferred option for the shoulder, hip and knee.

SYSTEMIC DISORDERS ASSOCIATED WITH OSTEONECROSIS

SICKLE-CELL DISEASE

This is a genetic disorder, limited to people of black Central and West African descent. Red cells containing abnormal haemoglobin (HbS) become distorted and sickle shaped; this is especially likely to occur with hypoxia (e.g. under anaesthesia or in extreme cold). Clumping of the sickle-shaped cells causes diminished capillary flow and repeated episodes of pain ('bone crises') or, if more severe, ischaemic necrosis. Almost any bone may be involved and there is a tendency for the infarcts to become infected, sometimes with unusual organisms such as *Salmonella*.

- *X-rays*: the tubular bones (including the phalanges) may show irregular endosteal destruction and medullary sclerosis, together with periosteal new bone formation. Not only does this resemble osteitis, but true infection is often superimposed on the infarct. In children, femoral head necrosis could be mistaken for Perthes' disease.
- *Treatment*: acute episodes are treated by rest and analgesics, followed by physiotherapy to minimize stiffness. Established necrosis is

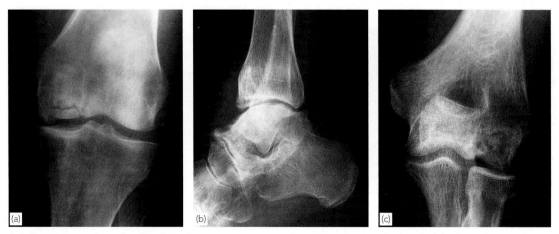

6.4 Osteonecrosis – distribution The most common site for osteonecrosis is the head of the femur but, as shown here, other sites can also be affected: e.g. (a) the medial condyle of the femur, (b) the talus and (c) the capitulum. All these areas are located beneath convex articular surfaces; osteonecrosis is very seldom seen beneath a concave articular surface.

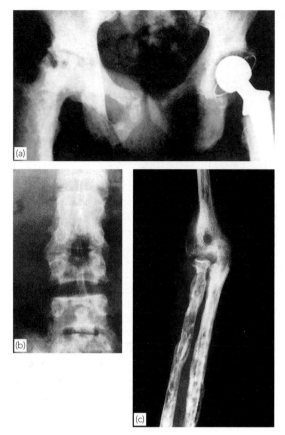

6.5 Sickle-cell disease (a) Typical changes in the femur due to marrow hyperplasia, with bone infarction and necrosis of the femoral head. (b) The spine also may be involved. (c) In severe cases infarctions of tubular bones may resemble osteomyelitis.

treated according to the principles on page 55, but with the emphasis on conservatism. Anaesthesia carries serious risks and may even precipitate vascular occlusion in the central nervous system, lungs or kidneys; moreover, the chances of postoperative infection are high.

CAISSON DISEASE

Decompression sickness (caisson disease) and osteonecrosis are important causes of disability in deep-sea divers and compressed-air workers building tunnels or underwater structures. Under increased air pressure the blood and other tissues (especially fat) become supersaturated with nitrogen; if decompression is too rapid the gas is released as bubbles, which cause local tissue damage and generalized embolic phenomena. The symptoms of decompression sickness are pain near

the joints ('the bends'), breathing difficulty and vertigo ('the staggers'). In the most acute cases there can be circulatory and respiratory collapse, severe neurological changes, coma and death. Bone necrosis may be due to capillary obstruction by gas bubbles and changes in marrow fat.

The patient complains of pain and loss of joint movement, but many lesions remain silent and are found only on routine x-ray examination.

■ *Management*: the aim is prevention; the incidence of osteonecrosis is proportional to the working pressure, the length of exposure, the rate of decompression and the number of exposures. Strict enforcement of suitable working schedules has reduced the risks considerably. The treatment of established lesions follows the principles already outlined.

GAUCHER'S DISEASE

Deficiency of the specific enzyme causes an abnormal accumulation of glucocerebroside in the reticuloendothelial system. The effects are seen chiefly in the liver, spleen and bone marrow, where the large, polyhedral 'Gaucher' cells accumulate.

Bone complications are common and osteonecrosis is among the worst of them. The hip is most frequently affected, but lesions also appear in the distal femur, talus and head of humerus. Bone ischaemia is usually attributed to the increase in medullary cell volume and capillary compression.

Symptoms may occur at any age; the patient complains of pain around one of the larger joints and movements may be restricted. There is a tendency for the Gaucher deposits to become infected and the patient may present with septicaemia. A diagnostic, though inconstant, finding is a raised serum acid phosphatase level.

■ *X-rays*: a special feature (due to replacement of myeloid tissue by Gaucher cells) is expansion of the tubular bones, especially the distal femur, producing a flask-like appearance. Osteonecrosis of the femoral head is common.
■ *Treatment*: the general disorder can now be treated by enzyme replacement. Management of the osteonecrosis follows the principles outlined on page 55. If joint replacement is contemplated, antibiotic cover is essential.

DRUG-INDUCED NECROSIS

Corticosteroids in high dosage may give rise to 'spontaneous' osteonecrosis; thus the condition

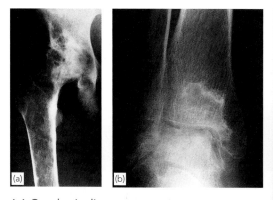

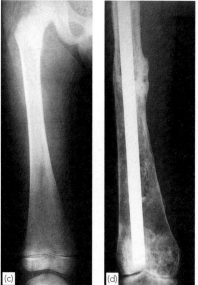

6.6 Gaucher's disease (a) Gaucher deposits are seen throughout the femur. The cortices are thin and there is osteonecrosis of the femoral head. (b) Bone infarction is seen in the distal end of the tibia and the talus. (c) The typical Erlenmeyer flask appearance is seen in the x-ray of this teenager. (d) 10 years later the bone changes are much more marked, the cortices are extremely thin and the patient has obviously suffered a pathological fracture.

is fairly common in renal transplant patients on immunosuppressive corticosteroids. Alcohol abuse is another potent cause. Both conditions result in widespread fatty changes and marrow infarction, which may be the cause of the bone necrosis. The sites usually affected are the femoral head, femoral condyles and the head of the humerus.

Pain may be present for many months before x-rays show any abnormality. MRI is the only reliable way of making an early diagnosis; typical changes are often discovered in asymptomatic joints.

■ *Treatment*: early changes, if not actually reversible, can be prevented from extending by stopping the cortisone or alcohol. Analgesics, weight-relief and physiotherapy are often all that is required. Decompression of the affected bone by drilling may relieve symptoms and even prevent progressive changes in very early cases. If the joint surface has collapsed, reconstructive surgery is required.

OSTEOCHONDROSIS ('OSTEOCHONDRITIS')

The term '*osteochondrosis*' or '*osteochondritis*' is applied to a group of conditions in which there is compression, fragmentation or separation of a small segment of bone, usually at the bone end and involving the attached articular surface. The affected portion of bone shows many of the features of ischaemic necrosis, including increased vascularity and reactive sclerosis in the surrounding bone. These conditions occur in children and adolescents, often during phases of rapid growth and increased physical activity.

The pathogenesis of these lesions is still not completely understood. Impact injuries can cause oedema or bleeding in the subarticular bone, resulting in capillary compression or thrombosis and localized ischaemia. The critical event may well be a small osteochondral fracture, too faint to show up on plain x-ray examination but often visible on MRI. If the crack fails to unite, the isolated fragment may lose its blood supply and become necrotic.

Clinical features

The condition usually occurs in adolescents and young adults and the classic example is *osteochondritis dissecans* of the lateral part of the *medial femoral condyle* at the knee. Similar lesions are seen at the *anteromedial corner of the talus*, the *superomedial part of the femoral head*, the *humeral capitulum (Panner's disease)*, the *head of the second metatarsal (Freiberg's disease)* and the *carpal lunate (Kienböck's disease)*.

The patient usually complains of intermittent pain; sometimes there is swelling and a small effusion in the joint. If the necrotic fragment becomes completely detached (not uncommon in osteochondritis dissecans) it may cause locking of the joint or episodes of 'giving way' in the knee or ankle.

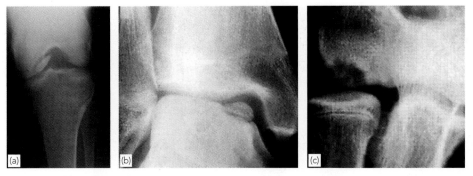

6.7 Osteochondrosis At the knee (a), the osteochondral fragment separates on the lateral side of the medial femoral condyle; other sites where this occurs are (b) the medial corner of the talus and (c) the capitulum at the elbow.

Imaging

The early changes (i.e. before demarcation of the ischaemic fragment) are best shown by *MRI*: there is decreased signal intensity in the area around the affected osteochondral segment. *Radionuclide scanning* with ^{99m}Tc-HDP shows markedly increased activity in the same area.

X-ray changes come later. The ischaemic or dissecting fragment is defined by a radiolucent line of demarcation. When it separates, the resulting 'crater' may be obvious.

Treatment

Treatment in the early stage consists of load reduction and restriction of activity. In young people complete healing may occur, though it can take up to 2 years. For a large joint like the knee, it is generally recommended that partially detached fragments be pinned back in position after roughening of the base, while completely detached fragments should be pinned back only if they are completely preserved.

Treatment of osteochondrosis at the elbow, wrist and metatarsal head is discussed in the relevant chapters.

CHAPTER 7

METABOLIC AND ENDOCRINE DISORDERS

BONE AND BONES

Bones as structural entities have three main functions, support, protection and leverage: they support and protect the soft tissues; transmit load and muscular force from one part of the body to another; and mediate movement and locomotion.

Bone as a tissue has an equally important role as a mineral reservoir which helps to regulate the composition – and in particular the calcium ion concentration – of the extracellular fluid.

For all its solidity, bone is in a continuous state of flux, its internal shape and structure changing from moment to moment in concert with the normal variations in mechanical function and mineral exchange. All modulations in bone structure and composition are brought about by cellular activity, which is regulated by hormones and local factors; these agents, in turn, are controlled by alterations in mineral ion concentrations. The metabolic bone disorders are conditions in which generalized skeletal abnormalities result from disruption of this complex interactive system.

BONE COMPOSITION AND STRUCTURE

Bone consists of a largely collagenous matrix which is impregnated with mineral salts and populated by cells – osteoclasts (concerned with bone resorption), osteoblasts (for bone formation) and osteocytes (resting bone cells which may have a function in communicating information about local stresses and strains to the other bone cells).

Newly formed bone tissue, which is unmineralized, is called *osteoid* and is usually seen only where active new-bone formation is taking place. Normally this soon becomes mineralized, but the immature tissue is somewhat disorganized, with collagen fibres arranged haphazardly and cells having no specific orientation; in this state it is called *woven bone* – typically seen in the early stages of fracture healing.

The mature tissue is *lamellar bone*, in which the collagen fibres are arranged parallel to each other to form multiple layers (or laminae) with the osteocytes lying between the lamellae. Almost one-half the bone volume is mineral matter – mainly calcium and phosphate in the form of *crystalline hydroxyapatite* – which is laid down in osteoid at the calcification front. The proportions of calcium and phosphate are constant and the molecule is firmly bound to collagen. *In living bone, 'demineralization' occurs only by resorption of the entire matrix.*

Lamellar bone exists in two structurally different forms: compact (cortical) bone and cancellous (trabecular) bone.

Compact bone is dense and strong and is found where support matters most: the outer walls (cortices) of all bones, but especially the shafts of tubular bones, and the subchondral plates supporting articular cartilage. It is made up of compact units – *haversian systems* or *osteons* – each of which consists of a central canal (the *haversian canal*) containing blood vessels, lymphatics and nerves, surrounded by closely packed, more or less concentric lamellae of bone. Seen in three dimensions, the haversian canals are long branching channels connecting extensively with each other and with the endosteal and periosteal surfaces by smaller channels called *Volkmann canals*.

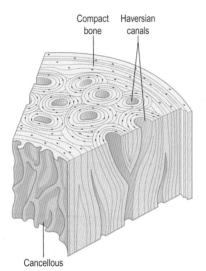

Compact bone   Haversian canals

Cancellous

7.1 Bone structure This picture represents a wedge taken from the cortex of a long bone. It shows the basic elements of compact bone: densely packed osteons each made up of concentric layers of bone and osteocytes around a central haversian canal which contains the vessels; outer laminae of subperiosteal bone; and similar laminae on the interior surface (endosteum) merging into a lattice of cancellous bone.

Cancellous (*trabecular*) *bone* has a honeycomb appearance; it makes up the interior meshwork of all bones and is particularly well developed in the ends of the tubular bones and in the vertebral bodies. Three-dimensionally the trabecular sheets are interconnected (like a honeycomb) and arranged according to the mechanical needs of the structure, the thickest and strongest along trajectories of compressive stress and the thinnest in the planes of tensile stress. Cancellous bone is obviously more porous than cortical bone. Though it makes up only one-quarter of the total skeletal mass, the trabeculae provide two-thirds of the total bone surface. It is easy to understand why the effects of metabolic disorders are usually seen first in trabecular bone.

Fully formed bones are covered (except at the articular ends) by a tough *periosteal membrane*, the deepest layer of which consists of potentially bone-forming cells. The inner, endosteal, surfaces are

irregular and lined by a fine *endosteal membrane* in close contact with the marrow spaces.

Bone has a rich *blood supply*. Vessels in the haversian canals form an anastomotic network between the medullary and periosteal blood supply. Blood flow in this capillary network is normally centrifugal – from the medullary cavity outwards – and it has long been held that the cortex is supplied entirely from this source. However, it seems likely that at least the outermost layers of the cortex are normally also supplied by periosteal vessels, and if the medullary vessels are blocked or destroyed the periosteal circulation can take over entirely. In cancellous bone, the spaces between the trabeculae contain marrow, fat and fine sinusoidal vessels that course through the tissue nourishing both marrow and bone.

Bone cells are of three types: osteoblasts, osteocytes and osteoclasts. *Osteoblasts* are concerned with bone formation and osteoclast activation. They develop from mesenchymal precursors in the bone marrow and beneath the periosteum. Differentiation is controlled by a number of interacting growth factors, including bone morphogenetic proteins (BMPs). The small mononuclear cells appear along the free surfaces of trabeculae and haversian systems where osteoid is laid down prior to calcification. Prompted by parathyroid hormone (PTH), osteoblasts also play an important role in the initiation and control of osteoclastic activity.

At the end of each bone-forming cycle the osteoblasts either remain on the newly formed bone surface as quiescent lining cells or they become embedded in the matrix as 'resting' *osteocytes*. However, these osteocytes are by no means inactive: they communicate with each other and they may, under the influence of PTH, participate directly in bone resorption.

Osteoclasts, considerably larger multi-nucleated cells, are the principal mediators of bone resorption. They develop from precursors in the haemopoietic marrow under the influence of local osteoblastic stromal cells that generate an essential osteoclast differentiating factor which is required to initiate osteoclast maturation and bone resorption. The mature osteoclasts are easily identified where they lie in shallow excavations – Howship's lacunae – along free bone surfaces on trabecular plates and in the central hollow of each expanding haversian system.

BONE DEVELOPMENT AND GROWTH

Bones develop in two different ways: by ossification of a prior cartilage model (*endochondral ossification*) and by direct *intramembranous ossification*.

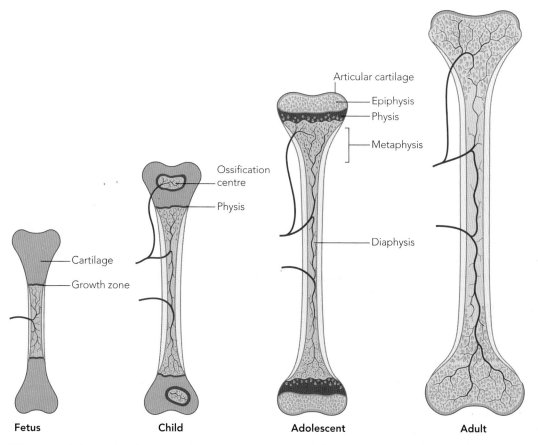

7.2 Stages in bone development Schematic representation of the stages in the development of a tubular bone showing the progress from diaphyseal ossification, through endochondral growth at the physis and increase in width of the diaphysis by subperiosteal appositional bone formation.

Endochondral ossification

This is the usual manner in which tubular bones develop. At birth the cartilage model is complete and ossification has already begun in the diaphysis; shortly afterwards ossification centres also appear in the epiphyses. For the next 15–20 years growth in length will take place in the still-cartilaginous zone between the ossifying diaphysis and the epiphysis.

This actively growing cartilage disc is called the *physis*. It consists of four distinct zones. Co-extensive with the epiphysis is a zone of *resting chondrocytes*; this merges into a *proliferative zone* where the chondrocytes are lined up longitudinally, multiplying by interstitial growth and so adding progressively to the overall length of the bone. As these cells mature they gradually enlarge and constitute a *hypertrophic zone* which gradually becomes calcified; this *zone of calcified cartilage* undergoes osteoclastic resorption and finally, with the ingrowth of new blood vessels from the bony diaphysis, ossification.

Intramembranous ossification

With the growth in length, the bone also has to increase in girth and, since a tubular bone is an open cylinder, this inevitably demands that the medullary cavity increase in size proportionately. New bone is added to the outside by direct ossification at the deepest layer of the periosteum where mesenchymal cells differentiate into osteoblasts (intramembranous, or 'appositional' bone formation); meanwhile 'old' bone is removed from the inside of the cylinder by osteoclastic endosteal resorption.

Bone resorption

Bone resorption is carried out by the osteoclasts under the influence of stromal cells (including osteoblasts) and both local and systemic activators. Although it has long been known that PTH promotes bone resorption, osteoclasts have no receptor for PTH, but the hormone acts indirectly through its effect on the vitamin D metabolite 1,25-dihydroxycholecalciferol (1,25-DHCC) and

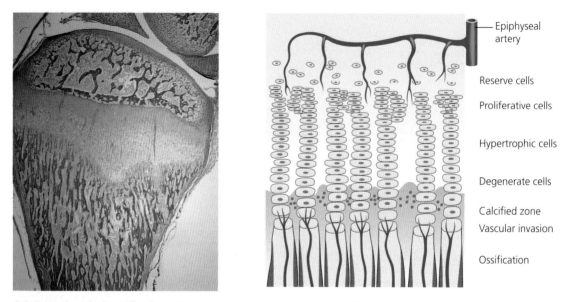

Epiphyseal artery

Reserve cells

Proliferative cells

Hypertrophic cells

Degenerate cells

Calcified zone
Vascular invasion

Ossification

7.3 Endochondral ossification Histological section of a growing endochondral bone with a schematic figure showing the layers of the growth disc (physis). (Reproduced from Bullough PG. *Atlas of Orthopaedic Pathology: With Clinical and Radiological Correlations* (2nd edition). Baltimore: University Park Press, 1985. Second figure by kind permission of Dr. Peter G. Bullough and Elsevier.)

on local osteoblasts which produce the essential osteoclast differentiating factor.

It is thought that osteoblasts first 'prepare' the resorption site by removing osteoid from the bone surface while other matrix constituents act as osteoclast attractors. In cancellous bone osteoclastic resorption results in thinning (and sometimes actual perforation) of existing trabeculae. In cortical bone the osteoclasts either enlarge an existing haversian canal or else burrow into the compact bone to create a cutting cone – like miners sinking a new shaft in the ground. During hyperactive bone resorption these processes are reflected in the appearance of hydroxyproline in the urine and a rise in serum calcium and phosphate levels.

Bone modelling and re-modelling

During growth the bone increases in size and changes in shape. The increase in length occurs at the physis where new bone is added by endochondral ossification. Increase in width takes place by subperiosteal new bone formation and expansion of the medullary cavity by endosteal resorption.

As the bone increases in length, the bulbous bone ends have to be continuously re-formed and sculpted into shape by alternating bone resorption and formation – a process known as *bone modelling*. However, it should not be thought that this process ceases when bone stops growing in size; the same process continues throughout adult life, but now it is directed not at the modelling of a particular shape but at the constant *re-modelling* of existing bone. This serves a crucial purpose in the renewal and preservation of skeletal structure: 'old bone' is continually replaced by 'new bone' and in this way the skeleton is protected from stress failure due to repetitive loading. At the same time *calcium homeostasis* is maintained by the constant turnover of the mineral deposits which would otherwise stay locked in bone.

At each *re-modelling site* work proceeds in an orderly and unvarying sequence: osteoclasts gather on a free bone surface and excavate a cavity; they disappear and, after a period of quiescence, are replaced by osteoblasts which proceed to fill in the excavation with new bone. Each cycle of bone turnover takes from 4 to 6 months. The annual rate of turnover is about 4% for cortical bone and 25% for trabecular bone.

During bone re-modelling, resorption and formation are *coupled*, the one ineluctably following the other. This ensures that, on average, a balance is maintained, though at any moment and at any particular site one or other process may predominate. Bone constantly adapts to the stresses imposed upon it and at any particular site cortical and trabecular thickness will be greatest in the trajectories of highest stress. This natural

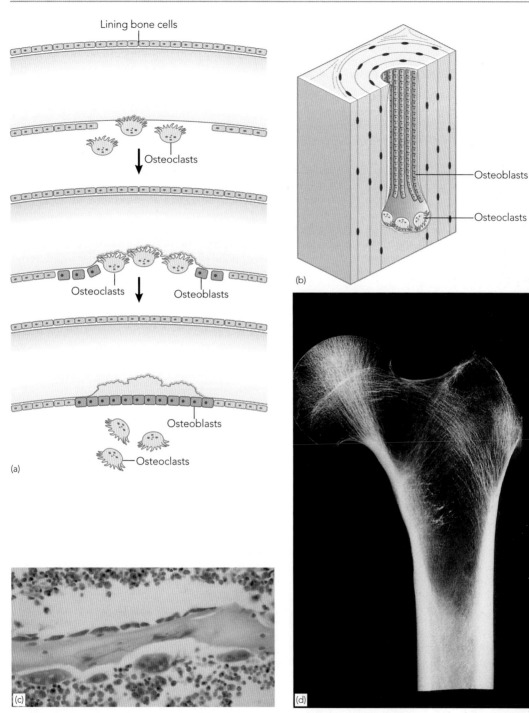

7.4 Bone re-modelling (a) Open trabecular surfaces are first excavated by osteoclasts and then lined and filled in again by a following train of osteoblasts. (b) In compact bone the osteoclasts burrow deeply into the existing bone with the osteoblasts following close behind to re-line the cavity with new bone. (c) Histological section showing a trabecula lined on its one surface by excavating osteoclasts and on the other surface by a string of much smaller osteoblasts. This process gradually reshapes the bone as well as the internal trabecular pattern (d), with the thickest trabecular spars arranged along the trajectories of greatest stress (Wolff's Law).

adaptation of bone structure to functional demands is known as *Wolff's Law*.

AGE-RELATED CHANGES IN BONE

During childhood and adolescence the entire bone increases in size and changes somewhat in shape. However, although the bones become bigger, the tissue of which they are made remains comparatively light and porous.

Between adolescence and 35 years of age the haversian canals and the spaces between trabeculae are gradually filled in and the cortices increase in thickness; i.e. the bones become heavier and stronger. Bone mass increases at the rate of about 3% per year and during the third decade each individual attains a state of *peak bone mass*.

From 35 to about 50 years there is a slow but inexorable loss of bone; haversian spaces enlarge, trabeculae become thinner, the endosteal surface is resorbed and the medullary space expands – i.e. year by year the bones become slightly more porous. The diminution in bone mass proceeds at a rate of about 0.3% per year in men and 0.5% per year in women up to the menopause.

From the onset of the menopause and for the next 10 years the rate of bone loss in women accelerates to about 3% per year, occurring predominantly in trabecular bone. This steady depletion is due mainly to excessive resorption, osteoclastic activity seeming to be released from the restraining influence of gonadal hormone; similar changes are seen in younger women about 5 years after oophorectomy. About 30% of white women will lose bone to the extent of developing postmenopausal osteoporosis; for reasons that are not fully understood, the degree of bone depletion is less marked in black than in white peoples.

From the age of 65 or 70 years the rate of bone loss gradually tails off and by the age of 75 years it is about 0.5% per year. This later phase of depletion is due mainly to diminishing osteoblastic activity.

Men are affected in a similar manner, but the phase of rapid bone loss occurs about 15 years later than in women, at the climacteric.

BONE MASS AND BONE STRENGTH

Bone mass refers to the actual amount of osseous tissue in any unit volume of bone. Throughout life, and regardless of whether bone mass increases or decreases, the degree of mineralization in normal people varies very little from age to age or from one person to another. With advancing years, as the bones become more porous there is a gradual loss of bone strength; but the loss of strength is out of proportion to the decrease in mass. This can be explained as follows: (a) with the diminution in bone mass, *interconnecting spars between the bone plates may be perforated or lost*; and (b) in old age there is a *decrease in bone cell activity*, which makes for a slow re-modelling rate, so that old bone takes longer to be replaced and microtrauma to be repaired. As a consequence, ageing is accompanied by increasing fragility.

REGULATION OF BONE TURNOVER AND MINERAL EXCHANGE

Over 98% of the body's calcium and 85% of its phosphorus is tightly packed in bone and can be released only by resorption of the entire tissue – a slow process. A small rapidly exchangeable component exists in the extracellular fluid and blood where their concentration is maintained within very narrow limits by homeostatic mechanisms involving intestinal absorption, renal excretion and mineral exchange in bone. Transient

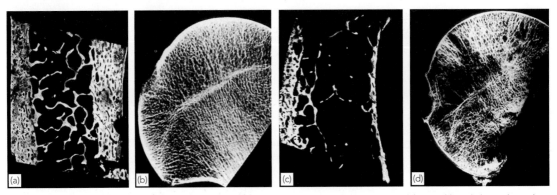

7.5 Age-related changes in bone These fine-detail x-rays of iliac crest biopsies and femoral head slices show the marked contrast between trabecular density in a healthy 40-year-old woman (a,b) and one of 75 years (c,d).

alterations in serum levels are accommodated quickly by changes in renal tubular reabsorption.

The control of calcium is much more critical than that of phosphate; thus, in persistent calcium deficiency the extracellular calcium ion concentration is maintained by drawing on bone, whereas phosphate deficiency simply leads to lowered serum phosphate concentration. The regulation of calcium exchange is therefore linked inescapably to that of bone formation and resorption. The complex balance between calcium exchange and bone re-modelling is controlled by an array of systemic and local factors.

Calcium

Calcium is essential for normal cell function and physiological processes such as nerve conduction and muscle contraction. The normal concentration in plasma and extracellular fluid is 2.2–2.6 mmol/L (8.8–10.4 mg/dL). Much of this is bound to protein; about half is ionized and effective in cell metabolism and the regulation of calcium homoeostasis.

The recommended daily intake of calcium is 800–1000 mg (20–25 mmol), and ideally this should be increased to 1500 mg (37.5 mmol) during pregnancy and lactation. About 50% of the dietary calcium is absorbed (mainly in the upper gut) but much of that is secreted back into the bowel and only about 200 mg (5 mmol) enters the circulation.

Calcium absorption is mediated by vitamin D metabolites and inhibited by excessive intake of phosphates (common in soft drinks), oxalates (found in tea and coffee), phytates (chapatti flour) and fats, as well as by the administration of corticosteroids; it is also reduced in malabsorption disorders of the bowel.

Urinary excretion varies between 2.5 and 5 mmol (100–200 mg) per 24 hours; if calcium intake is reduced, urinary excretion is adjusted by increasing tubular reabsorption. If calcium concentration is persistently reduced, calcium is drawn from the skeleton by increased bone resorption. These compensatory shifts in intestinal absorption, renal excretion and bone re-modelling are regulated by PTH and vitamin D metabolites.

Phosphorus

Phosphorus is needed for many important metabolic processes. Plasma concentration – almost entirely in the form of ionized inorganic phosphates – is 0.9–1.3 mmol/L (2.8–4.0 mg/dL). It is abundantly available in the diet and is absorbed in the small intestine, more or less in proportion to the amount ingested; however, absorption is reduced in the presence of antacids such as aluminium hydroxide, which binds phosphorus in the gut.

Phosphate excretion is extremely efficient, but 90% is reabsorbed in the proximal tubules. Tubular reabsorption is decreased (and overall excretion increased) by PTH.

Vitamin D

Vitamin D, through its active metabolites, is principally concerned with calcium absorption and transport and (acting together with PTH) bone re-modelling. Target organs are the small intestine and bone.

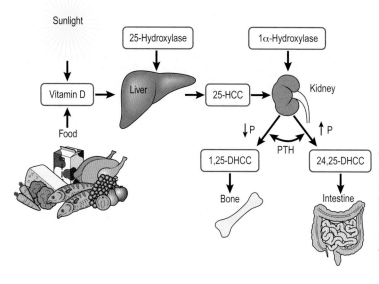
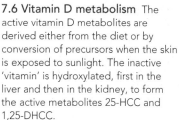

7.6 Vitamin D metabolism The active vitamin D metabolites are derived either from the diet or by conversion of precursors when the skin is exposed to sunlight. The inactive 'vitamin' is hydroxylated, first in the liver and then in the kidney, to form the active metabolites 25-HCC and 1,25-DHCC.

Naturally occurring vitamin D₃ (cholecalciferol) is derived from two sources: directly from the diet and indirectly by the action of ultraviolet light on the precursor 7-dihydrocholesterol in the skin. The normal requirement is about 400 IU per day. In most countries this is obtained mainly from exposure to sunlight.

Vitamin D itself is inactive. Conversion to active metabolites takes place first in the liver by 25-hydroxylation to form *25-hydroxycholecalciferol* (25-HCC), and then in the kidneys by further hydroxylation (mediated by PTH) to 1,25-DHCC.

The terminal metabolites, 1,25-DHCC (calcitriol) – and to a lesser extent 25-HCC – act on the *lining cells of the small intestine*, stimulating the absorption of calcium and phosphate. *In bone* they assist PTH to promote osteoclastic bone resorption; they also enhance calcium transport across the cell membrane and thus indirectly promote the process of mineralization.

Parathyroid hormone

PTH is the fine regulator of calcium exchange. It maintains the extracellular calcium concentration between very narrow limits; production and release are stimulated by a fall and suppressed by a rise in plasma ionized calcium.

Target organs are the kidney, bone and (indirectly) the gut. Acting on the *renal tubules*, PTH increases phosphate excretion by restricting its reabsorption, and conserves calcium by increasing its reabsorption. These responses rapidly compensate for any change in plasma ionized calcium. Acting on the *kidney parenchyma*, it controls hydroxylation of the vitamin D metabolite 25-HCC to form the active metabolite 1,25-DHCC. In the *intestine* an indirect effect is to promote calcium absorption. In *bone* PTH indirectly promotes osteoclastic resorption and the slow release of calcium and phosphate into the blood.

Calcitonin

Calcitonin, which is secreted by the C cells of the thyroid, does more or less the opposite of PTH: it suppresses osteoclastic bone resorption and increases renal calcium excretion.

Oestrogen

Oestrogen is thought to stimulate calcium absorption and to protect bone from the unrestrained action of PTH. Its withdrawal leads to osteoporosis; this occurs naturally at the menopause, but it also follows oophorectomy in younger women and a similar effect is seen in other amenorrhoeic states.

Adrenal corticosteroids

Corticosteroids administered in excess cause a pernicious type of osteoporosis due to a combination of increased bone resorption, diminished bone formation, decreased intestinal calcium absorption and increased calcium excretion; collagen synthesis may also be defective.

Local factors

Systemic hormones have a large-scale effect on bone turnover, but many of the cellular activities at the work-front where re-modelling takes place are mediated by local factors such as *insulin-like growth factor I (somatomedin C), transforming growth factors, interleukin-1 (IL-1), osteoclast-activating factor (OAF)* and *prostaglandins*.

Bone morphogenetic protein (BMP), which can be extracted from bone matrix, induces chondrogenesis and bone formation. This process – known as bone induction – may be important in fracture healing and bone graft replacement.

Mechanical stress

The effect of mechanical stress on bone re-modelling is embodied in Wolff's Law (pages 62–64). Positive influences on bone formation are produced by gravity, loadbearing, muscle action and vascular pulsation. Weightlessness, prolonged bed rest, lack of exercise, muscular weakness and limb immobilization are all associated with osteoporosis.

METABOLIC BONE DISORDERS

Most of the common metabolic bone disorders are associated with depletion of bone tissue, manifesting as: (1) *osteoporosis*, in which there is a quantitative diminution in bone mass; (2) *osteomalacia*, in which the osseous connective tissue (osteoid) is present in normal amounts but is insufficiently mineralized; and/or (3) *osteitis fibrosa*, in which an over-production of PTH leads to excessive bone resorption and replacement by fibrous tissue, as well as systemic changes due to hypercalcaemia.

Clinical assessment

Patients with metabolic bone disorders usually present with some of the following features: a child with below normal growth and deformities of the lower limbs (rickets); an elderly person with a fracture of the femoral neck or a vertebral body following comparatively minor trauma (postclimacteric osteoporosis); an elderly patient with bone pain and multiple compression fractures of the spine (osteomalacia); a middle-

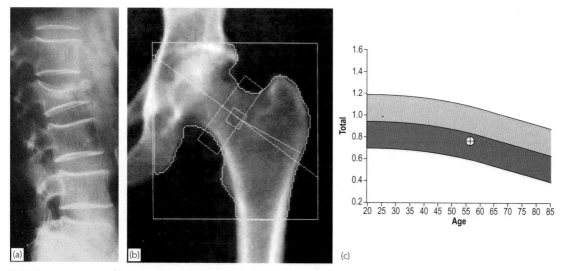

7.7 Measurement of bone mass (a) X-ray of the lumbar spine shows a compression fracture of L2. The general loss of bone density accentuates the cortical outlines of the vertebral body end plates. These features are characteristic of diminished bone mass, which can be measured accurately by dual-energy x-ray absorptiometry (b). In this case the value at the femoral neck was still within the normal range (c).

aged person with hypercalcaemia and pseudogout (hyperparathyroidism); or someone with multiple fractures and a history of prolonged corticosteroid treatment.

X-rays may show stress fractures, vertebral compression, cortical thinning, loss of trabecular structure or merely an ill-defined loss of radiographic density – osteopenia – which can signify either osteomalacia or osteoporosis.

These appearances are so common in ageing people that they seldom cause alarm. However, if someone under the age of 50 years has repeated fractures or bone deformities he or she should be referred for a full clinical, radiological and biochemical evaluation. Elderly people should also be investigated for signs of metastatic bone disease and myelomatosis.

Measurement of bone mass

X-ray signs of bone loss are late and unreliable; there are much more accurate ways of measuring bone mineral density (BMD) and bone mass. These are based on the principle that a beam of energy is attenuated as it passes through bone, and the degree of attenuation is related to the mass and mineral content of the bone. BMD is expressed in grams per unit area or unit volume and is recorded in comparison to the sex- and age-specific distribution of these values in the general population. The measurements are specific for each anatomical location (lumbar spine, femoral neck, distal radius and so on).

The most widely used technique is that of *dual-energy x-ray absorptiometry (DEXA)*. Precision and accuracy are excellent, x-ray exposure is not excessive and measurements can be obtained anywhere in the skeleton.

The main indication for using bone densitometry is to assess the degree and progress of bone loss in patients with clinically diagnosed metabolic bone disease. However, it is also useful as a screening procedure for perimenopausal women with multiple risk factors for osteoporotic fractures.

Biochemical tests

- *Serum calcium and phosphate* concentrations should be measured in the fasting state, and it is the ionized calcium fraction that is important.
- *Serum alkaline phosphatase* concentration is an index of osteoblastic activity; it is raised in osteomalacia and in disorders associated with high bone turnover (hyperparathyroidism, Paget's disease, bone metastases).
- *PTH activity* can be estimated from serum assays of the -COOH terminal fragment.
- *Vitamin D activity* is assessed by measuring the serum 25-HCC concentration. Serum 1,25-DHCC levels do not necessarily reflect vitamin uptake but are reduced in advanced renal disease.
- *Urinary calcium and phosphate* excretion can be

measured. Significant alterations are found in malabsorption disorders, hyperparathyroidism and other conditions associated with hypercalcaemia.

- *Urinary hydroxyproline* excretion is a measure of bone resorption. It may be increased in high-turnover conditions such as Paget's disease but it is not sensitive enough to reflect lesser increases in bone resorption.
- *Excretion of pyridinium compounds and telopeptides* derived from bone collagen cross-links is a much more sensitive index of bone resorption.

NB: Laboratory reports should always state the normal range for each test, which may be different for infants, children and adults.

OSTEOPOROSIS

In osteoporosis the bone is qualitatively normal but there is less of it than would be expected in a person of that age and sex. Generalized osteoporosis, as a clinical disorder, is characterized by an abnormally low bone mass and defects in bone structure, a combination which renders the bone unusually fragile and at greater than normal risk of fracture.

The term *osteopenia* is sometimes used to describe bone which appears to be less 'dense' than normal on x-ray, without defining whether the loss of density is due to osteoporosis or osteomalacia, or indeed whether it is sufficiently marked to be regarded as pathological. Other signs of osteoporosis are loss of trabecular definition, thinning of the cortices and insufficiency fractures. Compression fractures of the vertebral bodies, wedging at multiple levels and biconcave distortion of the vertebral end-plates due to bulging of intact intervertebral discs are typical of severe postmenopausal osteoporosis.

The clinical and radiographic diagnosis should be backed up by assessment of BMD as measured by DEXA of the spine and hips. In otherwise 'normal' women over the age of 50 years, anything more than 2 standard deviations below the average for the relevant population group may be taken as indicative of osteoporosis.

POSTMENOPAUSAL OSTEOPOROSIS

Symptomatic postmenopausal osteoporosis is an exaggerated form of the physiological bone depletion that normally accompanies ageing and loss of gonadal activity. Two overlapping phases are recognized: an early postmenopausal syndrome characterized by rapid bone loss due predominantly to increased osteoclastic resorption (high-turnover osteoporosis) and a less well-defined syndrome which emerges in elderly people and is due to a gradual slow-down in osteoblastic activity and the increasing effects of dietary insufficiencies, chronic ill health and reduced mobility (low-turnover osteoporosis).

Around the menopause, and for the next 10 years, bone loss normally accelerates to about 3% per year compared with 0.3% during the preceding two decades. This is due mainly to increased bone resorption, the withdrawal of oestrogen

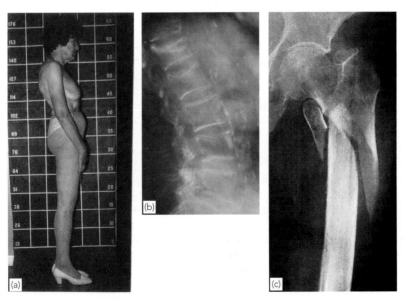

7.8 Osteoporosis (a) This woman noticed that she was becoming more and more round-shouldered; she also had chronic backache and her x-ray (b) shows obvious compression fractures of T12 and L1. Six years after this x-ray was obtained, she fell in her kitchen and sustained the fracture shown in (c).

Risk factors for postmenopausal osteoporosis
■ Caucasoid (white) or Asiatic ethnicity
■ Family history of osteoporosis
■ History of anorexia nervosa and/or amenorrhoea
■ Low peak bone mass in the third decade
■ Early onset of menopause
■ Unusually slim or emaciated build
■ Oophorectomy
■ Early hysterectomy
■ Nutritional insufficiency
■ Chronic lack of exercise
■ Cigarette smoking
■ Alcohol abuse

having removed one of the normal restraints on osteoclastic activity. Genetic influences play an important part in determining when and how this process becomes exaggerated, but a number of other risk factors have been identified.

Clinical features

A woman at or near the menopause develops back pain and increased thoracic kyphosis; she may give a history of previous Colles' fracture or a fracture of the ankle or femoral neck and x-rays of the spine may show compression of one or more vertebral bodies. DEXA may show significantly reduced bone density in the vertebral bodies or femoral neck.

Once the clinical diagnosis has been established, screening tests should be performed to rule out other causes of osteoporosis (e.g. hyperparathyroidism, malignant disease or hypercortisonism).

Prevention and treatment

Bone densitometry can be used to identify women who are at more than usual risk of suffering a fracture at the menopause, and prophylactic treatment of this group is sensible. However, routine DEXA screening is still not universally employed but is usually reserved for women with multiple risk factors and particularly those with suspected oestrogen deficiency (premature or surgically induced menopause).

Women approaching the menopause should be advised to maintain adequate levels of dietary calcium and vitamin D, to keep up a high level of physical activity and to avoid smoking and

excessive consumption of alcohol. If necessary, the recommended daily requirements should be met by taking calcium and vitamin D supplements.

Menopausal women with significant risk factors for osteoporosis, and more so those who have already suffered an 'osteoporotic fracture', should seek advice about using drug therapy.

Hormone replacement therapy

Until recently *hormone replacement therapy* (*HRT*) was the most widely used medication for postmenopausal osteoporosis. Taking oestrogen (or a combination of oestrogen and progesterone) for 5–10 years was shown convincingly to reduce the risk of osteoporotic fractures, though after stopping the medication the BMD gradually falls to the usual low level. Moreover, there was growing concern about the increased risks of thromboembolism, stroke, breast cancer and uterine cancer. As more experience has been gained with other antiresorptive drugs, the preference for HRT has waned.

Bisphosphonates

Bisphosphonates are now regarded as the preferred medication for postmenopausal osteoporosis. They act by suppressing osteoclastic bone resorption and thereby reduce the risk of vertebral and hip fractures. Alendronate can be administered by mouth in once-weekly doses for both prevention and treatment of osteoporosis. Gastrointestinal side-effects are a bother and suitable precautions should be taken; for patients who cannot tolerate the drug, pamidronate has been given intravenously at 3-monthly intervals.

Denosumab

A new approach to antiresorptive therapy employs a human monoclonal antibody which inhibits the receptor activator needed to activate osteoclast differentiation. Denosumab is administered by subcutaneous injection every 6 months. As with other antiresorptive drugs, it must be supplemented with calcium and vitamin D.

Management of fractures

Femoral neck and other long-bone fractures may need operative treatment. Methods are described in the relevant chapters in Part 3.

Vertebral fractures will call for analgesic treatment, partial rest and assistance with personal care as well as physiotherapy. Operative measures are occasionally needed to treat severe compression fractures.

POSTCLIMACTERIC OSTEOPOROSIS IN MEN

With the gradual depletion in androgenic hormones, men eventually suffer the same bone changes as postmenopausal women, only this occurs about 15 years later unless there is some specific cause for the hormone depletion. Osteoporotic fractures in men under 60 years of age should always arouse the suspicion of some underlying disorder: hypogonadism, metastatic bone disease, multiple myeloma, liver disease, alcohol abuse, malabsorption disorder, malnutrition, glucocorticoid medication or antigonadal hormone treatment for prostate cancer. Other causes of secondary osteoporosis are shown in *Table 7.1*.

Treatment is much the same as for post-menopausal osteoporosis.

> ⚠ Osteoporosis in middle-aged men – check for myelomatosis.

INVOLUTIONAL OSTEOPOROSIS

In advanced age the rate of bone loss decreases more slowly, yet the incidence of femoral neck and vertebral fractures rises steadily, and by the age of 75 years almost one-third of white women will have had at least one 'osteoporotic' fracture. The conclusion is that *qualitative changes* also contribute to bone fragility in old people. Causes would include a rising incidence of chronic illness, dietary deficiencies, lack of exposure to sunlight, muscular atrophy, loss of balance and an increased tendency to fall. It is well known that many old people suffer from vitamin D deficiency and develop some degree of osteomalacia on top of the postmenopausal osteoporosis.

Treatment is initially directed at managing the fracture; the sooner these patients are mobilized and rehabilitated the better. Patients with muscle weakness and/or poor balance will benefit from gait training and the use of walking aids and rail fittings in the home.

Causative factors must be addressed and if the patient is not already on vitamin D and calcium as well as antiresorptive medication, this should be started.

SECONDARY OSTEOPOROSIS

There are numerous causes of secondary osteoporosis (*Table 7.1*).

Table 7.1 Causes of secondary osteoporosis

Nutritional	Endocrine disorders
Malabsorption	Gonadal insufficiency
Malnutrition	Hyperparathyroidism
Scurvy	Thyrotoxicosis
Inflammatory disorders	Cushing's disease
Rheumatoid disease	**Malignant disease**
Ankylosing spondylitis	Carcinomatosis
Tuberculosis	Multiple myeloma
Drug induced	Leukaemia
Corticosteroids	**Other**
Excessive alcohol	Smoking
consumption	Chronic obstructive
Anticonvulsants	pulmonary disease
Heparin	Osteogenesis imperfecta
Immunosuppressives	Chronic renal disease

Hypercortisonism

Prolonged or excessive use of corticosteroids may cause severe osteoporosis, especially if the condition for which the drug is administered is itself associated with bone loss (e.g. rheumatoid arthritis). Bone resorption is markedly increased and formation is suppressed.

Treatment presents a problem, because the drug may be essential for the control of some generalized disease. However, corticosteroid dosage should be kept to a minimum; remember that topical and intra-articular preparations are absorbed and may have systemic effects if used repeatedly.

Preventive measures include the use of calcium supplements (at least 1500 mg per day) and vitamin D metabolites. In postmenopausal women and elderly men, bisphosphonates may also be effective in reducing bone resorption.

Thyrotoxicosis

Thyroxine speeds up the rate of bone turnover, but resorption exceeds formation. Osteoporosis is quite common in hyperthyroidism, but fractures usually occur only in older people who suffer the cumulative effects of the menopause and thyroid overload. In the worst cases osteoporosis may be severe with spontaneous fractures, a marked rise in serum alkaline phosphatase, hypercalcaemia and hypercalciuria. Treatment is needed for both the osteoporosis and the thyrotoxicosis.

Alcohol abuse

This is a common (and often neglected) cause of osteoporosis at all ages, with the added factor of an increased tendency to falls and other injuries. Bone changes are due to a combination of decreased calcium absorption, liver failure and a toxic effect on osteoblast function. Alcohol also has a mild glucocorticoid effect.

Multiple myeloma and carcinomatosis

Generalized osteoporosis, anaemia and a high erythrocyte sedimentation rate (ESR) are characteristic features of myelomatosis and metastatic bone disease. Bone loss is due to over-production of local OAFs. Bisphosphonates may help to reduce these effects.

Disuse

The worst effects of stress reduction are seen in states of weightlessness; bone resorption, unbalanced by formation, leads to hypercalcaemia, hypercalciuria and severe osteoporosis. Lesser degrees of osteoporosis are seen in bedridden patients, and regional osteoporosis is common after immobilization of a limb. The effects can be mitigated by encouraging mobility, exercise and weightbearing.

Other conditions

There are many other causes of secondary osteoporosis, including hyperparathyroidism (which is considered below), rheumatoid arthritis, ankylosing spondylitis and subclinical forms of osteogenesis imperfecta. The associated clinical features usually point to the diagnosis.

RICKETS AND OSTEOMALACIA

Rickets and osteomalacia are different expressions of the same disease: inadequate mineralization of bone. Osteoid throughout the skeleton is incompletely calcified, and the bone is therefore 'softened' (*osteomalacia*). In children there are additional effects on physeal growth and ossification, resulting in deformities of the endochondral skeleton (*rickets*).

The inadequacy may be due to defects anywhere along the metabolic pathway for vitamin D: nutritional lack, under-exposure to sunlight, intestinal malabsorption, decreased 25-hydroxylation (liver disease, anticonvulsants) and reduced 1α-hydroxylation (renal disease, nephrectomy, 1α-hydroxylase deficiency). The pathological changes may also be caused by calcium deficiency or hypophosphataemia.

Pathology

In *rickets* the characteristic pathological changes arise from the inability to calcify the intercellular matrix in the deeper layers of the physis. The proliferative zone is as active as ever, but the cells pile up irregularly and the entire physeal plate increases in thickness. The zone of calcification is poorly mineralized and bone formation is sparse in the zone of ossification. New trabeculae are thin and weak, and with joint loading the metaphysis becomes broad and cup shaped.

Further away from the physis the changes are essentially those of *osteomalacia*: thin

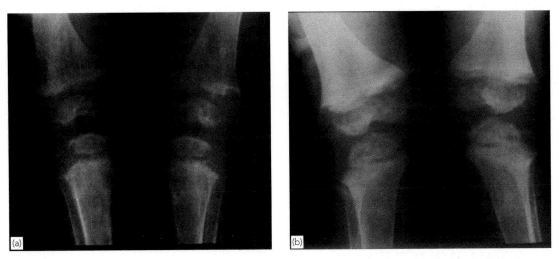

7.9 Rickets – x-rays X-rays obtained at two points during growth in a child with nutritional rickets. (a) Typical features of widening of the physis and flaring of the metaphysis are well marked. (b) After treatment the bones have begun to heal but the deformities are still noticeable.

trabeculae lined by unusually wide uncalcified osteoid seams; in severe cases the cortices also are thinner than normal and may show signs of new or older stress fractures. If the condition has been present for long, there may be widespread stress deformities of the bones: indentation of the pelvis, bending of the femoral neck (coxa vara) and bowing of the femora and tibiae. Even mild osteomalacia can increase the risk of fracture if it is superimposed on postmenopausal osteoporosis.

VITAMIN D DEFICIENCY RICKETS

Vitamin D deficiency rickets, once common in Northern Europe due to a combination of dietary lack and under-exposure to sunlight, is now seldom seen in its classic form. Infants may present with tetany or convulsions. There is failure to thrive, listlessness and muscular flaccidity.

Early bone changes are deformity of the skull (craniotabes) and thickening of the knees, ankles and wrists from physeal over-growth. Enlargement of the costochondral junctions ('rickety rosary') and lateral indentation of the chest (Harrison's sulcus) may also appear. Distal tibial bowing has been attributed to sitting or lying cross-legged.

Once the child stands, lower limb deformities increase and stunting of growth may be obvious. In severe rickets there may be spinal curvature, coxa vara and bending or fractures of the long bones.

X-rays

In active rickets there is thickening and widening of the physes, distortion of the metaphyses and, sometimes, bowing of the long bones. These changes often leave traces after healing.

Investigations

Serum calcium and phosphate concentrations as well as 25-HCC levels are diminished and alkaline phosphatase is increased. Urinary calcium excretion is diminished.

Treatment

The condition responds rapidly to vitamin D administration in the form of calciferol 400–1000 IU per day with calcium supplements. After normal growth, residual deformities are usually slight.

OSTEOMALACIA IN ADULTS

Osteomalacia may result from defects anywhere along the metabolic pathway for vitamin D: nutritional lack, under-exposure to sunlight, intestinal malabsorption or defective conversion to the active metabolites in the liver or kidney.

Clinical features

Symptoms usually appear insidiously; bone pain, backache and muscle weakness may be present for years before the diagnosis is made. Unexplained pain in the hip or one of the long bones may presage a stress fracture. Often the condition is suspected only when the patient is admitted to hospital with a vertebral compression fracture or an 'insufficiency fracture' of the femur or tibia.

Some of these patients have been living alone, on a poor diet and with little exposure to sunlight. Others are immigrants who have moved from sunny climates to countries with long winters, perhaps retaining traditional diets which are lacking in vitamin D. Others again suffer from intestinal malabsorption or disorders of the liver or kidney which affect conversion of vitamin D to the active metabolites. All of these diagnostic possibilities should be explored.

X-rays

Suspicious features are generalized rarefaction of bone and signs of previous fractures of the vertebrae, ribs, pubic rami or long bones. Almost pathognomonic is a poorly healing stress fracture which appears as a thin transverse band of rarefaction in the cortex – a so-called *Looser zone*. There may also be signs of secondary hyperparathyroidism.

Investigations

As in rickets, serum calcium and phosphate concentrations may be diminished and alkaline phosphatase raised. More significant are diminished values for 25-HCC and 1,25-DHCC. Biochemical changes are often insignificant and biopsy may be needed for diagnosis; excessive amounts of unmineralized osteoid can be demonstrated. Having made the diagnosis, it is still necessary to establish the cause. Patients should be investigated for malabsorption syndromes, liver disorders and renal disease.

Treatment

Treatment with vitamin D and calcium supplements is usually effective; elderly people may need very large doses (up to 2000 IU per day). Underlying disorders of the gut, liver or kidney will need treatment as well.

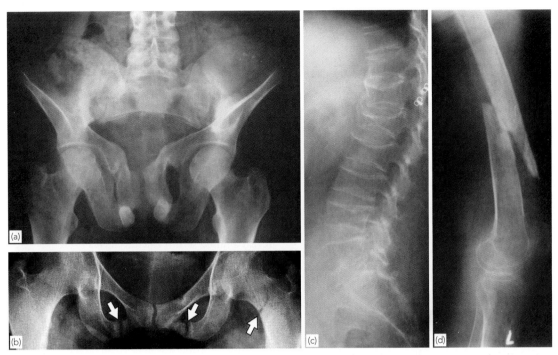

7.10 Osteomalacia Four characteristic features of adult osteomalacia: (a) indentation of the acetabula producing the trefoil or champagne glass pelvis; (b) Looser's zones (arrows) in the pubic rami and left femoral neck; (c) biconcave vertebrae; and (d) fracture in the mid-diaphysis of a long bone following low-energy trauma (the femoral cortices in this case are egg-shell thin).

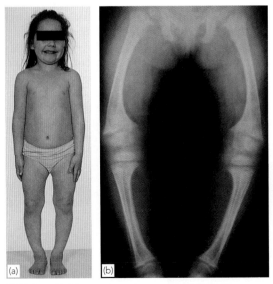

7.11 Familial hypophosphataemic rickets In countries with advanced health systems nutritional rickets is now uncommon. (a) This young girl has familial hypophosphataemic rickets. In addition to the obvious varus deformities of her legs, her lower limbs are disproportionately short compared to her upper body. (b) X-rays of another child with a similar condition.

HYPOPHOSPHATAEMIC RICKETS

Chronic hypophosphataemia occurs in a number of disorders in which there is impaired renal tubular reabsorption of phosphate. Calcium levels are normal but bone mineralization is defective.

Familial hypophosphataemic rickets (vitamin D-resistant rickets)

In many countries this is now the commonest form of rickets. It is an X-linked genetic disorder with dominant inheritance, starting in infancy or soon after and causing progressive bony deformity. The children are below normal height and deformities such as genu valgum or genu varum appear when they begin to walk. There is no myopathy.

X-rays show changes similar to those of vitamin D deficiency rickets, but often more marked. Serum calcium levels are normal but phosphate is reduced.

Treatment

Treatment is by large doses of vitamin D (50,000 IU or more) and up to 4 g of inorganic phosphate per day (with careful monitoring to prevent overdosage), continued until growth ceases.

73

Bony deformities may require bracing or osteotomy. If the child needs to be immobilized, vitamin D must be stopped temporarily to prevent hypercalcaemia from the combined effects of treatment and disuse bone resorption.

Adult hypophosphataemia

Although rare, this must be remembered as a cause of unexplained bone loss in adults. Patients may also complain of joint pains. The condition responds dramatically to treatment with phosphate, vitamin D and calcium.

HYPERPARATHYROIDISM

Excessive secretion of PTH may be *primary* (usually due to parathyroid adenoma or hyperplasia), *secondary* (due to persistent hypocalcaemia) or *tertiary* (when secondary hyperplasia leads to autonomous over-activity).

Pathology

The cardinal feature of hyperparathyroidism is a rise in serum calcium. Over-production of PTH enhances calcium conservation by stimulating tubular reabsorption and intestinal absorption as well as osteoclastic resorption of bone. The resulting hypercalcaemia so increases glomerular filtration of calcium that there is hypercalciuria despite the augmented tubular reabsorption. Urinary phosphate also is increased, due to suppressed tubular reabsorption.

The effects of these changes are seen in the *kidneys* (calcinosis, stone formation, recurrent infection and impaired function), the *bones* (osteoporosis and subperiosteal erosions) and in the general manifestations of *hypercalcaemia*, including calcification of soft tissues. In severe cases osteoclastic hyperactivity produces endosteal cavitation and replacement of the marrow spaces by vascular granulations and fibrous tissue (*osteitis fibrosa cystica*). Haemorrhage and giant-cell reaction within the fibrous stroma may give rise to brownish, tumour-like masses, whose liquefaction leads to fluid-filled cysts (*brown tumours*).

Clinical features

Primary hyperparathyroidism is quite common; the usual cause is a solitary adenoma in one of the small parathyroid glands.

Patients are middle-aged (40–65 years) and women are affected twice as often as men. Many remain asymptomatic and are diagnosed only because routine biochemistry tests unexpectedly reveal a raised serum calcium level.

Symptoms are due mainly to hypercalcaemia: anorexia, nausea, abdominal pain, depression, fatigue and muscle weakness. Patients may also develop polyuria, kidney stones or nephrocalcinosis due to chronic hypercalciuria. Some complain of joint symptoms, due to chondrocalcinosis. Only a minority (probably less than 10%) present with bone disease – and this is usually generalized osteoporosis rather than the classic features of osteitis fibrosa, bone cysts and pathological fractures.

X-rays

Typical features are osteoporosis (sometimes including vertebral collapse) and areas of cortical erosion. Hyperparathyroid 'brown tumours' should be considered in the differential diagnosis of atypical cyst-like lesions of long bones. However, the classical – and almost pathognomonic – feature, which should always be sought, is subperiosteal cortical resorption of the middle phalanges. Non-specific features of hypercalcaemia are renal calculi, nephrocalcinosis and chondrocalcinosis.

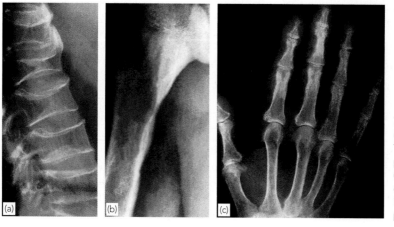

7.12 Hyperparathyroidism
(a) Spinal osteoporosis is typical. This patient also complained of pain in the right arm; an x-ray (b) showed cortical erosion of the humerus. Other signs included typical erosions of the phalangeal cortices (c).

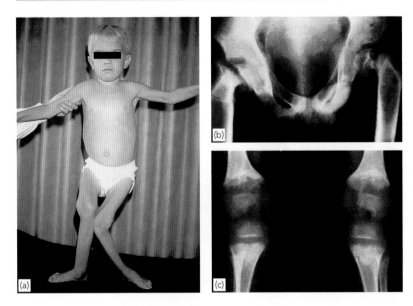

7.13 Renal glomerular osteodystrophy (a,b) This young boy with chronic renal failure developed severe deformities of the hips and knees. Note the displacement of the upper femoral epiphyses (c).

Investigations

Biochemical tests show hypercalcaemia, hypophosphataemia and a raised serum PTH concentration. Serum alkaline phosphatase may be raised.

Treatment

Treatment is usually conservative and includes adequate hydration and decreased calcium intake. If an adenoma is present it should be removed. The indications for parathyroidectomy are marked and unremitting hypercalcaemia, recurrent renal calculi, progressive nephrocalcinosis and severe osteoporosis.

Postoperatively there is a danger of severe hypocalcaemia due to brisk formation of new bone (the 'hungry bone syndrome'). This must be treated promptly, with one of the fast-acting vitamin D metabolites.

Secondary hyperparathyroidism

Secondary hyperparathyroidism is sometimes seen in rickets and osteomalacia, and accounts for some of the radiological features in these disorders. Treatment is directed at the primary condition.

RENAL OSTEODYSTROPHY

This condition must not be confused with renal tubular phosphate losing disorders which give rise to hypophosphataemic rickets (page 73).

Patients with *chronic renal failure* and lowered glomerular filtration rate are liable to develop diffuse bone changes due to a variable combination of rickets or osteomalacia, secondary hyperparathyroidism, osteoporosis and vertebral osteosclerosis. Uraemia and phosphate retention are accompanied by a fall in serum calcium which is due partly to the hyperphosphataemia and partly to 1,25-DHCC deficiency. In patients with end-stage renal failure the bone changes can be aggravated by aluminium retention or contamination of dialysing fluids.

Renal abnormalities precede the bone changes by several years. Children are clinically more severely affected than adults: they are stunted, pasty-faced and have marked rachitic deformities. Myopathy is common.

X-rays

Children show features similar to those of severe rickets. Those with long-standing disease may present with epiphyseal displacement (epiphyseolysis). Osteosclerosis is seen mainly in the axial skeleton and is more common in young patients. Signs of secondary hyperparathyroidism can be widespread and severe.

Biochemical features

Characteristic changes are low serum calcium, high serum phosphate and elevated alkaline phosphatase levels. Urinary excretion of calcium and phosphate is diminished. Plasma PTH levels may be raised.

Treatment

Renal failure, if irreversible, may require haemodialysis or renal transplantation. The osteodystrophy should be treated, in the first instance, with large doses of vitamin D (up to

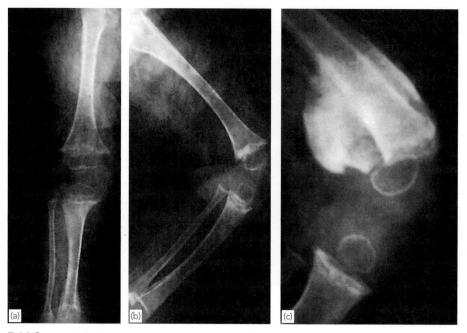

7.14 Scurvy (a,b) The epiphyseal ring sign and small subperiosteal haemorrhages; (c) the femoral epiphysis has displaced and the subperiosteal haemorrhage has calcified.

500,000 IU daily); in resistant cases, small doses of 1,25-DHCC may be effective. Epiphyseolysis may need internal fixation and residual deformities can be corrected once the disease is under control.

SCURVY

Vitamin C (ascorbic acid) deficiency causes failure of collagen synthesis and osteoid formation. The result is osteoporosis, which in infants is most marked in the juxtaepiphyseal bone. Spontaneous bleeding is common and may cause subperiosteal haematomas.

The infant is irritable and anaemic. The gums may be spongy and bleeding. Subperiosteal haemorrhage causes excruciating pain and tenderness near the large joints. Fractures or epiphyseal separations may occur.

X-rays show generalized bone rarefaction, most marked in the long-bone metaphyses. The normal calcification in growing cartilage produces dense bands in the juxtaepiphyseal metaphyses and around the ossific centres of the epiphyses (the 'ring sign'). The metaphyses may be deformed or fractured. Subperiosteal haematomas show as soft-tissue swellings or periosseous calcification.

Treatment with large doses of vitamin C produces prompt recovery.

FLUOROSIS

Fluorosis is fairly common in those parts of the world where fluorine appears in the soil and drinking water. Mottling of the teeth is a fairly common manifestation, and in areas where fluorine concentrations in the drinking water are particularly high, widespread skeletal abnormalities are occasionally encountered. Characteristic features in severe cases are subperiosteal new bone accretion and osteosclerosis, together with hyperostosis at the bony attachments of ligaments and tendons. Despite the apparent thickening and 'density' of the skeleton, the bones fracture more easily under bending and twisting loads.

Patients complain of backache, bone pain and joint stiffness. Sometimes the first clinical manifestation is a stress fracture.

The typical x-ray features are osteosclerosis, osteophytosis and ossification of ligamentous and fascial attachments. Changes are most marked in the spine and pelvis, where the bones become densely opaque.

There is no specific treatment for this condition. After exposure ceases it still takes years for bone fluoride to be excreted.

PAGET'S DISEASE (OSTEITIS DEFORMANS)

Paget's disease is characterized by enlargement and thickening of the bone, but the internal architecture is abnormal and the bone is unusually brittle. The condition has a curious ethnic and geographic distribution, being relatively common in North America, Britain, Germany and Australia (more than 3% of people aged over 40) but rare in Asia, Africa and the Middle East. The cause is unknown.

Pathology

Any bone may be affected; in the worst cases many are involved. Cortices are thickened but irregular, at one stage more porous than usual and at another more sclerotic. This is due to alternating phases of rapid bone resorption and formation. While resorption predominates (the 'vascular' stage) the bone is easily deformed; in the late stage the bone becomes increasingly sclerotic and brittle. The characteristic cellular change is a marked increase in osteoclastic and osteoblastic activity.

Clinical features

Paget's disease affects men and women equally. Only occasionally does it present in patients under 50 years, but from that age onwards it becomes increasingly common. The disease may for many years remain localized to a single bone, the pelvis and tibia being the commonest sites, and the femur, skull, spine and clavicle the next commonest.

Most people with Paget's disease are asymptomatic, the disorder being diagnosed when an x-ray is taken for some unrelated condition or after the incidental discovery of a raised serum alkaline phosphatase level. When pain occurs it is dull and constant.

Deformities are seen mainly in the lower limbs. The limb looks bent and feels thick, and the skin is unduly warm. If the skull is affected, it enlarges; the patient may complain that old hats no longer fit. The skull base may become flattened (platybasia), giving the appearance of a short neck. In generalized Paget's disease there may also be considerable kyphosis, so the patient becomes shorter and 'ape-like', with bent legs and arms hanging in front of them.

Cranial nerve compression may lead to impaired vision, facial palsy, trigeminal neuralgia or deafness. Vertebral thickening may cause spinal cord or nerve root compression.

X-rays

The appearances are so striking that the diagnosis is seldom in doubt. During the resorptive phase

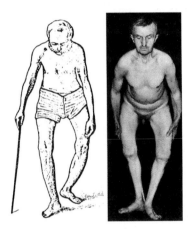

7.15 Paget's disease Paget's original case compared with a modern photograph.

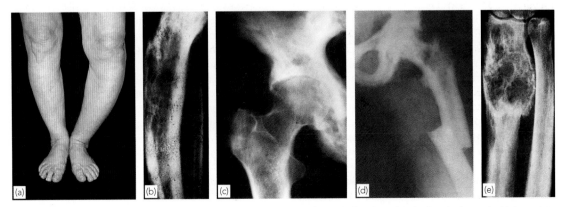

7.16 Paget's disease (a) Deformity of the tibia due to Paget's disease. (b) X-ray shows that the bone is thickened, coarsened and bent. Complications include (c) erosive arthritis in a nearby joint; (d) fracture; and (e) osteosarcoma of the affected bone.

there may be localized areas of osteolysis; later the bone becomes thick and sclerotic, with coarse trabeculation. Occasionally the diagnosis is made only when the patient presents with a pathological fracture.

Investigations

Serum calcium and phosphate levels are usually normal. The most useful test is measurement of the serum alkaline phosphatase level, which correlates with the activity and extent of disease.

Twenty-four hour urinary excretion of pyridinoline cross-links is a good indicator of disease activity and bone resorption.

Complications

- *Fractures*: common, especially in the weightbearing bones. The fracture line is usually partly transverse and partly oblique, like the line of section of a felled tree. In the femur there is a high rate of non-union; for femoral neck fractures prosthetic replacement and for shaft fractures early internal fixation are recommended.
- *Nerve compression and spinal stenosis*: occasionally this is the first abnormality to be detected, and may call for definitive surgical treatment.
- *Bone sarcoma*: osteosarcoma arising in an elderly patient is almost always due to malignant transformation in Paget's disease. The frequency of malignant change is probably around 1%. It should always be suspected if a known site of Paget's disease becomes more painful, swollen or tender. The prognosis is extremely grave.
- *High-output cardiac failure*: though rare, this is an important general complication. It is due to prolonged, increased bone blood flow.
- *Hypercalcaemia*: patients who are immobilized for long periods may develop hypercalcaemia.

Treatment

Most patients with Paget's disease never have any symptoms and require no treatment. Indeed, there is no specific therapy, but drugs such as calcitonin and bisphosphonates can control the disease by suppressing bone turnover. Patients should be examined regularly for signs of increased bone activity, such as local tenderness and warmth, or a rise in the alkaline phosphatase level.

The indications for specific treatment are: (1) persistent bone pain; (2) repeated fractures; (3) neurological complications; (4) high-output cardiac failure; (5) hypercalcaemia due to immobilization; and (6) preparation for major bone surgery where there is a risk of excessive haemorrhage.

Calcitonin is the most widely used therapy. It reduces bone resorption by decreasing both the activity and the number of osteoclasts; serum alkaline phosphatase and urinary hydroxyproline levels are lowered. Maintenance injections once or twice weekly may have to be continued indefinitely, but some authorities advocate stopping the drug and resuming treatment if symptoms recur.

Bisphosphonates bind to hydroxyapatite crystals, inhibiting their rate of growth and dissolution. It is claimed that the reduction in bone turnover following their use is associated with the formation of lamellar rather than woven bone and that, even after treatment is stopped, there may be prolonged remission of disease. Etidronate can be given orally (always on an empty stomach) but dosage should be kept low lest impaired bone mineralization results in osteomalacia. The newer bisphosphonates, such as pamidronate and alendronate, are more effective and produce remissions even with short courses of 1 or 2 weeks.

Operative treatment may be needed for a pathological fracture. An osteosarcoma, if detected early, may be resectable, but generally the prognosis is grave.

ENDOCRINE DISORDERS

The endocrine system plays an important part in skeletal growth and maturation, as well as the maintenance of bone turnover. The anterior lobe of the pituitary gland directly affects growth; it also controls the activities of the thyroid, the gonads and the adrenal cortex, each of which has its own influence on bone. Thus endocrine abnormalities may cause problems at several levels: (a) local effects due to glandular enlargement (e.g. pressure on cranial nerves from a pituitary adenoma); (b) over-secretion or under-secretion of hormone by the primarily affected gland; and (c) over- or under-activity of other glands which are controlled by the primary dysfunctional gland.

For the sake of clarity, the descriptions which follow have been somewhat simplified.

PITUITARY DYSFUNCTION

The *posterior lobe* of the pituitary gland has no influence on the musculoskeletal system. The *anterior lobe* is responsible for the secretion of pituitary growth hormone, as well as thyrotropic, gonadotropic and adrenocorticotropic hormones.

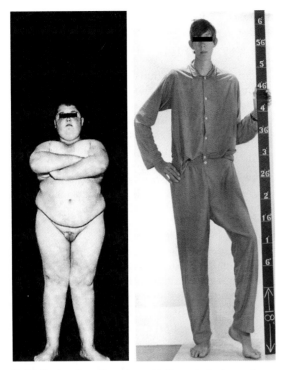

7.17 Endocrine disorders (a) Hypopituitarism: a boy of 12 years with the unmistakable build of Fröhlich's syndrome. (b) Hyperpituitarism: this 16-year-old 'giant' suffered from a pituitary adenoma.

Hypopituitarism

Anterior pituitary hyposecretion may be caused by *intrinsic disorders* (such as infarction, haemorrhage and intrapituitary tumours) or by *extrinsic lesions* (such as a craniopharyngioma) which press on the anterior lobe of the pituitary. Space-occupying lesions are likely to have other intracranial pressure effects.

In *children and adolescence* two distinct clinical disorders are encountered. In the *Lorain syndrome* the predominant effect is on growth: the child fails to grow but the body proportions are normal. In *Fröhlich's syndrome* delayed skeletal maturation is associated with adiposity and hypogonadism. Weakness of the physes combined with disproportionate adiposity may result in slipping of the proximal femoral or proximal tibial epiphyses.

In *adults* panhypopituitarism causes a variety of symptoms and signs, including those of cortisol and sex hormone deficiency. The only important skeletal effect is premature osteoporosis.

Treatment

Treatment will depend on the cause and the degree of dwarfism. If a tumour is identified (e.g. a craniopharyngioma), it can be removed or ablated.

Growth hormone deficiency has been successfully treated by the administration of biosynthetic growth hormone (somatotropin). The response should be checked by serial plots on the growth chart.

Hyperpituitarism

Over-secretion of pituitary growth hormone is usually due to an acidophil adenoma. The effects vary according to the age of onset.

Gigantism

Growth hormone over-secretion in childhood and adolescence causes excessive growth of the entire skeleton. The condition may be suspected quite early, and it is important to track the child's development by regular clinical and x-ray examination. In addition to being excessively tall, patients may develop deformity of the hip due to epiphyseal displacement. *Treatment* is directed at early removal of the pituitary tumour.

Acromegaly

Over-secretion of pituitary growth hormone in adulthood causes enlargement of the bones and soft tissues, but without the very marked elongation which is seen in gigantism. The bones are thickened, rather than lengthened; there is also hypertrophy of articular cartilage, which leads to enlargement of the joints. Bones such as the mandible, the clavicles, ribs, sternum and scapulae, which develop secondary growth centres in late adolescence or early adulthood, may go on growing longer than usual. Thickening of the skull, prominence of the orbital margins, over-growth of the jaw and enlargement of the nose, lips and tongue produce the characteristic facies of acromegaly. The chest is broad and barrel shaped and the hands and feet are large. Thickening of the bone ends may cause secondary osteoarthritis. About 10% of acromegalics develop diabetes and cardiovascular disease is more common than usual.

Treatment

The indications for operation are the presence of a tumour in childhood and cranial nerve pressure symptoms at any age. Trans-sphenoidal surgery has a high rate of success, provided the diagnosis is made reasonably early and the tumour is not too large.

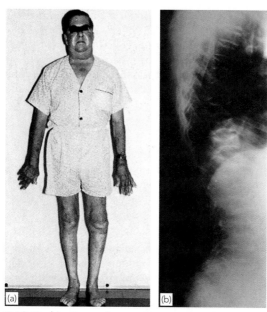

7.18 Cushing's syndrome (a) A patient with rheumatoid arthritis on long-term corticosteroid treatment. (b) On x-ray the bones look washed-out and there are compression fractures at multiple levels.

ADRENOCORTICAL DYSFUNCTION

The adrenal cortex secretes both mineralocorticoids (aldosterone) and glucocorticoids (cortisol). The latter has profound effects on bone and mineral metabolism, causing suppression of osteoblast activity, reduced calcium absorption, increased calcium excretion and enhanced PTH activity. Bone resorption is increased and formation is suppressed.

Hypercortisonism (Cushing's syndrome)

Glucocorticoid excess may be caused by increased pituitary secretion of adrenocorticotropic hormone (ACTH) (the original Cushing's disease), by independent over-secretion by the adrenal cortex (usually due to a steroid-secreting tumour) or by prolonged or excessive treatment with glucocorticoids (probably the commonest cause). Whatever the cause, the clinical picture is much the same and is generally referred to as *Cushing's syndrome*.

Clinical features

Patients have a characteristic appearance: the face is rounded and looks somewhat puffy ('moon face') and the trunk is obese, often with abdominal striae. However, the legs are quite thin and there may be proximal wasting and weakness.

X-rays

This is one of the causes of generalized osteoporosis; compression fractures of the vertebrae are common. Computed tomography may show an adrenal tumour.

Complications

Wounds and fractures heal slowly, bones provide little purchase for internal fixation and postoperative infection is more common than usual. A common complication of high-dosage corticosteroid therapy is avascular necrosis (see Chapter 6).

Management

Systemic corticosteroids should be used only when essential and in low dosage. If treatment is prolonged, calcium supplements (at least 1500 mg per day) and vitamin D should be given.

THYROID DYSFUNCTION

Hypothyroidism

Congenital hypothyroidism (cretinism)

Cretinism may be caused by developmental abnormalities of the thyroid, but it also occurs in endemic form in areas of iodine deficiency. Unless the condition is treated immediately (and diagnosis at birth is not easy!) the child becomes severely dwarfed and mentally retarded. X-rays may show irregular epiphyseal ossification. *Treatment* with thyroid hormone is essential.

Hyperthyroidism

Hyperthyroidism in adults may give rise to osteoporosis. Treatment of the primary disorder results in improved bone mass.

CHAPTER 8

GENETIC DISORDERS, DYSPLASIAS AND MALFORMATIONS

Abnormal development of the musculoskeletal system may give rise to a variety of physical defects which are described as *skeletal dysplasias* (abnormal bone growth and/or modelling), *malformations* (e.g. absence or duplication of certain parts) or structural *defects of connective tissue*; in some a specific *metabolic abnormality* has been identified.

In many cases the main determinant of the abnormality is a genetic defect. Such conditions can be broadly divided into three categories: *chromosome disorders*, *single gene disorders* and *polygenic* or *multifactorial disorders*. Some anomalies may also result from injury to the formed embryo.

CHROMOSOMES AND GENES

Each cell (apart from germ cells) in the human body contains within its nucleus 46 *chromosomes*, each of which consists of a single molecule of *deoxyribonucleic acid* (DNA); unravelled, this life-imparting molecule would be several centimetres long, a double-stranded chain along which thousands of segments are defined and demarcated as *genes*. These are the basic units of inherited biological information, each gene coding for the synthesis of a specific protein. Working as a set (or *genome*) they tell the cells how to develop, differentiate and function in specialized ways.

Chromosomes can be identified and numbered by microscopic examination of suitably prepared blood cells or tissue samples; the *cell karyotype* defines its chromosomal complement. *Somatic (diploid) cells* should have 46 chromosomes: 44 (numbers 1–22), called *autosomes*, are disposed in 22 homologous pairs, one of each pair being derived from the mother and one from the father and both carrying the same type of genetic information; the remaining two chromosomes are the *sex chromosomes*, females having two X chromosomes (one from each parent) and males having one X chromosome from the mother and one Y chromosome from the father. Thus *germ line cells* (eggs and sperm) have a *haploid* number of chromosomes (22 plus either an X or a Y).

Genes are distributed along the DNA chains, each gene at a specific point, or *locus*, on a specific chromosome. The chromosomes being paired, there will be two forms, or *alleles*, of each gene (one maternal, one paternal) at each locus; if the two alleles coding for a particular trait are identical, the person is said to be *homozygous* for that trait; if they are not identical, the individual is *heterozygous*.

The full genetic make-up of an individual is called the genotype. The finished person – a product of inherited traits and environmental influences – is the phenotype.

An important part of the unique human genotype is the *major histocompatibility complex* (MHC), also known as the *HLA system* (after human leucocyte antigen). This is a cluster of genes on chromosome 6 that is responsible for immunological specificity.

Genetic mutation

Mutation is any permanent change in DNA sequencing or structure. Such changes in a somatic cell are characteristic of malignancy. In a germ-line cell, mutations contribute to generational diversity:

■ *Point mutations*: the substitution of one nucleotide for another is the most common type of mutation. The effect varies from production of a more useful protein to a new but functionless protein, or an inability to form any protein at all; the result may be compatible with an essentially normal life or it may be lethal.
■ *Deletions/insertions*: deletion or insertion of a segment in the gene chain can result in an unusual protein being synthesized, perhaps a more advantageous one but maybe one that is non-functional or one that has a dire effect on tissue structure and function.

Single gene disorders

Gene mutation may occur by insertion, deletion, substitution or fusion of amino acids or nucleotides in the DNA chain. This can have profound consequences for cartilage growth, collagen structure, matrix patterning and marrow cell metabolism. The abnormality is then passed on to future generations according to simple mendelian rules (see below). There are literally thousands of single gene disorders, accounting for over 5% of child deaths, yet it is rare to see any one of them in an orthopaedic practice.

Chromosome disorders

Additions, deletions or changes in chromosomal structure usually have serious consequences, the affected fetuses being either stillborn or developing with severe physical and mental abnormalities, e.g. Down's syndrome in which there is one extra chromosome 21 (trisomy 21). Unlike genetic disorders, these conditions are not transmitted in future generations.

Polygenic and multi-factorial disorders

Many normal traits (body build, for example) derive from the interaction of multiple genetic and environmental influences. Likewise, certain diseases have a polygenic background, and some occur only when a genetic predisposition combines with an appropriate environmental 'trigger'. Gout, for example, is more common than usual in families with hyperuricaemia: the uric acid level is a polygenic trait, reflecting the interplay of multiple genes; it is also influenced by diet and may be more than usually elevated after a period of over-indulgence; finally, a slight bump on the toe acts as the proximate trigger for an acute attack of gout.

Embryonal damage

Many fetal abnormalities result from injury to the developing embryo. Most are of unknown aetiology but some are due to specific teratogenic agents which damage the embryo or the placenta during the first few months of gestation. Suspected or known teratogens include viral infections (e.g. rubella), certain drugs (e.g. thalidomide) and ionizing radiation. The resulting defects are usually asymmetrical and localized, ranging from mild anatomical faults to severe malformations such as non-development of an entire limb.

PATTERNS OF INHERITANCE

If it is certain that both parents of a child with a genetic disorder are normal, the defect must have been caused by a *mutant gene*. From then the genetic abnormality will be transmitted to future offspring according to well-defined patterns of inheritance, which may be either *autosomal* or *X-linked*, and *dominant* or *recessive*.

Autosomal dominant transmission means that the abnormality is inherited even if only one allele of a pair is abnormal, i.e. only one parent need have been affected and the condition is *heterozygous* (e.g. hereditary multiple exostoses). In that case one-half of the children of either sex are likely to develop the disease, though it may appear in varying degrees of severity (*variable expressivity*).

Autosomal recessive transmission means that both alleles of a pair have to be abnormal for the child to be affected, i.e. the condition is *homozygous*. Each parent contributes a faulty gene, though if both are heterozygous they themselves will be clinically normal. Theoretically one in four of their children will then be homozygous sufferers, two out of four will be *heterozygous carriers* of the faulty gene and one will be completely normal. It is easy to see why the rare recessive disorders are seen mainly in the children of consanguineous marriages or in closed communities where many people are related to each other.

X-linked disorders are caused by a faulty gene in the X chromosome. Characteristically, therefore, they never pass directly from father to son because the father's X chromosome inevitably goes to the daughter and the Y chromosome to the son. *X-linked dominant disorders* (e.g. hypophosphataemic rickets) pass from an affected mother to one-half of her daughters and one-half of her sons, or from an affected father to all of his daughters but none of his sons. (Not surprisingly, these conditions are twice as common in girls as in boys.) *X-linked recessive disorders* – of which the most notorious is haemophilia – have a highly distinctive pattern of inheritance: an affected male will pass the gene only to his daughters, who will become unaffected heterozygous carriers; they, in turn, will transmit it to one-half of their daughters (who will likewise be carriers) and one-half of their sons (who will be bleeders).

In-breeding

All types of genetic disease are more likely to occur in the children of consanguineous marriages or in closed communities where many people are related to each other. The rare recessive disorders, in particular, are seen in these circumstances, where there is an increased risk of a homozygous pairing between two mutant genes.

Genetic heterogeneity

The same phenotype (i.e. a patient with a characteristic set of clinical features) can result from widely different gene mutations. For example, there are four different types of osteogenesis imperfecta (brittle bone disease), some showing autosomal dominant and some autosomal recessive inheritance. Where this occurs, the recessive form is usually the more severe. This must be borne in mind when counselling parents.

Genetic markers

Many common disorders show an unusually close association with certain blood groups, tissue types or other serum proteins that occur with higher than expected frequency in the patients and their relatives. These are referred to as genetic markers. A good example is ankylosing spondylitis: over 90% of patients and 60% of their first-degree relatives are positive for HLA-B27.

Gene mapping

With advancing recombinant DNA technology, the genetic disorders are gradually being mapped to specific loci. In some cases (e.g. Duchenne muscular dystrophy) the mutant gene itself has been cloned, holding out the possibility of effective treatment in the future.

DIAGNOSIS

Prenatal diagnosis

Many genetic disorders can be diagnosed before birth, thus giving the parents the choice of selective abortion. *High-resolution ultrasound imaging* is harmless and is now done almost routinely. On the other hand, tests that involve *amniocentesis* or *chorionic villus sampling* carry a risk of injury to the fetus and are therefore used only when there is an increased likelihood of some abnormality.

Gender prediction at 7 weeks gestation by testing maternal blood for cell-free fetal DNA indicating the presence of Y chromosome fragments is now being offered and is reported to be over 98% accurate.

Diagnosis in childhood

Physical abnormalities may be obvious *at birth*; for example, disproportionately short limbs suggesting achondroplasia. *During infancy* the reasons for presentation are failure to grow normally, disproportionate shortness of the limbs, delay in walking or repeated fractures.

Older children are more obviously abnormal. Features which attract attention are retarded growth, deformities of the spine and/or limbs, unusual facial characteristics and a history of repeated fractures. There is a remarkable consistency about the deformities, which makes for a disturbing similarity of appearance in members of a particular group.

X-ray examination is important even if the physical features look familiar. A limited radiographic survey should include a postero-anterior view of the chest, anteroposterior views of the pelvis, knees and hands, additional views of one arm and one leg, a lateral view of the thoracolumbar spine and standard views of the skull. Fractures, bent bones, exostoses, epiphyseal dysplasia and spinal deformities may be obvious, especially in the older child. Sometimes a complete survey is needed and it is important to note which portion of the long bones (epiphysis, metaphysis or diaphysis) is affected. If there are *multiple fractures in different stages of healing*, or *features of several old healed fractures*, consider the possibility of *non-accidental injury* (the 'battered baby' syndrome).

The family history may reveal a characteristic pattern of inheritance. However, even an apparently normal parent may be very mildly affected, a fact which will not come to light if one relies entirely on the 'history', without the benefit of direct observation. *Racial background* is sometimes important: some diseases are particularly common in specific communities, e.g. sickle-cell disease in some black peoples and Gaucher's disease in Ashkenazi Jews.

Special investigations may be indicated to identify specific enzyme or metabolic abnormalities. *Direct testing for gene mutations* is already available for a number of conditions and is rapidly being extended to others.

Presentation in adults

Dysmorphic individuals who reach adulthood may lead fulfilling lives and have children of their own. Nevertheless, they often seek medical advice for problems such as abnormally short stature, local bone deformities, spinal stenosis, repeated fractures, secondary osteoarthritis or joint instability. As in children, family history and special investigations for enzyme or metabolic abnormalities are important.

PRINCIPLES OF MANAGEMENT

Rare developmental disorders are best treated in a centre that offers a 'special interest' team consisting of a paediatrician, medical geneticist, orthopaedic surgeon, psychologist, social worker, occupational therapist, orthotist and prosthetist. Management must be influenced by goals for adult life and not just the short-term goals of childhood. Patients and family members should be handled with sensitivity; terms such as 'dwarf' and 'dwarfism' should be avoided as they are often felt to be insulting.

Counselling

Patients and families may need expert counselling about: (a) the likely outcome of the disorders; (b) what will be required of the family; and (c) the risk of siblings or children being affected. Where there are severe deformities or mental disability, the entire family will need counselling.

Intrauterine surgery

The concept of operating on the unborn fetus is already a reality; however, it is too early to say whether the advantages (e.g. prenatal skin closure for dysraphism) will outweigh the risks.

Specific medication

The ideal form of treatment would be modification or replacement of the abnormal gene. For the present, however, treatment is directed mainly at identifying the faulty protein or enzyme and then, where possible, administering the essential ingredient that will restore physiological function or counteract the pathological effects of the abnormality. One example is the treatment of Gaucher's disease by administering the missing enzyme, alglucerase.

Gene therapy is still at the experimental stage. A carrier molecule or vector (often a virus that has been genetically modified to carry some normal human genetic material) is used to deliver the therapeutic material into the abnormal target cells where the DNA is 'uploaded' allowing, for example, functional protein production to be resumed.

Prevention and correction of deformities

Realignment of the limb, correction of ligamentous laxity and joint reconstruction can improve joint stability and gait. Anomalies such as coxa vara, genu valgum, club-foot, radial club-hand or scoliosis (and many others outside the field of orthopaedics) are amenable to corrective surgery. Short-limbed patients may benefit from lengthening operations; however, the risks should be carefully explained. One should bear in mind that cosmetic improvement is not always accompanied by any significant functional change. Conservative measures such as physiotherapy and splinting still have an important role to play.

Several developmental disorders are associated with potentially dangerous spinal anomalies, e.g. spinal stenosis and cord compression in achondroplasia and severe kyphoscoliosis in various types of vertebral dysplasia. Cord decompression or occipitocervical fusion are feasible but spinal operations carry considerable risks and should be undertaken only in specialized units. *Bear in mind that patients with spinal dysplasia undergoing any procedure under anaesthesia should be examined beforehand for odontoid hypoplasia and atlantoaxial instability.*

CLASSIFICATION

There is no completely satisfactory classification of developmental disorders. The same genetic abnormality may be expressed in different ways, while a variety of gene defects may cause almost identical clinical syndromes. The grouping presented in *Table 8.1* is no more than a convenient way of cataloguing the least rare of the clinical syndromes. Only a few representative conditions will be described in this chapter.

Table 8.1 A practical grouping of generalized developmental disorders

1. Genetic disorders of cartilage and bone growth (chondro-osteodystrophies)

Dysplasias with predominantly epiphyseal changes
   Multiple epiphyseal dysplasia
   Spondyloepiphyseal dysplasia
Dysplasias with predominantly physeal and metaphyseal changes
   Hereditary multiple exostosis
   Achondroplasia
   Metaphyseal chondrodysplasia
   Dyschondroplasia (enchodromatosis, Ollier's disease)
Dysplasias with predominantly diaphyseal changes
   Osteopetrosis (marble bones, Albers–Shönberg disease)
   Diaphyseal dysplasia (Engelmann's disease, Camurati's disease)

2. Collagen disorders

Osteogenesis imperfecta (brittle bones)
   Mild Lethal Severe Moderate
Generalized joint laxity
Ehlers–Danlos syndrome

3. Enzyme defects and metabolic disorders

Mucopolysaccharidoses
   Hurler's syndrome (MPS I)
   Hunter's syndrome (MPS II)
   Morquio–Brailsford syndrome (MPS IV)
Gaucher's disease

4. Chromosome disorders

Down's syndrome

CHONDRO-OSTEODYSTROPHIES

The chondro-osteodystrophies, or skeletal dysplasias, are a large group of disorders characterized by abnormal cartilage and bone growth. Only a few of the least rare conditions are discussed here. They are presented in clinical rather than aetiological groups:

- Those with predominantly epiphyseal changes.
- Those with predominantly physeal and metaphyseal changes.
- Those with mainly diaphyseal changes.
- Those with a mixture of abnormalities.

DYSPLASIAS WITH PREDOMINANTLY EPIPHYSEAL CHANGES

MULTIPLE EPIPHYSEAL DYSPLASIA

Multiple epiphyseal dysplasia (MED) varies in severity from a trouble-free disorder with mild anatomical abnormalities to a severe crippling condition. There is widespread involvement of the epiphyses but the vertebrae are not at all, or only mildly, affected.

Clinical features

MED is a familial disorder (autosomal dominant in most cases) in which the long-bone epiphyses develop abnormally. Children may present with stunted growth or with joint pain and progressive deformity. The face, skull and spine are normal. In adult life, residual bone defects may lead to joint incongruity and secondary osteoarthritis.

X-rays

Abnormal features are apparent from early childhood. Epiphyseal ossification is irregular or abnormal in outline. In the growing child the epiphyses are misshapen, and in the hips this may be mistaken for bilateral Perthes' disease. The vertebral ring epiphyses may be affected, but only mildly. At maturity the femoral heads and femoral condyles are flattened and secondary osteoarthritis may ensue; if the changes are mild, the underlying abnormality may be missed and the patient is regarded as 'just another case of osteoarthritis'. If many joints are involved, the patient can be severely disabled.

Diagnosis

MED is often confused with other childhood disorders which are associated with either lower-limb shortness or Perthes'-like changes in the epiphyses:

- Achondroplasia: marked by severe diminution in height and characteristic facial changes.
- Perthes' disease: is confined to the hips and shows a typical cycle of changes from epiphyseal irregularity to fragmentation, flattening and healing.
- Hypothyroidism: if untreated, causes progressive and widespread epiphyseal dysplasia. However, these children have other clinical and biochemical abnormalities and have learning difficulties.

Management

Children may complain of slight pain and limp, but little can (or need) be done about this. At maturity, deformities around the hips, knees or

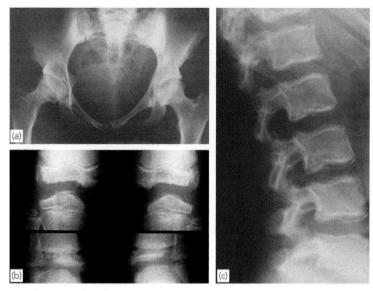

8.1 Multiple epiphyseal dysplasia (a,b) X-rays show epiphyseal distortion and flattening at multiple sites, in this case the hips, knees and ankles. (c) The ring epiphyses of the vertebral bodies also may be affected and in spondyloepiphyseal dysplasia this is the dominant feature.

ankles sometimes require corrective osteotomy. In later life, secondary osteoarthritis may call for reconstructive surgery.

SPONDYLOEPIPHYSEAL DYSPLASIA

Spondyloepiphyseal dyplasia (SED) comprises a heterogeneous group of disorders in which MED is associated with well-marked vertebral changes: delayed ossification, flattening of the vertebral bodies (platyspondyly), irregular ossification of the ring epiphyses and indentations of the end-plates. The mildest of these disorders is indistinguishable from MED; the more severe forms have characteristic appearances.

SED congenita

This autosomal dominant disorder can be diagnosed in infancy: the limbs are short, but the trunk is even shorter and the neck hardly there. Older children develop a dorsal kyphosis and a typical barrel-shaped chest; they stand with the hips flexed and the lumbar spine in marked lordosis. By adolescence they often have scoliosis.

X-rays show widespread epiphyseal dysplasia and the characteristic vertebral changes including odontoid hypoplasia.

Management may involve corrective osteotomies for severe coxa vara or knee deformities. Odontoid hypoplasia increases the risks of anaesthesia.

SED tarda

SED tarda, an X-linked recessive disorder, is less common and less severe than SED congenita, usully becoming apparent only after the age of 5 years when the child fails to grow normally and develops a kyphoscoliosis. Clinical features are similar to those of SED congenita.

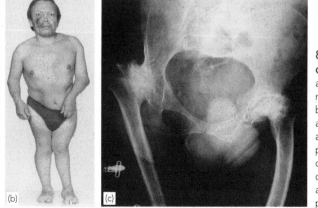

8.2 Spondyloepiphyseal dysplasia The x-ray features are similar to those in multiple epiphyseal dysplasia, but are usually more marked and affecting the vertebrae as well. (a,b) As adults these patients may be severely deformed. Note the barrel chest, deformity of all limbs and severe changes in the pelvic x-ray (c).

Treatment may be needed for backache or for secondary osteoarthritis of the hips.

DYSPLASIAS WITH PREDOMINANTLY PHYSEAL AND METAPHYSEAL CHANGES

HEREDITARY MULTIPLE EXOSTOSIS (DIAPHYSEAL ACLASIS)

This, the most common of all skeletal dysplasias, is a congenital disorder in which multiple exostoses appear at the long-bone metaphyses and the apophyseal borders of the scapula and pelvis. It is inherited by autosomal dominant transmission and starts with unrestrained lateral growth of the cartilaginous physis and defective modelling at the physeal/metaphyseal junction. Each exostosis is covered by a cartilage cap and can go on growing as long as endochondral growth normally proceeds; *any enlargement after that may herald malignant change to a chondrosarcoma.* The failure of modelling results in deformities of the long bones.

Clinical features

The condition is usually discovered in childhood; hard lumps appear near the ends of the long bones and along the edges of the scapula and pelvis. The child may be slightly short, with bowing of the forearms and valgus knees. Occasionally one of the lumps becomes tender or causes trouble due to pressure on a tendon.

X-rays show the pathognomonic exostoses as well as broadening and imperfect modelling of the metaphyses.

Management

If an exostosis is troublesome (and certainly if it starts to 'grow' after the parent bone has stopped) it should be removed. Long-bone deformities may call for corrective osteotomy.

ACHONDROPLASIA

This is the classic example of chondrodysplasia, and the commonest form of abnormally short stature. It is inherited as an autosomal dominant trait, but because most of the affected individuals do not have children, new cases usually appear sporadically due to gene mutation.

Clinical features

Severe, disproportionate shortening of the limb bones may be diagnosed by x-ray before birth. The abnormality is certainly obvious in childhood: growth is severely stunted, the limbs (particularly

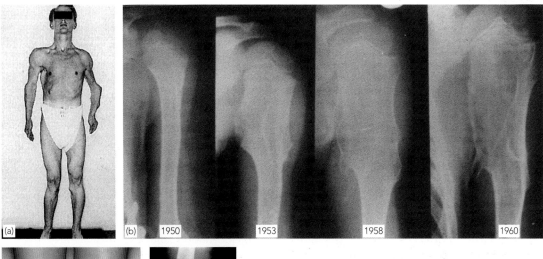

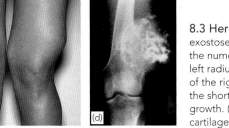

8.3 Hereditary multiple exostosis (a) Adult with multiple exostoses and typical deformities of the arms and legs. Note the numerous small 'bumps' in the limb bones, bowing of the left radius, shortening of the left forearm and valgus deformity of the right knee. (b) Serial x-rays showing the evolution of the shortened left humerus and the wide metaphysis during growth. (c,d) Patient with a large lump above the knee due to a cartilage-capped exostosis.

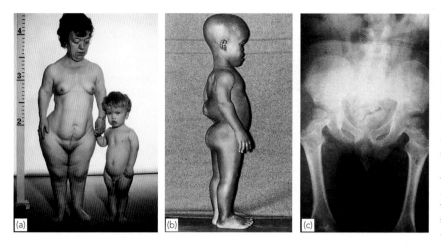

8.4 Achondroplasia (a) Mother and child with achondroplasia, showing the typical disproportionate shortening of the tubular bones, particularly the proximal segments of the upper and lower limbs. (b) Other features are seen in this child: lumbar lordosis, a prominent thoracolumbar gibbus and bossing of the forehead. (c) X-ray showing the flat pelvis and short femora.

the proximal segments) are disproportionately short and the skull is quite large with a prominent forehead and saddle-shaped nose. The fingers appear stubby and somewhat splayed (trident hands). The trunk seems too long by comparison with the limbs and the posture when standing is typical: the back is excessively lordotic, the buttocks prominent, the hips flexed, the legs bowed and the elbows bent. In infancy there is often a thoracolumbar gibbus, which disappears after a few years.

These features are more striking in adults, whose height is usually around 122 cm (48 inches). In addition, shortening of the vertebral pedicles may lead to lumbar spinal stenosis.

X-rays show the short but thick bones, an unusually small pelvic cavity and flaring of the iliac wings, producing almost horizontal acetabular roofs. Changes in the spine may produce narrowing of the spinal canal. The epiphyses are quite normal.

Diagnosis

Achondroplasia should not be confused with other types of short-limbed dwarfism. In some (e.g. Morquio's disease) the shortening affects distal segments more than proximal and there may be widespread associated abnormalities. Others (e.g. the epiphyseal dysplasias) are distinguished by the fact that the head and face are quite normal whereas the epiphyses show characteristic changes on x-ray examination.

Management

During childhood, operative treatment may be needed for lower limb deformities (usually genu varum). Occasionally the thoracolumbar kyphosis fails to correct itself; if there is significant deformity (angulation of more than 40 degrees) by the age of 5 years, there is a risk of cord compression and operative correction may be needed.

During adulthood, spinal stenosis may require decompression. Intervertebral disc prolapse superimposed on a narrow spinal canal should be treated as an emergency.

Advances in methods of external fixation have made lower limb lengthening a feasible option. However, there are drawbacks: complications, including non-union, infection and nerve palsy, may be disastrous – and the cosmetic effect of long legs and short arms may be less pleasing than anticipated.

DYSCHONDROPLASIA (ENCHONDROMATOSIS, OLLIER'S DISEASE)

This is a rare, but easily recognized, disorder in which there is defective transformation of physeal cartilage columns into bone. No consistent inheritance pattern has been identified.

Clinical features

Typically the disorder is unilateral; indeed only one limb or even one bone may be involved. An affected limb is short, and if the growth plate is asymmetrically involved the bone grows bent; bowing of the distal end of the femur or tibia is not uncommon and the patient may present with valgus or varus deformity at the knee and ankle. Shortening of the ulna may lead to bowing of the radius and, sometimes, dislocation of the radial head. The fingers or toes frequently contain multiple enchondromata. A rare variety of dyschondroplasia is associated with multiple haemangiomata (Maffucci's disease).

The condition is not inherited; it is probably an embryonal rather than a genetic disorder.

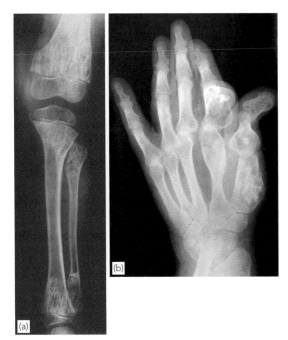

8.5 Dyschondroplasia (a) X-ray features in the femur and tibia. (b) The condition also appears as multiple chondromas.

X-rays

The characteristic change in the long bones is radiolucent streaking extending from the physis into the metaphysis – the appearance of persistent, incompletely ossified cartilage columns trapped in bone. If only one-half of the physis is affected, growth is asymmetrically retarded and the bone becomes curved. With maturation the radiolucent columns eventually ossify but the deformities remain. In the hands and feet the cartilage islands characteristically produce multiple enchondromata. Any change in the appearance of the lesions after the end of normal growth may be a sign of malignant change, which occurs in 5–10% of cases.

Treatment

Bone deformity may need correction, but this should be deferred until growth is complete; otherwise it is likely to recur.

DYSPLASIAS WITH MAINLY DIAPHYSEAL CHANGES

Most of the 'diaphyseal dysplasias' appear to be the result of defective bone modelling. Unlike the physeal and epiphyseal disorders, dwarfing is not a feature. Only the most common example will be described.

OSTEOPETROSIS (MARBLE BONES, ALBERS–SCHÖNBERG DISEASE)

Osteopetrosis is one of several conditions that are characterized by sclerosis and thickening of the bones which then appear unusually 'dense' on x-ray.

Osteopetrosis tarda

The common form of osteopetrosis is a fairly benign, autosomal dominant disorder that seldom causes symptoms and may only be discovered in adolescence or adulthood after a pathological fracture or when an x-ray is taken for other reasons – hence the designation *tarda*. Shape and function are unimpaired unless there are complications: pathological fracture or cranial nerve compression due to bone encroachment on foramina. Sufferers are also prone to bone infection, particularly of the mandible after tooth extraction.

X-rays show increased density of all the bones: cortices are widened, leaving narrow medullary

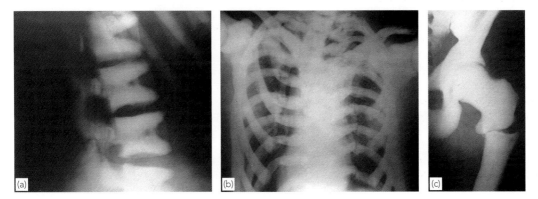

8.6 Osteopetrosis (a–c) Despite the remarkable density, the bones fracture easily. Typical x-ray features in the spine, ribs and femur.

canals; sclerotic vertebral end-plates produce a striped appearance ('football-jersey spine'); the skull is thickened and the base densely sclerotic, carrying the risk of foraminal occlusion and cranial nerve entrapment.

Treatment is required only if complications occur.

Osteopetrosis congenita

This rare, autosomal recessive form of osteopetrosis is present at birth and causes severe disability. Bone encroachment on marrow results in pancytopenia, haemolysis, anaemia and hepatosplenomegaly. Foraminal occlusion may cause optic or facial nerve palsy. Osteomyelitis following, for example, tooth extraction or internal fixation of a fracture is quite common. Repeated haemorrhage or infection usually leads to death in early childhood.

Treatment has focused on methods of enhancing bone resorption and haematopoeisis, e.g. by transplanting marrow from normal donors and by long-term treatment with gamma-interferon.

CONNECTIVE-TISSUE DISORDERS

Heritable defects of collagen synthesis give rise to a number of disorders involving either the soft connective tissues or bone, or both. In many cases the specific collagen defect has now been identified.

GENERALIZED JOINT LAXITY

About 5% of people have hypermobile joints, as defined by a positive score of more than 5 (the Beighton score) in the following tests:

- Passive hyperextension of the metacarpophalangeal joints to beyond 90 degrees (score 2).
- Passive stretching of the thumb to touch the radial border of the forearm (score 2).
- Hyperextension of the elbows (score 2).
- Hyperextension of the knees (score 2).
- Ability to bend forward and place the hands flat on the floor with the knees held perfectly straight (score 1).

This trait runs in families and is inherited as a mendelian dominant. The condition is not in itself disabling but it may predispose to congenital dislocation of the hip in the newborn or recurrent dislocation of the patella or shoulder in later life. Transient joint pains are common and there is an increased risk of ankle sprains.

MARFAN'S SYNDROME

This is a generalized autosomal dominant disorder affecting the bones, joint ligaments, eyes and cardiovascular structures. It is thought to be due to a cross-linkage defect in collagen and elastin.

Clinical features

Patients are tall, with disproportionately long legs and arms; typically, arm span exceeds height. The digits are unusually long, giving rise to the term 'arachnodactyly' or 'spider fingers'. Spinal abnormalities include spondylolisthesis and scoliosis. There is an increased incidence of slipped upper femoral epiphysis. Generalized joint laxity is usual and patients may develop flat-feet or dislocation of the patella or shoulder. Associated abnormalities include a high arched palate, hernias, lens dislocation, retinal detachment, aortic aneurysm and mitral or aortic incompetence.

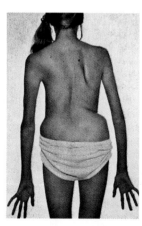

8.8 Marfan's syndrome The combination of disproportionately long arms, 'spider fingers' and scoliosis is characteristic.

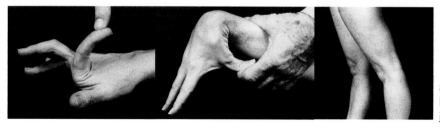

8.7 Generalized joint laxity Simple tests for joint hypermobility.

Management

Patients occasionally need treatment for progressive scoliosis or flat-feet. The heart should be carefully checked before operation.

EHLERS–DANLOS SYNDROME

Ehlers–Danlos syndrome (EDS) designates a heterogeneous group of connective tissue disorders characterized by joint hypermobility, skin laxity and (in some cases) blood vessel fragility. The syndrome comprises at least 10 distinct types; almost all cases are associated with autosomal dominant inheritance.

Classic EDS (Types I and II)

These account for about 80% of cases. Babies show marked hypotonia. Hypermobility persists and older patients are often capable of bizarre feats of contortion. The skin is soft, hyperelastic and easily damaged. Deformities to look for are sloping shoulders and ribs and thoracolumbar scoliosis.

Type III EDS

In this condition there is marked joint laxity but almost normal skin. Joint dislocation (usually shoulder or patella) is common.

Type IV EDS

These patients usually have neither joint hypermobility nor skin laxity; the effects are seen in blood vessels and internal organs and include arterial rupture, intracranial bleeding, bowel rupture and even uterine rupture. Tissue fragility makes repair of visceral ruptures very difficult.

Other types of EDS

A number of patients show combinations of the above features in conditions that include odd recessive and X-linked disorders.

Management

Complications (e.g. recurrent dislocation or scoliosis) may need treatment. However, if joint laxity is marked, soft-tissue reconstruction usually fails to cure the tendency to dislocation. Blood vessel fragility may cause severe bleeding at operation, and wound healing is often poor.

Joint instability may lead to osteoarthritis, which will require treatment in later life.

OSTEOGENESIS IMPERFECTA (BRITTLE BONES)

Osteogenesis imperfecta (OI) is one of the commonest of the heritable bone disorders, with an estimated incidence of 1 in 20,000. It is due to defective synthesis of type I collagen with generalized involvement of the bones, teeth, ligaments, sclerae and skin. It is a heterogeneous condition and there are at least four sub-groups showing variations in phenotype and pattern of inheritance. What they have in common are: (1) osteopenia; (2) proneness to fracture; and (3) laxity of ligaments. About two-thirds of patients have (4) blue sclerae and about one-half have (5) 'crumbling teeth' (*dentinogenesis imperfecta*).

Clinical features

The clinical features vary considerably, according to the severity of the condition. The most striking abnormality is the propensity to fracture, generally after minor trauma and often without much pain or swelling. In the classic case fractures are discovered during infancy and they recur frequently throughout childhood. Callus formation is florid; however, the new bone is also abnormal and it remains 'pliable' for a long time, thus predisposing to malunion and an increased risk of further fracture. By the age of 6 years there may be severe deformities of the long bones, and vertebral compression fractures often lead to kyphoscoliosis. After puberty fractures occur less frequently.

The skin is thin and somewhat loose and the joints are hypermobile. Blue or grey sclerae, when they occur, are due to uveal pigment showing through the hypertranslucent cornea. The teeth may be discoloured and carious.

In milder cases fractures develop a year or two after birth – perhaps when the child starts to walk; they are also less frequent and deformity is not a marked feature.

In the most severe types of OI, fractures are present before birth and the infant is either stillborn or lives only for a few weeks, death being due to respiratory failure, basilar indentation or intracranial haemorrhage following injury.

X-rays

There is generalized osteopenia, thinning of the long bones, fractures in various stages of healing, vertebral compression and spinal deformity. After puberty, fractures occur less frequently, but in those who survive the incidence rises again after the climacteric. It is thought that very mild

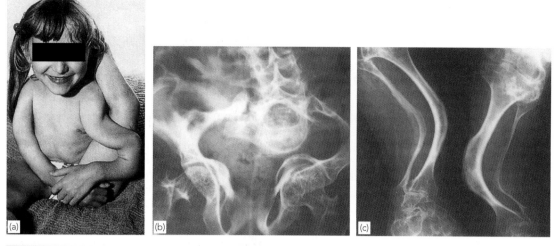

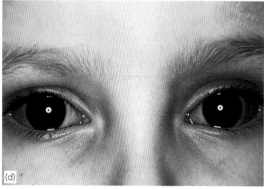

8.9 Osteogenesis imperfecta (a) This young girl had severe deformities of all her limbs, the result of multiple mini-fractures of the long bones over time. This is the classic (Type III) form of osteogenisis imperfecta (OI). (b,c) X-ray features in a slightly older patient with the same condition. (d) Blue sclerae usually occur in the milder, Type I OI.

('subclinical') forms of OI may account for some cases of recurrent fractures in adults.

In older children with atypical features it is essential to look for evidence of physical abuse.

Classification

Four clinical sub-groups of OI have been identified: mild, lethal, severe and moderately severe.

OI Type I (mild)

This, the commonest variety, is a comparatively mild autosomal dominant disorder. Fractures occur throughout life but deformity is uncommon. Characteristically the sclerae are blue and the joints are hypermobile.

OI Type II (lethal)

This severe, recessive disorder may be diagnosed before birth by x-ray or ultrasound imaging. Some infants are stillborn, and those who survive have multiple fractures and deformities of the long bones.

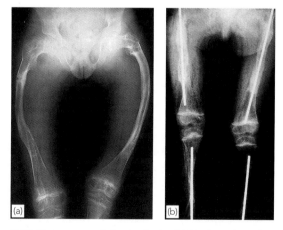

8.10 Osteogenesis imperfecta (a) Moderately severe (type IV) disease. These deformities can be corrected by multiple osteotomies and 'rodding' (b).

OI Type III (severe, deforming)

This is the classic, though not the commonest, form of OI. It is sometimes diagnosed at birth and by the age of 6 years the child has had numerous fractures and has usually developed severe deformities. It is not as severe as Type II, but few of the children survive into adulthood; those who do are markedly dwarfed and disabled.

OI Type IV (moderately severe)

This autosomal dominant disorder is similar to Type I but the sclerae are only a pale blue and they become normal in colour in adult life.

Management

The most severe forms of OI defy treatment and none is indicated apart from sympathetic nursing care. For other types of OI, treatment is aimed at: (1) gentle nursing of infants to prevent fractures as far as possible; (2) prompt splinting when fractures do occur, to prevent unnecessary deformity; (3) mobilization to prevent further osteoporosis; and (4) correction of deformities, if necessary by multiple osteotomies, bone realignment and intramedullary fixation.

NEUROFIBROMATOSIS

Neurofibromatosis is one of the commonest single gene disorders affecting the skeleton. Two types are recognized: *Type 1* (NF-1) – also known as *von Recklinghausen's disease* – has an incidence of about 1 in 3500 live births. The abnormality is located in the gene which codes for neurofibromin, on chromososme 17. It is transmitted as autosomal dominant, with almost 100% penetrance, but more than 50% of cases are due to new mutation. The most characteristic lesions are neurofibromata (Schwann cell tumours) and patches of skin pigmentation (*café-au-lait spots*), but other features are remarkably protean and musculoskeletal abnormalities are seen in almost one-half of those affected. *Type 2* (NF-2) is very rare and is seldom associated with skeletal defects.

Clinical features of NF-1

Almost all patients have the typical widespread patches of skin pigmentation and multiple cutaneous neurofibromata which usually appear before puberty. Less common is a single large plexiform neurofibroma, or an area of soft-tissue over-growth in one of the limbs.

The orthopaedic surgeon is most likely to encounter the condition in a child or adolescent who presents with *scoliosis*; the most suggestive deformity is a very short, sharp curve. *Local tumours* in the spine can cause symptoms resembling those of disc prolapse and x-rays may show scalloping of the posterior aspects of the vertebral bodies, erosion of the pedicles or intervertebral foraminal enlargement.

Congenital tibial dysplasia and *pseudarthrosis* are rare conditions, but almost 50% of patients with these lesions have some evidence of neurofibromatosis.

Malignant change occurs in 2–5% of affected individuals and is the most common complication in elderly patients.

Treatment

A local tumour causing nerve compression should be removed. Treatment may be needed also for

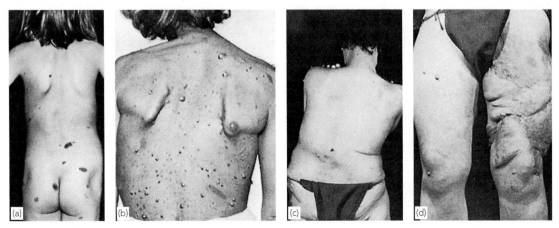

8.11 Neurofibromatosis (a) Café-au-lait spots. (b) Multiple neurofibromata and slight scoliosis. (c,d) A patient with scoliosis and soft-tissue over-growth ('elephantiasis').

associated conditions such as scoliosis or tibial pseudarthrosis.

STORAGE DISORDERS

Many single gene disorders are expressed as under-secretion of an enzyme that controls a specific stage in the metabolic chain; the undegraded substrate accumulates and may be stored, with harmful effects, in various tissues. All these inborn errors of metabolism are inherited as recessive traits. Two examples involving the musculoskeletal system are the mucopolysaccharidoses and Gaucher's disease.

MUCOPOLYSACCHARIDOSES

The mucopolysaccharidoses (MPS) are a group of metabolic disorders in which, because of a deficiency of certain essential lysosomal enzymes, there is incomplete breakdown (and therefore excessive storage) of glycosaminoglycans (GAGs). Partially degraded GAGs accumulate in the liver, spleen, bones and other tissues and spill over into the blood and urine where they can be detected by suitable biochemical tests. Almost all the clinical forms of these inborn errors of metabolism are inherited as autosomal recessive traits.

Clinical features

Depending on the specific enzyme deficiency and the type of GAG storage, at least 10 clinical syndromes have been defined. Most of the typical changes appear in *Morquio–Brailsford's syndrome* (MPS IV). In this condition the infant looks normal at birth but during the next 2 or 3 years walking is delayed and the child is seen to be under-sized with increasing kyphosis, a short neck and protuberant sternum. There is marked joint laxity and progressive genu valgum. Suitable tests may reveal a conductive hearing loss. However, unlike those with some of the other mucopolysaccharidosis syndromes (e.g. *Hurler's syndrome*, MPS I), the face is unaffected and intelligence is normal.

X-rays of the spine show ovoid, hypoplastic vertebral bodies which end up abnormally flat (platyspondyly); odontoid hypoplasia is usual. A marked manubriosternal angle (almost 90 degrees) is pathognomonic. By the age of 5 years the femoral head epiphyses are under-developed and flattened, and the acetabula abnormally shallow. The long bones are of normal width but the metacarpals may be short and broad, and pointed at their proximal ends.

The diagnosis can be confirmed by testing for abnormal GAG excretion or demonstrating the enzyme deficiency in blood cells or cultured skin fibroblasts.

Management

There is, as yet, no specific treatment for the mucopolysaccharide disorder. Enzyme replacement and gene manipulation are possible in the future. Bone marrow transplantation has been used: when successful it halts progression of central nervous

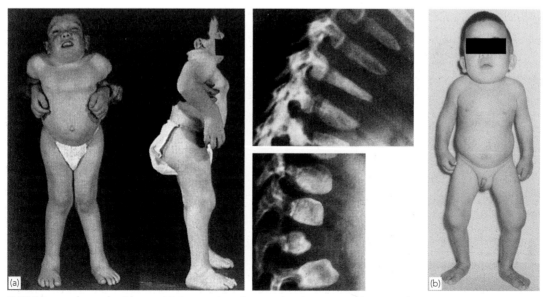

8.12 Mucopolysaccharidoses (a) A young boy showing the characteristic features of Morquio–Brailsford syndrome. (b) A child with Hunter's syndrome.

system disease and some of the clinical features but it cannot reverse neurological damage that has already developed and it does not prevent progression of bone and joint disease.

Enzyme replacement therapy is successful in mild cases of MPS I (*Hurler's syndrome*) but it does not cross the blood–brain barrier. This condition generally has a very poor prognosis.

Morquio's syndrome presents several orthopaedic problems. Genu valgum may need correction by femoral osteotomy, though this should be delayed until growth has ceased. Coxa valga and subluxation of the hips, if symmetrical, may cause little disability; unilateral subluxation may need femoral or acetabular osteotomy. Atlantoaxial instability may threaten the cord and require occipitocervical fusion.

GAUCHER'S DISEASE

The genetic disorder described by Gaucher over 100 years ago is caused by lack of a specific enzyme which is responsible for the breakdown and excretion of cell membrane products from defunct cells. This is a classic example of a lipid storage disease with secondary effects in bone.

When cells die a glucocerebroside is released from the cell membrane; before it can be excreted, the glycoside bond holding the glucose molecule has to be split by a specific enzyme – glucosylceramide β-glucosidase. If this enzyme is lacking, the glucocerebroside cannot be excreted and instead is stored in the lysosomal bodies of macrophages of the reticuloendothelial system, notably in the marrow, spleen and liver. Accumulation of these abnormal macrophages leads to enlargement of the spleen and liver, and secondary changes in the marrow and bone. Like other storage disorders, Gaucher's disease is transmitted as an autosomal recessive trait.

Most patients suffer from a chronic form of the disorder, with changes predominantly in the marrow, bone and spleen, and varying degrees of pancytopenia (*Type I*). A rare form of the disease affecting the central nervous system (*Type II*) appears in infancy and usually causes death within 1 year. *Type III* is a subacute disorder characterized by the appearance of hepatosplenomegaly in childhood and skeletal and neurological abnormalities during adolescence.

Clinical features

Children usually present with pain, and sometimes loss of movement, in one of the larger joints. The spleen may be enlarged (or it may already have been removed!). Older patients may develop back pain due to vertebral osteopenia and compression fractures; femoral neck fractures also are not uncommon. A suggestive finding (when positive) is elevation of the serum acid phosphatase level.

A common complication is *osteonecrosis*, usually of the femoral head. The patient (often a child or adolescent) may present with an acute 'bone crisis': unrelenting pain, local tenderness and restriction of movement accompanied by pyrexia, leucocytosis and an elevated erythrocyte sedimentation rate (ESR). The clinical features

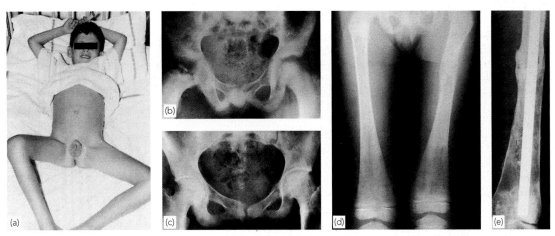

8.13 Gaucher's disease (a) A distressed young boy during an acute Gaucher crisis. The right hip is intensely painful and abduction is restricted. The x-ray (b) shows avascular necrosis of the right femoral head. (c) X-ray of an older patient with a sclerotic left femoral head, the result of previous ischaemic necrosis. (d) Bilateral failure of femoral tubularization (the Erlenmeyer flask appearance). (e) Pathological fractures sometimes occur and can be treated by internal fixation. The sclerotic patches in the interior part of the bone are typical of old medullary infarcts.

resemble those of osteomyelitis or septic arthritis; diagnosis is further confused by the fact that Gaucher's disease predisposes to true bone infection.

Imaging

X-rays may show the distinctive feature of an expanded distal half of femur (the so-called Erlenmeyer flask appearance). Typical signs of osteonecrosis sometimes appear in the femoral head, femoral condyles, talus or humeral head.

A radio-isotope bone scan may help to distinguish a crisis episode from infection: the former is usually 'cold', the latter 'hot'.

Magnetic resonance imaging is the most reliable way of defining marrow involvement.

Treatment

Bone pain may need symptomatic treatment. For the acute crisis, analgesic medication and bed rest followed by a period of non-weightbearing is recommended. Specific therapy is available (albeit costly) in the form of the replacement enzyme, alglucerase. This has been shown to reverse the blood changes and reduce the size of the liver and spleen. The bone complications also are diminished.

Osteonecrosis of the femoral head may require operative treatment (see Chapter 6). However, most patients manage quite well with symptomatic treatment.

CHROMOSOME DISORDERS

Chromosome disorders are common but they usually result in fetal abortion. Of the non-lethal conditions, several produce bone or joint abnormalities. Three of the less rare conditions are described here.

DOWN'S SYNDROME (TRISOMY 21)

This condition results from having an extra copy of chromosome 21. It is much more common than any of the skeletal dysplasias, with an overall incidence of 1 per 800 live births – and 1 in 250 if the mother is over 37 years of age. Affected infants can be recognized at birth: the head is foreshortened and the eyes slant upwards, with prominent epicanthic folds; the nose is flattened, the lips are parted and the tongue protrudes. There may be abnormal palmar creases, clinodactyly and spreading of the

first and second toes. The babies are unusually floppy (hypotonic) and skeletal development is delayed. Children are short and, because of their characteristic facial appearance, they tend to resemble each other. They show varying degrees of learning difficulty. Joint laxity may lead to sprains or subluxation (e.g. of the patella).

Associated anomalies, particularly cardiac defects, are common, and there is diminished resistance to infection. The average life expectancy is about 50 years.

There is no specific treatment but surgery can offer considerable cosmetic improvement. Attentive care will allow many of these individuals to pursue a pleasant and productive life.

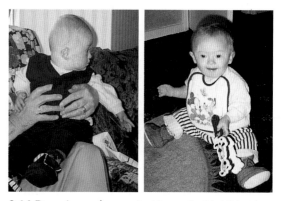

8.14 Down's syndrome An 11-month-old child with Down's syndrome. Note the shape of the head.

TURNER'S SYNDROME

Congenital female hypogonadism is a rare abnormality caused by a defective or non-functioning X chromosome. Those affected are phenotypically female, with a normal vagina and uterus, but the ovaries are markedly hypoplastic or absent. Patients are short, with webbing of the neck, barrel chest and increased carrying angle of the elbows.

Cardiovascular and renal abnormalities are common. Women have primary amenorrhoea, and hypogonadism leads to early-onset osteoporosis.

Treatment consists of oestrogen replacement from puberty onwards.

KLINEFELTER'S SYNDROME

Klinefelter's syndrome, a form of male hypogonadism, occurs in about 1 per 1000 males. Those affected have more than one X chromosome (as well as the usual Y chromosome). They are recognizably male, but they have eunuchoid proportions, with gynaecomastia and under-developed testicles. The condition should be borne in mind as a cause of osteoporosis in men.

Treatment with androgens may improve bone mass.

LOCALIZED MALFORMATIONS

Localized malformations of the vertebrae or limbs are common. The majority cause no disability and may be discovered incidentally during investigation of some other disorder. Some have a genetic background and similar malformations are seen in association with generalized skeletal dysplasia. Most are sporadic and probably non-genetic – i.e. caused by injury to the developing embryo, especially during the first 3 months of pregnancy. In some cases there is a known teratogenic agent: for example, maternal infection or drug administration. Usually, however, the exact cause is unknown. Local examples are dealt with in Part 2 of the book.

VERTEBRAL ANOMALIES

These are of three main kinds of vertebral anomaly: *agenesis* – complete absence of one or more vertebrae; *dysgenesis* – errors of segmentation causing hemivertebrae, with or without vertebrae fused together; and *dysraphism* – deficiencies of the neural arch (e.g. spina bifida).

Associated visceral anomalies (lower intestinal and urogenital defects) are common in sacral dysgenesis and dysraphism.

CONGENITAL SHORT NECK (KLIPPEL–FEIL SYNDROME)

This condition (also known as *cervical-vertebral synostosis*) is due to failure of vertebral segmentation. Associated anomalies are common and include hemivertebrae, posterior arch defects, cervical meningomyelocele, thoracic defects, scapular elevation and visceral abnormalities involving the renal and cardiorespiratory systems. Occasionally, a familial pattern of inheritance is noted, suggesting a genetic aetiology.

X-rays may show fusion of the lower cervical vertebrae and various combinations of the associated disorders, together with scoliosis or kyphosis. The natural history of the condition often depends on the severity of the visceral anomalies.

Orthopaedic treatment is usually unnecessary. However, cervical instability in an adjacent hypermobile segment may call for surgical fusion.

SPRENGEL'S DEFORMITY

This condition, which usually occurs sporadically, represents a failure of scapular descent from the cervical spine. The high scapula may still be attached to the spine by a tough fibrous band or a cartilaginous bar (the omovertebral bar). Associated vertebral or rib anomalies are quite common.

Treatment is required only if shoulder movements are severely limited or if the deformity is particularly unsightly. Operation is best performed before the age of 6 years. The vertebroscapular muscles are released from the spine, the supraspinous part of the scapula is excised together with the omovertebral bar and the scapula is repositioned by tightening the lower muscles. Great care is needed as there is a risk of injury to the accessory nerve or the brachial plexus.

THORACOSPINAL ANOMALIES

Segmentation defects in the thoracic region usually involve the ribs as well; for example, hemivertebrae may be associated with fusion of adjacent ribs or other types of dysplasia. Some of these disorders are of autosomal dominant inheritance.

Clinically, patients present in childhood with scoliosis or kyphoscoliosis, sometimes leading to paraplegia. X-rays may show various combinations of thoracic vertebral fusion or dysgenesis and rib anomalies, together with scoliosis and marked distortion of the thorax.

Operative treatment may be needed for threatened cord compression.

SACRAL AGENESIS

This term describes a group of conditions in which part or all of the distal spine is missing. Variable motor deficiencies are noted below the lowest level of normal spine but sensation is often preserved more distally. Other deformities of the lower limb may be present and, as with congenital scoliosis, there may be associated cardiac, visceral and renal abnormalities. Some cases of sacral agenesis appear to be inherited in either an autosomal or sex-linked dominant fashion.

Spina bifida is the commonest vertebral anomaly. This condition is dealt with on page 127.

LIMB ANOMALIES

Localized malformations of the limbs include extra bones, absent bones, hypoplastic bones and fusions. Most of the anomalies involving limb reductions are due to embryonal insults between the 4th and 6th weeks of gestation. Some are genetically determined and these usually have an autosomal dominant pattern of inheritance. Only the more important and less rare conditions will be described here.

Complete absence of a limb is called *amelia*, almost complete absence *phocomelia* and partial absence *ectromelia*; defects may be transverse or axial. In the hands and feet *brachydactyly, syndactyly, polydactyly* and *symphalangism* are among the many possibilities.

Always remember that function may be satisfactory even if the appearance is not. Before any surgical treatment is considered one must review what side-effects there might be and how to achieve the most acceptable balance between *function, appearance* and *pain*. A hand that functions better but is painful may not be useful to a particular patient.

PSEUDARTHROSIS OF THE CLAVICLE

The child usually presents with a lump over the midclavicular region, almost always on the right side except in cases of dextrocardia! Sometimes there is obvious mobility at the pseudarthrosis site and over time this may become painful.

While occasional familial autosomal dominant cases have been described, the true aetiology is unknown; other theories such as external compression from the subclavian artery or a failure of coalescence of the two intramembranous centres of ossification have been proposed.

TRANSVERSE DEFICIENCY OF THE ARM

Transverse deficiency of the distal part of the arm will leave a simple stump below a normal elbow. This can be managed by fitting a prosthesis with a mechanical facility for grasp.

RADIAL DEFICIENCY

The forearm is short and bowed; the hand is under-developed and markedly deviated towards the radial side (*radial club-hand*) and the thumb may be missing. The elbow too is often abnormal. In about one-half of cases the condition is bilateral.

The clinical deformity may look bizarre but children often acquire excellent function. If this seems unlikely, operative reconstruction may be advisable. This could involve pollicization of a digit and other complex reconstructive procedures.

In a young child simple stretching and splinting may help to improve hand and wrist position until further options need to be considered.

ULNAR DEFICIENCY

Hypoplasia of the distal end of the ulna is usually seen as part of a generalized dysplasia, but occasionally it occurs alone. The radius is bowed (as if growth is tethered on the ulnar side) and the radial head may dislocate; the wrist is deviated medially. Only if function is severely disturbed should wrist stabilization be advised.

Congenital absence of the ulna is extremely rare; overall function is severely restricted. Operative reconstruction may provide some improvement.

RADIOULNAR SYNOSTOSIS

This is often associated with a posterolateral dislocation of the radial head. Clinically there is complete loss of pronation and supination. This movement cannot be regained with surgery but improvement in the resting position of the forearm (and hence of the hand) can be achieved.

DIGITAL ANOMALIES

A variety of anomalies can occur, ranging from simple soft-tissue 'extra digits' (which are easy to excise) to complex syndactylies that restrict hand function. They may occur alone or in conjunction with more generalized skeletal dysplasias.

FEMORAL DEFICIENCY (CONGENITAL SHORT FEMUR)

In its most benign form, femoral dysplasia consists merely of shortening of the bone with a normal hip and knee. This can be dealt with by limb lengthening procedures or, if shortening is very marked, by adding a distal orthosis. More severe grades of proximal femoral dysplasia are encountered, some associated with coxa vara. The most widely used classification is that of Aitkin, as illustrated in Figure 8.15.

Coxa vara with moderate shortening of the shaft can be dealt with by corrective osteotomy and limb lengthening. Severe degrees of coxa vara, sometimes associated with pseudoarthrosis of the femoral neck, may result in marked shortening of the femur.

In the worst cases most of the femoral shaft is missing, the knee is situated at thigh level and the foot hangs where the knee is normally expected to be. If the deformity is bilateral and symmetrical,

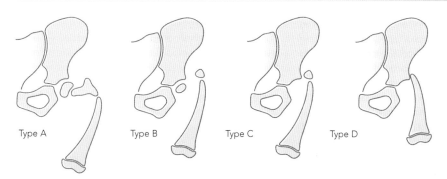

8.15 Proximal femoral dysplasia The most widely used classification of proximal femoral focal deficiency is that of Aitkin. *Type A*: the child is born with a 'gap' between the proximal part of the femur and the diaphysis but this usually ossifies by the end of growth. *Type B*: the femoral head is present (though hypoplastic) but there is a 'gap' which fails to ossify. *Type C*: the femoral head and neck are absent and the acetabulum is under-developed. *Type D*: the acetabulum and proximal femur are absent. Congenital coxa vara is not included in this classification although it may also be a variant of the same disorder (see Chapter 19).

walking is possible and some individuals acquire remarkable agility; however, they may still seek treatment to overcome the severe cosmetic problem. Unilateral deformities are not only unsightly but also very disabling. Effective limb lengthening is out of the question, and fitting a prosthesis to a short limb with flexion deformities of the 'hip' and knee and a foot jutting forwards where the knee-hinge of the prosthesis will lie is a daunting prospect. One alternative is to fuse the knee in a functional position, amputate the foot and fit a suitable prosthesis. The earlier this is done the better.

TIBIAL DEFICIENCY

Tibial dysplasia is very rare: several forms exist and the condition may be associated with other limb anomalies. Prognosis, and hence treatment, depend on the quality of the knee joint: if there is no ability for knee extension, a proximal amputation must be

considered. If the ankle cannot be reconstructed a distal amputation may be required.

FIBULAR DEFICIENCY

This is the most common long-bone deficiency. Mild fibular dysplasia causes little shortening or deformity; however, complete absence of the fibula leads to considerable shortening of the leg, bowing of the tibia and valgus deformity of the unsupported ankle. There may also be absence of the fourth and fifth rays of the foot and under-development of the entire limb. Sometimes, if only the distal fibula is absent, there is a fibrous band in its place. Excision of this remnant may permit correction of the valgus deformity.

In severe cases, management is dictated by the quality of the foot and by the percentage growth inhibition. This can be calculated by a variety of methods and allows good prediction of final limb length discrepancy at skeletal maturity. Once this is

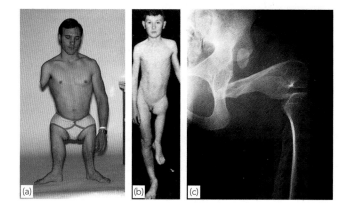

8.16 Proximal femoral dysplasia (a) This man was born with transverse deficiency of the right arm and bilateral proximal femoral focal deficiency. Though unhappy with his appearance, because the lower limb defects were symmetrical he was able to get about remarkably well. (b) By contrast, this young man with a similar but unilateral dysplasia was severely disabled. (c) X-ray showing the proximal femoral deficiency.

known, treatment can be planned. Options range from partial amputation and the use of a prosthetic limb to epiphyseodesis of the longer limb and one or more limb lengthening procedures involving distraction osteogenesis techniques and ring external fixators. Reconstructive techniques such as these rely on a high degree of compliance from the child and their family over a long time-span. In contrast, modern advances in amputation prosthetics may provide a more acceptable outcome.

CONGENITAL PSEUDARTHROSIS OF THE TIBIA

This rare condition is usually diagnosed in early infancy. The child may be born with a fractured tibia, or the bone may be attenuated and then fracture some months later. In either case, the fracture fails to unite, or heals very poorly only to fracture again shortly afterwards. By the age of 2 years the leg is noticeably short and bowed anterolaterally. By then it has become obvious that this is an intractable condition which will not yield to ordinary forms of fracture treatment.

X-rays shows a gap, or marked thinning, of the tibial shaft. Sometimes the fibula also is affected.

Treatment is likely to be prolonged and fraught with difficulty. Simple immobilization will certainly fail, and internal fixation with bone grafting succeeds only occasionally. Better results have been achieved by excising the affected segment of bone, correcting the deformity and closing the gap gradually by bone transport in a circular external fixator (the Ilizarov technique).

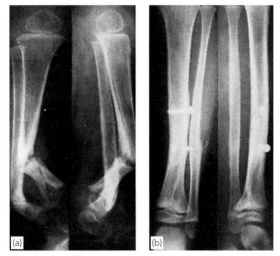

8.17 Congenital pseudarthrosis (a) The tibia is the most common site; in this case bone grafting was successful (b).

CHAPTER 9

TUMOURS AND TUMOUR-LIKE LESIONS

Some non-neoplastic lesions are included here because of their similarity to true bone tumours, though they are usually omitted from pathological classifications. *Table 9.1* shows one such listing, based on the Revised World Healthy Organization (WHO) Classification of bone tumours. A few caveats are worth mentioning:

- The most pervasive tissue is not necessarily the tissue of origin.
- There is not necessarily any connection between conditions in the 'benign' category and the corresponding 'malignant' category.
- There is often no relationship between benign and malignant lesions with similar tissue elements (e.g. osteoma and osteosarcoma).
- By far the commonest malignant lesions in bone are metastatic tumours, which are not, strictly speaking, 'bone' tumours, i.e. not of mesenchymal origin.

Only the more common conditions are discussed in this chapter.

DIAGNOSIS

Most tumours cause *pain, lumpy swelling* and local *tenderness*; occasionally a lesion is discovered accidentally during x-ray examination, or as the result of a *pathological fracture*.

If there is a lump, where does it arise? Is it discrete or ill-defined? Is it soft or hard, or pulsatile? And is it tender? Examine the area of lymphatic drainage. Exclude conditions that can mimic a tumour, e.g.

a haematoma, bone infection, a stress fracture or a healing fracture.

It is not always easy to tell whether a bone tumour is benign or malignant, but rapid growth, warmth, tenderness and an ill-defined edge suggest malignancy. If treatment is to be rational, we must know the precise diagnosis and also the extent of the lesion, its relationship to local blood vessels and the likelihood of distant spread. Therefore, in all cases of suspected malignancy (and sometimes even with unusual benign lesions), investigations should include high-quality radiography, computed tomography (CT) or magnetic resonance imaging (MRI), bone scanning and a carefully planned biopsy before definitive treatment begins.

Imaging

Plain x-rays are the most useful of all imaging techniques. There may be an obvious abnormality in the bone – a lump, bone destruction, cortical thickening or something that looks like a 'cyst' in the bone. The site of the lesion, whether solitary or multiple and whether well defined or ill defined are all helpful clues to the diagnosis.

Remember that 'cystic' lesions are not necessarily hollow cavities: any radiolucent material (e.g. a fibroma or a chondroma) may look like a cyst. If the boundary of the 'cyst' is sharply defined it is probably benign; if it is hazy and diffuse it suggests an invasive tumour. Stippled calcification inside a vacant area is characteristic of cartilage tumours.

Look carefully at the bone surfaces and beyond: periosteal new bone formation and extension of

Table 9.1 A classification of bone tumours. Modified after Revised WHO Classification – Schajowicz (1994)

Predominant tissue	Benign	Malignant
Bone forming	Osteoma Osteoid osteoma Osteoblastoma	Osteosarcoma: central peripheral parosteal
Cartilage forming	Chondroma Osteochondroma Chondroblastoma ?Chondromyxoid fibroma	Chondrosarcoma: central peripheral juxtacortical clear-cell mesenchymal
Fibrous tissue	Fibroma Fibromatosis	Fibrosarcoma
Mixed	?Chondromyxoid fibroma	
Giant-cell tumours	Benign osteoclastoma	Malignant osteoclastoma
Marrow tumours		Ewing's tumour Myeloma
Vascular tissue	Haemangioma Haemangiopericytoma Haemangioendothelioma	Angiosarcoma Malignant haemangiopericytoma
Other connective tissue	Fibroma Fibrous histiocytoma Lipoma	Fibrosarcoma Malignant fibrous histiocytoma Liposarcoma
Other tumours	Neurofibroma Neurilemmoma	Adamantinoma Chordoma

the tumour into the soft tissues are suggestive of malignant change.

For all its informative detail, the x-ray alone can seldom be relied on for a definitive diagnosis. With some notable exceptions, in which the appearances are pathognomonic (osteochondroma, non-ossifying fibroma, osteoid osteoma), further investigations will be needed.

CT and *MRI* are useful for assessing the true extent of the tumour and its relationship to surrounding structures. *Radionuclide scanning* with ^{99m}Tc-HDP shows non-specific reactive changes in bone; this can be helpful in revealing the site of a small tumour (e.g. an osteoid osteoma) or the presence of skip lesions or silent secondary deposits.

> ⚠ All imaging studies should be completed before undertaking a biopsy, which may itself distort the appearances.

Biopsy

With few exceptions, biopsy is essential for both diagnosis and planning of treatment. If sufficient expertise is available, the biopsy can be done with a *large-bore needle*; however, *open biopsy* is more reliable.

The site is selected so that it can be included in any subsequent ablative operation. As little as possible of the tumour is exposed and a block of tissue is removed – ideally in the boundary zone, so as to include normal tissue, pseudocapsule and abnormal tissue. A *frozen section* should be examined – not so much as to make a definitive diagnosis but to ensure that representative tissue has been obtained. If necessary, several samples can be taken. If bone is removed the raw area is covered with bone wax or methylmethacrylate cement. If a tourniquet is used, it should be released and full haemostasis achieved before closing the wound. Drains should be avoided, so as to minimize the risk of tumour contamination.

Tumour biopsy should never be regarded as a 'minor' procedure. Complications include haemorrhage, wound breakdown, infection and pathological fracture. The person doing the biopsy should have a clear idea of what may be done next and where operative incisions or skin flaps will be placed. Errors and complications are far less likely if the biopsy is performed at a specializing centre.

For tumours that are almost certainly benign, an *excisional biopsy* is permissible (the entire lesion is removed); with cysts, representative tissue can be obtained by careful curettage.

When dealing with tumours that could be malignant, there is a strong temptation to perform the biopsy as soon as possible; as this may alter the CT and MRI appearances, it is important to delay the operation until all the imaging studies have been completed.

Differential diagnosis

Chronic osteomyelitis typically causes pain and swelling and x-rays may show an area of bone destruction in the metaphysis and periosteal new bone formation. If systemic features have been suppressed by antibiotics, these changes may be mistaken for those of a destructive tumour. Tissue should be submitted for both *bacteriological* and *histological* examination.

Stress fractures are another source of misdiagnosis. The patient is often a young adult with localized pain near a large joint; x-rays show a dubious area of cortical 'destruction' and overlying periosteal new bone; if a biopsy is performed the healing callus may show histological features resembling those of osteosarcoma. Proper consultation

between surgeon, radiologist and pathologist should prevent any error.

A gouty tophus occasionally takes on the appearance of an excavating tumour.

PRINCIPLES OF TREATMENT

BENIGN, ASYMPTOMATIC LESIONS

If the diagnosis is beyond doubt one can temporize: treatment may never be needed. Otherwise a biopsy is advisable, either an excisional biopsy or curettage.

BENIGN, SYMPTOMATIC OR ENLARGING TUMOURS

Painful lesions and tumours that continue to enlarge after the end of normal bone growth always require biopsy and confirmation of the diagnosis. Unless they are unusually aggressive, they can generally be removed by complete local excision.

SUSPECTED MALIGNANT TUMOURS

If there is any suspicion that the lesion could be a primary malignant tumour, the patient is admitted for detailed assessment in order to: (a) confirm the diagnosis; (b) establish the grade of malignancy; and (c) define precisely how far the tumour has spread. The various treatment options can then be discussed; they include local excision, wide excision with limb sparing, amputation and different types of adjuvant therapy. The patient must be fully informed about the 'pros and cons' of each.

Tumours are graded according to cytological

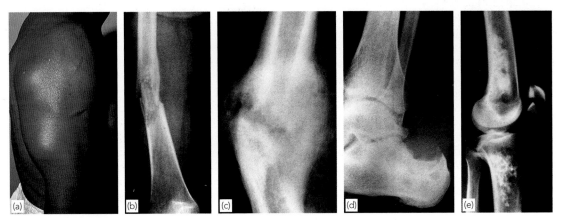

9.1 Tumours – differential diagnosis (a) This huge swelling was simply a clotted haematoma. (b) Bone infection with pathological fracture. (c) Florid callus in an ununited fracture. (d) Large erosion in the calcaneum by a gouty tophus. (e) Bone infarcts.

characteristics which indicate how aggressive they are; i.e. the likelihood of recurrence and spread after surgical removal. *Benign lesions*, by definition, occupy the lowest grade and are usually amenable to local (marginal) excision with little risk of recurrence. *Sarcomas* are divided into *low-grade* and *high-grade*; the former are only moderately aggressive (the estimated risk of metastasis is less than 25%) and take a long time to metastasize (e.g. secondary chondrosarcoma or parosteal osteosarcoma), while the latter are usually very aggressive and metastasize early (e.g. osteosarcoma or fibrosarcoma).

Assuming that there are no metastases, the local extent of the tumour is the most important factor in deciding how much tissue has to be removed. This is best shown by CT and MRI. *Intracompartmental lesions* (those that are confined to an enclosed tissue space such as a single bone or a muscle group within its fascial envelope) are more amenable to complete excision than *extracompartmental lesions* (those that extend into interfascial or extrafascial planes with no natural barrier to proximal or distal spread).

In general terms, low-grade lesions which are still intracompartmental can be treated by wide excision without exposing the tumour. High-grade sarcomas confined to bone may need more radical excision, with or without bone graft or prosthetic replacement; and high-grade lesions with extracompartmental spread need either radical excision and prosthetic replacement or amputation. In addition, the patient may need chemotherapy to reduce the risk of metastasis.

Limb-sparing surgery

Limb salvage seems preferable to amputation, provided there are no skip lesions and the limb is still functional. However, it should only be undertaken where advanced surgical facilities for bone grafting and endoprosthetic replacement at various sites are available. The first step consists of wide excision of the tumour with preservation of the neurovascular structures. The resulting defect is then dealt with in one of several ways. Short diaphyseal segments can be replaced by *vascularized* or *non-vascularized bone grafts*. Longer gaps may require *custom-made implants*. Osteoarticular segments can be replaced by *large allografts, endoprostheses* or *allograft–prosthetic composites*; however, large allografts carry a high risk of infection and fracture. In growing children, *extendible implants* have been used in order to avoid the need for repeated operations; however, they may need to be replaced at the end of growth. Other procedures, such as *grafting* or *distraction osteosynthesis*, are suitable for some situations.

The complication rate is considerable (e.g. wound breakdown, infection and prosthetic failure). If there is any doubt about the extent or aggressiveness of the tumour, *amputation* may be the better option.

Amputation

Preoperative planning and the definitive operation are best carried out in a specialized unit, so as to minimize the risk of complications and permit early rehabilitation. The operation may be curative but it is sometimes performed essentially to achieve local control of a tumour which is resistant to chemotherapy and radiation therapy.

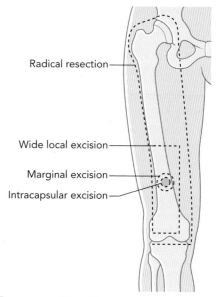

9.2 Tumour excision The more aggressive a tumour is, and the wider it has spread, the more widely it needs to be excised. Local excision is suitable only for low-grade tumours that are confined to a single compartment. Radical resection may be needed for high-grade tumours and this often means amputation at a level above the compartment involved.

Multi-agent chemotherapy

Multi-agent chemotherapy is now the preferred neoadjuvant and adjuvant treatment for malignant bone and soft-tissue tumours. For sensitive tumours, modern chemotherapy regimens reduce the size of the primary lesion, prevent metastatic seeding and improve the chances of survival. When combined with surgery for osteosarcoma and Ewing's tumours, the long-term disease-free survival rate in the best series is now about 60%.

Drugs currently in use are methotrexate, doxorubicin (Adriamycin), cyclophosphamide, vincristine and cis-platinum. Treatment is started 8–12 weeks preoperatively and the effect is assessed by examining the resected tissue for tumour necrosis; greater than 90% necrosis is taken as a good response. If there is little or no necrosis, a different drug may be selected for postoperative treatment. Maintenance chemotherapy is continued for another 6–12 months.

Radiotherapy

For highly sensitive tumours (such as Ewing's sarcoma) radiotherapy offers an alternative to amputation; it is then combined with adjuvant chemotherapy. The same combination can be used as adjunctive treatment for high-grade tumours, for tumours in inaccessible sites, lesions that are inoperable because of their size, proximity to major blood vessels or advanced local spread, for marrow-cell tumours such as myeloma and malignant lymphoma, for metastatic deposits and for palliative local tumour control where no surgery is planned. Radiotherapy may also be employed postoperatively when a marginal or intralesional excision has occurred, so as to 'sterilize' the tumour bed.

The main *complications* are the occurrence of postirradiation spindle-cell sarcoma and pathological fracture in weight-bearing bones, particularly in the proximal half of the femur.

BENIGN BONE LESIONS

NON-OSSIFYING FIBROMA (FIBROUS CORTICAL DEFECT)

This, the commonest benign lesion of bone, is a developmental defect in which a nest of fibrous tissue appears within the bone and persists for some years before ossifying. It is asymptomatic and is almost always encountered in children as an incidental finding on x-ray. The usual sites are the metaphyses of long bones; occasionally there are multiple lesions.

X-rays

The appearance is unmistakable. There is a more or less oval radiolucent area in or adjacent to the cortex. Although it looks cystic on x-ray, it is a solid lesion consisting of unremarkable fibrous tissue. As the bone grows the defect becomes less obvious and it eventually heals spontaneously. However, it sometimes enlarges and there may be a pathological fracture.

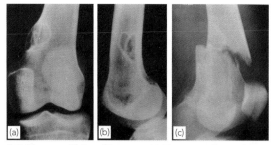

9.3 Non-ossifying fibroma (a) The x-ray always shows a cortical defect, although in some projection planes this looks deceptively like a medullary 'cyst' (b). The bone may fracture through the weakened area (c).

Treatment

Except for a pathological fracture, treatment is unnecessary.

FIBROUS DYSPLASIA

Fibrous dysplasia is a developmental disorder in which areas of trabecular bone are replaced by fibrous tissue, osteoid and woven bone. At operation the lesional tissue has a coarse, gritty feel, due to the specks of immature bone. The condition may affect one bone (*monostotic*), one limb (*monomelic*) or many bones (*polyostotic*). Malignant transformation to fibrosarcoma occurs in 5–10% of patients with polyostotic lesions, but only rarely in monostotic lesions.

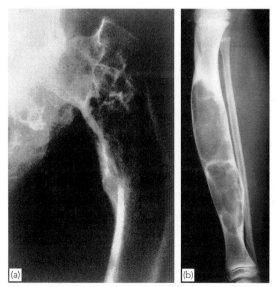

9.4 Fibrous dysplasia (a) The large cyst-like lesion in the proximal femur has resulted in a so-called shepherd's crook deformity. (b) X-ray showing the typical ground-glass appearance of fibrous dysplasia in the tibia.

Clinical features

Small, single lesions are asymptomatic. Large, monostotic lesions may cause pain and bone deformity, or may be discovered only when the patient develops a pathological fracture.

X-rays

Cyst-like areas in the metaphysis or shaft have a hazy (so-called ground-glass) appearance. The weight-bearing bones may be bent, and one of the classic features is the 'shepherd's crook' deformity of the proximal femur.

Pathology

The histological picture is of cellular fibrous tissue with patches of woven bone and scattered giant cells.

Treatment

Small lesions need no treatment. Those that are large and painful or threatening to fracture (or have fractured) can be curetted and grafted, but there is a strong tendency for the abnormality to recur. Deformities may need correction by suitably designed osteotomies.

OSTEOID OSTEOMA

This is a benign tumour consisting of osteoid and newly formed bone. It is small (usually less than 1 cm in size), round or oval in shape and is encased in dense bone. It is usually seen in patients aged under 30 years, and over one-half of the cases occur in the femur or tibia.

The leading symptom is pain, which is sometimes severe and is usually relieved by aspirin but not by rest.

X-rays

The important feature is a tiny radiolucent area, the so-called 'nidus'. In the diaphysis the nidus is surrounded by dense bone and the cortex is thickened. Lesions in the metaphysis show less cortical thickening. It is sometimes difficult to distinguish an osteoid osteoma from a small Brodie's abscess without biopsy.

Treatment

The only effective treatment is complete removal of the nidus. The lesion is carefully localized by x-ray and/or CT and then excised in a small block of bone; the specimen should be x-rayed immediately to confirm that it does contain the little tumour.

CHONDROMA (ENCHONDROMA)

Islands of cartilage may persist in the metaphyses of bones formed by endochondral ossification; sometimes they grow and take on the characteristics of a benign tumour. The lesional tissue is indistinguishable from normal hyaline cartilage, but there is often a central area of degeneration and calcification.

Clinical features

Chondromas are usually asymptomatic and discovered incidentally on x-ray or after a pathological fracture. They are seen at any age (mostly in young people) and in any bone preformed in cartilage. Lesions may be solitary or multiple and part of a generalized dysplasia.

X-rays

The tumour appears as a central, sometimes expanded, radiolucent area near the bone end. What distinguishes it from other cyst-like lesions is

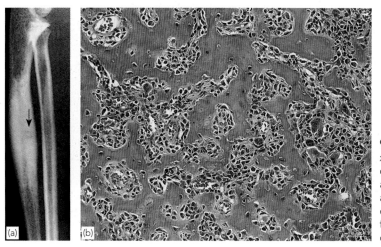

9.5 Osteoid osteoma (a) Typical x-ray appearance: a small lucent cavity with a dense central nidus, and reactive bone thickening around it. (b) Histology shows sheets of pink-staining osteoid in a fibrovascular stroma. Giant cells and osteoblasts are prominent (×300).

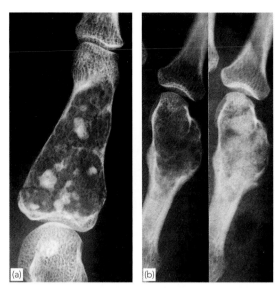

9.6 Chondroma The hand is a common site. Though the lesion in (a) looks like a cyst, it is in fact a solid but radiolucent tumour with central patches of calcification – a typical feature of chrondroma. The lesion in (b) was treated by curettage and bone grafting.

the appearance of tiny flecks of calcification within the lucent area.

Treatment

If the tumour is painful or is enlarging, or if it presents as a pathological fracture, it should be removed as thoroughly as possible by curettage; the defect is filled with bone graft.

Prognosis

There is a small but significant risk of *malignant change*; suspicious features in adult patients are:

(1) the onset of pain; (2) enlargement of the lesion; and (3) cortical erosion. If these features are present, and especially in older patients, the tumour should be treated as a low-grade malignancy.

OSTEOCHONDROMA (CARTILAGE-CAPPED EXOSTOSIS)

Pathology

This, one of the commonest 'tumours' of bone, is a developmental lesion which starts as a small over-growth of cartilage at the edge of the physeal plate and develops by endochondral ossification into a bony protuberance still covered by the cap of cartilage. Any bone that develops in cartilage may be involved; the commonest sites are the fast-growing ends of long bones and the crest of the ilium. Multiple lesions may develop as part of a heritable disorder – *hereditary multiple exostosis* – in which there is abnormal bone growth resulting in characteristic deformities (see page 87).

There is a small risk of malignant transformation. This is seen most often with pelvic exostoses – not because they are inherently different but because considerable enlargement may, for long periods, pass unnoticed. The exact incidence is difficult to assess because troublesome lesions are usually removed before they show histological features of malignancy; estimates range from 1% for solitary lesions to 6% for multiple.

Clinical features

The patient is usually a teenager or young adult when the lump is first discovered. The exostosis may go on enlarging up to the end of the normal

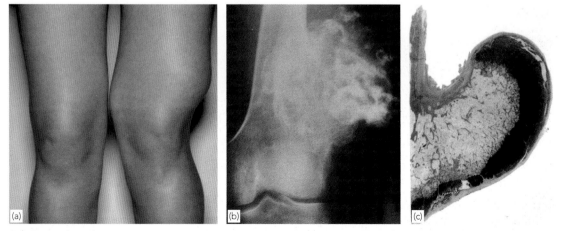

9.7 Osteochondroma (a) A young girl presented with this lump on her leg. It felt bony hard. (b) X-ray examination showed the typical features of a large cartilage-capped exostosis; of course the cartilage cap does not show on x-ray unless it is calcified. (c) Histological section of an exostosis with its dark stained cartilage cap.

growth period for that bone; *any further enlargement after that is suggestive of malignant change.*

X-rays

What is seen on x-ray is a well-defined bony protuberance (exostosis) emerging from the metaphysis. It looks smaller than it feels because the cartilage cap does not show on x-ray; however, large lesions undergo cartilage degeneration and calcification and then the x-ray shows the bony exostosis surrounded by blotches of calcified material.

Treatment

If the tumour causes symptoms it should be excised; if, in an adult, it has recently become bigger or painful then operation is urgent, for these features suggest malignancy, even if the histology looks 'benign'.

CHONDROBLASTOMA

This rare tumour of immature cartilage cells is one of the very few lesions to appear primarily in the epiphysis, usually of the proximal humerus, femur or tibia. The presenting symptom is aching and tenderness adjacent to the joint. The characteristic *x-ray* appearance is of a well-demarcated radiolucent area in the epiphysis.

Treatment

In children the risk of damage to the physis makes it risky to remove the lesion. In adults this is not a problem; however, there is a high risk of recurrence after incomplete removal, and if this happens repeatedly there may be serious damage to the nearby joint.

CHONDROMYXOID FIBROMA

Like other benign cartilaginous lesions, this is seen mainly in adolescents and young adults. It may occur in any bone but is more common in those of the lower limb.

Patients seldom complain and the lesion is usually discovered by accident or after a pathological fracture.

On x-ray examination this looks like an ovoid cyst situated eccentrically in the metaphysis. However, it is a solid tumour of mixed cartilage, fibrous and myxomatous tissues.

Where feasible, the lesion should be excised but often one can do no more than a thorough curettage – followed by autogenous bone grafting.

SIMPLE BONE CYST

This is a true solitary or unicameral bone cyst. It appears during childhood, typically in the metaphysis of one of the long bones and most commonly in the proximal humerus or femur. It is not a tumour, tends to heal spontaneously and is seldom seen in adults.

The condition is usually discovered after a pathological fracture or as an incidental finding on x-ray.

X-rays

The appearance on x-ray is of a large bubble inside the bone. It may occupy the entire metaphysis but it does not extend beyond the physeal plate.

9.8 Cyst-like lesions (a) *Simple bone cyst*: fills the medullary cavity but does not expand the bone. (b) *Chondromyxoid fibroma*: looks cystic but is actually a radiolucent benign tumour; always in the metaphysis; hard boundary tailing off towards the diaphysis. (c) *Aneurysmal bone cyst*: expansile cystic tumour, always on the metaphyseal side of the physis. (d) *Giant-cell tumour*: hardly ever appears before the epiphysis has fused; pathognomonic feature is that it extends right up to the subarticular bone plate; sometimes malignant.

Treatment

Asymptomatic lesions in older children can be left alone but the patient should be cautioned to avoid injury which might cause a fracture. 'Active' cysts (those in young children, usually abutting against the physeal plate and obviously enlarging in sequential x-rays) should be treated, in the first instance, by aspiration of fluid and injection of 80–160 mg of methylprednisolone. This has been found to stop further enlargement and promote healing of the cyst; however, there is doubt as to whether it is the prednisolone or the act of injection which does the trick. If the cyst goes on enlarging, or if there is a pathological fracture, the cavity should be curetted and then packed with bone chips.

ANEURYSMAL BONE CYST

Pathology

This is a cystic tumour-like lesion which occurs chiefly in the spine and the metaphyses of long bones, usually affecting young adults. It may expand the bone and cause marked thinning of the cortex. When the cyst is opened it is found to contain clotted blood, and during curettage there may be considerable bleeding from the fleshy lining membrane. Histologically the membrane consists of fibrous tissue with vascular spaces, deposits of haemosiderin and multinucleated giant cells. There is no risk of malignant transformation.

X-rays

In a growing tubular bone the cyst is always situated in the metaphysis and may resemble a simple cyst. In adults it can be mistaken for a giant-cell tumour but, unlike the latter, its boundary stops well short of the articular margin (see Figure 9.8(c)).

Treatment

The cyst should be thoroughly curetted and then packed with bone grafts. Sometimes the grafts are resorbed and the cyst recurs, necessitating a second or third operation.

GIANT-CELL TUMOUR

Pathology

Giant-cell tumour is a lesion of uncertain origin that appears after the end of bone growth, most commonly in the distal femur, proximal tibia, proximal humerus and distal radius. The tumour has a reddish, fleshy appearance; it comes away in pieces quite easily when curetted but is difficult to remove completely from the surrounding bone.

Aggressive lesions have a poorly-defined 'floor' and appear to extend into the surrounding bone. Histologically the striking feature is an abundance of multinucleated giant cells scattered on a background of stromal cells with little or no visible intercellular tissue.

About one-third of these tumours remain truly benign; one-third become locally invasive and one-third metastasize.

Clinical features

The patient is usually a young adult who complains of pain at the end of a long bone; sometimes there is slight swelling. Pathological fracture occurs in 10–15% of cases.

Imaging

Although this is a solid tumour, it appears on x-ray as a 'cystic' (i.e. radiolucent) area situated eccentrically at the end of a long bone. *Unlike any of the other 'cystic' lesions, it always extends right up to the subchondral bone plate* (see Figure 9.8(d)). The endosteal margin is usually clear-cut, but in invasive lesions it is ill defined.

Considering the tumour's potential for aggressive behaviour, detailed staging procedures are essential. CT scans and MRI will reveal the extent of the tumour, both within the bone and beyond. It is important to establish whether the articular surface has been broached; arthroscopy may be helpful. Biopsy is essential.

Treatment

Well-confined, slow-growing lesions with benign histology can safely be treated by thorough curettage and 'stripping' of the cavity with burrs and gouges, followed by swabbing with hydrogen peroxide or by the application of liquid nitrogen;

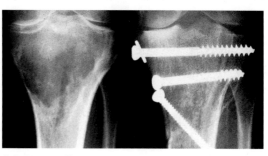

9.9 Giant-cell tumour – treatment Giant-cell tumour of the proximal tibia, treated by block resection and replacement with a large corticocancellous allograft.

the cavity is then packed with bone chips. More aggressive tumours, and recurrent lesions, should be treated by excision followed, if necessary, by bone grafting or prosthetic replacement.

PRIMARY MALIGNANT BONE TUMOURS

OSTEOSARCOMA

Pathology

In its classic form, osteosarcoma is a highly malignant tumour arising within the bone and spreading rapidly outwards to the periosteum and surrounding soft tissues. The histological appearances show considerable variation. Some areas may consist of characteristic spindle cells in an osteoid matrix; others may contain cartilage cells or fibroblastic tissue with little or no osteoid.

Clinical features

Osteosarcoma occurs predominantly in children and adolescents. It may affect any bone but most commonly the long-bone metaphyses, especially around the knee and at the proximal end of the humerus. Pain is usually the first symptom; it is constant, worse at night and gradually increases in severity. Sometimes the patient presents with a lump. On examination there may be some swelling and local tenderness. In late cases there is a palpable mass and the overlying tissues may look inflamed. The erythrocyte sedimentation rate (ESR) is usually raised and there may be an increase in serum alkaline phosphatase.

Imaging

On *x-ray*, some tumours are entirely osteolytic, others show alternating areas of lysis and increased bone density. The tumour margins are poorly defined. Often the cortex is breached and the tumour extends into the adjacent tissues; when this happens, streaks of new bone appear, radiating outwards from the cortex – the so-called 'sunburst' effect. Where the tumour emerges from the cortex, reactive new bone forms in the angle between periosteum and cortex (Codman's triangle). While both the sunburst appearance and Codman's triangle are typical of osteosarcoma, they can also be seen in other rapidly growing tumours.

Other imaging studies are essential for staging purposes. *Radio-isotope* scans may reveal skip lesions, but a negative scan does not exclude them. *CT* and *MRI* reliably show the extent of the tumour. Chest x-rays are done routinely, but *pulmonary CT* is a much more sensitive detector of lung metastases. *About 10% of patients have pulmonary metastases by the time they are first seen.*

Diagnosis

In most cases the diagnosis can be made on the x-ray appearances. However, atypical lesions can be mistaken for more benign conditions, and non-neoplastic conditions such as chronic bone

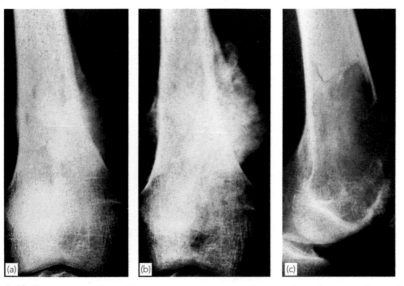

9.10 Osteosarcoma (a) Characteristic x-ray appearances, with sunburst spicules and Codman's triangle where the periosteum begins to be lifted away from the shaft; (b) after radiotherapy; (c) a predominantly osteolytic tumour.

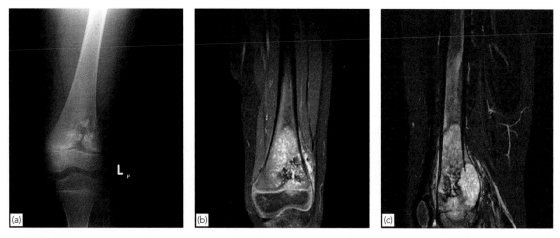

9.11 Osteosarcoma – imaging (a) X-ray of a distal femoral osteosarcoma in a child. (b,c) MRI examination: coronal and sagittal scans showing the intra- and extraosseous extensions of the tumour and its proximity to the neurovascular bundle at the back of the knee.

infection, large gouty tophi and stress fractures sometimes masquerade as malignant lesions.

A biopsy should always be performed before commencing treatment; it must be planned to allow for complete removal of the track when the tumour is excised.

Treatment

The principles of treatment are outlined on page 103. Multi-agent chemotherapy is given for 8–12 weeks and then, provided the tumour is resectable and there are no skip lesions, a wide resection is carried out. *It is important to eradicate the primary lesion completely; the mortality rate after local recurrence is far worse than following effective ablation at the first encounter.* Depending on the site of the tumour, preparations would have been made to replace that segment of bone with either a large bone graft or a custom-made implant; in some cases an amputation may be more appropriate.

The pathological specimen is examined to assess the response to preoperative chemotherapy. If tumour necrosis is marked (more than 90%), chemotherapy is continued for another 6–12 months; if the response is poor, a different chemotherapeutic agent is substituted.

Pulmonary metastases, especially if they are small and peripherally situated, may be completely resected with a wedge of lung tissue.

Outcome

Long-term survival after wide resection and chemotherapy is higher than 60%. Tumour-replacement implants usually function well. There

is a fairly high complication rate (mainly wound breakdown and infection) but in patients who survive, the risk of aseptic loosening at 10 years is around 10% for hip prostheses and 30% for prostheses around the knee.

Paget's sarcoma

Paget's disease of bone occasionally undergoes malignant transformation; most osteosarcomas appearing after the age of 50 years fall into this category. This tumour is, if anything, even more malignant than classic osteosarcoma and extracompartmental spread is more likely. Most patients have pulmonary metastases by the time the tumour is diagnosed.

Even with radical resection or amputation and chemotherapy the 5-year survival rate is low. If the lesion is definitely extracompartmental, palliative treatment by radiotherapy may be preferable; chemotherapy is usually difficult because of the patient's age and uncertainty about renal and cardiac function.

CHONDROSARCOMA

Pathology

Chondrosarcoma occurs either as a primary tumour or as a secondary change in a pre-existing benign chondroma or osteochondroma. Cartilage-capped exostoses of the pelvis and scapula seem to be more susceptible than others to malignant change, but perhaps this is simply because at these sites the tumour can grow without being detected and removed at an early stage.

A *low-grade chondrosarcoma* may show histological features no different from those of an aggressive benign cartilaginous lesion.

High-grade tumours are more cellular, and there may be abnormal features such as cellular plumpness, hyperchromasia and mitoses.

Clinical features

Chondrosarcomas have their highest incidence in the fourth and fifth decades, and men are affected more often than women. The tumours are slow growing and are usually present for many months before being discovered. Patients may complain of a dull ache or a gradually enlarging lump. Medullary lesions may present as a pathological fracture.

Imaging

Primary chondrosarcoma can occur in any bone that develops in cartilage but is usually seen in the metaphysis of one of the tubular bones. *X-ray examination* shows a radiolucent area with central flecks of calcification. Some lesions look like benign chondromas; others are associated with unmistakable features of bone destruction.

Secondary chondrosarcoma usually arises in the cartilage cap of an osteochondroma that has been present since childhood. Large osteochondromas with widespread calcification in the cartilage cap should be viewed with suspicion, and any osteochondroma that increases in size after the end of normal bone growth should be regarded as definitely malignant; in that case *CT and MRI should be performed before biopsy.*

Treatment

Chondrosarcomas are usually slow-growing and metastasize late. They present the ideal case for wide excision and prosthetic replacement, provided it is certain that the lesion can be completely removed without exposing the tumour and without causing an unacceptable loss of function. Otherwise amputation may be a safer option. The tumour does not respond to either radiotherapy or chemotherapy.

EWING'S SARCOMA

Pathology

Ewing's sarcoma is believed to arise from endothelial cells in the bone marrow. It occurs most commonly between the ages of 10 and 20 years, usually in a tubular bone and especially in the tibia, fibula or clavicle. Macroscopically the tumour is lobulated and often fairly large. Microscopically, sheets of small, dark polyhedral cells with no regular arrangement and no ground substance are seen.

Clinical features

The patient presents with pain – often throbbing in character – and swelling. Generalized illness and pyrexia, together with a warm, tender swelling and a raised ESR, may suggest a diagnosis of osteomyelitis.

Imaging

X-ray usually shows an area of bone destruction which, unlike that in osteosarcoma, is predominantly in the mid diaphysis. New bone formation may extend along the shaft and sometimes it appears as fusiform layers of bone around the lesion – the so-called '*onion-peel*' effect. *CT and MRI* will reveal any large extraosseous

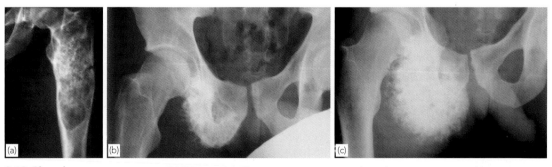

9.12 Chondrosarcoma – x-rays (a) Primary chondrosarcoma appears as a large lucent area encroaching upon or expanding the cortex. A characteristic feature is patchy calcification in the centre of the lesion, well demonstrated in this case. Note that the lateral cortex has fractured. (b,c) Secondary chondrosarcoma usually arises in the cartilage cap of an osteochondroma. In this case the tumour started in the right inferior pubic ramus and went on enlarging after the end of the normal growth period. Although the first biopsy looked benign, continued tumour growth was highly suspicious and a second biopsy showed features of malignancy.

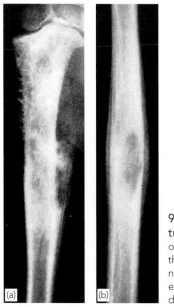

9.13 Ewing's tumour (a,b) X-rays of Ewing's tumour in the humerus. In (b) note the 'onion-peel' effect in the mid diaphysis.

component and *radio-isotope scans* may disclose multiple lesions elsewhere in the skeleton.

Diagnosis

The condition which should be excluded as rapidly as possible is bone infection. On biopsy the essential step is to recognize this as a malignant round-cell tumour, distinct from osteosarcoma. Other round-cell tumours that may resemble Ewing's are *reticulum-cell sarcoma* and *metastatic neuroblastoma*.

Treatment

The prognosis is always poor and surgery alone does little to improve it. Radiotherapy has a dramatic effect on the tumour but overall survival is not much enhanced. Chemotherapy is more effective, offering a 5-year survival rate of about 50%. The best results are achieved by a combination of all three methods: a course of preoperative neo-adjuvant chemotherapy; then wide excision if the tumour is in a favourable site, or radiotherapy followed by local excision if it is less accessible; and then a further course of chemotherapy for 1 year.

MULTIPLE MYELOMA

Pathology

Multiple myeloma is a malignant B-cell lymphoproliferative disorder of the marrow, with plasma cells predominating. The effects on bone are due to marrow cell proliferation and increased osteoclastic activity, resulting in *osteoporosis* and the appearance of discrete *lytic lesions* throughout the skeleton (*myelomatosis*). A particularly large colony of plasma cells may form what appears to be a solitary tumour (*plasmacytoma*) in one of the bones, but sooner or later most of these cases turn out to be examples of the same widespread disease.

At operation the affected bone is soft and crumbly. The typical microscopic picture is of sheets of plasmacytes with a large eccentric nucleus containing a spoke-like arrangement of chromatin.

Clinical features

The patient, typically aged 45–65 years, presents with weakness, backache, bone pain or a patho-logical fracture. Hypercalcaemia may cause symptoms such as thirst, polyuria and abdominal pain.

Associated features of the marrow cell disorder are *plasma protein abnormalities*, *increased blood viscosity* and *anaemia*. Bone resorption leads to *hypercalcaemia* in about one-third of cases. Late secondary features are due to *renal dysfunction* and *spinal cord or root compression* caused by vertebral collapse.

The prognosis in established cases is poor, with a median survival of 2 or 3 years.

X-rays

X-rays often show nothing more than generalized osteoporosis; but remember that *myeloma is one of the commonest causes of osteoporosis and vertebral compression fracture in men over the age of 45 years.* The 'classical' lesions are multiple punched-out defects in the skull, pelvis and proximal femur, a crushed vertebra, or a solitary lytic tumour in a large-bone metaphysis.

Investigations

Mild anaemia is common, and an almost constant feature is a high ESR. Blood chemistry may show a raised creatinine level and hypercalcaemia. Over one-half the patients have Bence–Jones protein in their urine, and serum protein electrophoresis shows a characteristic abnormal band. A sternal marrow puncture may show plasmacytosis, with typical 'myeloma' cells.

Diagnosis

If the only x-ray change is osteoporosis, the differential diagnosis must include all the *other causes of bone loss*. If there are lytic lesions, the features can be similar to those of *metastatic bone disease*.

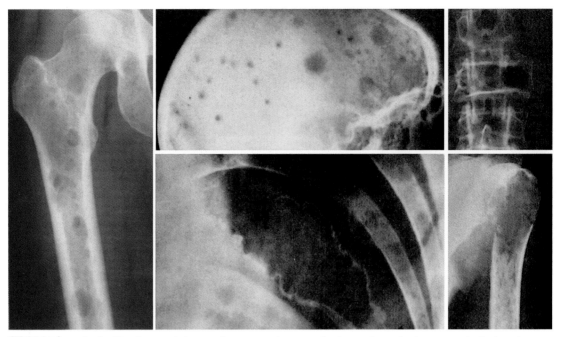

9.14 Myelomatosis The characteristic x-ray features are bone rarefaction and punched-out areas in the long bones, ribs and skull.

Paraproteinaemia is a feature of other (benign) *gammopathies*; it is wise to seek the help of a haematologist before reaching a clinical diagnosis.

Treatment

The immediate need is for pain control and, if necessary, treatment of pathological fractures. General supportive measures include correction of fluid balance and treatment for hypercalcaemia.

Limb fractures are best managed by internal fixation and packing of cavities with methylmethacrylate cement (which also helps to staunch the profuse bleeding that sometimes occurs). Perioperative antibiotic prophylaxis is important as there is a higher than usual risk of infection and wound breakdown.

Spinal fractures carry the risk of cord compression and need immediate stabilization – either by effective bracing or by internal fixation. Unrelieved cord pressure may need decompression.

Specific therapy is with alkylating cytotoxic agents (e.g. melphalan). Corticosteroids are also used – especially if bone pain is marked – but this probably does not alter the course of the disease. Solitary plasmacytomas can be treated by radiotherapy.

The prognosis in established cases is poor, with a median survival rate of only 2–5 years.

METASTATIC BONE DISEASE

In patients over 50 years, bone metastases are seen more frequently than all primary malignant bone tumours together. The commonest source is carcinoma of the breast; next in frequency are carcinomas of the prostate, kidney, lung, thyroid, bladder and gastrointestinal tract. In about 10% of cases no primary tumour is found.

The commonest sites for bone metastases are the vertebrae, pelvis, the proximal half of the femur and the humerus.

Metastases are usually osteolytic, and pathological fractures are common. Bone resorption is due either to the direct action of tumour cells or to tumour-derived factors that stimulate osteoclastic activity. Osteoblastic lesions are uncommon; they usually occur in prostatic carcinoma.

Clinical features

The patient is usually aged 50–70 years; with any destructive bone lesion in this age group, the differential diagnosis must include metastasis.

Pain is the commonest – and often the only – clinical feature. The sudden appearance of backache or thigh pain in an elderly person (especially someone known to have been treated for carcinoma in the past) is always suspicious. If

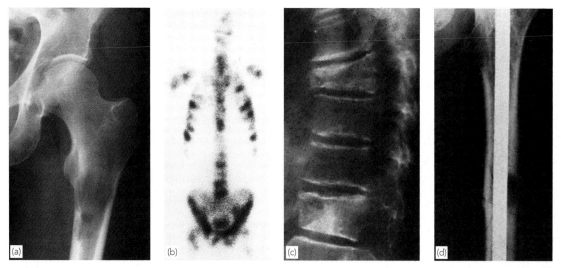

9.15 Metastatic tumours (a) This patient presented with pain in the right thigh. X-ray showed what appeared to be a single metastasis in the upper third of the femur. However, the radio-isotope scan revealed many deposits in other parts of the skeleton (b). (c) Patients over 60 years with vertebral compression fractures should always be investigated for metastatic bone disease and myelomatosis. (d) Prophylactic nailing for a femoral metastasis.

x-rays do not show anything, a radionuclide scan might.

Some deposits remain clinically silent and are discovered incidentally on x-ray, or after a pathological fracture. Sudden collapse of a vertebral body or a fracture of the midshaft of a long bone in an elderly person are ominous signs; if there is no history and no clinical clue pointing to a primary carcinoma, a biopsy of the fracture area is essential.

Symptoms of hypercalcaemia may occur (and are often missed) in patients with skeletal metastases. These include anorexia, nausea, thirst, polyuria, abdominal pain, general weakness and depression.

Imaging

On x-ray examination skeletal deposits usually appear as rarefied areas in the medulla or patches of bone destruction in the cortex. Vertebral collapse is also common. Osteoblastic deposits are seen in late cases of prostatic carcinoma. *Radioscintigraphy*, using ^{99m}Tc-HDP, is the most sensitive method of detecting 'silent' metastatic deposits in bone; areas of increased activity are selected for x-ray examination.

Special investigations

The ESR may be increased and the haemoglobin concentration is usually low. The serum alkaline phosphatase concentration is often increased, and in prostatic carcinoma the acid phosphatase also is elevated.

Treatment

By the time a patient has developed secondary deposits, the prognosis for survival is almost hopeless. Occasionally, radical treatment (by combined surgery and radiotherapy) of a solitary secondary deposit and of its parent primary may be rewarding and even apparently curative. This applies particularly to hypernephroma and thyroid tumours; but in the great majority of cases, and certainly in those with multiple secondaries, treatment is entirely symptomatic. For that reason, elaborate witch-hunts to discover the source of an occult primary tumour are avoided, though it may be worthwhile investigating for tumours that are amenable to hormonal manipulation.

Despite the ultimately hopeless prognosis, patients deserve to be made comfortable, to enjoy (as far as possible) their remaining months or years, and to die in a peaceful and dignified way. The active treatment of skeletal metastases contributes to this in no small measure. In addition, patients need sympathetic counselling and practical assistance with their material affairs.

Control of pain and metastatic activity

Most patients require *analgesics*, but the more powerful narcotics should be reserved for the terminally ill.

Unless specifically contraindicated, *radiotherapy* is used both to control pain and to reduce metastatic

115

growth. This is often combined with other forms of treatment (e.g. internal fixation).

Secondary deposits from breast or prostate can often be controlled by *hormone therapy*: stilboestrol for prostatic secondaries and androgenic drugs or oestrogens for breast carcinoma. Disseminated secondaries from breast carcinoma are sometimes treated by oophorectomy combined with adrenalectomy or by hypophyseal ablation.

Hypercalcaemia may have serious consequences, including renal acidosis, nephrocalcinosis, unconsciousness and coma. It should be treated by ensuring adequate hydration, reducing the calcium intake and, if necessary, administering bisphosphonates.

Treatment of fractures

Surgical timidity may condemn the patient to a painful lingering death, so shaft fractures should almost always be treated by internal fixation and (if necessary) packing with methylmethacrylate cement. Pain is immediately relieved, nursing is made easier and the patient can get up and about or attend for other types of treatment without unnecessary discomfort. The fractures usually unite satisfactorily.

In most cases intramedullary nailing is the most effective method; fractures near joints (e.g. the distal femur or proximal tibia) may need fixation with plates or blade-plates. Fractures of the femoral neck rarely, if ever, unite and are best treated by prosthetic replacement.

Postoperative irradiation is essential to prevent further extension of the metastatic lesion.

Prophylactic fixation

Large deposits that threaten to result in fracture should be treated by internal fixation while the bone is still intact. A preoperative radionuclide scan will show whether other lesions are present in that bone, thus calling for more extensive fixation and postoperative radiotherapy.

Spinal stabilization

Vertebral fractures usually require some form of support. If the spine is stable, a well-fitting brace may be sufficient. However, spinal instability may cause severe pain, making it almost impossible for the patient to sit or stand – with or without a brace. For these patients, operative stabilization is indicated – usually a posterior spinal fusion – followed by radiotherapy.

Preoperative assessment should include CT or MRI, and sometimes myelography, to establish whether the cord is threatened; if it is, spinal decompression should be carried out at the same time.

If there are overt symptoms and signs of cord compression, treatment is urgent. If the patient is expected to live for some time, surgical decompression and fusion are indicated. However, if the patient is in a terminal stage, it may be more humane to give radiotherapy, alone or together with corticosteroids and narcotics, to control oedema and pain.

NEUROMUSCULAR DISORDERS

Of the vast range of neurological disorders, those which most commonly give rise to orthopaedic problems are:

■ Cerebral palsy and stroke (upper motor neuron, spastic disorders).
■ Compressive lesions of the spinal cord.
■ Neural tube defects (spina bifida).
■ Anterior poliomyelitis.
■ Degenerative motor neuron disorders.
■ Nerve root disorders.
■ Peripheral neuropathies.

This chapter also deals with two types of 'muscle disorder':

■ Arthrogryposis.
■ Muscular dystrophy.

NERVES AND MUSCLES

NEURONS

The *neuron* is the defining unit of the nervous system. This is a specialized cell, capable of electrical excitation and conduction of electrochemical impulses (action potentials) along its thread-like extensions. It consists of a *cell body* with branching processes – *dendrites* – that can receive signals from other neuronal terminals. A finer, longer branch – the *axon* – carries the action potentials to or from excitable target organs. Further signal transmission to the dendrites of another neuron, or neuroexcitable tissue like muscle, occurs at a *synapse* where the axon terminal releases a chemical *neurotransmitter* – typically acetylcholine.

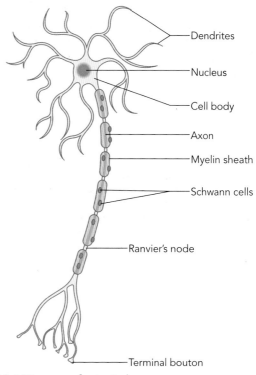

Dendrites

Nucleus

Cell body

Axon

Myelin sheath

Schwann cells

Ranvier's node

Terminal bouton

10.1 Diagram of a typical neuron.

All motor axons and the larger sensory axons serving touch, pain and proprioception are covered by a sheath – the *neurilemma* – and coated with *myelin*, a multi-layered lipoprotein substance which serves as an insulator and allows impulses to be propagated much faster than is the case in unmyelinated nerves. Depletion of the myelin sheath causes slowing – and eventually complete blocking – of axonal conduction.

NERVOUS PATHWAYS

Neurological structures can be divided into the *central nervous system* (CNS), comprising the brain and tracts within the spinal cord, and the *peripheral nervous system* (PNS) which includes the cranial and spinal nerves. Both the CNS and the PNS have a somatic component and an autonomic component.

The *somatic nervous system* provides efferent (motor) and afferent (sensory) pathways to and from peripheral parts of the body serving, respectively, voluntary muscle contraction and sensibility. *Upper motor neurons* (UMNs) are those between the brain and the spinal cord; *lower motor neurons* (LMNs) are those between the anterior horn of the spinal cord and the peripheral muscles. Axons conveying sensory impulses from receptors in the skin and other peripheral structures enter the dorsal nerve roots, with their cell bodies in the dorsal root (or cranial nerve) ganglia, and end in synapses within the CNS. Sensory areas (dermatomes) corresponding to the spinal nerve roots are shown in Figure 10.4.

The *autonomic system* controls involuntary reflex and homeostatic activities of the various bodily organs and peripheral structures. Its two components, *sympathetic* and *parasympathetic* divisions, serve more or less opposing functions.

REFLEX ACTIVITY AND TONE

Sudden stretching of a muscle (e.g. by tapping sharply over the tendon) induces an involuntary muscle contraction – the stretch reflex. The sharp change in muscle fibre length is detected by the muscle spindle; the impulse is transmitted rapidly along myelinated afferent (sensory) neurons which synapse directly with the corresponding motor neurons in the spinal cord, triggering efferent signals which stimulate the muscle to contract. This is the basis of the familiar clinical tests for tendon reflexes, and is also the mechanism for maintaining normal muscle tone.

Normally this reflex activity is regulated by UMN impulses passing from the brain down the spinal cord; interruption of these pathways results in undamped reflex muscle contraction, clinically seen as *spastic paralysis* and hyperactive tendon reflexes. Interruption of the LMN pathways results in *flaccid paralysis*.

AUTONOMIC FUNCTIONS

The autonomic system is involved with the regulation of involuntary activities of cardiac muscle and smooth (unstriated) muscle in the lungs, gastrointestinal tract, kidneys, bladder, genital organs, sweat glands and small blood vessels. Afferent (sensory) and efferent (motor) pathways constitute a continuously active reflex arc.

The autonomic system is divided into sympathetic and parasympathetic pathways, both of which comprise efferent and afferent neurons. *Sympathetic neurons* leave the spinal cord with the ventral nerve roots at all levels from T1 to L1, enter the paravertebral sympathetic chain of ganglia and synapse with postganglionic neurons that spread out to all parts of the body. Important functions are the reflex control of heart rate, blood flow and sweating, as well as other responses associated with conditions of 'fight and flight'. *Parasympathetic neurons* leave the CNS (from the brainstem) with cranial nerves

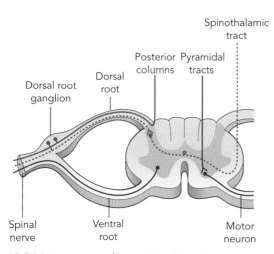

10.2 Main nerve pathways Simplified diagram showing the main neurological pathways to and from a typical thoracic spinal cord segment. Fibres carrying touch, sharp pain and temperature impulses (- - - - -) decussate, in some cases over several spinal segments, and ascend in the contralateral spinothalamic tracts; those carrying vibration and proprioceptive impulses (——) enter the ipsilateral posterior columns. Motor neurons (——) arise in the anterior horn of the grey matter and innervate ipsilateral muscles.

III, VII, IX and X and with the nerve roots of S2, 3 and 4 to reach ganglia where they synapse with postganglionic neurons close to their target organs.

PERIPHERAL NERVES

Peripheral nerves are bundles of axons conducting efferent (motor) impulses from cells in the anterior horn of the spinal cord to the muscles, and afferent (sensory) impulses from peripheral receptors via cells in the posterior root ganglia to the cord. They also convey sudomotor and vasomotor fibres from ganglion cells in the sympathetic chain. Some nerves are predominantly motor, some predominantly sensory; the larger trunks are mixed, with motor and sensory axons running in separate bundles. Peripheral nerve structure is described in Chapter 11.

SKELETAL MUSCLE

Each skeletal muscle belly consists of thousands of *muscle fibres*, separated into bundles (or

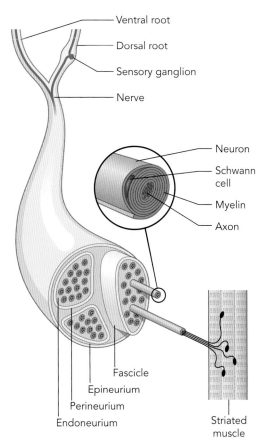

Ventral root
Dorsal root
Sensory ganglion
Nerve

Neuron
Schwann cell
Myelin
Axon

Fascicle
Epineurium
Perineurium
Endoneurium
Striated muscle

10.3 Nerve structure Diagram of the structural elements of a peripheral nerve.

fascicles). Each fascicle is surrounded by a flimsy perimysium which envelops anything up to about 100 muscle fibres. Large muscles concerned with mass movement, like the glutei or quadriceps, have a large number of fibres in each fascicle, while muscles used for precision movements (like those of the hand) have a much smaller number in each bundle.

Muscle fibres are of different types: *type I fibres* contract slowly and are not easily fatigued; their prime function is postural control; *type II fibres* are fast contracting but they fatigue rapidly, so they are ideally suited to intense activities of short duration. All muscles consist of a mixture of fibre types, the balance depending mainly on genetic disposition, basic muscle function and degree of training: thus long-distance runners have a greater proportion of type I fibres than the average.

Muscle contraction is a complex activity. Individual myofibrils respond to electrical stimuli in much the same way as do motor neurons. When the fibres contract, internal tension in the muscle increases. In *isometric contraction* there is increased tension without actual shortening of the muscle or movement of the joint controlled by that muscle. In *isotonic contraction* the muscle shortens and moves the joint.

Muscle tone is the state of tension in a resting muscle when it is passively stretched: tone is increased in UMN lesions (spastic paralysis) and decreased in LMN lesions (flaccid paralysis).

Muscle contracture (as distinct from contraction) is the change that occurs when a normally innervated muscle is held immobile in a shortened position for a long time; for example, if a joint is habitually held flexed it may be impossible to straighten it passively without injuring the muscle. Active exercise will eventually overcome the muscle contracture, unless the muscle has been permanently damaged.

Muscle wasting follows either disuse or denervation. In the former, the fibres are intact but thinner; in the latter, they degenerate and are replaced by fibrous tissue or fat.

Muscle fasciculation – or muscle twitch – is a local involuntary muscle contraction of a small bundle of muscle fibres. It is usually benign but can be due to motor neuron disease or dysfunction.

CLINICAL ASSESSMENT

HISTORY

Age at presentation is important. Certain disorders are obvious at birth (e.g. spina bifida and arthrogryposis).

Cerebral palsy presents during infancy; poliomyelitis usually occurs in childhood; spinal cord lesions and peripheral neuropathies are more common in adults. However, the residual effects of neurological disease, such as muscle weakness and deformity, may need attention throughout life.

Numbness or *paraesthesia* is often the main complaint among adults. It is important to establish its exact distribution to help localize the level of the lesion. The rate of onset and the relationship to posture may, similarly, suggest the cause.

Muscle weakness may be due to UMN or LMN lesions (spastic versus flaccid paralysis) but it may also be due to a primary muscle problem. Ask about the type and degree of weakness, the rate of onset, whether it affects part of a limb, a whole limb, upper or lower limb, one side of the body or both sides.

Deformity is a common complaint in long-standing disorders. It arises as a result of muscle imbalances that may be very subtle and the deformity (such as 'claw-toes') may not be recognized until it is pointed out to the patient.

EXAMINATION

Neurological examination is described in Chapter 1. Attention should be paid to the patient's mental state, natural posture, gait, sense of balance, involuntary movements, muscle wasting, muscle tone and power, reflexes, skin changes, the various modes of sensibility and autonomic functions such as sphincter control, peripheral blood flow and sweating. The back should always be carefully examined as it holds the key to many neurological disorders.

Gait and posture

Typical patterns can often be recognized:

- *Dystonia* refers to abnormal posturing that may affect any part of the body and is often aggravated when the patient is concentrating on a particular motor task such as walking.
- *A spastic gait* is stiff and jerky, often with the feet in equinus, the knees somewhat flexed and the hips adducted ('scissoring').
- *A drop-foot gait* is due to peripheral neuropathy or injury of the nerves supplying the dorsiflexors of the ankle. During the swing phase the foot falls into equinus ('drops') and if it were not lifted higher than usual the toes would drag along the ground.
- *A high-stepping* gait signifies either bilateral foot-drop or a problem with proprioception and balance.

- *A waddling gait*, in which the trunk is thrown from side to side with each step, may be due to dislocation of the hips or to weakness of the abductor muscles.
- *Ataxia* produces a more obvious and irregular loss of balance, which is compensated for by a broad-based gait, or sometimes uncontrollable staggering.

Table 10.1 Nerve root supply and muscle actions

Sternomastoids	Spinal accessory C2, 3, 4
Trapezius	Spinal accessory C3, 4
Diaphragm	C3, 4, 5
Deltoid	C5, 6
Supra- and infraspinatus	C5, 6
Serratus anterior	C5, 6, 7
Pectoralis major	C5, 6, 7, 8
Elbow flexion	C5, 6
extension	C7
Supination	C5, 6
Pronation	C6
Wrist flexion	C6, (7)
extension	C6, 7, (8)
Finger flexion	C7, 8, T1
extension	C7, 8, T1
ab- and adduction	C8, T1
Hip flexion	L1, 2, 3
extension	L5, S1
adduction	L2, 3, 4
abduction	L4, 5, S1
Knee extension	L(2), 3, 4
flexion	L5, S1
Ankle dorsiflexion	L4, 5
plantarflexion	S1, 2
inversion	L4, 5
eversion	L5, S1
Toe extension	L5
flexion	S1
abduction	S1, 2

Muscle weakness

Muscle power is usually graded on the Medical Research Council Scale (see Box). Partial loss of power is called *paresis* and complete loss of power *paralysis*. The type of weakness is important: *spastic weakness* suggests an UMN lesion while *flaccid weakness* could be due to either a LMN lesion or some muscle disorder.

the child sits and sleeps, works and eats in a good position and with good posture. Splints can prevent muscle contractures, maintain joint position and improve movement and hence function.

Operative treatment plays a crucial role. The indications for surgery are: (1) a spastic deformity which cannot be controlled by conservative measures; (2) fixed deformity that interferes with function; and (3) secondary complications such as bony deformities, dislocation of the hip and joint instability. Weak muscles can be augmented by tendon transfers but it requires considerable expertise to avoid the opposing problems of transferring a muscle that is too weak or else one that produces over-correction because of its increased tone. Correction of bony deformity may also be important.

The timing of surgical intervention is often crucial. Development of the CNS and the gait pattern matures around the age of 7–8 years and thus many orthopaedic surgeons advocate delaying surgery until this age and then doing all the necessary operations at one or two sittings. Others still prefer the older approach of 'little and often' surgery.

Patients with *hemiplegia* respond well to both conservative and operative treatment, and all of them should eventually be able to walk unaided. Those with *diplegia* are more difficult to manage but most of them will eventually be able to walk. Patients with *total body involvement* have a poor prognosis for walking, yet even in this group surgery may be needed to improve spinal stability. Low intelligence is no bar to surgery.

For a regional survey of corrective operations the reader is referred to *Apley's System of Orthopaedics and Fractures*, 9th edition, Hodder Arnold (2010).

ADULT ACQUIRED SPASTIC PARESIS

Cerebral damage following a stroke may cause persistent spastic paresis in the adult; disturbance of proprioception and stereognosis may co-exist.

In the early recuperative stage, physiotherapy and splintage are important in preventing fixed contractures; all affected joints should be put through a full range of movement every day, and deformities should be corrected and splinted until controlled muscle power returns. Proprioception and co-ordination can be improved by occupational therapy. Once maximal motor recovery has been achieved – usually by 9 months – residual deformity

or joint instability may need surgical correction or permanent splinting. In general treatment is similar to that of spastic deformity in the child, and is summarized in *Table 10.2.*

Table 10.2 Treatment of principal deformities of the limbs

	Deformity	Splintage	Surgery
Foot	Equinus	Spring-loaded dorsiflexion	Lengthen tendo Achillis
	Equinovarus	Bracing in eversion and dorsiflexion	Lengthen tendo Achillis and transfer lateral half of tibialis anterior to cuboid
Knee	Flexion	Long caliper	Hamstring release
Hip	Adduction	–	Obturator neurectomy Adductor muscle release
Shoulder	Adduction	–	Subscapularis release
Elbow	Flexion	–	Release elbow flexors
Wrist	Flexion	Wrist splint	Lengthen or release wrist flexors; may need fusion or carpectomy
Fingers	Flexion	–	Lengthen or release flexors

LESIONS OF THE SPINAL CORD

With lesions of the spinal cord, patients complain of muscle weakness, numbness or loss of balance; bladder and bowel control may be impaired and men may complain of impotence. Examination reveals a spastic UMN paresis, with exaggerated reflexes and a Babinski response. There may be a fairly precise boundary of sensory change, suggesting the level of cord involvement. Extradural compression may also involve nerve roots and cause LMN signs.

Patterns of cord dysfunction

The pattern of motor and sensory impairment suggests the level of cord involvement:

- Cervical cord: LMN weakness and sensory loss in arms; UMN signs in the lower limbs.

- Thoracic cord: UMN paresis in lower limbs; variable sensory impairment.
- Lumbar cord: combination of UMN and LMN signs in lower limbs.
- Cauda equina: LMN signs and sensory loss in lower limbs, plus urinary retention with overflow.
- Spinal shock: acute cord lesions may present with a flaccid paralysis which resolves over time, usually to reveal the typical UMN signs associated with cord injury.

Diagnosis and management

The more common causes of spinal cord dysfunction are listed in *Table 10.3*. Traumatic and compressive lesions are the ones most likely to be seen by orthopaedic surgeons. Plain x-rays will show structural abnormalities of the spine; cord

Table 10.3 Causes of spinal cord dysfunction

Acute injury

Vertebral fractures
Fracture–dislocation

Infection

Epidural abscess
Poliomyelitis

Intervertebral disc prolapse

Sequestrated disc
Disc prolapse in spinal stenosis

Vertebral canal stenosis

Congenital stenosis
Acquired stenosis

Spinal cord tumours

Neurofibroma
Meningioma

Intrinsic cord lesions

Tabes dorsalis
Syringomyelia
Other degenerative disorders

Miscellaneous

Spina bifida
Vascular lesions
Multiple lesions
Multiple sclerosis
Haemorrhagic disorders

compression can be visualized by myelography, alone or combined with CT. Intrinsic lesions of the cord require further investigation by blood tests, CSF examination and MRI.

Acute compressive lesions require urgent diagnosis and treatment if permanent damage is to be prevented. *Bladder dysfunction is ominous: whereas motor and sensory signs may improve after decompression, loss of bladder control, if present for more than 24 hours, is usually irreversible.*

With chronic lesions one can afford to temporize. Once the diagnosis is certain, appropriate treatment can be applied.

Epidural abscess is a surgical emergency. The patient rapidly develops acute pain and muscle spasm, with fever, leucocytosis and elevation of the erythrocyte sedimentation rate (ESR). X-rays may show disc space narrowing and bone erosion. Treatment is by immediate decompression and antibiotics.

Acute disc prolapse usually causes unilateral symptoms and signs. However, complete lumbar disc prolapse may present as a cauda equina syndrome. Spinal canal obstruction is demonstrated by MRI. Operative discectomy is urgent.

Chronic discogenic disease is often associated with narrowing of the intervertebral foramina and compression of nerve roots. Diagnosis is usually obvious on x-ray and MRI. Operative decompression may be needed.

Spinal stenosis produces a typical clinical syndrome, due partly to direct pressure on the cord or nerve roots and partly to vascular obstruction and ischaemic neuropathy during hyperextension of the lumbar spine. The patient complains of pain and paraesthesia in one or both lower limbs after standing or walking for a few minutes, symptoms that are relieved by bending forward, sitting or crouching so as to flex the lumbar spine. Congenital narrowing of the spinal canal is rare, except in developmental disorders such as achondroplasia. Treatment calls for bony decompression of the nerve structures.

Vertebral disease, such as tuberculosis or metastatic disease, may cause cord compression and paraparesis. The diagnosis is usually obvious on x-ray, but a needle biopsy may be necessary for confirmation. Management is usually by anterior decompression and, if necessary, internal stabilization.

Spinal cord tumours are a comparatively rare cause of progressive paraparesis. X-rays may show bony erosion, widening of the spinal canal or flattening of the vertebral pedicles. Widening of the intervertebral foramina is typical of neurofibromatosis. Treatment usually involves operative removal of the tumour.

Intrinsic lesions of the cord produce slowly progressive neurological signs. Two conditions in particular – *tabes dorsalis* and *syringomyelia* – may present with orthopaedic problems because of neuropathic joint destruction. In syringomyelia a long cavity (the syrinx) filled with CSF develops within the spinal cord, most commonly in the cervical region. Symptoms and signs are most noticeable in the upper limbs. The expanding cyst presses on the anterior horn cells, producing weakness and wasting of the hand muscles. Destruction of the spinothalamic fibres in the centre of the cord produces a characteristic dissociated sensory loss in the upper limbs: impaired response to pain and temperature but preservation of touch. CT may reveal an expanded cord and the syrinx can be defined on MRI. Deterioration may be slowed down by decompression of the foramen magnum.

SPINA BIFIDA

Spina bifida is a congenital disorder in which the two halves of the posterior vertebral arch (or several arches) have failed to fuse. This is often associated with maldevelopment of the neural tube and the overlying skin; the combination of faults is called dysraphism. It usually occurs in the lumbar or lumbosacral region. If neural elements are involved there may be paralysis and loss of sensation and sphincter control.

Spina bifida occulta

In the mildest forms of dysraphism there is a midline defect between the laminae and nothing more; hence the term *occulta* (meaning secret). However, there may be tell-tale defects in the overlying skin: a dimple, a pit or a tuft of hair.

Spina bifida cystica

In severe forms of dysraphism the vertebral laminae are missing and the contents of the vertebral canal prolapse through the defect – either as a CSF-filled meningeal sac or *meningocele* or as a sac containing part of the spinal cord and nerve roots, a *myelomeningocele* (the commonest lesion). The cord may be in its primitive state, the unfolded neural plate forming part of the roof of the sac; this is an 'open' myelomeningocele or rachischisis. In a 'closed' myelomeningocele the neural tube is fully formed and covered by membrane and skin.

Hydrocephalus

Distal tethering of the cord may cause herniation of the cerebellum and brainstem through the foramen magnum, resulting in obstruction to CSF circulation and hydrocephalus. The ventricles dilate and the skull enlarges by separation of the cranial sutures. Persistently raised intracranial pressure may cause cerebral atrophy and mental retardation.

Neurological dysfunction

Myelomeningocele is always associated with neurological deficit below the level of the lesion. This may also occur – though less frequently and much less severely – in spina bifida occulta.

Incidence and screening

Isolated laminar defects are seen in over 5% of lumbar spine x-rays. By comparison, cystic spina bifida is rare at 2–3 per 1000 live births, but if one child is affected the risk for the next child is 10 times greater.

Neural-type defects are associated with high levels of alpha-fetoprotein in the amniotic fluid and serum. This offers an effective method of antenatal screening during the 15th to 18th week of pregnancy.

Clinical features

Antenatal tests and scans may already have revealed the defect.

Spina bifida occulta, marked by isolated laminar defects, is often seen in normal people and can usually be ignored. However, a posterior midline dimple, a tuft of hair or a pigmented naevus is

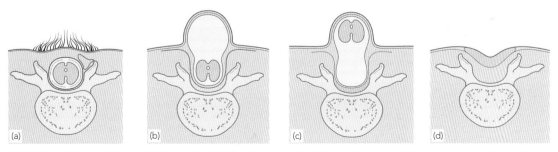

10.7 Dysraphism (a) Spina bifida occulta. (b) Meningocele. (c) Myelomeningocele. (d) Open myelomeningocele.

more serious; patients may present at any age with neurological symptoms and signs.

Spina bifida cystica is obvious at birth in the shape of a sacular lesion over the lumbar spine. It may be covered only with membrane, or with membrane and skin. In *open myelomeningoceles* the neural elements form the roof of the cyst. *Hydrocephalus* is common.

The baby's posture may suggest the type of paralysis and sometimes indicates its neurological level. There is generally a flaccid weakness of muscle groups in the lower limbs; sensibility is impaired and there may be urinary and bowel incontinence. The precise neurological deficit varies according to the level of the lesion. Deformities such as hip dislocation, genu recurvatum and talipes may also be present at birth, or they may develop later due to muscle imbalance.

In about one-third of infants with myelomeningocele there is complete LMN paralysis and loss of sensation and sphincter control below the affected level; in one-third there is a complete lesion at some level but a distal segment of cord is preserved, giving a mixed neurological picture with intact segmental reflexes and spastic muscle groups; in the remaining one-third the cord lesion is incomplete and some movement and sensation are preserved.

X-rays and CT will show the extent of the bony lesion as well as other vertebral anomalies. MRI may be helpful to define the neurological defects.

Management

Folic acid, taken daily before conception and continuing through the first 12 weeks of pregnancy, reduces the risk of neural tube defects in the fetus.

Selection of patients for operative closure of the spinal lesion is ethically controversial. Most centres avoid urgent operation if the neurological level is high (above L1), if spinal deformities are severe or if there is marked hydrocephalus. In the remainder (about one-half) the skin lesion is closed within 48 hours in order to prevent drying and ulceration.

A few weeks later, when the back has healed, the degree of hydrocephalus is assessed. Most children also have the Arnold–Chiari malformation with displacement of the posterior fossa structures through the foramen magnum and will require management of their real or potential hydrocephalus in the form of a ventriculoperitoneal shunt (VP shunt) to reduce the risk of further damage to their CNS. A chronically raised intracranial pressure may be associated with learning difficulties and other problems. Later, if the child's neurological status changes unexpectedly, shunt problems such as infection or blockage should be considered. Ventriculoperitoneal drainage can be maintained for 5 or 6 years, by which time the tendency to hydrocephalus usually ceases.

Subsequent management may involve urological surgery (for bladder incontinence or urinary retention and hydronephrosis) and orthopaedic surgery (for muscle imbalance and joint deformity). Surgical treatment must however always be backed up by prolonged and skilled physiotherapy, occupational therapy and splintage, preferably carried out in a specialized centre.

Except in the mildest cases, the late functional outcome cannot be predicted with any confidence until the child's neuromuscular condition is assessed at the age of 3 or 4 years. Most patients with myelomeningocele will never be functionally independent. More important than walking is the development of upper limb function and intellectual skills and the ability to cope with the basic activities of daily living. These objectives can be achieved from a wheelchair just as well as from unsteady legs.

Joint deformities should be corrected – initially by gentle physiotherapy (beware of causing

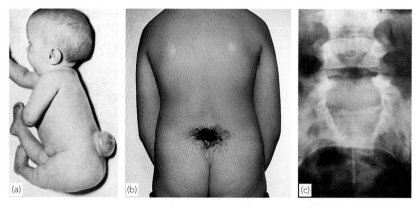

(a) (b) (c)

10.8 Spina bifida (a) Baby with spina bifida cystica (a myelomeningocele). (b) Tuft of hair over the lumbosacral junction; x-ray in this case showed a sacral defect (c).

iatrogenic fractures!) and later by splintage with lightweight orthoses. Surgical correction may be needed if these measures fail. Prolonged immobilization carries the risk of pathological fracture and should therefore be avoided.

Spinal deformity (scoliosis and/or kyphosis) is common in children with myelomeningocele, due to a combination of muscle weakness, associated congenital vertebral anomalies and the tethered cord syndrome. Indications for operative release of the tethered cord are increasing pain and neurological dysfunction or progressive spinal deformity.

Kyphosis may be severe enough to need localized vertebral resection and arthrodesis. Paralytic scoliosis is usually progressive and makes sitting particularly difficult. It is unlikely to respond to the use of a brace. Moulded seat inserts for the wheelchair are essential to aid sitting balance and independence and may help reduce the rate of curve deterioration. Surgery via an anterior, a posterior or a combined approach is often necessary and fusion to the pelvis may be required. The operation is always difficult and carries a high risk of complications, particularly postoperative infection and implant failure.

Hip problems may also call for operative treatment. However, if the neurological level of the lesion is above L1, all muscle groups are flaccid and splintage is the only option; in the long term, the child will probably use a wheelchair. With lesions below S1 a hip flexion contracture is the most likely problem, and this can be corrected by elongation of the psoas tendon combined with detachment of the flexors from the ilium (the Soutter operation). For children with 'in between' lesions, many hips (up to 50%) will subluxate or dislocate by early childhood. Retaining hip movement may be more useful than striving for hip reduction by multiple operations, with their attendant complications and uncertain prognosis. There is little evidence to suggest that function is improved significantly by operative hip relocation.

Unlike the hip, the knee usually presents few problems. Children with lesions below L4 will have quadriceps control and active knee extension; they should therefore be encouraged to walk. In others the objective is simple: a straight knee suitable for wearing calipers and using gait-training devices. Children with high lumbar lesions may start off walking with the aid of lower limb braces but they will eventually opt for a wheelchair.

In older children prolonged sitting may result in fixed flexion. If stretching fails to correct this deformity, one or more of the hamstrings may be lengthened, divided or reinserted into the femur or patella.

Foot deformities are among the most common problems. The aim of treatment is a mobile foot, with healthy skin and soft tissues that will not break down easily, that can be held or braced in a plantigrade position. Flail feet are relatively easy to treat and only require the use of accurately made orthoses. Equinovarus deformity is likely to be more severe (and more resistant to treatment) than the 'ordinary' club-foot. This subject is dealt with in the section on talipes equinovarus in Chapter 21.

POLIOMYELITIS

Poliomyelitis is an acute infectious viral disease. In a small percentage of cases the CNS is involved, the effects falling on the anterior horn cells in the spinal cord and brainstem, leading to flaccid (LMN) paralysis of isolated groups of muscles.

Clinical features

Following a trivial and often unrecognized minor illness (a sore throat or diarrhoea), the patient develops symptoms resembling those of meningitis. He or she lies curled up with the joints flexed; the muscles are painful and tender and passive stretching provokes painful spasms.

Soon muscle weakness appears; it reaches a peak in the course of 2–3 days and may give rise to difficulty with breathing and swallowing. If the patient does not succumb from respiratory paralysis, pain and pyrexia subside after 7–10 days and the patient enters the convalescent stage but may continue to be infective for at least 4 weeks from the onset of illness.

Some anterior horn cells will have been destroyed by the virus; others, merely damaged by oedema, survive, and the muscles they supply can regain their lost power. Such recovery may continue for about 2 years but after that any residual weakness is permanent.

If recovery is not complete the patient is left with some degree of asymmetrical flaccid paralysis or unbalanced muscle weakness that can lead to joint deformity and growth defects. If the trunk muscles were involved, he or she may have respiratory difficulty and/or scoliosis. An affected limb often looks bluish, wasted and deformed; there are frequently extensive chilblains and the skin feels cold. However, sensation is unaffected.

Paralysis may be obvious, but lesser degrees of weakness are discovered only by systematic examination.

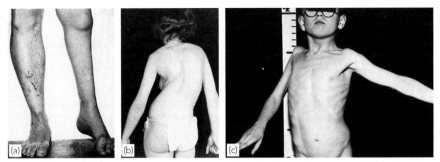

10.9 Poliomyelitis (a) Shortening and wasting of the left leg, with equinus of the ankle. (b) This long curve is typical of a paralytic scoliosis. (c) Paralysis of the right deltoid and supraspinatus makes it impossible for this boy to abduct his right arm.

Principles of treatment

In some countries immunization has been so successful that poliomyelitis has become a rare disease. However, the victims of earlier epidemics continue to pose challenging problems.

During the acute phase the patient is isolated and kept at complete rest, with symptomatic treatment for pain and muscle spasm. Active movement is avoided but gentle passive stretching helps to prevent contractures. Respiratory paralysis calls for artificial respiration.

During the period of recovery physiotherapy is stepped up and every effort is made to regain maximum power; because of the associated trophic changes, hydrotherapy also is useful. Between exercise periods splintage may be needed to prevent fixed deformities. Muscle charting (see page 121) is carried out at regular intervals until no further recovery is detected.

In the late stage orthopaedic treatment comes into its own. Six types of problem in particular may need attention:

- *Isolated muscle weakness without deformity* may affect important movements and joint stability. Quadriceps paralysis may make weightbearing and walking impossible; it can be managed by using a splint or calliper which holds the knee straight. Elsewhere isolated weakness (e.g. of thumb opposition) may be treated by tendon transfer. Muscle charting is essential: a muscle usually loses one grade of power when it is transferred, so to be really useful it should have grade 4 or 5 power; however, even a grade 3 muscle may act as a kind of tenodesis and reduce the deformity caused by gravity.
- *Passively correctible deformity* (due to unbalanced paralysis) can at first be counteracted by splintage. However, an appropriate tendon transfer may solve the problem permanently.

- *Fixed deformities* cannot be corrected by either splintage or tendon transfer alone; alignment must be restored operatively to stabilize the joint (if necessary, by arthrodesis). This is especially applicable to fixed deformities of the ankle and foot, but the same principle applies in treating paralytic scoliosis. Occasionally fixed deformity is an advantage; e.g. a stable equinus foot may help to compensate mechanically for quadriceps weakness and, if so, it should not be corrected.
- *A flail joint*, because it causes no deformity, may need no treatment. However, if the joint is unstable it must be stabilized, either by permanent splintage or by arthrodesis.
- *Leg length inequality* of up to 3 cm can be compensated for by building up the shoe. Anything more is unsightly and operative

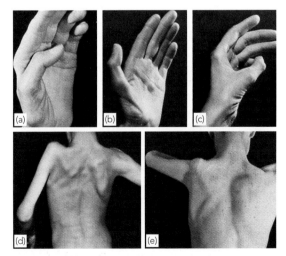

10.10 Poliomyelitis – treatment (a–c) Superficialis tendon transfer for opponens paralysis. In (b) the tendon can be seen in action at the start of thumb opposition (c). (d,e) Arthrodesis of the left shoulder to restore abduction after paralysis of the deltoid.

lengthening of the femur or tibia (or shortening of the opposite limb) might be preferable.

- *Vascular dysfunction* may need treatment. Sensation is intact but the paralysed limb is often cold and blue. Large chilblains sometimes develop and sympathectomy may be needed.

For a detailed regional survey consult *Apley's System of Orthopaedics and Fractures*, 9th edition, Hodder Arnold (2010) (now CRC Press).

MOTOR NEURON DISORDERS

Rare degenerative disorders of the CNS motor neurons and/or anterior horn cells of the cord cause progressive and sometimes fatal paralysis.

Spinal muscular atrophy

This term applies to a rare group of heritable disorders in which there is *widespread anterior horn cell degeneration* leading to progressive lower motor neuron weakness. In the worst cases the infant is weak and floppy at birth and death usually occurs within 1 year. In less severe forms adolescents or young adults present with limb weakness, proximal muscle wasting and 'paralytic' scoliosis. Patients may live to 30–40 years of age but are usually confined to a wheelchair. Spinal braces are used to improve sitting ability; if this cannot prevent the spine from collapsing, operative instrumentation and fusion is advisable.

Motor neuron disease (amyotrophic lateral sclerosis)

Motor neuron disease *affects both UMNs and anterior horn cells*, causing widespread symptoms and signs. Patients may present in middle age with muscle weakness (e.g. clumsy hands or unexplained foot-drop) and wasting in the presence of exaggerated reflexes. Sensation and bladder control are normal. The disease is progressive and incurable. Patients usually end up in a wheelchair and have increasing difficulty with speech and eating. Most of them die within 5 years from a combination of respiratory weakness and aspiration pneumonia. Supportive treatment includes nursing, occupational therapy and the use of various mechanical and electronic aids to assist in essential activities.

PERIPHERAL NEUROPATHIES

Disorders of the peripheral nerves may affect motor, sensory or autonomic functions, may be localized to a short segment or may involve the full length of the nerve fibres. In some cases spinal cord tracts are involved as well.

There are over 100 types of neuropathy; here we consider those conditions that are of most interest to orthopaedic surgeons.

Classification

Classification by anatomical level and distribution is the simplest. In over 40% of cases no specific cause has been found!

- *Radiculopathy* – involvement of nerve roots, most commonly by vertebral trauma, intervertebral disc herniation and nerve root infections like herpes zoster.
- *Plexopathy* – e.g. brachial plexus injury or viral infection (neuralgic amyotrophy).
- *Distal neuropathy* – involvement of neurons in distinct peripheral nerves:
  - Mononeuropathy – involvement of a single nerve, (e.g. nerve injury, or nerve compression).
  - Multiple mononeuropathy – involvement of several nerves (e.g. leprosy).
  - Polyneuropathy – widespread symmetrical dysfunction (e.g. diabetic neuropathy, alcoholic neuropathy and various hereditary neuropathies).

Pathology

Abnormalities may be predominantly sensory (e.g. diabetic polyneuropathy), predominantly motor (e.g. peroneal muscular atrophy) or mixed. Chronic motor loss with no sensory component is usually due to anterior horn cell disease rather than more esoteric pathology.

There are three basic types of peripheral neuronal pathology: (1) acute interruption of axonal continuity; (2) chronic axonal degeneration; and (3) demyelination. In all three, conduction is disturbed or completely blocked, with consequent loss of motor and/or sensory and/or autonomic functions.

Acute axonal interruption occurs most typically after nerve division and is described in Chapter 11. Loss of motor and sensory functions is immediate and complete. The distal segments of axons that are crushed or severed will degenerate – as will the muscle fibres which are supplied by motor neurons – if nerve conduction is not restored within 2 years. Axonal regeneration, when it occurs, is slow (the new axon grows by about 1 mm per day) and is often incomplete.

Chronic (non-traumatic) axonal degeneration is slow and typically progressive. Most large-fibre disorders affect both sensory and motor neurons causing 'stocking' and 'glove' numbness, altered postural reflexes and ataxia as well as muscle weakness and wasting, beginning distally and progressing proximally. Symptoms tend to appear in the feet and legs before the hands and arms. Some disorders are predominantly either motor or sensory.

Demyelinating neuropathies occur most commonly in nerve entrapment syndromes and blunt soft-tissue trauma. The main effects are slowing of conduction and sometimes complete nerve block, causing sensory and/or motor dysfunction distal to the lesion. These changes are potentially reversible; recovery usually takes less than 6 weeks, and in some cases only a few days. Demyelinating polyneuropathies are rare, with the exception of Guillain–Barré syndrome. Other conditions include the heritable motor and sensory neuropathies.

Clinical features

Patients usually complain of 'pins and needles' (paraesthesiae), numbness or 'restless legs'. They may also notice weakness or loss of balance in walking. Occasionally (in the predominantly motor neuropathies) the main complaint is of progressive deformity; for example, claw-hand or cavus foot.

The onset may be rapid (over a few days) or very gradual (over weeks or months). Sometimes there is a history of injury, infection, a known disease such as diabetes or malignancy, alcohol abuse or nutritional deficiency.

Examination may reveal weakness in a particular muscle group and/or loss of peripheral sensation. In the polyneuropathies the limbs are involved symmetrically, usually legs before arms and distal before proximal parts. In mononeuropathy, sensory loss follows the 'map' of the affected nerve. In polyneuropathy, there is a symmetrical 'glove' or 'stocking' distribution.

Trophic skin changes may be present. Deep sensation is also affected and some patients develop ataxia. If pain sensibility and proprioception are depressed there may be joint instability or breakdown of the articular surfaces (neuropathic joint disease or 'Charcot joints').

Clinical examination alone may establish the diagnosis. Further help is provided by EMG (which may suggest the type of abnormality) and nerve conduction studies (which may show exactly where the lesion is).

The mononeuropathies (mainly nerve injuries and entrapment syndromes) are dealt with in Chapter 11. Some of the more common polyneuropathies are described below.

DIABETIC NEUROPATHY

Diabetes is one of the commonest causes of peripheral neuropathy. The metabolic disturbance associated with hyperglycaemia interferes with axonal and Schwann cell function, leading to mixed patterns of demyelination and axonal degeneration. Autonomic dysfunction and vascular disturbance also play a part.

The onset is insidious and the condition often goes undiagnosed until patients start complaining of numbness and paraesthesiae in the feet and lower legs. Even at that early stage there may be areflexia and diminished vibration sense. Another suspicious pattern is an increased susceptibility to nerve entrapment syndromes. Later, muscle weakness becomes more noticeable in proximal parts of the limbs. In advanced cases trophic complications can arise: neuropathic ulcers of the feet, regional osteoporosis, insufficiency fractures of the foot bones, or Charcot joints in the ankles and feet.

Treatment starts with proper control of the underlying disorder. Local measures consist of skin care, management of fractures and splintage or arthrodesis of grossly unstable or deformed joints. Management of the diabetic foot is discussed on page 301.

NEURALGIC AMYOTROPHY (ACUTE BRACHIAL NEURITIS)

This unusual cause of severe shoulder girdle pain and weakness is believed to be due to a parainfectious disorder of one or more of the cervical nerve roots and the brachial plexus, sometimes producing a pseudomononeuropathic pattern (e.g. scapular winging or wrist-drop). There is often a history of an antecedent viral infection or antiviral inoculation; sometimes a small epidemic occurs among several residents of an institution.

The history alone often suggests the diagnosis. Pain in the shoulder and arm is typically sudden in onset, intense and unabating; the patient can often recall the exact hour when symptoms began. Pain may extend into the neck and down as far as the hand; usually it lasts for 2 or 3 weeks. Other symptoms are paraesthesiae in the arm or hand and weakness of the muscles of the shoulder, forearm and hand.

Winging of the scapula (due to serratus anterior weakness), wasting of the shoulder girdle muscles, and occasionally involvement of more distal arm muscles may be profound, becoming evident as the pain improves. Shoulder movement is initially limited by pain but this is superseded by weakness due to muscle atrophy. Sensory loss and paraesthesiae in one or more of the cervical dermatomes are not uncommon. Involvement of overlapping root territories of the brachial plexus is a feature that helps to distinguish neuralgic amyotrophy from an acute cervical disc herniation which is monoradicular.

There is no specific treatment; pain is controlled with analgesics. The prognosis is usually good but full neurological recovery may take months or years.

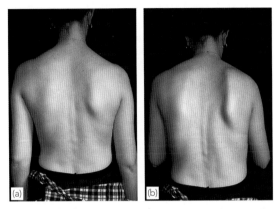

10.11 Neuralgic amyotrophy A common feature of neuralgic amyotrophy is winging of the scapula due to serratus anterior weakness. Even at rest (a) the right scapula is prominent in this young woman. When she thrusts her arms forwards against the wall (b) the abnormality is more pronounced.

GUILLAIN–BARRÉ SYNDROME

Guillain–Barré syndrome describes an acute demyelinating motor and sensory polyneuropathy. It can occur at any age and usually appears 2 or 3 weeks after an upper respiratory or gastrointestinal infection – probably as an autoimmune reaction.

The typical history is of aching and weakness in the legs, often accompanied by numbness and paraesthesiae, which steadily progresses upwards over a period of hours, a few days or a few weeks. Symptoms may stop when the thigh and pelvic muscles are reached, and then gradually retreat, or may go on ascending to involve the upper limbs, facial muscles and diaphragm, resulting in quadriplegia and respiratory failure. In the established case there will be areflexia and loss of position sense. In severe cases patients may develop features of autonomic dysfunction.

CSF analysis may show a characteristic pattern: elevated protein concentration in the presence of a normal cell count (unlike an infection, in which the cell count would also be elevated). Neurophysiological studies may show conduction slowing or block; in severe cases there may be EMG signs of axonal damage.

Treatment consists essentially of bed rest, pain-relieving medication and supportive management to monitor, prevent and deal with complications such as respiratory failure and difficulty with swallowing. In severe cases specific treatment with intravenous immunoglobulins or plasmapheresis should be started as soon as possible. Once the acute disorder is under control, physiotherapy and splintage will help to prevent deformities and improve muscle power.

Most patients recover completely, though this may take 6 months or longer; about 10% are left with long-term disability and about 3% are likely to die.

LEPROSY

Although uncommon in Europe and North America, this is still a frequent cause of peripheral neuropathy in Africa and Asia.

Mycobacterium leprae, an acid-fast organism, causes a diffuse inflammatory disorder of the skin, mucous membranes and peripheral nerves. Depending on the host response, several forms of disease may evolve.

The most severe neurological lesions are seen in *tuberculoid leprosy*. Anaesthetic skin patches develop over the extensor surfaces of the limbs; loss of motor function leads to weakness and deformities of the hands and feet. Thickened

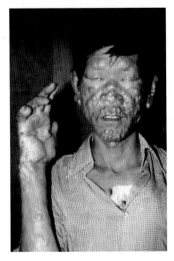

10.12 Leprosy – ulnar nerve paralysis Ulnar nerve paralysis is relatively common in long-standing leprosy. This patient has the typical ulnar claw-hand deformity.

nerves may be felt as cords under the skin or where they cross the bones (e.g. the ulnar nerve behind the medial epicondyle of the elbow). Trophic ulcers are common and may predispose to osteomyelitis. *Lepromatous leprosy* is associated with a symmetrical polyneuropathy, which occurs late in the disease.

Treatment by combined chemotherapy (mainly rifampicin and dapsone) is continued for 6 months to 2 years, depending on the response. Muscle weakness, particularly intrinsic muscle paralysis due to ulnar nerve involvement, may require multiple tendon transfers.

HEREDITARY NEUROPATHIES

These rare disorders present in childhood and adolescence, usually with muscle weakness and deformity.

Hereditary sensory neuropathy

Congenital insensitivity to pain and temperature is inherited as either a dominant or a recessive trait. Patients are prone to painless injury and may develop ulceration of the feet or neuropathic joint disease.

Hereditary motor and sensory neuropathy (HMSN)

This is a group of conditions which includes peroneal muscular atrophy and Charcot–Marie–Tooth disease, the commonest of the inherited neuropathies, which are usually passed on as autosomal dominant disorders.

HMSN Type I is seen in children who have difficulty walking and develop claw-toes and pes cavus or cavovarus. There may be severe wasting of the legs and (later) the upper limbs, but often the signs are quite subtle. Spinal deformity may occur in severe cases. This is a demyelinating disorder; nerve conduction velocity is markedly slowed and the diagnosis can be confirmed by finding demyelination on sural nerve biopsy.

HMSN Type II occurs in adolescents and young adults and is less disabling than Type I. It affects only the lower limbs, causing mild pes cavus and wasting of the peronei. Nerve conduction velocity is only slightly reduced, indicating primary axonal degeneration.

Treatment during the early stages of HMSN may call for foot and ankle orthoses. If the deformities are progressive or disabling, operative correction may be indicated. Claw-toes (due to intrinsic muscle weakness) can be corrected by transferring the toe flexors to the extensors, with or without fusion of the interphalangeal joints. Clawing of the big toe is best corrected by transfer of the

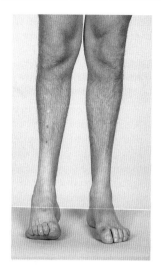

10.13 Hereditary neuropathies This patient with peroneal muscular atrophy has the typical wasting of the legs, cavus feet and claw-toes.

extensor hallucis longus to the metatarsal neck and fusion of the interphalangeal joint (the Robert Jones procedure). The cavus deformity needs treatment only if it causes pain; it can be improved by calcaneal or dorsal midtarsal osteotomy or (in severe cases) triple arthrodesis.

Friedreich's ataxia

This autosomal recessive condition is the classic archetype of a large group of genetic disorders – the spinocerebellar ataxias – characterized by spinocerebellar dysfunction, but there may also be degeneration of the posterior root ganglia and peripheral nerves. Many of these disorders have now been genotypically defined. Patients generally present at around the age of 6 years with gait ataxia, lower limb weakness and deformities similar to those of severe Charcot–Marie–Tooth disease. The muscle weakness, which may also involve the upper limbs and the trunk, is progressive; by the age of 20 years the patient has usually taken to a wheelchair and is likely to die of cardiomyopathy before the age of 45. Despite the potentially poor prognosis, surgical correction of deformities is worthwhile.

ARTHROGRYPOSIS MULTIPLEX CONGENITA

This unwieldy term is applied to a group of rare congenital disorders characterized by multiple (often symmetrical) non-progressive soft-tissue contractures and restriction of joint movement. Deformities and contractures develop in utero and remain largely unchanged throughout life. Myopathic and neuropathic features may co-exist in the same muscle.

The incidence is said to be about 1 in 3000 live births; in some cases a genetic linkage has been demonstrated. A more proximate cause may be an intrauterine lack of sufficient room for movement during fetal development.

Three major categories are recognized: (1) children with total body involvement (the condition traditionally known as arthrogryposis multiplex congenita and now termed *amyoplasia*); (2) those with predominantly hand or foot involvement – *distal arthrogryposis*; and (3) patients with *pterygia syndromes*: conditions characterized by arthrogrypotic joint contractures with soft-tissue webs, usually across the flexor aspects of the knees and ankles.

Clinical features

Involved joints are tubular and featureless and although the normal skin creases are absent there are often deep dimples over the joints. Muscle mass is markedly reduced. In some cases there is true muscle weakness.

In the classic form of *amyoplasia* the shoulders are adducted and internally rotated, the elbows usually extended and the wrists/hands flexed and deviated ulnarwards. In the lower limbs, the hips are flexed and abducted, the limbs externally rotated, the knees usually extended and the feet showing equinovarus or vertical talus deformities.

Distal arthrogryposis often manifests an autosomal dominant pattern of inheritance. Common deformities are ulnar deviation of the metacarpophalangeal joints, fixed flexion of the proximal interphalangeal joints and tightly adducted thumbs. Foot deformities are likely to be resistant forms of equinovarus or vertical talus.

Treatment

Treatment begins soon after birth and initially consists of gentle manipulation and muscle stretching exercises, later combined with splintage to prevent (or slow down) recurrence of joint contractures. If progress is slow, tendon release, tendon transfers and osteotomies may become necessary. In the pterygia syndromes, physiotherapy can be tried but early release of the popliteal contractures should be considered. Great care is needed to avoid injury to tight neurovascular structures.

Arthrogrypotic club-foot usually demands operative correction. Dislocation of the hip, likewise, often defies conservative treatment and open reduction is needed. Whatever the form of treatment, parents should be warned that recurrent deformity is common. Remember that the aims of treatment are to provide these children with the ability to walk and upper limb function adequate to the needs of their most important daily activities, rather than the restoration of full movement.

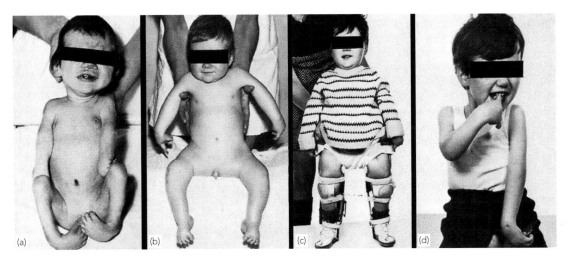

10.14 Arthrogryposis multiplex congenita (a,b) Severe deformities are present at birth. In this case all four limbs are affected. (c,d) Operative treatment is often worthwhile. In this young boy the lower limbs were tackled first and the feet and knees are held in splints. In the upper limbs, the minimum aim is to enable a hand to reach the mouth.

MUSCULAR DYSTROPHY

The muscular dystrophies are a group of about 30 extremely rare inherited disorders characterized by progressive muscle weakness and wasting. Pathological changes include malformation of muscle fibres, death of muscle cells and replacement of muscle by fibrous tissue and fat. Only one of them will be considered here: *pseudohypertrophic muscular dystrophy (Duchenne dystrophy)*. This is a progressive disease of sex-linked inheritance with recessive transmission. It is therefore seen only in boys, affecting 1 in 3500 male births. A defect at locus p21 on the X chromosome results in failure to code for the dystrophin gene, which is essential for maintaining the integrity of cardiac and skeletal muscle cells. Absence of functional dystrophin leads to cell membrane leakage, muscle fibre damage and replacement by fat and fibrous tissue.

Clinical features

The condition is usually unsuspected until the child starts to walk. He has difficulty standing, he cannot run properly and he falls frequently. A characteristic feature is the boy's method of rising from the floor by climbing up his own legs (Gowers' sign); this is due to weakness of the gluteus maximus and thigh muscles.

Shoulder girdle weakness follows about 5 years after the clinical onset of the disease. By the age of 10 the child has usually lost the ability to walk and has to use a wheelchair; from then on there is rapid deterioration in spinal posture with the development of scoliosis and, subsequently, further deterioration in lung function. Cardiopulmonary failure is the usual cause of death, generally before the age of 30 years.

The diagnosis is usually based on the clinical features and family history and by testing for serum creatinine phosphokinase levels which are 200–300 times the normal in the early stages of the disease. Muscle biopsy and genetic testing confirms the diagnosis.

Family counselling is important. Up to 20% of families already have a younger affected sibling by the time the proband is diagnosed.

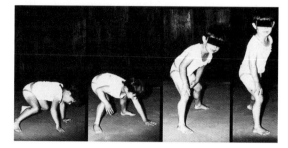

10.15 Muscular dystrophy This boy with a Duchenne type of dystrophy has to climb up his legs in order to achieve the upright position.

Treatment

While the child can still walk, physiotherapy and splintage or tendon operations may help to prevent or correct joint deformities and so prolong the period of mobility. Corticosteroids are useful in preserving muscle strength but there are significant side-effects such as osteoporosis, increased risk of fractures and cataract formation.

If scoliosis is marked (more than 30 degrees), instrumentation and spinal fusion helps to maintain pulmonary function and improves quality of life. Preoperative cardiac and pulmonary function should be reviewed.

CHAPTER 11

PERIPHERAL NERVE INJURIES

Peripheral nerves are bundles of *axons* conducting efferent (motor) impulses from cells in the anterior horn of the spinal cord to the muscles, and afferent (sensory) impulses from peripheral receptors, via cells in the posterior root ganglia, to the cord. They also convey sudomotor and vasomotor fibres from ganglion cells in the sympathetic chain. Some nerves are predominantly motor, some predominantly sensory; the larger trunks are mixed, with motor and sensory axons running in separate bundles.

A single motor neuron supplies ten to several thousand muscle fibres, the ratio depending on the degree of dexterity demanded of the particular muscle (the smaller the ratio, the finer the movement). Similarly, the peripheral branches of each sensory neuron may serve anything from a single muscle spindle to a comparatively large patch of skin; here again, the fewer the end receptors served by a single axon, the greater the degree of discrimination.

The signal, or action potential, carried by motor neurons is transmitted to the muscle fibres by the release of a chemical transmitter, acetylcholine, at the terminal bouton of the nerve. Sensory signals are similarly conveyed to the dorsal root ganglia and from there up the ipsilateral column of the spinal cord, through the brainstem and thalamus, to the opposite (sensory) cortex. Proprioceptive impulses from the muscle spindles and joints bypass this route and are carried to the anterior horn cells as part of a local reflex arc. The economy of this system ensures that 'survival' mechanisms such as balance and sense of position in space are activated with great speed.

In the peripheral nerves, all motor axons and the large sensory axons serving touch, pain and proprioception are coated with *myelin*, a multi-layered lipoprotein membrane derived from the accompanying *Schwann cells*. Every few millimetres the myelin sheath is interrupted, leaving short segments of bare axon called the *nodes of Ranvier*. Nerve impulses leap from node to node with the speed of electricity, much faster than would be the case if these axons were not insulated by the myelin sheaths. Depletion of the myelin sheath causes slowing – and eventually complete blocking – of axonal conduction.

Most axons – in particular the small-diameter fibres carrying crude sensation and the efferent sympathetic fibres – are unmyelinated but wrapped in Schwann cell cytoplasm. Damage to these axons causes unpleasant or bizarre sensations and various sudomotor and vasomotor effects.

Outside the Schwann cell membrane the axon is covered by a connective tissue stocking, the *endoneurium*. The axons that make up a nerve are separated into bundles (fascicles) by fairly dense membranous tissue, the *perineurium*. In a transected nerve, these fascicles are seen pouting from the cut surface, their perineurial sheaths well defined and strong enough to be grasped by fine instruments. The groups of fascicles that make up a nerve trunk are enclosed in an even thicker connective tissue coat, the *epineurium*.

The nerve is richly supplied by *blood vessels*

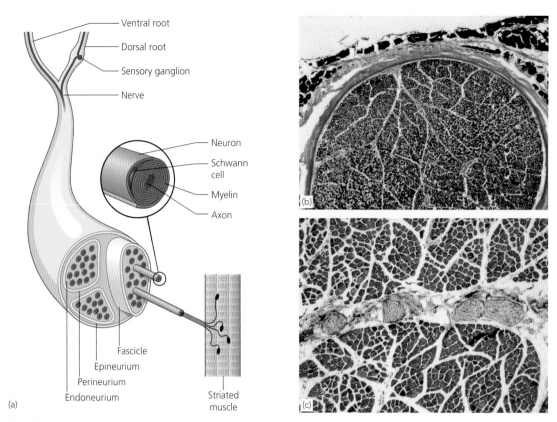

11.1 Nerve structure (a) Diagram of the structural elements of a peripheral nerve. (b) Histological section through a large nerve. The epineurium and perineurial septa are well defined; axons appear as tiny black dots. (c) High-power view, showing blood vessels in the perineurium.

that run longitudinally in the epineurium before penetrating the various layers to become the *endoneurial capillaries*. These fine vessels may be damaged by stretching or rough handling.

PATHOLOGY OF NERVE INJURIES

Nerves can be injured by ischaemia, compression, traction, laceration or burning. Damage varies in severity from transient and quickly recoverable loss of function to complete interruption and degeneration.

Transient ischaemia

Acute nerve compression causes numbness and tingling within 15 minutes, loss of pain sensibility after 30 minutes and muscle weakness after 45 minutes. Relief of compression is followed by intense paraesthesiae lasting up to 5 minutes (the familiar 'pins and needles' after a limb 'goes to sleep'); feeling is restored within 30 seconds and full muscle power after about 10 minutes. These

changes are due to transient endoneurial anoxia and they leave no trace of nerve damage.

Neurapraxia

Herbert Seddon, in 1943, coined the term 'neurapraxia' to describe a reversible block to nerve conduction in which there is loss of sensation and muscle power, followed by spontaneous recovery after a few days or weeks. The nerve is intact but mechanical pressure has caused demyelination of axons in a limited segment. This reversible lesion is also called a 'first-degree' injury.

Axonotmesis

This is a more severe form of injury in which there is interruption of the axons in a segment of nerve. It is seen typically after closed fractures and dislocations. There is loss of conduction but the nerve is in continuity and the neural tubes are intact. Distal to the lesion, and for a few millimetres proximal to it, axons disintegrate and are resorbed by phagocytes. This *Wallerian degeneration* (named after the physiologist Augustus Waller) takes only a few days and is accompanied by proliferation of Schwann cells and fibroblasts lining the endoneurial tubes. The denervated motor end-plates and sensory receptors gradually atrophy and if they are not re-innervated within 2 years they will never recover.

Axonal regeneration starts within hours of nerve damage. The proximal stumps sprout numerous unmyelinated tendrils, many of which find their way into the cell-clogged endoneurial tubes. These new axonal processes grow at a speed of 1–2 mm per day, the larger fibres slowly acquiring a new myelin coat. Eventually they join to the denervated end-organs, which enlarge and start functioning again.

Depending on the degree of damage within the axonotmesis, there may be full recovery (second-degree injury), partial recovery (third-degree) or no recovery (fourth-degree).

Neurotmesis

In Seddon's original classification, neurotmesis meant division of the nerve trunk, such as may occur in an open wound. It is now recognized that severe

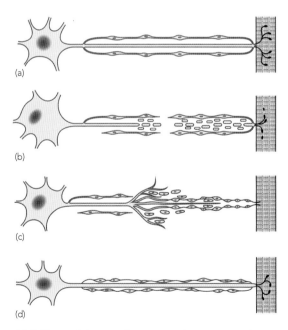

11.2 Nerve injury and regeneration (a) Normal axon and target organ (striated muscle). (b) Following nerve injury, the distal part of the axon disintegrates and the myelin sheath breaks up. (c) New axonal tendrils grow into the mass of proliferating Schwann cells. One of the tendrils will find its way into the old endoneurial tube and (d) the axon will slowly regenerate.

injury can be inflicted without actually dividing the nerve; in such cases there may be degrees of damage between that of axonotmesis, which is potentially recoverable, and complete neurotmesis which will never recover without surgical intervention. It may therefore be called a fifth-degree injury. As in axonotmesis there is rapid Wallerian degeneration, but here the endoneurial tubes are destroyed over a variable segment and scarring thwarts any hope of regenerating axons entering the distal segment and regaining their target organs. Instead, regenerating fibres mingle with proliferating Schwann cells and fibroblasts in a jumbled knot, or 'neuroma', at the site of injury. Even after surgical repair many new axons fail to reach the distal segment; those that do may not find suitable Schwann tubes, or may not reach the correct end-organs in time, or may remain incompletely myelinated. Function may be adequate but is never normal.

CLINICAL FEATURES

Acute nerve injuries are easily missed, especially if associated with fractures or dislocations, the symptoms of which may overshadow those of the nerve lesion. *Always test for nerve injuries following any significant trauma. And test again after manipulation or operation, in case the nerve has been damaged during treatment!*

Ask the patient if there is numbness, tingling or muscle weakness in the target area. Then examine the injured limb systematically for signs of abnormal posture (e.g. a wrist-drop in radial nerve palsy), weakness in specific muscle groups and changes in sensibility. The pattern of change is usually sufficiently characteristic to provide an anatomical diagnosis (see *Table 10.1* and Figure 10.1).

If a nerve injury is present, it is crucial also to look for an accompanying vascular injury.

Diagnosis
■ Are there neurological symptoms?
■ Are there neurological signs?
■ What is the level of the lesion?
■ What type of lesion is it?
■ Are there signs of nerve recovery?

Diagnosis

Having established the presence of a *nerve injury* and, in most cases, the likely anatomical *level* of the injury, it is still necessary to diagnose the *type* of injury and the *degree* of damage. Nerve loss in low-energy injuries is likely to be due to neurapraxia, and in high-energy injuries and open wounds to axonotmesis or neurotmesis. In doubtful cases, one may have to wait a few weeks to see if signs of recovery appear, which would exclude complete nerve division. Muscles supplied by the nerve should be tested repeatedly: assuming that nerve regeneration occurs at the rate of 1 mm per day, one can estimate the expected time of recovery in muscles closest to the site of injury. With open wounds, however, early exploration is the best policy.

Testing for muscle power

Motor power should be recorded using the Medical Research Council scale:

- 0 = No contraction.
- 1 = A flicker of muscle activity.
- 2 = Muscle contraction but inability to overcome gravity.
- 3 = Contraction able to overcome gravity.
- 4 = Contraction and movement against resistance.
- 5 = Normal power.

Tinel's sign

A classic sign of progressive nerve recovery is peripheral tingling provoked by percussing the nerve at the site of injury (where regenerating axons are most sensitive). After a delay of a few weeks, the sensitive spot should begin to advance down the limb at a rate of about 1 mm per day. Failure of Tinel's sign to advance suggests a severe degree of nerve injury and the need for operative exploration.

Two-point discrimination

The density of sensory axonal recovery can be determined by measuring the ability to sense the distance between two pin-points or the pressure applied through fine filaments.

Stereognosis

The ability to recognize objects by touch alone can also be gauged asking the patient to handle a number of small commonly used items.

Electrodiagnostic tests

Nerve conduction tests and electromyography may help to establish the level and severity of the injury, as well as the progress of nerve recovery. Remember, though, that these tests are not very accurate during the first few weeks after nerve injury.

PRINCIPLES OF TREATMENT

Open injuries

The earlier a nerve is repaired, the better the recovery. Nerve injuries associated with an open wound (even a small stab wound) should be explored and, if necessary, repaired as part of the patient's primary treatment. If the nerve is cleanly divided, end-to-end suture may be possible. A ragged cut will need paring of the stumps with a sharp blade. If this leaves too large a gap, or if the nerve stumps have retracted so that they cannot be brought together without tension, some slack can be gained by mobilizing the nerve, but if it is still difficult to bring the ends together without tension, nerve grafts (usually from the sural nerve) are inserted with special glue or very fine sutures; an alternative is to use artificial nerve conduits to span the interval. This is specialized surgery, which must be performed under magnification.

Postoperatively, physiotherapy is applied to retain joint movement. However, if there is the least doubt about tension on the nerve, the limb should be splinted in a position which keeps the nerve relaxed for about 2 weeks before starting physiotherapy.

Closed injuries

With closed nerve lesions it is more difficult to decide what to do, especially during the first few

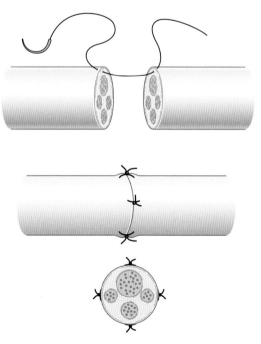

11.3 Nerve repair The stumps are correctly oriented and attached by fine sutures through the epineurium.

weeks after injury. In most cases, if the history suggests that the force of injury was low, the nerve sheath is likely to be intact (neurapraxia or axonotmesis), so one can afford to wait at least until the muscle whose nerve supply arises just below the injury should have recovered (see pages 139–140, Diagnosis). If at that time there is still no sign of recovery, the nerve should be explored. If the history suggests a higher degree of force, or if the nerve could be trapped, for example in a fracture, then early exploration should be considered because the earlier a nerve is repaired, the better its recovery.

Delayed repair

Late repair – i.e. weeks or months after the injury – may be indicated because: (1) a closed injury was left alone but showed no sign of recovery at the expected time; (2) the diagnosis was missed and the patient presented late; or (3) primary repair has failed. The options must be weighed carefully: if the patient has adapted to the functional loss, if it is a high lesion and re-innervation is unlikely within the critical 2-year period, or if there is a pure motor loss which can be treated by tendon transfer, it may be best to leave well alone. Excessive scarring and intractable joint stiffness may, likewise, make nerve repair questionable; yet in the hand it is still worthwhile simply to regain protective sensation.

The lesion is exposed under high magnification, working from normal tissue above and below towards the scarred area. If the nerve is in continuity, only slightly thickened and soft, or if there is conduction across the lesion, resection is not advised; if the nerve is scarred and there is no conduction on electrical stimulation, the scar should be resected, paring back the stumps until healthy fascicles are exposed. Nerve suture or grafting is then performed as described above.

Care of paralysed parts

While recovery is awaited, the skin must be protected from friction damage and burns. The joints should be moved through their full range twice daily to prevent stiffness and minimize the work required of muscles when they recover.

Tendon transfers

Motor recovery may not occur if the regenerating axons fail to reach the muscle within 18–24 months of injury. In such circumstances, tendon transfers should be considered. The following principles must be observed: (1) the donor muscle should be expendable and have adequate power;

(2) the recipient site must be mobile and stable; (3) the transferred tendon should be routed subcutaneously in a straight line of pull; (4) the patient should be well motivated; and (5) dedicated physiotherapy is important.

NERVE INJURIES AFFECTING THE UPPER LIMB

BRACHIAL PLEXUS INJURIES

The brachial plexus is formed by the confluence of nerve roots from C5 to T1. The network is most vulnerable to injury where the nerves run from the cervical spine, between the muscles of the neck and beneath the clavicle en route to the arm – either a stab wound or severe traction caused by a fall on the side of the neck or the shoulder. *Supraclavicular lesions* typically occur in motorcycle accidents. *Infraclavicular lesions* are usually associated with fractures or dislocations of the shoulder. Fractures of the clavicle rarely damage the plexus, and then only if caused by a direct blow.

The injury may affect any level of the plexus. *Preganglionic lesions* (i.e. disruption of nerve roots proximal to the dorsal root ganglion) cannot recover and are surgically irreparable. *Postganglionic lesions* can be repaired and are capable of recovery. Lesions in continuity have a better prognosis than complete ruptures.

Clinical features

Clinical examination should establish: (a) the level of the lesion; (b) whether it is preganglionic or postganglionic; and (c) the type of damage.

The level of the lesion

Upper plexus injuries (C5 and 6) cause paralysis of the shoulder abductors and external rotators and the forearm supinators; typically the arm hangs close to the body and internally rotated. Sensation is lost along the outer aspect of the arm and forearm.

Pure lower plexus injuries are rare; the intrinsic hand muscles are paralysed, resulting in clawing, and sensation is lost along the inner (ulnar) aspect of the arm.

Total plexus lesions result in paralysis and numbness of the entire limb.

Preganglionic or postganglionic

It is important to establish whether the lesion is proximal or distal to the dorsal root ganglion: the former is irreparable; the latter can be repaired and may recover. Features suggesting

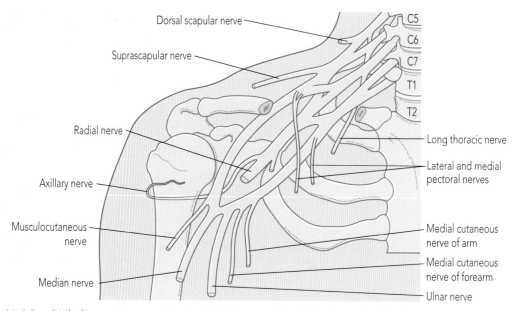

11.4 Brachial plexus Diagram of the brachial plexus and its relationship to the clavicle.

preganglionic root avulsion are: (1) burning pain in an anaesthetic hand; (2) paralysis of scapular muscles or diaphragm; (3) Horner's syndrome; (4) severe vascular injury; (5) associated fractures of the cervical spine; and (6) spinal cord dysfunction.

The *histamine test* is helpful. Intradermal injection of histamine normally causes a reflex triple response in the surrounding skin (central capillary dilatation, a wheal and a surrounding flare). If the flare reaction persists in an anaesthetic area of skin, the lesion must be proximal to the posterior root ganglion – i.e. it is probably a root avulsion. With a postganglionic lesion, the test will be negative because nerve continuity between the skin and the dorsal root ganglion is interrupted.

Computed tomography (CT) myelography or *magnetic resonance imaging (MRI)* may show pseudomeningoceles produced by root avulsion.

The type of damage

In postganglionic lesions it helps to know how severely the nerve has been damaged. With low-velocity injuries, a period of observation is justified; neurapraxia and axonotmesis should show signs of recovery by 6 or 8 weeks. If neurotmesis seems likely, early operative exploration is called for.

Management

The patient is likely to be admitted to a general unit where fractures and other injuries will be given priority. Emergency surgery is required for brachial plexus lesions associated with penetrating wounds, vascular injury or severe (high-energy) soft-tissue damage, whether open or closed; clean-cut nerves should be repaired or grafted. This is best performed by a team specializing in this kind of work.

All other closed injuries are left until detailed examination and special investigations have been completed. Patients with root avulsion or severe, mutilating injuries of the limb will be unsuitable for nerve surgery, at least until the prognosis for limb function becomes clear.

Progress of the neurological features is carefully monitored. As long as recovery proceeds at the expected rate, watchful observation is in order. If recovery falters, or if special investigations suggest neurotmesis, the patient should be referred to a special centre for surgical exploration of the brachial plexus and nerve repair, grafting or a nerve transfer procedure. The sooner this decision is made, the better: during the early days, operative exposure is easier and the response to repair more reliable. Repairs performed after 2 or 3 months are much less likely to succeed.

Prognosis

Pure upper plexus lesions have the best prognosis. Hand function is spared and muscles innervated from the upper roots often recover after plexus repair or nerve transfer. With avulsion of C7, C8 and T1, even if shoulder and elbow movements are restored, the loss of hand function causes severe disability.

Late reconstruction

If the patient is not seen until very late after injury, or if plexus reconstruction has failed, tendon transfers may restore a moderate level of function.

OBSTETRICAL BRACHIAL PLEXUS INJURIES

Obstetrical palsy is caused by excessive traction on the brachial plexus during childbirth. Three patterns are seen: (1) upper root injury (*Erb's palsy*), typically in overweight babies with shoulder dystocia at delivery; (2) lower root injury (*Klumpke's palsy*), usually after breech delivery of smaller babies; and (3) *total plexus injury*.

> ⚠️ **Prolonged labour and/or shoulder dystocia:**
> Examine for brachial plexus injury.

Clinical features

The diagnosis is usually obvious at birth: after a difficult delivery the baby has a floppy or flail arm. Further examination a day or two later will define the type of brachial plexus injury.

Erb's palsy is caused by injury of C5, C6 and (sometimes) C7. The abductors and external rotators of the shoulder as well as the forearm supinators are paralysed. The arm is held to the side, internally rotated and pronated.

Klumpke's palsy is due to injury of C8 and T1. The baby lies with the arm supinated and the elbow flexed; there is loss of intrinsic muscle power in the hand. Reflexes are absent and there may be a unilateral Horner's syndrome.

With a *total plexus injury* the baby's arm is flail and pale; all finger muscles are paralysed and there may also be vasomotor impairment and a unilateral Horner's syndrome.

X-rays should be obtained to exclude fractures of the shoulder or clavicle, which can be mistaken for obstetrical palsy.

Management

Over the next few weeks, one of the following may happen:

- *Paralysis may recover completely.* Upper root lesions often recover spontaneously. A reliable indicator is return of biceps activity by the third month.
- *Paralysis may improve and then remain static.* A total lesion may partially resolve, leaving the infant with either an upper or a complete root syndrome which is unlikely to change.
- *Paralysis may remain unaltered.* This is more likely with complete lesions, especially in the presence of Horner's syndrome.

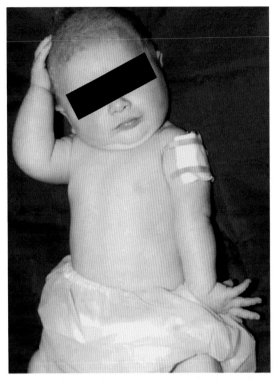

11.5 Erb's palsy Paralysis of the abductors and external rotators of the shoulder, as well as the forearm supinators, results in the typical posture demonstrated in this baby with Erb's palsy of the left arm.

While waiting for recovery, physiotherapy is applied to keep the joints mobile.

Treatment

If there is no biceps recovery by 3 months, operative intervention should be considered. Unless the roots are avulsed, it may be possible to excise the scar and bridge the gap with free sural nerve grafts; if the roots are avulsed, nerve transfer may give a worthwhile result. This is advanced surgery which should be undertaken only in specialized centres.

The shoulder is prone to fixed internal rotation and adduction deformity. If diligent physiotherapy does not prevent this, a subscapularis release will be needed, sometimes supplemented by a tendon transfer. In older children, the deformity can be treated by rotation osteotomy of the humerus.

LONG THORACIC NERVE

The nerve to serratus anterior may be damaged in shoulder or neck injuries, or by carrying heavy loads on the shoulder.

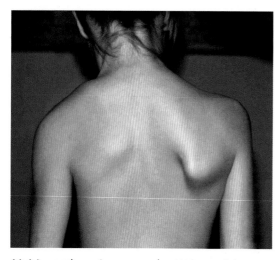

11.6 Long thoracic nerve palsy Winging of the scapula is demonstrated by the patient pushing forwards against the wall. If the serratus anterior is paralysed, the scapula cannot be held firmly against the rib-cage.

The classic sign of serratus anterior palsy is winging of the scapula. This is displayed by asking the patient to push forwards forcefully against a wall.

Except after direct injury or division, the nerve usually recovers spontaneously, though this may take a year or longer.

SPINAL ACCESSORY NERVE

The spinal accessory nerve supplies the sternomastoid muscle and then runs obliquely across the posterior triangle of the neck to innervate the upper half of the trapezius. Because of its superficial course, it is easily injured in stab wounds and operations in the posterior triangle of the neck.

Following an open wound or operation, the patient complains of pain in the shoulder and weakness on abduction of the arm. There is mild winging of the scapula on active abduction against resistance. In late cases there may be wasting of the trapezius and drooping of the shoulder.

Stab injuries and operative injuries should be explored immediately and the nerve repaired. If the exact cause of injury is uncertain, it is prudent to wait for 6 weeks for signs of recovery. If this does not occur, the nerve should be repaired or grafted.

AXILLARY NERVE

The axillary nerve (C5) is sometimes injured during shoulder dislocation or fractures of the humeral neck. The patient cannot abduct the shoulder (even when pain subsides) owing to deltoid weakness. There may be a small patch of numbness over the deltoid (C5 dermatome).

The nerve usually recovers spontaneously, but if there is no sign of recovery by 8 weeks and electrodiagnostic tests suggest denervation, the nerve should be explored and grafted. A good result can be expected if surgery is performed within 12 weeks of injury.

RADIAL NERVE

The radial nerve may be injured at the elbow, in the upper arm or in the axilla.

Low lesions are usually due to fractures or dislocations at the elbow, or an open wound or surgical accident. The patient cannot extend the metacarpophalangeal joints.

High lesions occur with fractures of the humerus or after prolonged tourniquet pressure. They are also seen in patients who fall asleep with the arm dangling

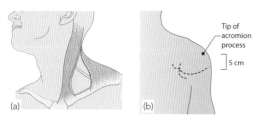

11.7 Dangerous landmarks (a) The accessory nerve runs across the middle of the posterior triangle of the neck and is easily damaged during lymph node biopsy in this area. (b) The axillary nerve runs from behind the shoulder around the outer aspect of the arm about 5 cm below the tip of the acromion process. Incisions across the top of the shoulder must stop short of this level if injury to the axillary nerve is to be avoided.

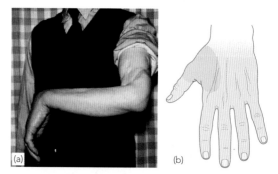

11.8 Radial nerve palsy (a) This man developed a complete drop-wrist palsy following a severe open fracture of the humerus and division of the radial nerve. (b) The typical area of sensory loss.

over the back of a chair (Saturday night palsy). There is an obvious wrist-drop due to weakness of the wrist extensors and a small patch of sensory loss on the back of the hand at the base of the thumb.

Very high lesions are usually due to pressure in the axilla ('crutch palsy'). The triceps muscle is wasted and paralysed.

For injuries caused by pressure (a crutch, tourniquet, Saturday night palsy, fractured humerus), the lesion is usually an axonotmesis and spontaneous recovery is the rule. One can therefore afford to wait. However, if there is no sign of recovery by 8–12 weeks, the nerve should be explored and repaired or grafted.

Open wounds should be explored and the nerve repaired or grafted as soon as possible.

With a fractured humerus, if it is certain that there was no nerve injury on admission and the signs appear only after manipulation or operative treatment, the chances of an iatrogenic injury are high and the nerve should be explored and repaired.

In all cases, while recovery is awaited, the wrist should be splinted in extension and the metacarpophalangeal and finger joints kept moving.

In radial nerve lesions that do not recover, the disability can be largely overcome by suitable tendon transfers.

ULNAR NERVE

Injuries of the ulnar nerve are usually either near the wrist or near the elbow, although open wounds may damage it at any level.

Low lesions may be caused by pressure (e.g. from a deep ganglion) or a laceration at the wrist. There is hypothenar wasting and the hand is clawed due to paralysis of the intrinsic muscles. Finger abduction is weak, and the loss of thumb adduction makes pinch difficult (see Figure 11.9(c) for Froment's test). Sensation is lost over the ulnar one and a half fingers.

High lesions occur with elbow fractures; they are also seen (much later) if malunion produces marked cubitus valgus with tension on the nerve where it skirts the medial epicondyle. Remember that ulnar nerve symptoms can also be caused by nerve entrapment in the cubital tunnel, especially in patients lying for long periods with the elbows flexed and pressing on the bed. Curiously, the visible deformity is not marked, because the ulnar half of flexor digitorum profundus is paralysed and the fingers are therefore less 'clawed'. Otherwise motor and sensory loss are the same as in low lesions.

Exploration and suture of a divided ulnar nerve are more easily achieved than with most other nerves; large gaps can be bridged because one can gain length by transposing the nerve to the front of the elbow. If recovery does not occur, hand function is significantly impaired because of the loss of power in metacarpophalangeal flexion, finger abduction, pinch and grip. Tendon transfers are possible, but usually restore only a modest level of function.

MEDIAN NERVE

The median nerve is commonly injured near the wrist or high up in the forearm.

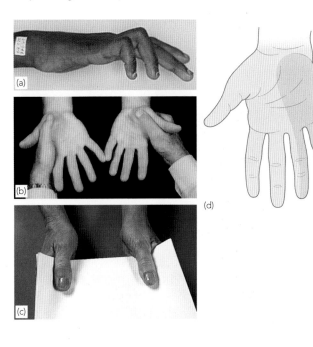

11.9 Ulnar nerve palsy (a) Clawing of the ring and little fingers and wasting of the intrinsic muscles. (b) A good test for interosseous muscle weakness. Ask the patient to spread their fingers (abduct) as strongly as possible and then force the hands together with the little fingers apposed; the weaker side will collapse (the left hand in this case). (c) Froment's sign: the patient is asked to grip a card firmly between thumbs and index fingers; normally this is done using the thumb adductors while the interphalangeal joint is held extended. In the right hand, because the adductor pollicis is weak, the patient grips the card only by acutely flexing the interphalangeal joint of the thumb (flexor pollicis longus is supplied by the median nerve). (d) Typical area of sensory loss.

Low lesions may be caused by cuts in front of the wrist or by carpal dislocations. The thenar eminence is wasted and thumb abduction and opposition are weak. Sensation is lost over the radial three and a half digits, and trophic changes may be seen.

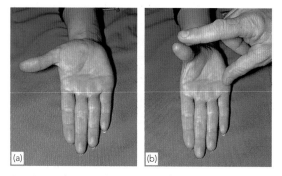

11.10 Median nerve – testing for abductor power (a) The hand must remain flat, palm upwards. (b) The patient is told to point the thumb towards the ceiling against the examiner's resistance.

High lesions are generally due to forearm fractures or elbow dislocation, but stabs and gunshot wounds may damage the nerve at any level. The signs are the same as those of low lesions but, in addition, the long flexors to the thumb, index and middle fingers are paralysed.

If the nerve is divided, suture should always be attempted; if this cannot be done without producing tension, nerve grafts can be placed in the gap. If no recovery occurs, disability is severe – mainly because of sensory loss. Tendon transfer can restore thumb opposition, but useful function depends on having sensation as well.

NERVE INJURIES AFFECTING THE LOWER LIMB

FEMORAL NERVE

The femoral nerve may be injured by a gunshot wound, by traction during an operation or by bleeding into the thigh. There is weakness of knee extension (quadriceps) and numbness of the anterior thigh and medial aspect of the leg. The knee jerk is depressed.

This is a disabling lesion and early treatment is essential. A thigh haematoma may need to be evacuated. A clean cut of the nerve may be treated successfully by careful suturing or grafting.

SCIATIC NERVE

Division of the main sciatic nerve is rare except in gunshot wounds or operative (iatrogenic) accidents. Traction and compression are more common and occur with local trauma.

The patient complains of foot-drop, numbness and paraesthesia in the leg and foot; if there has been direct injury to the nerve, the limb may also be painful. Muscles below the knee are paralysed and sensation is absent in most of the leg. If only the deep (peroneal) component of the nerve is affected, paralysis is incomplete and the signs are easily mistaken for those of a common peroneal nerve injury. Late features are wasting of the calf and trophic ulcers.

If the nerve injury follows hip dislocation or fracture, this must be attended to urgently. Open wounds should be explored and the nerve repaired. While recovery is awaited, a drop-foot splint should be fitted.

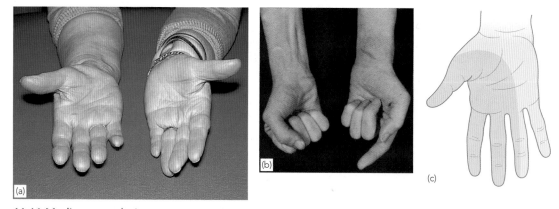

11.11 Median nerve lesions (a) Wasting of the thenar eminence on the right side. (b) In high median nerve lesions, the long flexors to the thumb and index fingers are also paralysed and the patient shows the 'pointing index sign'. (c) Typical area of sensory loss.

The chances of recovery are generally poor and, at best, it will be long delayed and incomplete. Partial lesions can sometimes be managed by tendon transfers. However, if there is no recovery whatever, amputation may be preferable to a flail, deformed, insensitive limb.

Iatrogenic lesions

Sciatic nerve palsy is one of the recognized complications of hip replacement. Usually it is a partial lesion, which is sometimes misdiagnosed as a common peroneal compression injury. There is little to guide one as to whether the sciatic injury is due to direct trauma or to traction on the nerve. If direct injury is suspected, the nerve should be explored. Otherwise it is best to wait for spontaneous recovery, which may take several weeks. In all cases the foot should be splinted to prevent a permanent equinus deformity.

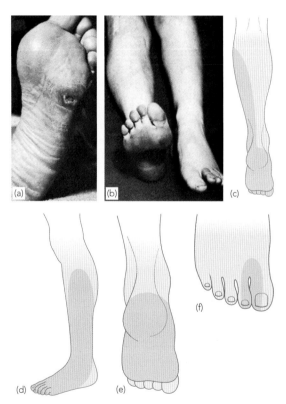

11.12 Sciatic and peroneal nerve lesions (a) One of the late complications is trophic ulceration due to loss of sensibility in the foot. (b) Loss of dorsiflexion causes foot-drop. Characteristic areas of sensory loss are shown: (c) complete sciatic nerve injury; (d) common peroneal nerve injury; (e) posterior tibial nerve injury; and (f) anterior tibial (deep peroneal) nerve injury.

PERONEAL NERVES

The *common peroneal nerve* may be damaged in lateral ligament injuries when the knee is forced into varus, or by pressure from a splint or a plaster cast, or from lying with the leg externally rotated. The patient develops a drop-foot in which both dorsiflexion and eversion are weak, causing a tendency to trip and fall while walking. Sensation is lost over the front and outer half of the leg and the dorsum of the foot.

If only the *superficial branch* is involved, the peroneal muscles are paralysed and eversion is lost, but dorsiflexion is intact. There is loss of sensation over the outer side of the leg and foot.

The *deep branch* may be threatened in an anterior compartment syndrome (see page 353). The patient complains of pain, abnormal sensation and weakness of dorsiflexion; on testing, there may be an area of sensory loss around the first web space on the dorsum of the foot.

Treatment depends on the local circumstances. A threatened compartment syndrome must be treated as an emergency and may need immediate decompression. If there is an open wound, the nerve should be explored and sutured.

While recovery is awaited, a splint is worn to control the foot-drop; the skin must be protected against ulceration. If recovery does not occur, disability can be improved by transferring the tibialis posterior tendon to the dorsum of the foot (so that it acts as a dorsiflexor); alternative solutions are operative stabilization of the hindfoot or else permanent splintage.

> ⚠ Following hip surgery, symptoms and signs of 'peroneal nerve injury' are usually, in fact, due to partial sciatic nerve injury.

NERVE ENTRAPMENT SYNDROMES

Wherever peripheral nerves traverse fibro-osseous tunnels, they are at risk of entrapment or compression, especially if the soft tissues increase in bulk, as they may in pregnancy, myxoedema or rheumatoid arthritis, or if there is a local obstruction (e.g. a ganglion or osteophytic spur). The most common sites are the *carpal tunnel* at the wrist (median nerve) and the *cubital tunnel* at the elbow (ulnar nerve). Less common sites are the *radial tunnel* in the forearm as the posterior interosseous nerve enters supinator muscle, the *tarsal tunnel* below the ankle (posterior tibial nerve) and the lateral part of the *inguinal ligament* (lateral cutaneous nerve of the thigh). A special case is the *thoracic outlet*, where the subclavian vessels and trunks of the brachial plexus cross the first rib between the scalenus anterior and medius muscles. In these cases there may be vascular as well as neurological signs in the upper limb.

Patients with long-standing, mild, possibly unrecognized, polyneuropathies (for example due to diabetes or alcohol abuse) are particularly prone to symptoms of localized nerve compression. A general neurological assessment is therefore advisable in all patients with features of local nerve compression.

Clinical features

The patient complains of unpleasant tingling or pain or numbness in the territory of the compressed nerve. Symptoms are usually intermittent and related to specific postures which compromise the nerve. Areas of altered sensation, motor weakness and muscle wasting are so characteristic that the diagnosis and the site of compressive trauma are immediately suggested. The clinical features of altered peripheral nerve function are described in the preceding pages.

The likely site of compression should be carefully examined for any local cause – for example in ulnar nerve entrapment a long-standing valgus deformity of the elbow, or in the carpal tunnel syndrome an old Colles' fracture.

The diagnosis may be confirmed by measuring nerve conduction velocity, which is likely to be impaired in the affected segment of the nerve. It is well to remember, though, that this test is not infallible and it should not be used as substitute for careful clinical assessment.

Treatment

In early cases, simple measures such as advising the patient to avoid compromising postures of the affected limb, or preventing flexion of the wrist or elbow with a light-weight splint, may help. If an inflammatory disorder is suspected, corticosteroid injection into the entrapment area can reduce local tissue swelling. The condition is often self-limiting, so there is no hurry about operative treatment. If symptoms persist, or if there is muscle weakness and wasting, operative decompression is indicated. Once axonal degeneration occurs, tunnel decompression may fail to give complete relief.

CARPAL TUNNEL SYNDROME

This is the most common compressive neuropathy, caused by compression of the median nerve beneath the transverse carpal ligament. It is described in detail in Chapter 15.

ULNAR NERVE COMPRESSION

At the elbow

Compression of the ulnar nerve usually occurs behind the medial epicondyle at the elbow. It usually occurs spontaneously, more commonly in middle-aged men (as opposed to carpal tunnel syndrome which is more common in women). It is sometimes associated with a post-traumatic valgus deformity of the elbow or swelling from arthritis. Most patients complain only of a tingling sensation in the fifth and the ulnar side of the fourth finger; this is most likely to occur when the elbow is held flexed for long periods or when leaning on the inner side of the flexed elbow.

On examination there is usually a positive Tinel's sign when percussing the nerve behind the elbow (but beware: even normal people may experience sharp 'tingling' when they suffer a bump on the 'funny bone' at the medial edge of the elbow – so always examine the normal side for comparison). Objective numbness and weakness in the ulnar nerve distribution denotes axonal damage; in that case the nerve should be decompressed, and sooner rather than later.

Treatment may simply be a matter of avoiding the provocative posture; in more refractory cases, and always if there is established numbness or muscle wasting, the nerve should be released through an incision behind the epicondyle. If the nerve is unstable it can be gently transposed in front of the epicondyle.

At the wrist

The ulnar nerve is occasionally compressed as it runs in front of the wrist just radial to the pisiform. The cause is usually a ganglion from the underlying joint, but neurological symptoms may also be produced by external pressure – e.g. in cyclists who lean too heavily on their handlebars. MRI may define a local compressive lesion; the nerve can then be carefully explored and any causal pathology removed.

THORACIC OUTLET SYNDROME

Neurological and vascular symptoms and signs in the upper limbs may be produced by compression of the lower trunk of the brachial plexus (C8 and T1) and subclavian vessels between the clavicle and the first rib. These neurovascular structures are made taut when the shoulders are braced back and the arms held tightly to the sides; an extra rib (or its fibrous equivalent extending from a large costal process) exaggerates this effect by forcing the vessel and nerve upwards. Such anomalies are present at birth, yet symptoms are rare before the age of 30. This is probably because, with increasing age, the shoulders sag, thus putting more traction on the neurovascular bundle.

Clinical features

The patient, typically a woman in her 30s, complains of pain and paraesthesiae extending from the shoulder, down the ulnar aspect of the arm and into the medial two fingers. Symptoms tend to be worse at night and are also aggravated by bracing the shoulders (wearing a back-pack) or working with the arms above shoulder height. Examination may show weakness and slight wasting of the intrinsic muscles in the hand. Vascular signs are uncommon, but there may be cyanosis, coldness of the fingers and increased sweating.

Symptoms and signs can sometimes be reproduced by certain provocative manoeuvres. In *Adson's test* the patient's neck is extended and turned towards the affected side while he or she breathes in deeply; this compresses the interscalene space and may cause paraesthesia and obliteration of the radial pulse. In *Wright's test* the arms are abducted and externally rotated; again, the symptoms recur and the pulse disappears on the abnormal side.

Investigations

X-rays of the neck occasionally demonstrate a cervical rib or an abnormally long C7 transverse process. However, similar features are sometimes encountered as purely incidental findings in asymptomatic people, and the demonstration of a cervical rib should not be taken as 'proof positive' of a thoracic outlet problem. Equally important are x-rays of the lungs (is there an apical tumour?) and the shoulders (to exclude any local lesion).

Electrodiagnostic tests are helpful mainly to exclude peripheral nerve lesions such as ulnar or median nerve compression which may confuse the diagnosis.

Angiography and *venography* are reserved for the few patients with vascular symptoms.

Diagnosis

The diagnosis of thoracic outlet syndrome is not easy. Indeed, some clinicians doubt its very existence as a pathological entity!

Tumours of the lower cervical cord or cervical vertebrae and compressive lesions affecting the lower cervical nerve roots must always be excluded. The presence of Horner's syndrome is a valuable clue.

Cervical spondylosis is sometimes discovered on x-ray. However, this seldom involves the T1 nerve root.

Pancoast's syndrome, due to apical carcinoma of the bronchus with infiltration of the structures at the root of the neck, includes pain, numbness and weakness of the hand. A hard mass may be palpable in the neck, and x-ray of the chest shows a characteristic opacity.

Ulnar nerve compression can be excluded by electromyography and nerve conduction studies.

Treatment

Conservative treatment suffices for most patients: exercises to strengthen the shoulder-girdle muscles; postural training; instruction in work practices; and other ways of preventing shoulder droop and muscle fatigue. Analgesics may be needed for pain.

Operative treatment is indicated if pain is severe, if muscle wasting is obvious or if there are vascular disturbances. The thoracic outlet is decompressed by removing the first rib (or the cervical rib). This can be accomplished by either a supraclavicular approach or a transaxillary approach.

CHAPTER 12

PRINCIPLES OF OPERATIVE TREATMENT

The art and skill of orthopaedic surgery is directed not to constructing a particular arrangement of parts but to restoring function to the whole. The operation is only part of this exercise; orthopaedic 'surgery' also involves careful preoperative preparation and planning as well as postoperative rehabilitation.

PREOPERATIVE PREPARATION

General assessment of the patient

The need for general assessment of the patient and their ability to tolerate the operation goes without saying. It is important also to evaluate the risk of complications such as thromboembolism and infection in the particular individual and, where necessary, to start prophylactic treatment before the operation.

Planning the operation

Operations must be carefully planned in advance, when accurate measurements can be made and the bones and joints can be compared for symmetry with those of the opposite side. X-rays, magnetic resonance imaging (MRI) and computed tomography (CT) (if necessary with three-dimensional re-formation) are helpful; templates may be needed to help select the appropriate shape and size of a prosthetic implant; complex corrective osteotomies should ideally be simulated on paper cut-outs or manipulation of x-ray images before the operation is undertaken; best of all is a rehearsal of the operation using artificial bones and joints.

The operating environment

Short operating times and limiting the number of people in the theatre will reduce the likelihood of infection. Long and complex operations, joint replacement procedures and all operations in which the risk of tissue contamination or infection is considered to be high, should be performed in ultra-clean laminar airflow theatres and prophylactic antibiotics should be administered before, during and after the operation.

Some types of fracture surgery require intraoperative traction. Operating tables designed for this purpose, as well as intraoperative limb manipulation and positioning, should be available.

Surgical equipment

The minimum requirements for orthopaedic operations are drills (for boring holes), osteotomes (for cutting cancellous bone), saws (for cutting cortical bone), chisels (for shaping bone), gouges (for removing bone) and plates, screws, wires and screwdrivers (for fixing bone).

Operations such as joint replacement, spinal fusion and internal fixation require special implants and instruments. It is very unwise to attempt these operations without gaining familiarity with the equipment and practising beforehand on dry specimens. Equally important, it is the surgeon's responsibility to ensure that all

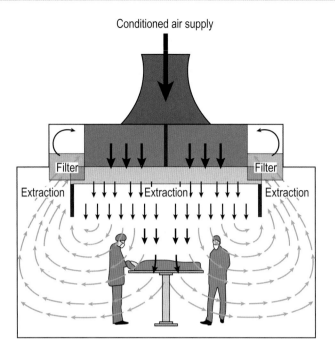

Conditioned air supply

Filter

Filter

Extraction

Extraction

Extraction

12.1 Ultra-clean operating theatre ventilation This is an important theatre environment for implant surgery in orthopaedics. Conditioned air is cleaned by high efficiency particulate air (HEPA) filters; an air flow and extraction stream is created to ensure that ingress of air from outside is resisted and there are at least 25 air exchanges per hour.

the special equipment needed for the intended procedure is available in the theatre before starting the operation. The types, sizes and right/left side conformance of implants should be checked well before the operation day.

Intraoperative radiography

Intraoperative radiography and image intensification are often helpful and sometimes essential. Fracture reduction, osteotomy alignments and the positioning of implants and fixation devices can be checked during the operation and often again at the end of the procedure.

Magnification

Magnification is an integral part of peripheral nerve and hand surgery. The improved view minimizes the trauma of surgery and allows more accurate apposition of tissues during reconstruction. Operating loupes or microscopes can be used for nerve repair or vascular anastomoses.

The 'bloodless field'

Many operations on limbs can be performed more rapidly and accurately if bleeding is prevented by the application of a tourniquet. Only a *pneumatic cuff* is suitable. Rubber bandages are potentially dangerous; the pressure beneath the bandage cannot be controlled and there is a risk of damage to the underlying nerves and muscle. A layer of wool bandage beneath the pneumatic cuff will distribute the pressure and prevent wrinkling of the underlying skin.

Adequate exsanguination of the tissues can usually be achieved by elevating the limb to 60 degrees above horizontal for 30 seconds before inflating the tourniquet cuff. If a completely bloodless field is required then an Esmarch rubber bandage wrapped from distal to proximal is effective. A Rhys Davies rubber tubular exsanguinator is equally effective.

Tourniquet pressure should not exceed 150 mmHg above systolic for the lower limb and 100 mmHg above systolic for the upper limb.

Tourniquet time should not exceed 2 hours. Time can be saved by ensuring that the limb is shaved, prepared, draped and marked before inflating the cuff. Whenever practicable the tourniquet should be removed before the wound is closed, so that bleeding can be controlled and a 'silent' postoperative haematoma avoided. *Excessive or prolonged pressure can cause permanent nerve or muscle damage.*

A tourniquet should not be used if the patient has peripheral vascular disease.

The WHO Surgical Safety Checklist

The World Health Organization (WHO) has issued a surgery checklist which should be performed in three stages: when the patient arrives for anaesthesia, just before the start of the operation and just after completion – time-points designated as 'sign in', 'time out' and 'sign out'.

The risks of inaccurate siting of the operation, harm from retention of instruments or swabs, patient allergies, blood loss or anaesthetic issues and absence of relevant imaging are significantly reduced by adopting this system. The list is easily available online.

Infection prophylaxis

Use of prophylactic antibiotics is routine for almost all orthopaedic procedures and is one of the items in the WHO surgical safety checklist. General measures including skin cleaning with antiseptic solutions such as 2% chlorhexidine in 70% alcohol, impermeable drapes, appropriate surgical attire and keeping the patient warm during the operation.

Thromboembolism prophylaxis

Deep vein thrombosis (DVT) is the commonest complication of lower limb surgery and – in a small percentage of cases – the prelude to *pulmonary embolism* (PE) which can be fatal. Some patient groups are at greater risk than others: elderly people with hip fractures; those who are obese or immobile; those with a previous history of thrombosis; or those with active cancer. This subject is dealt with on page 162.

OPERATIONS ON BONES

FIXATION OF BONE SEGMENTS AND FRACTURES

Fixation of separated bone segments – whether produced intentionally (osteotomy) or by trauma (fracture) – is a fundamental part of bone surgery. It provides stability, assists segmental re-union,

holds anatomical position and enables the patient to resume activity (although not necessarily weightbearing). This can be performed by either *internal fixation* or *external fixation*.

Internal fixation

Fixation is achieved by using screws, plates (held on by screws), intramedullary nails, stiff wires or malleable cerclage wires. Compression plates are designed to hold the segments forcibly together; bridging plates simply align the segments.

Internal fixation is particularly useful for treating fractures in elderly patients, for multiple injuries and for fractures which are prone to displacement and malunion. Scrupulous asepsis and meticulous technique are imperative.

Intramedullary nails are metal rods inserted into the medullary canal across two bone segments. There are two varieties; those with holes through which screws can be inserted to lock the nail to the bone segment (interlocking nails) and those without. Interlocking nails are the standard type but non-interlocking nails are sometimes used in paediatric practice, e.g. flexible intramedullary nails and telescopic nails.

External fixation

Fractures associated with severe soft-tissue injuries are often best managed by external fixation. The principles are straightforward: metal pins or tensioned wires are driven through the bone above and below the fracture; the fracture is reduced and the pins or wires are attached to external bars or rings which hold the system rigidly while leaving the soft tissues exposed and accessible for treatment. There are numerous variations in pin and frame configuration, aiming to provide

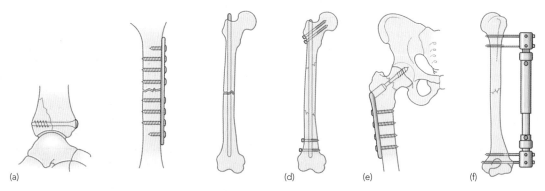

12.2 Bone fixation Several methods of fixation are used, depending on site and circumstances. (a) A lag screw for interfragmentory compression. (b) Plate and screws. (c) Intramedullary nail. (d) Locked intramedullary nail. (e) Dynamic hip screw. (f) External fixator.

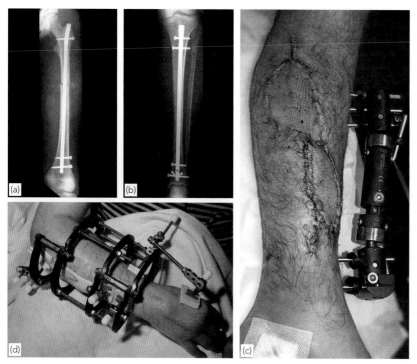

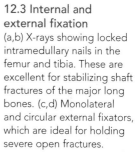

12.3 Internal and external fixation (a,b) X-rays showing locked intramedullary nails in the femur and tibia. These are excellent for stabilizing shaft fractures of the major long bones. (c,d) Monolateral and circular external fixators, which are ideal for holding severe open fractures.

the best mechanical structure for the particular problem. Modifications in design have extended the use of external fixation to the management of non-union, bone elongation, repair of bone defects and correction of deformities (see page 155).

OSTEOTOMY

Osteotomy may be used to correct deformity, to change the shape of the bone, or to relieve pain in arthritis by redirecting the load trajectories. Preoperative planning is essential, with precise measurements of the patient and the x-rays. The site of the osteotomy, the amount of bone to be removed (if any), the degree of angular and rotational correction and the proposed method of fixation should be firmly established beforehand.

To change an angular deformity a wedge of bone may have to be removed (a 'closing wedge' which slightly shortens a long bone) or inserted (an 'opening wedge' which slightly lengthens the bone). A 'neutral' effect can be achieved by making the osteotomy dome shaped (see Figure 12.4). The size of the wedge should be calculated accurately and reproduced precisely by using suitable templates. The bone segments are then fixed in the new position, either with a plate and screws or (at the proximal and distal ends of the femur) with an angled blade-plate and screws.

When correcting severe deformities, care should be taken not to put excessive tension on the soft tissues as this may cause nerve damage. *Postoperatively a careful watch should be kept for signs of compartment compression due to oozing from the cut bone surfaces into the surrounding tissues* (see page 353). Partial weightbearing is allowed if fixation is stable; otherwise it is deferred until healing is sufficiently advanced.

An alternative approach is to divide the bone and then apply an adjustable external fixation device which will permit progressive correction over time (see below).

BONE GRAFTS

Bone grafts are both *osteoinductive* and *osteoconductive*, i.e. they are able to stimulate osteogenesis and they also provide linkage across defects and a scaffold upon which new bone can form.

Osteoinduction is a property carried by stem cells and growth promoters from bone marrow content in the graft; the cells differentiate (and stimulate other stem cells in the receiving area to do the same) into osteoprogenitor cells which form bone.

The conductive capability is through the collagen scaffold within bone. Cancellous grafts are more rapidly incorporated into host bone than

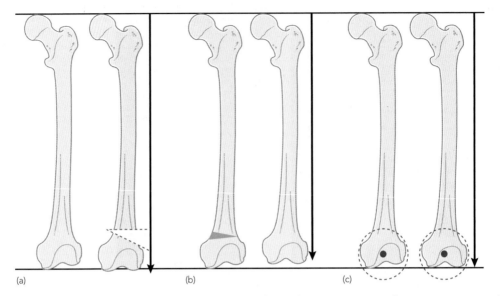

12.4 Corrective osteotomy Angular corrections can be performed by creating a cut and (a) prising open a wedge (open wedge), (b) removing a wedge of bone (closing wedge) or (c) making a curved cut and rotating one segment to achieve angular correction (dome osteotomy). Open wedge osteotomies increase the overall length of the bone, closing wedge procedures reduce length and dome osteotomies have no residual effect (a neutral 'wedge').

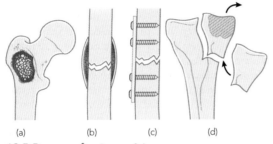

12.5 Bone grafts Some of the more common applications are illustrated. (a) Chip grafts to fill a cavity. (b) On-lay strips of cancellous bone (Phemister technique). (c) On-lay cortical graft. (d) Cadaveric osteocartilaginous graft obtained fresh and sterile from an organ donor. Vascularized grafts can be transferred from one part of the skeleton to another.

Cancellous autografts can be obtained from the thicker portions of the ilium, the greater trochanter, the proximal metaphysis of the tibia, the lower radius, the olecranon, or from an excised femoral head. Bone marrow aspirates from the iliac crest are also used for their osteoinductive function. The number of stem cells decreases with age and more so in females. Centrifugation of the aspirate in order to concentrate the cells shows an improved effect in animal studies.

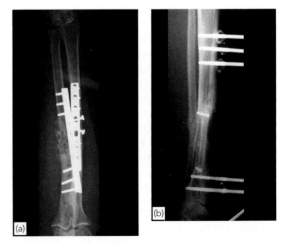

12.6 Bone grafts X-rays showing: (a) autogenous chips filling a defect in the ulna; and (b) a vascularized fibular graft used to fill a long defect in the tibia.

cortical grafts, but sometimes the greater strength of cortical bone is needed to provide structural integrity.

Autografts

In these, bone is taken from one site to another in the individual. They are the most commonly used grafts and serve to induce new bone formation and bridge defects. This form of grafting is highly successful as long as the harvested bone is of good quality and the recipient area is clean, vascular and has tissue that will respond to the graft.

Cortical grafts can be harvested from any convenient long bone or from the iliac crest; they usually need to be fixed with screws, sometimes reinforced by a plate, and can be placed on the host bone, or inlaid.

The ideal autograft is one with an intact blood supply. Bone is transferred complete with its blood vessels, which are anastomosed to vessels at the recipient site. The technique is difficult and time consuming, requiring microsurgical skill. Available donor sites include the iliac crest (complete with one of the circumflex arteries), the fibula (with the peroneal artery) and the radial shaft. Vascularized grafts remain completely viable and become incorporated by a process analogous to fracture healing.

Allografts (homografts)

This bone is transferred from an individual (alive or dead) to another of the same species. It is available in large quantities, can take the form of anatomically preserved bone segments (e.g. whole segments of femur) and can be held in a bone bank for use when needed. Control over sterility, transfer of infection and antigenicity (being from a different individual) are issues that need to be overcome. Antigenicity is believed to be reduced by freezing or freeze-drying, by demineralization or by ionizing radiation.

In practice, allografts are used in revision joint replacement surgery (where loss of bone stock is a common problem) and for reconstruction after bone tumour excision. The graft must always be harvested under sterile conditions and the donor must be cleared for malignancy, venereal disease, hepatitis and human immunodeficiency virus (HIV).

Synthetic substitutes

Calcium-derived pastes or granules are available for use to stimulate healing across defects. These usually consist of calcium sulphate, calcium phosphate or calcium hydroxyapatite. Almost all are primarily osteoconductive and they vary in strength properties and their rate of reabsorption. They are often mixed with autografts to increase the bulk of graft or improve their osteoinductive capability. A new use for these synthetic grafts is as a depot for antibiotics; the grafts are mixed with antibiotics and placed into cavities which then receive high antibiotic concentrations over a period through elution.

Bone morphogenetic protein (BMP) is a synthetic osteoinductive agent. BMP-2 and BMP-7 are available for use in non-unions and open fractures but remain costly.

DISTRACTION HISTIOGENESIS AND LIMB RECONSTRUCTION

Distraction histiogenesis is a technique for creating new bone in response to gradual distraction applied across an osteotomy or fracture site. It was discovered and researched by Gavril Ilizarov in Russia in the 1960s and has become established as the *Ilizarov method*. This is now used: (a) for limb lengthening; (b) to fill a gap in the bone by gradually 'transporting' a healthy segment of bone to a new position while new bone forms in its wake; or (c) to correct intractable deformities.

Patients should be warned that these procedures take months rather than weeks and carry a risk of complications such as pin-track infection, angulatory deformity, fracture and non-union.

Ilizarov techniques should be employed only by surgeons who have undergone training in this method.

Bone lengthening

A neat fracture is created through the bone, followed by a short wait (5–10 days) before the young callus is gradually distracted by traction on the bone via a circular or monolateral external fixator. Distraction proceeds at 1 mm a day, with small (usually 0.25 mm) increments spaced out evenly. New callus can be seen on the x-ray after 3 weeks; in optimum conditions, it forms an even column in the gap between the bone fragments (this is called the *regenerate*). If the distraction rate is too fast, or the osteotomy performed poorly, the regenerate may be thin with an hourglass appearance; conversely if distraction is too slow it may appear bulbous, or worse still, may consolidate prematurely, thereby preventing any further lengthening. When the desired length is reached, a second waiting period follows which allows the regenerate callus to consolidate and harden. The external fixator remains in place and weightbearing is permitted throughout this period. When cortices of even thickness appear in the regenerate, the fixator can be removed. Throughout treatment, physiotherapy is important to preserve joint movement and avoid contractures.

In children, bone lengthening can be achieved by distracting the physis (chondrodiatasis). No osteotomy is needed and the distraction rate is slower, usually 0.25 mm twice daily. Although a wide, even column of regenerate is usually seen, the fate of the physis is sealed; it frequently closes after the process and for this reason the technique is best reserved for children close to the end of growth.

155

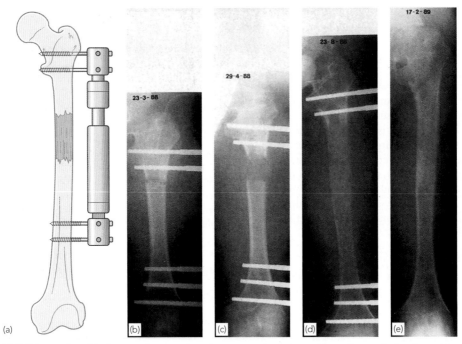

12.7 Distraction histiogenesis Bone lengthening can be achieved by callotasis (callus 'stretching'). (a) A distracting external fixator is applied; the bone is then osteotomized and the fragments are gradually dragged apart over a period of months. (b–e) Serial x-rays show the progress over a period of 11 months. In this case, lengthening of 10 cm was achieved.

Bone transport

The same principle is applied as a means of treating non-union and filling defects in bone. *Bone transport* allows a defect (or gap) to be filled in gradually by creating a 'floating' segment of bone through a corticotomy either proximal or distal to the defect, and slowly moving the isolated segment of bone across the gap. As the segment is transported from the corticotomy site to the new docking site, it leaves a trail of regenerate new bone behind it. An external fixator provides stability during this process.

Correcting bone deformities and joint contractures

Angular bone deformities can usually be corrected by carefully planned closing or opening wedge osteotomies. However, the degree of correction

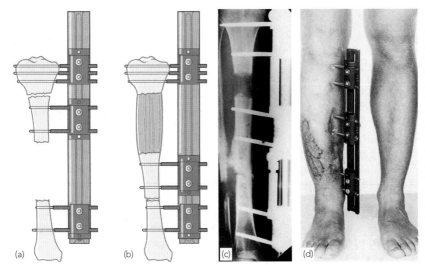

12.8 Bone transport
(a) Bone loss may leave a gap in the shaft. Proximal osteotomy and callotasis allows a segment of the diaphysis to be moved distally until it 'docks' with the distal fragment (b). The resulting gap gradually fills first with callus and then with new bone. (c) The x-ray shows the situation at the end of transport and docking. (d) The entire system is stabilized by some type of external fixation and the patient is able to walk about during the long transport period.

is limited by the effect on soft-tissue tension, in particular nerves. With the Ilizarov method, it is now possible to undertake large corrections with much lower risk to the soft tissues. Length, rotation and translation deformities can be dealt with simultaneously by adjusting the traction wires and frame. Even intractable club-foot deformities can now be treated in this manner.

LEG LENGTH EQUALIZATION

Inequality of leg length may result from many causes, including congenital anomalies, malunited fractures, epiphyseal and physeal injuries, infections and paralysis. Inequality of less than 2.5 cm may be accepted by the patient or can be managed by fitting a small shoe-raise. Larger inequalities usually require some type of surgical correction – shortening the longer leg or lengthening the shorter leg.

Shortening the longer leg

During childhood, growth in the normal leg can be stopped by arresting the activity of the growth plates around the knee; this can be temporary, using removable staples fixed across the physes, or permanent, by excavating the physes and replacing them with bone grafts (epiphysiodesis). Timing of surgery is vital: the expected rate of change in leg length difference can be predicted by reference to suitable charts or tables and the operation is timed to provide limb length equality at skeletal maturity.

In adults a piece of bone can be excised and the approximated ends held by internal fixation. Shortening should be advised only if the patient's residual height will still be acceptable. It should also be remembered that, since the longer leg is usually the normal one, if a serious complication such as non-union ensues, the patient may end up worse off than before.

Lengthening the shorter leg

Limb lengthening by the Ilizarov method is an appropriate solution for predicted length discrepancies of greater than 5 cm. Major length corrections can be tackled by staging the treatment process over several years. Patients should be warned that treatment will be prolonged and often painful.

OPERATIONS ON JOINTS

INJECTIONS

It is often necessary to enter a joint with a sterile needle, either to aspirate fluid or to instil something into the joint. This barely qualifies as an 'operation'; however, it is an invasive procedure and it is well to remember that it carries some of the same risks as a 'real' operation, especially the risk of infection.

Aspiration may be purely diagnostic (e.g. in the management of suspected joint infection) or partly therapeutic (e.g. relief of a tense haemarthrosis).

Injection also is used for diagnostic purposes (e.g. the instillation of radio-opaque fluid for arthrography); usually, though, it means injection of an antibiotic or corticosteroid preparation into an infected or inflamed joint, or around neighbouring soft tissues. Corticosteroid injections should not be repeated more than three times over a period of 6 months. Although the injected preparation is regarded as a 'depot steroid', some of it is absorbed and systemic effects are usual. *All intra-articular injections should be performed with full aseptic precautions.*

ARTHROSCOPY

Arthroscopy is performed for both diagnostic and therapeutic purposes. Almost any joint can be reached but the procedure is most usefully employed

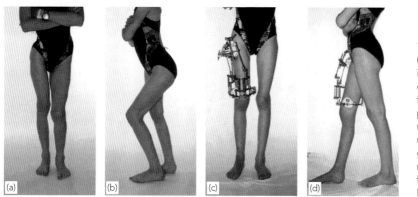

12.9 Leg lengthening (a,b) Following a childhood infection of the right hip and destruction of the proximal femoral epiphysis, this patient ended up with marked shortening of the right femur and an awkward gait. (c,d) Here she is seen, markedly improved, after femoral lengthening by the Ilizarov method.

157

in the shoulder, elbow, wrist, finger joints, knee, and hip. If a definite abnormality is demonstrated, and is amenable to corrective surgery, it can often be dealt with at the same sitting without the need for an open operation. However, arthroscopy is an invasive procedure and its mastery requires skill and practice; it should not be used simply as an alternative to clinical examination and imaging.

The instrument is basically a rigid telescope fitted with fibreoptic illumination. Tube diameter ranges from about 2 mm (for small joints) to 4–5 mm (for the knee). It carries a lens system that gives a magnified image. The eyepiece allows direct viewing by the arthroscopist, but it is more convenient to fit a small, sterilizable solid-state television camera which produces a picture of the joint interior on a television monitor.

The procedure is best carried out under general anaesthesia. The joint is distended with fluid and the arthroscope is introduced percutaneously. Instruments such as probes, curettes, forceps and nibblers can be inserted through other skin portals and used to help expose less accessible parts of the joint, to obtain biopsies and to perform operations such as soft-tissue releases, joint debridement, meniscal and labral tears and capsular repairs. At the end of the procedure the joint is washed out and the small skin wounds are sutured. The patient is usually able to return home later on the same day.

Arthroscopy is safe but not entirely free of complications, the commonest of which are haemarthosis, thrombophlebitis, infection and joint stiffness.

ARTHROTOMY

Arthrotomy (opening a joint) may be indicated: (1) to inspect the interior or perform a synovial biopsy; (2) to drain a haematoma or an abscess; (3) to remove a loose body or damaged structure (e.g. a torn meniscus); and (4) to excise inflamed synovium. The intra-articular tissues should be handled with care, and if postoperative bleeding is expected (e.g. after synovectomy) a drain should be inserted. Following the operation the joint should be rested for a few days, but thereafter movement should be encouraged.

JOINT FUSION (ARTHRODESIS)

Painful, worn or unstable joints can be treated by fusion; indeed, this is often the treatment of choice if the resulting rigidity will not severely compromise function. Examples include the spine, tarsus, wrist and interphalangeal joints. Even major joints like the knee, hip or shoulder are suitable for fusion if a joint replacement is unsafe or unpredictable in outcome, e.g. in flail joints where muscle control is absent.

The operative principles are straightforward: the joint surfaces are denuded of cartilage and sometimes the subchondral bone is 'feathered' to increase the contact area; then the prepared surfaces are apposed in the optimum position and held rigidly by some form of internal or external fixation. Sometimes (especially in large joints) bone grafts are added to promote osseous bridging. The area is protected from excessive load stresses until union is complete (3–6 months).

The main *complication* is non-union and the formation of a pseudoarthrosis. Rigid fixation lessens this risk; where feasible (e.g. the knee and ankle), the bony parts are squeezed together by compression–fixation devices.

Arthrodesis of the hip carries the risk of late 'secondary' complications due to abnormal loading of the knee (especially if the hip is fused in a little too much adduction or abduction) and chronic backache due to compensatory postural changes which compensate for the loss of hip movement.

JOINT REPLACEMENT

Total joint replacement has been one of the triumphs of modern orthopaedic surgery. From the

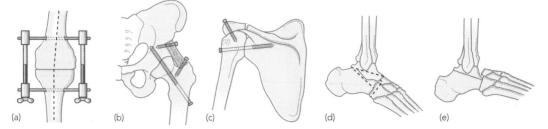

12.10 Arthrodesis (a) Compression arthrodesis. (b) Screw plus bone graft. (c) Similar technique using the acromion. (d,e) Subtalar and midtarsal fusion.

earliest development of total hip replacement in the 1950s by McKee and Farrar, and its perfection by Charnley 10 years later, this was envisaged as the ideal way of treating painful, destructive joint disorders. Several difficult problems had to be overcome: the prosthetic implants had to replicate the joint anatomy; they had to be durable; they had to move with minimal friction; they had to be firmly fixed to the skeleton; and they had to be made of inert materials which would not provoke any unwanted reaction in the tissues. The usual low frictional articular combinations are metal on high density polyethylene, metal on ceramic, or ceramic on ceramic.

Fixation is achieved in one of two ways: (a) putty-like methylmethacrylate cement is applied firmly to the exposed metaphyseal bone surface and the implant is then embedded in the cement and held there until the methylmethacrylate polymerizes and hardens; the cement acts as a grouting material which fills the spaces between the implant and the bone and penetrates into interstices on the bone surface; (b) the alternative method is to prepare the bone bed to a predetermined shape and size and then press-fit the implant snugly to the bone without cement. In neither case is there a true bond between implant and bone. Various modifications of implant design and surface coating have helped to reduce the long-term problem of implant loosening, but most important of all is sound technique.

Total joint replacement has been most successful in the hip and knee. Similar principles have been applied to replacement operations for the shoulder, elbow and ankle, with less satisfactory long-term results.

Partial joint replacement is sometimes preferred. Only one articular surface is replaced, the implant then articulating with an unmodified opposite articular surface; or one compartment of the joint (e.g. the medial compartment of the knee is replaced if only that part is affected).

EXCISION ARTHROPLASTY

Sometimes the elected option is to excise the articular ends of the bones forming a joint, without implanting any type of prosthetic replacement. This sounds drastic and in practice excision arthroplasty is reserved for situations where a more anatomical solution is either unnecessary (e.g. excision of the trapezium for carpometacarpal osteoarthritis – page 195) or inadvisable, perhaps because of intractable joint infection. Sufficient bone is excised to create a gap where movement can occur. In Girdlestone's arthroplasty of the hip (a 'last resort' when previous operations have failed or the joint has been irremediably destroyed), the femoral head and neck are excised, leaving a false articulation (pseudarthrosis) between the upper end of the femur and the side wall of the pelvis. The 'joint' is obviously unstable but, because of local fibrosis and the stabilizing effect of powerful surrounding muscles, the patient can still take weight on that side and can walk about, albeit with a marked limp.

SOFT-TISSUE OPERATIONS

RELEASE OF JOINT CONTRACTURES

Joint contractures can be apparent at birth (e.g. in a club-foot deformity) or may occur after prolonged disuse of a limb (e.g. in paralytic disorders) or inappropriate splintage. If mild and not long-standing, they can be corrected by physiotherapy and regular stretching exercises. More established or severe contractures require open release of the joint capsule and lengthening of tendons that traverse the joint on the affected side.

Tendon lengthening is performed by creating a step-cut division of the tendon or by dividing that portion of the tendon that lies within the muscle belly.

TENDON TRANSFERS

Tendon transfers are used to restore movement that has been lost because of muscle injury or paralysis. An adjacent tendon with function that can be more easily sacrificed can be re-routed; even one serving antagonistic movement (e.g. a normal flexor to replace a paralysed extensor) may be acceptable, although postoperative rehabilitation is at first more difficult.

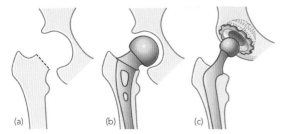

12.11 Arthroplasty The main varieties, as applied to the hip, are illustrated here. (a) Excision arthroplasty (Girdlestone); (b) partial replacement with an Austin–Moore prosthesis; (c) total replacement using a polyethylene implant for the socket and a metal implant for the femoral head and neck.

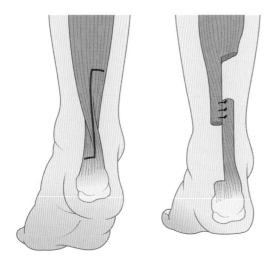

12.12 Tendon lengthening Tendons can be lengthened by performing a step-cut division of the main tendon and allowing the two parts to slide along each other.

Tendon transfers work best if the muscle is strong, the transfer is performed in as direct a route as possible and the function is complementary with that of the replaced tendon.

REPAIR OF NERVES, TENDONS AND LIGAMENTS

Lacerations, avulsions and ruptures of nerves, tendons and ligaments can follow sharp and blunt injuries. Direct repair is possible if the two ends can be approximated without tension. If this is not feasible, a graft is interposed between the two ends (intercalary graft).

Ligaments are more usually repaired late and may need to be reconstructed using a substitute material, whether this be a tendon graft or artificial material. A common example is reconstruction of the anterior cruciate ligament of the knee.

MICROSURGERY

Microsurgical techniques are used in repairing nerves and vessels, transplanting bone with a vascular pedicle, and – occasionally – for re-attaching a severed digit or part of a limb. Essential prerequisites are an operating microscope, special instruments, microsutures, a chair with arm supports and – most of all – a surgeon well practised in microsurgical techniques.

For *replantation*, the severed part should be kept cool during transport. The more muscle in the amputated part, the shorter the period it will last; a finger tip may survive for 24 hours, a forearm only a few hours. Two teams dissect, identify and mark each artery, nerve and vein of the stump and the limb. Following careful debridement the bones are shortened to reduce tension and fixed together by wires, nails or plates. Next the vessels are sutured – veins first and (if possible) two veins for each artery. A vessel of 1 mm diameter needs seven or eight circumferential sutures! Nerves and tendons next need suturing; only healthy ends of approximately equal diameter should be joined; tension, kinking and torsion must be prevented. Decompression of skin and fascia, as well as thrombectomy, may be needed in the postoperative period.

Replantation surgery is time consuming, expensive and often unsuccessful. It should be carried out only in centres specially equipped, and by teams specially trained, for this work.

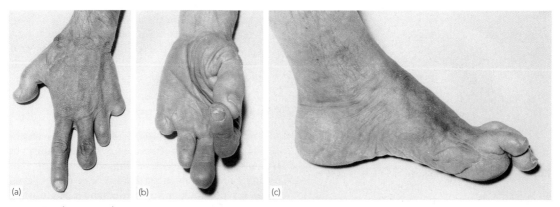

(a)   (b)   (c)

12.13 Replantation by microsurgery This guillotine operator lost several fingers and (most importantly) his thumb. The crucial prehensile functions – pinch and grasp – were restored by transplanting his left big toe to the remaining thumb stump (a,b), with minimal loss of function in the foot (c).

COMPLICATIONS OF ORTHOPAEDIC OPERATIONS

Patients most vulnerable to postoperative complications are the very young and the elderly. Infants are susceptible to hypothermia and surgery in very young babies calls for steps to prevent heat loss. Internal fixation of femoral neck fractures and joint replacement operations are most often performed on older people, who are likely to have other medical disorders, usually respiratory or cardiac; this increases the risk of postoperative problems.

Swelling

This is common after limb surgery and may be aggravated by prolonged tourniquet use. Tight bandages and casts make it worse. Steps should be taken to prevent this problem:

■ See that dressings are snug but not tight.
■ Avoid using circumferential casts after operation – a split cast or plaster slab is better.
■ Keep the limb elevated.
■ Encourage early movement of neighbouring joints.

Be on the watch for a *compartment syndrome*, which will necessitate emergency surgery (see page 353).

Haematoma formation

A haematoma can interfere with wound healing and poses an increased risk of infection. Haemostasis (checking that the operation field is dry just prior to wound closure) is an important step. A tourniquet can be deflated just before wound closure and all bleeding points dealt with. Some surgeons may prefer to close the wound with the tourniquet inflated but it is important that they deal with any cut vessels during the procedure to minimize bleeding after tourniquet deflation, even if there is a snug bandage applied over the wound. Suction drainage after limb surgery is a mixed blessing and its true efficacy is still uncertain; while it may reduce the development of a haematoma it also increases the risk of infection. If drains are used, they should be removed after 24 hours and no later.

Delayed wound healing

Causes of delayed healing are a poor peripheral circulation, dissection through scarred areas, wound closure under tension, haematoma formation, and poor nutritional status of the patient.

Infection

Although the incidence of infection is low, this is the most serious complication. If related to an implant (internal fixation or joint replacement) it may herald failure of the procedure and require a revision operation. This subject is dealt with in Chapter 2.

Thromboembolism

Venous thromboembolism (VTE), the commonest complication of lower limb surgery, comprises three

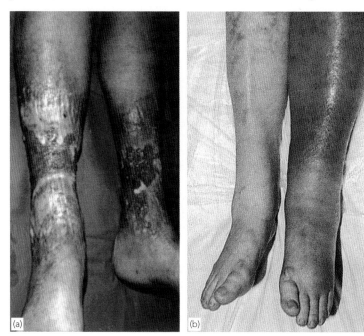

(a) (b)

12.14 Venous thromboembolism
(a) Chronic venous insufficiency.
(b) Acute thrombophlebitis.

associated disorders: *DVT*, *PE* and the late onset of *chronic venous insufficiency*. If preventative measures are not used, the incidence of symptomatic DVT/PE after joint replacement surgery is probably in the region of 5%, and of *fatal pulmonary embolism* (FPE) between 0.25 and 0.5%. In major trauma and in elderly patients with hip fractures the risk of FPE is greater – probably around 1%. It occasionally occurs after major shoulder and elbow surgery but is vanishingly rare after hand and wrist surgery. It sometimes also occurs after knee arthroscopy and in patients wearing a below-knee plaster cast.

The most important *general risk factors* are a family history, increasing age, obesity, and a history of previous thrombosis.

Pathophysiology

Thrombosis results from an interaction between vessel wall damage, alterations in blood components and venous stasis. Following major orthopaedic operations, there is activation of the coagulation cascade and restricted fibrinolysis lasting for several days. During hip replacement, femoral vein blood flow is temporarily interrupted when the acetabulum and femoral medulla are exposed. There is also more prolonged stasis as the patient recovers from surgery and begins to mobilize.

DVT most often affects the veins of the calf, and less often the proximal veins of the thigh and pelvis. It is from the larger thrombi that fragments sometimes break off and get carried (i.e. embolize) to the lungs, where they may result in sudden death.

Clinical features and diagnosis

Asymptomatic DVT is probably quite common. When clinical features appear, they usually consist of pain in the calf or thigh but the first sign may be sudden shortness of breath or even death from PE. Following trauma or operation, even those patients who do not complain should be examined regularly for swelling, soft-tissue tenderness and a sudden slight increase in temperature and pulse rate. The diagnosis can be confirmed by ascending venography, but this is an invasive procedure; nowadays duplex ultrasound scanning is regarded as the diagnostic technique of choice.

Patients with symptomatic DVT, and also asymptomatic patients who develop pain in the chest, shortness of breath or haemoptysis, should be examined for signs of PE. The diagnosis can be confirmed by ventilation–perfusion (V/Q) scanning or preferably by spiral CT.

Chronic venous insufficiency occurs some years after a symptomatic DVT; it is caused by reflux of blood through the damaged veins. The patient presents with leg discomfort, swelling, skin changes and/or frank ulceration. The diagnosis is usually obvious. This is a debilitating condition which places huge demands on health resources.

Prevention

The risk of DVT and PE can be reduced by both physical and pharmacological methods.

Physical methods vary from simple routines such as elevation of the foot of the bed, use of graduated elastic stockings and early mobilization to more sophisticated contrivances like the application of *intermittent plantar venous compression by foot-pump* or *intermittent pneumatic compression of the leg*. The use of *spinal or epidural anaesthesia* also reduces the incidence of DVT by improving venous blood flow and possibly by a local fibrinolytic effect.

Pharmacological methods can effectively reduce the risk of VTE but must be used with care to avoid the equally troublesome alternative problem of bleeding. *Low-molecular-weight heparin* has, until recently, been the preferred pharmacological method for most surgeons. It is given subcutaneously a few hours postoperatively and continued until the patient is fully weightbearing and no longer at risk of VTE. Dose adjustment and monitoring are not required. Randomized studies have shown that it effectively reduces the prevalence of venographic DVT in hip and knee replacement surgery, knee arthroscopy and in patients with plaster casts. *Warfarin* has been widely used in the past; it is much less popular now in Europe although it still has a keen following in the USA. Drawbacks are the difficulty in establishing appropriate dosage levels and the need for constant monitoring; there is also a risk of interaction with other drugs and alcohol. *Aspirin* probably provides a small reduction in the rate of PE after surgery; used alone it is ineffective.

There are now oral agents which interfere directly in the clotting cascade by inhibiting Factor Xa or thrombin. These drugs are very effective in reducing VTE after major joint surgery, are easy to give by daily tablet and require no monitoring. They are becoming the agents of choice.

The risk of thrombosis persists for at least 5 weeks after hip surgery and 2 weeks after knee surgery; the death rate after hip replacement does not return to 'normal' until 3 months. Thromboprophylaxis should be prolonged until the risk of VTE has diminished, which usually means after discharge from hospital.

Treatment of thromboembolism

Whenever possible, the clinical diagnosis of DVT or PE should be confirmed by imaging – ideally ultrasound (otherwise venography) for DVT, and spiral CT (otherwise V/Q) for PE – before treatment is started. This is important because the clinical diagnosis of these complications is notoriously unreliable and full therapeutic anticoagulation carries a high complication rate soon after major surgery.

Once the diagnosis of DVT has been confirmed, treatment is started with a loading dose of 5000 units of heparin intravenously. This is followed by a daily weight-adjusted dose of low-molecular-weight heparin subcutaneously. Warfarin is started with a loading dose of 10 mg daily for 3 days. Thereafter the dose is adjusted until the international normalized ratio (INR) is prolonged and stable at 2.0–3.0 times the control value; the heparin is then discontinued. If low-molecular-weight heparin is not available, unfractionated heparin can be given by continuous intravenous infusion, or twice daily subcutaneously, adjusted to maintain the activated partial thromboplastin time (APTT) at 1.5–2 times normal. The new oral agents are likely to provide an alternative way of treating VTE.

Acute, severe PE demands cardiorespiratory resuscitation, vasopressors for shock, oxygen, and a large intravenous dose (15,000 units) of heparin. Streptokinase is used both to dissolve clots and to prevent more forming. Emergency pulmonary thrombectomy may be considered. Anticoagulant treatment is continued for at least 6 months.

COMPLICATIONS ASSOCIATED WITH JOINT REPLACEMENTS

Hip and knee replacements are usually performed on older patients, many of whom have generalized arthritis or systemic disorders. Consequently the *general complication rate* is by no means trivial; DVT is more common than with other types of surgery. There are also a number of *local complications* which are peculiar to total hip replacement. Factors that may contribute to their development include previous hip operations, severe deformity and inadequate 'bone stock'.

Intra-operative complications include bone perforation or even fracture of the femur or acetabulum. Special care should be taken with patients who are very old or osteoporotic.

Sciatic nerve palsy (usually due to traction but occasionally caused by direct injury) occurs in about 2% of patients undergoing total hip replacement. Most patients recover spontaneously but if there is reason to suspect nerve damage the area should be explored.

Postoperative dislocation is rare if the prosthetic components are correctly placed.

Heterotopic bone formation around the hip is seen in about 20% of patients 5 years after joint replacement. The cause is unknown, but patients with skeletal hyperostosis and ankylosing

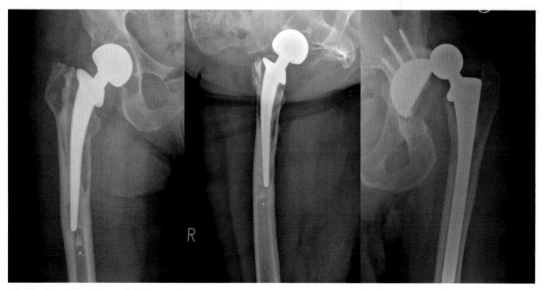

12.15 Complications of joint replacements X-rays showing examples of infection, loosening and dislocation following hip joint replacements. (Courtesy of Mr G. Kumar.)

spondylitis are particularly at risk. In severe cases this is associated with pain and stiffness. Ossification can be prevented in high-risk patients by giving either a course of non-steroidal anti-inflammatory drugs for 3–6 weeks postoperatively or a single dose of irradiation to the hip.

Aseptic loosening of one or both components occurs mainly in the hip and (to a lesser extent) in the knee. With modern methods of implant fixation, there is likely to be radiographic evidence of loosening in about 10% of patients 10 years after operation. At microscopic level many stable implants show cellular reaction and membrane formation at the bone–cement interface; fortunately, only a fraction of these are symptomatic. Pain may be a feature, especially when first taking weight on the leg after sitting for a while, but the diagnosis usually rests on x-ray signs of progressively increasing radiolucency around the implant, fracturing of cement, movement of the implant or periprosthetic bone resorption. Radionuclide scanning shows increased activity in the bone around the implant. If symptoms are marked, and particularly if there is evidence of progressive bone resorption, the implant and cement should be painstakingly removed and a new prosthesis inserted – either cemented or uncemented, depending on the condition of the bone.

Aggressive osteolysis is sometimes seen. It is associated with granuloma formation at the interface between cement (or implant) and bone. This is evidently due to a severe cellular reaction stimulated by shedding of cement, polyethylene or metal particles that find their way into the boundary zone around the implant and into the surrounding soft tissues, causing bone resorption and soft-tissue necrosis. Revision is usually necessary and this may have to be accompanied by impaction bone grafting.

Infection is the most serious postoperative complication. With adequate prophylaxis the risk should be less than 1%, but it is higher in the very old, in patients with rheumatoid disease or psoriasis, and in those on immunosuppressive therapy (including corticosteroids). Other predisposing factors are prolonged wound exposure, tissue damage and local haematoma formation. Haematogenous spread from a distant site may cause late infection.

Early wound infection sometimes responds to antibiotics. Later infection does so less well and may need operative 'debridement' followed by irrigation with antibiotic solution for 3–4 weeks, as well as systemic antibiotic treatment. Once the infection has cleared, a new prosthesis can be inserted, preferably without cement. An alternative, more applicable to 'mild' or 'dubious' infection, is a one-stage exchange arthroplasty using gentamicin-impregnated cement. The results of revision arthroplasty for infection are only moderately good. If all else fails, the implants and cement may have to be removed, leaving an excisional (Girdlestone) arthroplasty.

AMPUTATIONS

INDICATIONS

Colloquially speaking, the indications for amputation are remembered as the three Ds: *Dead, Dangerous and Damned nuisance.*

- *Dead or dying*: peripheral vascular disease accounts for almost 90% of all amputations. Other causes of tissue death are severe trauma, burns and frostbite.
- *Dangerous*: 'dangerous' disorders are malignant tumours, potentially lethal sepsis and crush injury. In crush injury, releasing the compression may result in renal failure (the crush syndrome).
- *Damned nuisance*: retaining the limb may be worse than having no limb at all – because of pain, gross malformation, recurrent sepsis or severe loss of function.

TYPES OF AMPUTATION

A *provisional amputation* may be necessary because primary healing is unlikely. The limb is amputated as distal as seems appropriate; skin flaps sufficient to cover the deep tissues are cut and sutured loosely over a pack. Re-amputation is performed when the stump condition is favourable.

Definitive endbearing amputation is performed when weight is to be taken through the end of a stump. Therefore the scar must not be terminal, and the bone end must be solid, not hollow, which means it must be cut through or near a joint. Examples are through-knee and through-ankle (Syme's) amputations.

Definitive non-endbearing amputations are the commonest variety. All upper limb and most lower limb amputations come into this category. Because weight is not to be taken at the end of the stump, the scar can be terminal.

AMPUTATIONS AT THE SITES OF ELECTION

Most lower limb amputations are for ischaemic disease and are performed through the site of

Look

- *Skin*: scars or sinuses are noted; don't forget the axilla!
- *Shape*: asymmetry of the shoulders, winging of the scapula, wasting of the deltoid or short rotators and acromioclavicular dislocation are best seen from behind; joint swelling or wasting of the pectoral muscles is more obvious from in front. Ask the patient to flex the elbow: the appearance of an unnatural bulge over the deltoid muscle is the classic sign of a ruptured biceps tendon.
- *Position*: if the arm is held persistently internally rotated, think of posterior dislocation of the shoulder.

Feel

Because the joint is well covered, inflammation rarely influences skin temperature. The soft tissues and bony points are carefully palpated, following a mental picture of the anatomy. Start with the sternoclavicular joint, then follow the clavicle laterally to the acromioclavicular joint, onto the anterior edge of the acromion and around the acromion to the back of the joint. The supraspinatus tendon lies just below the anterior edge of the acromion. Tenderness and crepitus can often be accurately localized to a particular structure.

Move

Active movements: the patient is asked to raise both arms sideways until the fingers point to the ceiling. Abduction may be: (1) difficult to initiate; (2) diminished in range; (3) altered in rhythm, the scapula moving too early and creating a shrugging effect.

If movement is painful, the arc of pain must be noted; pain in the mid range of abduction suggests

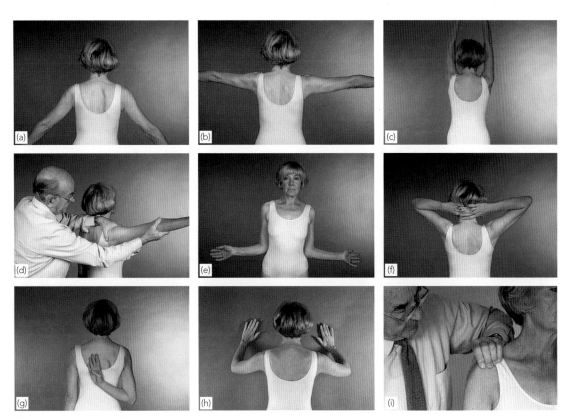

13.1 Examination Active movements are best examined from behind the patient, paying careful attention to symmetry and the co-ordination between scapulothoracic and glenohumeral movements. (a) Abduction; (b) limit of glenohumeral abduction; (c) full abduction and elevation, a combination of scapulothoracic and glenohumeral movement. (d) The range of true glenohumeral movement can be assessed by blocking scapular movement with a hand placed firmly on the top edge of the scapula. (e) External rotation. (f,g) Complex movements involving abduction, rotation and flexion or extension of the shoulder. (h) Testing for serratus anterior weakness. (i) Feeling for supraspinatus tenderness.

a rotator cuff tear or supraspinatus tendinitis; pain at the end of abduction is often due to acromioclavicular arthritis.

Flexion and extension are examined, asking the patient to raise the arms forwards and then backwards. To test adduction they are asked to move the arm across the front of the body. Rotation is tested: first, with the arms close to the body and the elbows flexed to 90 degrees, the hands are separated as widely as possible (external rotation) and brought together again across the body (internal rotation); then the patient is asked to clasp their fingers behind their neck (external rotation in abduction); then to reach up the back with their fingers (internal rotation in adduction).

Passive movements: these can be deceptive because even with a stiff shoulder the arm can be raised to 90 degrees by scapulothoracic movement. To test true glenohumeral abduction the scapula must first be anchored; this is done by pressing firmly down on the top of the shoulder with one hand while the other hand moves the patient's arm.

Power: the deltoid is examined while the patient abducts against resistance. To test serratus anterior (long thoracic nerve) ask the patient to push forcefully against a wall with both hands; if the muscle is weak, the scapula is not stabilized on the thorax and stands out prominently (*winged scapula*). Pectoralis major is tested by having the patient thrust both hands firmly into the waist. Any difference in muscle bulk between the two sides is noted at the same time.

Other systems: the cervical spine should be examined as it is a common source of referred pain. If the shoulder feels unstable, look for generalized joint laxity. If weakness is the main complaint, a neurological examination is needed.

IMAGING

At least two x-ray views should be obtained: an anteroposterior in the plane of the glenoid, and an axillary projection with the arm in abduction to show the relationship of the humeral head to the glenoid. Look for evidence of subluxation, or dislocation, joint space narrowing, bone erosion and calcification in the soft tissues. Special views can show the acromioclavicular joint and the subacromial space.

Magnetic resonance imaging (MRI) is useful to identify osteonecrosis of the humeral head, or a bone tumour. It can also identify labral tears and rotator cuff tears although the accuracy for these latter two is enhanced by combining the scan with arthrography. *Computed tomography (CT)* arthrography is an alternative.

Ultrasound is a simple and accurate test for identifying rotator cuff tears and calcific tendinitis. It can also be useful in guiding injections or aspirating calcific deposits in the rotator cuff.

ARTHROSCOPY

Arthroscopy is useful for diagnosing and treating subacromial impingement, intra-articular lesions, detachment of the glenoid labrum and rotator cuff tears.

DISORDERS OF THE ROTATOR CUFF

The commomest causes of pain around the shoulder are disorders of the rotator cuff, chiefly the rotator cuff syndrome, calcific tendinitis and adhesive capsulitis.

THE ROTATOR CUFF SYNDROME

The rotator cuff is a sheet of conjoined tendons closely applied over the shoulder capsule and inserting mainly into the greater tuberosity of the humerus (subscapularis is inserted into the lesser tuberosity). The cuff is made up of subscapularis in front, supraspinatus above and infraspinatus and teres minor behind (the 'rotator' muscles) which have an important function in stabilizing the head

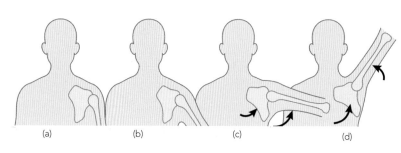

(a)   (b)   (c)   (d)

13.2 Abduction and elevation (a–c) During the early phase of abduction, most of the movement takes place at the glenohumeral joint. As the arm rises the scapula begins to rotate on the thorax (c). In the last phase of abduction, the movement is almost entirely scapulothoracic (d).

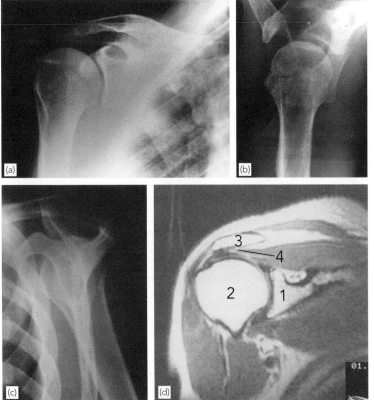

13.3 Imaging (a) Normal anteroposterior x-ray. (b) Axillary view showing the humeral head opposite the shallow glenoid fossa. (c) True lateral view; the head of the humerus should lie where the corocoid process, the spine of the scapula and the blade of the scapula meet. (d) MRI. Note: (1) the glenoid; (2) the head of the humerus; (3) the acromion process; and (4) the supraspinatus. The high signal in the supraspinatus suggests degenerative change.

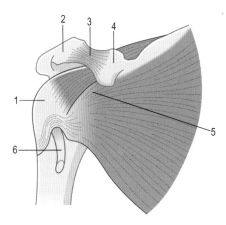

13.4 Anatomy The tough coracoacromial ligament stretches from the coracoid to the underside of the anterior third of the acromion process; the humeral head moves beneath this arch during abduction and the rotator cuff may be irritated or damaged as it glides in this confined space. (1, Rotator cuff; 2, acromion process; 3, coracoacrominal ligament; 4, coracoid process; 5, suscapularis; 6, long head of biceps.)

of the humerus by pulling it firmly into the glenoid whenever the deltoid lifts the arm forwards or sideways.

Arching over the cuff is a fibro-osseous canopy – the coracoacromial arch – formed by the acromion process posterosuperiorly, the coracoid process anteriorly and the coracoacromial ligament joining them. Separating the tendons from the arch and allowing them to glide, is the subacromial bursa. Normally, when the shoulder is abducted, the conjoint tendon passes under the arch. There should be enough room for it to do so, but if there is not, due to either pathology within the tendon (e.g. swelling from inflammation) or to narrowing of the space (e.g. by osteoarthritis of the acromioclavicular joint) then pain or awkward shoulder movement may result.

The commonest cause of pain around the shoulder is a disorder of the rotator cuff – the so-called *rotator cuff syndrome* – which comprises several conditions with distinct clinical features and natural history: *subacute tendinitis (painful arc syndrome); chronic tendinitis (impingement syndrome);* and *rotator cuff tears.*

171

Pathology

The differing clinical pictures stem from three basic pathological processes: degeneration, trauma and vascular reaction.

Degeneration: with advancing age, the cuff degenerates; minute tears develop, and there may be scarring, fibrocartilaginous metaplasia or calcium deposition. The common site is the 'critical zone' of the supraspinatus, the relatively avascular region near its insertion.

Trauma and impingement: the supraspinatus tendon is liable to injury if it contracts against firm resistance; this may occur when lifting a weight, or when using the arm to save oneself from falling. This is much more likely if the cuff is already degenerate. An insidious type of trauma is attrition of the cuff due to impingement against the coracoacromial arch during abduction. The long head of biceps also may be abraded to the point of rupture. Small tears of the cuff or the long head of biceps are found at autopsy in almost everyone aged over 60 years.

Vascular reaction: in an attempt to repair a torn tendon or to revascularize a degenerate area, new blood vessels grow in and calcium deposits are resorbed. This vascular reaction may cause congestion and pain.

These three pathological processes can be summed up as *'wear'*, *'tear'* and *'repair'*. In the young patient 'repair' is vigorous; consequently, healing is relatively rapid but (because the repair process itself causes pain) it is accompanied by considerable distress. The older patient has more 'wear' but less vigorous 'repair'; healing will be

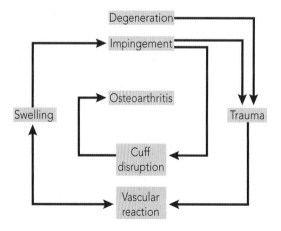

13.5 Pathological progression of rotator cuff lesions

slower but pain less severe. Thus acute tendinitis (which affects younger patients) is intensely painful but rapidly better; chronic tendinitis (a middle group) is only moderately painful but takes many months to recover and may be complicated by partial tears; and a complete tear (which generally occurs in the elderly) becomes painless soon after injury, but never mends.

Symptoms and signs

In all these conditions the patient is likely to complain of pain and/or weakness during certain movements of the shoulder. Pain may have started recently, sometimes quite suddenly, after a particular type of exertion; the patient may know precisely which movements now re-ignite the pain and which to avoid, providing a valuable clue to its origin. 'Rotator cuff' pain typically appears over the front and lateral aspect of the shoulder during activities with the arm abducted and medially rotated, but it may be present even with the arm at rest. Tenderness is felt at the anterior edge of the acromion.

Pain and tenderness directly in front along the deltopectoral boundary could be associated with the biceps tendon. Localized pain over the top of the shoulder is more likely to be due to acromioclavicular pathology, and pain at the back along the scapular border may come from the cervical spine. All these sites should be inspected for muscle wasting, carefully palpated for local tenderness and constantly compared with the opposite shoulder.

If there is weakness with some movements but not with others, then one must rule out a partial or complete tendon rupture; here again, as with pain, localization to a specific site is the key to diagnosis. In both cases clinical examination should include provocative tests to determine the source of the patient's symptoms:

- *The painful arc*: on active abduction scapulohumeral rhythm is disturbed and pain is aggravated as the arm traverses an arc between 60 and 120 degrees. Repeating the movement with the arm in full external rotation may be much easier for the patient and relatively painless.
- *Neer's impingement sign*: the scapula is stabilized with one hand while with the other hand the examiner raises the affected arm to the full extent in passive flexion, abduction and internal rotation, thus bringing the greater tuberosity directly under the coracoacromial arch. The test is positive when pain, located to the

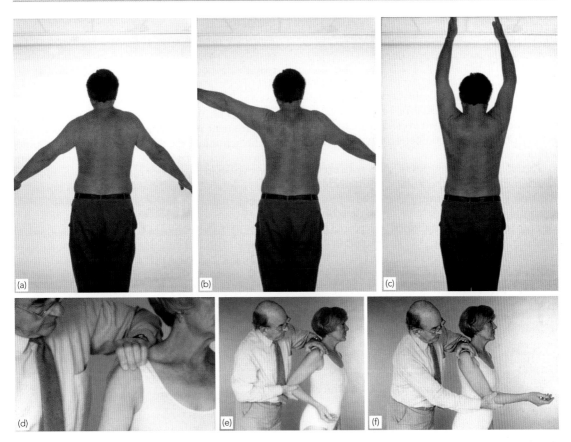

13.6 Supraspinatus tendinitis (a–c) The painful arc. During active abduction, the scapulohumeral rhythm is disturbed on the right and the patient starts to experience pain at about 60 degrees (a). As the arm passes beyond 120 degrees (b) the pain eases and the patient is able to abduct and elevate up to the full 180 degrees (c). (d–f) The tender spot is at the anterior edge of the acromion process. With the shoulder extended (e) tenderness is more acute. When the shoulder is flexed (f) the painful tendon disappears under the acromion process and tenderness disappears.

subacromial space or anterior edge of acromion, is elicited by this manoeuvre. If the previous manoeuvre is positive, it may be repeated after injecting 10 mL of 1% lidocaine into the subacromial space; if the pain is abolished (or significantly reduced), this will help to confirm the diagnosis.

Subacute tendinitis (painful arc syndrome)

The patient develops anterior shoulder pain after vigorous or unaccustomed activity, e.g. competitive swimming or a weekend of house decorating. The shoulder looks normal but is acutely tender along the anterior edge of the acromion. Point tenderness is most easily elicited by palpating this spot with the arm held in extension, thus placing the supraspinatus tendon in an exposed position anterior to the acromion

process; with the arm held in flexion the tenderness disappears.

Chronic tendinitis

The patient, usually aged between 40 and 50 years, gives a history of recurrent attacks of subacute tendinitis, the pain settling down with rest or anti-inflammatory treatment, only to recur when more demanding activities are resumed.

Characteristically pain is worse at night; the patient cannot lie on the affected side and often finds it more comfortable to sit up out of bed. Pain and slight stiffness of the shoulder may restrict even simple activities such as hair grooming or dressing. The physical signs for cuff impingement pain described above should be elicited.

A disturbing feature is coarse crepitation or palpable snapping over the rotator cuff when the shoulder is passively rotated; this may signify a partial tear or marked fibrosis of the cuff.

Rotator cuff tears

The most advanced stage of the disorder is progressive fibrosis and disruption of the cuff, resulting in either a partial or full thickness tear. The patient is usually aged over 45 years and gives a history of refractory shoulder pain with increasing stiffness and weakness.

Partial tears are not easily detected, even on direct inspection of the cuff. Continuity of the remaining cuff fibres permits active abduction with a painful arc, making it difficult to tell whether chronic tendinitis is complicated by a partial tear. If the diagnosis is in doubt, pain can be eliminated by injecting a local anaesthetic into the subacromial space. If active abduction is now possible the tear must be only partial. If active abduction remains impossible, then a complete tear is likely.

A *full thickness tear* may follow a long period of chronic tendinitis, but occasionally it occurs spontaneously after a sprain or jerking injury of the shoulder. There is sudden pain and the patient is unable to abduct the arm.

If some weeks have elapsed since the injury the two types are more easily differentiated. With a complete tear, pain has by then subsided and the clinical picture is unmistakable: active abduction is impossible and attempting it produces a characteristic shrug; but passive abduction is full and once the arm has been lifted above a right angle the patient can keep it up by using the deltoid (the 'abduction paradox'); when they lower it sideways it suddenly drops (the 'drop arm sign').

In long-standing cases of partial or complete rupture, secondary osteoarthritis of the shoulder may supervene and movements are then severely restricted.

Imaging

X-rays are usually normal in the early stages of the cuff dysfunction, but with chronic tendinitis there may be erosion, sclerosis or cyst formation at the site of cuff insertion on the greater tuberosity, or over-growth of the anterior edge of the acromion, thinning of the acromion process and upward displacement of the humeral head. Osteoarthritis of the acromioclavicular joint is common in older patients and in late cases the glenohumeral joint also may show features of osteoarthritis. Sometimes there is calcification of the supraspinatus but this is coincidental and not the cause of the pain.

MRI can effectively show cuff pathology but it should be remembered that up to one-third of asymptomatic individuals also have abnormalities of the rotator cuff on MRI. Changes on MRI always need to be correlated with the clinical examination.

Ultrasonography has comparable accuracy to MRI for identifying and measuring the size of full thickness and partial thickness rotator cuff tears, but is not as accurate in predicting the reparability of the tendons.

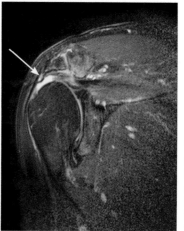

13.8 Rotator cuff tear – MRI High signal on MRI, indicating a full-thickness tear of the rotator cuff.

13.7 Acute calcification of supraspinatus The dense mass in the tendon (a) is gradually resorbed or dispersed into the subdeltoid bursa (b).

Treatment of rotator cuff syndrome

Conservative treatment

Uncomplicated impingement syndrome (or tendinitis) is often self-limiting and symptoms settle down once the aggravating activity is eliminated. Patients should be taught ways of avoiding the 'impingement position'. Physiotherapy, including ultrasound and active exercises in the 'position of freedom', may tide the patient over the painful healing phase. A short course of non-steroidal anti-inflammatory medication sometimes brings relief. If all these methods fail, and before disability becomes marked, the patient should be given one or two injections of depot corticosteroids into the subacromial space. In most cases this will relieve the pain and it is then important to persevere with protective modifications of shoulder activity for at least 6 months.

Healing is slow, and a hasty return to full activity will often precipitate further attacks of tendinitis.

Surgical treatment for impingement

If the patient has a useful range of movement, adequate strength and well-controlled pain, non-operative measures are adequate. If symptoms do not subside after 3 months of conservative treatment, or if they recur persistently after each period of treatment, an operation is considered preferable to prolonged and repeated treatment with anti-inflammatory drugs and local corticosteroids. The indication is more pressing if there are signs of a partial rotator cuff tear and in particular if there is good clinical evidence of a full thickness tear in a younger patient. The object is to decompress the rotator cuff (acromioplasty) by removing the structures pressing upon it – the coracoacromial ligament, the anterior part of the acromion process and osteophytes at the acromioclavicular joint. This can be achieved by open surgery or arthroscopically. If tears are encountered they can be repaired.

Arthroscopy allows good visualization inside the glenohumeral joint and therefore detection of other abnormalities which may cause shoulder pain. This

procedure also allows earlier rehabilitation than open surgery because there is no need to detach the deltoid muscle.

Repair of rotator cuff tears

The indications for operative repair of the rotator cuff are chronic pain, weakness of the shoulder and significant loss of function. The younger and more active the patient, the greater is the justification for surgery. The operation always includes acromioplasty as described above. The repair can be performed either by open techniques or by arthroscopy. Advantages of the arthroscopy include less soft-tissue damage, faster rehabilitation and a better cosmetic appearance.

Massive tears which cannot be approximated might be treated by decompression and debridement alone, or with tendon transfer or tendon grafts.

CALCIFIC TENDINITIS

Acute calcific tendinitis

Calcium hydroxyapatite crystals are deposited in the supraspinatus tendon, probably due to fibrocartilaginous metaplasia from local ischaemia. Calcification alone is probably not painful; symptoms, when they occur, are due to the florid vascular reaction which produces swelling and tension in the tendon. Resorption of the calcific material is rapid and it may soften or disappear entirely within a few weeks.

Clinical features

The condition affects 30–50 year olds. Aching, sometimes following over-use, develops and increases in severity within hours, rising to an agonizing climax. After a few days, pain subsides and the shoulder gradually returns to normal. In some patients the process is less dramatic and recovery slower. During the acute stage the arm is held immobile; the joint is usually too tender to permit palpation or movement.

X-rays

Calcification just above the greater tuberosity is always present. As pain subsides, the dense blotch lightens and may then disappear.

Treatment

If symptoms are not very severe the arm is rested in a sling and the patient is given a short course of non-steroidal anti-inflammatory medication. If pain is more intense then corticosteroid is injected into the subacromial space. Extracorporeal shockwave

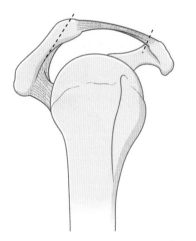

13.9 Impingement syndrome – surgical treatment The coracoacromial ligament and underside of the anterior third of the acromion are removed to enlarge the space for the rotator cuff. This can be performed by open surgery or arthroscopically.

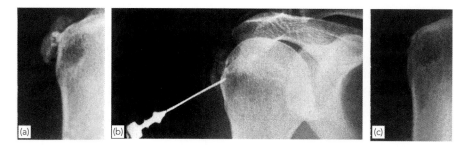

13.10 Acute calcification (a) Calcific deposit in the subdeltoid bursa. (b) Treatment by needle aspiration; best done under ultrasound control. (c) X-ray after treatment.

therapy, to disintegrate the calcium crystals, is also an effective option.

An alternative approach is to drain the pasty calcium deposit under ultrasound guidance (a process known as 'barbotage').

For patients with disabling or recurrent symptoms unresponsive to conservative measures, relief can be obtained by an operation to remove the calcific material. While this can be performed by open surgery, arthroscopy is preferable.

Chronic calcification

Asymptomatic calcification of the rotator cuff is common and often appears as an incidental finding in shoulder x-rays. When it is seen in association with the impingement syndrome, it is tempting to attribute the symptoms to the only obvious abnormality – supraspinatus calcification. However, the connection is spurious and treatment should be directed at the impingement lesion rather than the calcification.

ADHESIVE CAPSULITIS ('FROZEN SHOULDER')

The term *frozen shoulder* should be reserved for a well-defined disorder characterized by progressive pain and stiffness which usually resolves spontaneously

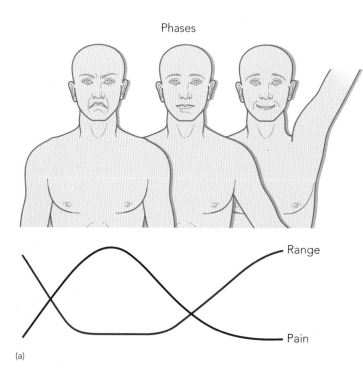

Phases

Range

Pain

(a)

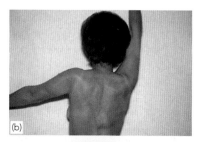

(b)

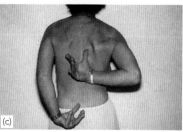

(c)

13.11 Frozen shoulder (a) Natural history of frozen shoulder. The face tells the story. (b,c) This patient has hardly any abduction but manages to lift her arm by moving the scapula. She cannot reach her back with her left hand.

after about 18 months. The cause and pathogenesis are still topics of heated debate.

The process probably starts in the same way as a chronic tendinitis but it then spreads to involve the entire cuff and joint capsule.

Clinical features

The patient, aged 40–60 years, may give a history of trauma, often trivial, followed by pain. Gradually it increases in severity and often prevents sleeping on the affected side. After several months it begins to subside, but as it does so stiffness becomes more and more of a problem. Untreated, stiffness persists for another 6–12 months. Gradually movement is regained, but may not return to normal.

Usually there is nothing to see except slight muscle wasting; there may also be some tenderness, but movements are always limited and in a severe case the shoulder is extremely stiff.

X-rays are normal. The main role of an x-ray is to exclude other causes of pain and stiffness.

Differential diagnosis

Post-traumatic stiffness

After any severe shoulder injury, stiffness (without much pain) may persist for some months. It is maximal at the start and gradually lessens, unlike the pattern of a frozen shoulder.

Disuse stiffness

If the arm is nursed overcautiously (e.g. following a wrist fracture) the shoulder may stiffen. Again, the characteristic pain pattern of a frozen shoulder is absent.

Regional pain syndrome

This condition, formerly known as *reflex sympathetic dystrophy*, may follow acute trauma; it is also seen in patients with myocardial infarction or a stroke. The features can be similar to those of a frozen shoulder.

Arthritis

Both rheumatoid arthritis and osteoarthritis can affect the shoulder, and either of these can develop bilaterally. The diagnosis is usually obvious on x-ray. In the case of rheumatoid arthritis, there may also be characteristic generalized symptoms and signs.

Treatment

Conservative treatment with analgesics, anti-inflammatory drugs, local heat and exercise aims at relieving pain and preventing further stiffening while recovery is awaited. The role of physiotherapy and steroid injections is unproven. Once the acute pain has subsided, manipulation under anaesthesia often hastens recovery. This can be accompanied by distending the joint with saline until the capsule ruptures. Active exercises should recommence immediately afterwards.

Operative treatment is occasionally called for. Arthroscopic division of the interval between supraspinatus and infraspinatus may dramatically improve the range of movement.

LESIONS OF THE BICEPS TENDON

TENDINITIS

Though not part of the rotator cuff, the tendon of long head of biceps lies adjacent to the rotator cuff and may be involved in the impingement syndrome. Rarely, it presents as an isolated problem in young people after unaccustomed shoulder strain. Pain and tenderness are sharply localized to the bicipital groove. Stressing the biceps tendon (resisted elbow flexion and supination) will provoke the pain.

Rest, local heat and deep transverse frictions usually bring relief; if recovery is delayed, a corticosteroid injection will help. For refractory cases, surgery is considered.

TORN LONG HEAD OF BICEPS

Degeneration and disruption of the tendon of long head of biceps is fairly common and is often associated with rotator cuff problems. The patient is usually middle-aged or elderly. While lifting a heavy object, he or she feels something snap; the

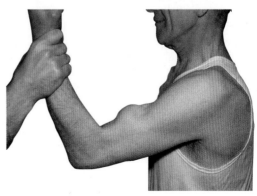

13.12 Ruptured long head of biceps The lump in the front of the arm becomes even more prominent when the patient contracts the biceps against resistance.

shoulder, which previously felt normal, aches for a time and bruising appears over the front of the arm. Soon the ache subsides and good function returns, but when the elbow is flexed actively the belly of the muscle contracts into a prominent lump. Sometimes the initial episode passes unremarked and the patient presents for the first time with a 'lump' in the arm, which is easily mistaken for tumour. Ask the patient to flex the elbow against resistance; this will show that the 'lump' is actually the bunched-up belly of biceps.

Function is usually so little disturbed that treatment is unnecessary, unless the associated rotator cuff symptoms need attention.

Avulsion of the distal attachment of the biceps is discussed in Chapter 14.

'SLAP' LESIONS

A fall on the outstretched arm can sometimes damage the superior part of the glenoid labrum anteriorly and posteriorly (SLAP). There is usually a history of a fall followed by pain in the shoulder. As the initial acute symptoms settle, the patient continues to experience a painful 'click' on lifting the arm above shoulder height, together with loss of power when using the arm in that position. He or she may also complain of an inability to throw with that arm.

MRI arthrography is the modality of choice, though the diagnosis is best confirmed by arthroscopic examination; at the same time the lesion is treated by re-attachment or debridement.

CHRONIC INSTABILITY OF THE SHOULDER

The shoulder achieves its uniquely wide range of movement at the cost of stability. The glenoid socket is very shallow and the joint is held secure by the fibrocartilaginous glenoid labrum and the surrounding ligaments and muscles. If these structures give way the shoulder becomes unstable and prone to recurrent dislocation or subluxation.

Anterior dislocation (the most common) usually follows an acute injury in which the arm is forced into abduction, external rotation and extension (see page 366). In *recurrent dislocation* the labrum and capsule are often detached from the anterior rim of the glenoid (the classic Bankart lesion).

Anterior subluxation may follow and alternate with episodes of dislocation. The joint feels as if it 'pops out' momentarily during certain actions (e.g. serving at tennis) but in reality it becomes only partially displaced.

Posterior dislocation is rare; when it occurs it is usually due to a violent jerk in an unusual position, e.g. following an epileptic fit or a severe electric shock. Recurrent posterior instability is almost always a *subluxation*, with the humeral head riding back on the posterior lip of the glenoid.

Atraumatic instability is associated with capsular and ligamentous laxity, and sometimes with weakness of the shoulder muscles. This type of joint laxity is not the same as true instability.

ANTERIOR INSTABILITY

This is far and away the commonest type of instability, accounting for over 95% of cases. It usually occurs as sequel to acute anterior dislocation of the shoulder, with detachment or stretching of the glenoid labrum and capsule (see page 366). In those over 50 years, dislocation is often associated with a rotator cuff tear.

Clinical features

The typical patient is a young man who describes an initial episode of the shoulder coming out of joint following an injury; he may even remember that his arm was suddenly forced into abduction and external rotation. Thereafter, he complains of the shoulder repeatedly 'coming out of joint' during over-arm movements (lifting the arm in abduction, extension and external rotation), and each time having to have it manipulated back into position. An initial, acute episode of dislocation goes on to *recurrent dislocation* in over one-third of patients under the age of 30 years and in about one-fifth of those over 50 years.

Recurrent subluxation is less obvious. The patient may describe a 'catching' sensation (rather than complete displacement), followed by 'numbness' or 'weakness' – the so-called dead arm syndrome – when attempting to throw a ball or serve at tennis.

Between episodes the diagnosis rests on demonstrating the *apprehension sign*. With the patient seated, the examiner cautiously lifts the arm into abduction, external rotation and then extension; at the crucial moment the patient senses that the humeral head is about to slip out anteriorly and his body tautens in apprehension.

Imaging

The classic *x-ray* feature is a depression in the posterosuperior part of the humeral head (the Hill–Sachs lesion), where the bone has been damaged by repeated impact with the anterior rim of the glenoid. Subluxation is more difficult to demonstrate; an axillary view may show the

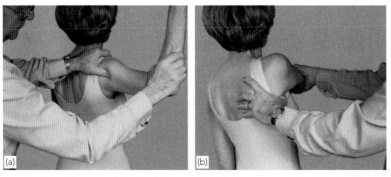

13.13 Shoulder instability – the apprehension test (a) This is the apprehension test for anterior subluxation or dislocation. Abduct, externally rotate and extend the patient's shoulder while pushing on the head of the humerus. If the patient feels that the joint is about to dislocate, she will forcibly resist the manoeuvre. (b) Posterior dislocation can be tested for in the same way by drawing the arm forward and across the patient's body (adduction and internal rotation).

humeral head riding on the anterior lip of the glenoid.

MRI arthrography may reveal a detached glenoid labrum (the Bankart lesion) and/or the Hill–Sachs lesion.

Treatment

If dislocation recurs only at long intervals, the patient may choose to put up with the inconvenience. Indications for *operative treatment* are: (1) frequent dislocations, especially if these are painful; and (2) a fear of recurrent subluxation or dislocation sufficient to prevent participation in everyday activities, including sport.

Surgery nowadays aims to restore the anatomy. The glenoid labrum is re-attached, together with tightening of the anterior capsule. This is usually achieved by open operation, although with advanced equipment and specialized sutures, arthroscopic repair is an option.

POSTERIOR INSTABILITY

Posterior instability sometimes persists after an acute posterior dislocation (see page 368). It usually takes the form of recurrent subluxation rather than full-blown dislocation. The shoulder subluxates when the arm is held in flexion and internal rotation.

Treatment is usually conservative – muscle strengthening exercises and voluntary control of the joint. Operative reconstruction is indicated only if disability is marked, there is no gross joint laxity and a structural abnormality is found on investigation with CT or MRI.

ATRAUMATIC INSTABILITY

In this condition the patient complains of the shoulder going 'out of joint' with remarkable ease. This can occur in athletes such as swimmers and throwers who overload and fatigue the stabilizing muscles around the shoulder, leading to pain and

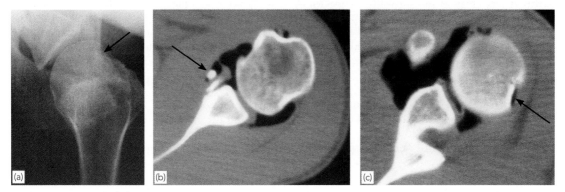

13.14 Anterior instability – imaging (a) The plain x-ray shows a large depression in the posteriosuperior part of the humeral head (the Hill–Sachs sign). (b,c) MRI shows both a Bankart lesion, with a flake of bone detached from the anterior edge of the glenoid, and the Hill–Sachs lesion (arrows).

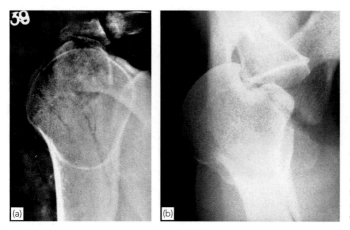

13.15 Posterior dislocation (a) In the anteroposterior view the humeral head looks globular – the so-called 'light bulb' appearance. (b) In the lateral view one can see the humeral head is lying behind the glenoid fossa, with an impaction fracture on the anterior surface of the head.

subluxation in various directions. This is usually treated by physiotherapy to strengthen the muscles and to restore proprioception. Just occasionally surgery is needed to tighten the capsule.

Another form of atraumatic instability is associated with individuals who are able to voluntarily subluxate or dislocate their shoulders (often demonstrated as a 'party trick'). This can then become involuntary. Treatment requires physiotherapy and sometimes even psychological counselling. *Surgery should be avoided.*

DISORDERS OF THE GLENOHUMERAL JOINT

TUBERCULOUS ARTHRITIS

Tuberculosis of the shoulder is uncommon. It usually starts as an osteitis but is rarely diagnosed until arthritis has supervened. This may proceed to abscess and sinus formation; in some cases fibrous ankylosis develops. Patients are usually adults. They complain of a constant ache and stiffness lasting many months. The striking feature is wasting of the muscles around the shoulder. In neglected cases a sinus may be present. There is diffuse warmth and tenderness, and all movements are limited and painful. Axillary lymph nodes may be enlarged.

X-rays

Early signs are generalized rarefaction of bone on both sides of the joint and erosion of the joint surfaces. In late cases there may be 'cystic' destruction of the humeral head and/or glenoid fossa.

Treatment

In addition to systemic treatment with antituberculous drugs, the shoulder should be rested until acute symptoms have settled.

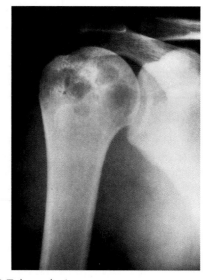

13.16 Tuberculosis X-ray of the shoulder showing tuberculous abscesses in the head of the humerus.

Thereafter movement is encouraged and, provided the articular cartilage is not destroyed, the prognosis for painless function is good. If there are repeated flares, or if the articular surfaces are extensively destroyed, the joint should be arthrodesed.

RHEUMATOID ARTHRITIS

The acromioclavicular joint, the glenohumeral joint and the various synovial pouches around the shoulder are frequently involved in rheumatoid disease. Chronic synovitis leads to rupture of the rotator cuff and progressive joint erosion.

Clinical features

The patient, who usually has generalized arthritis, complains of pain in the shoulder and difficulty

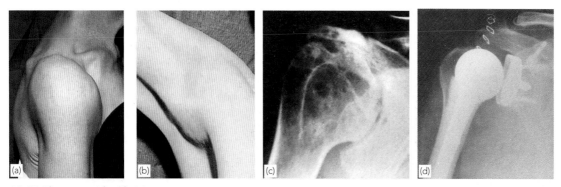

13.17 Rheumatoid arthritis (a) Large synovial effusions cause easily visible swelling; small ones are likely to be missed, especially if they are present in the axilla (b). (c) X-rays show progressive erosion of the joint. (d) X-ray appearance after total joint replacement.

with tasks such as combing the hair or washing the back.

Active movements are limited, and passive movements are painful and accompanied by marked crepitus. If the supraspinatus is involved the features are similar to those of post-traumatic cuff lesions.

X-rays

There are three patterns – wet (periarticular erosions, rapid progress, early cuff rupture), dry (subchondral sclerosis, osteophytes, slow progress, cuff intact) and resorptive (marked bone loss, few erosions). Often the acromioclavicular joint is involved. Although it may start on one side, the condition usually becomes bilateral.

Treatment

If general measures do not control the synovitis, corticosteroid may be injected into the joint and the subacromial bursa. If synovitis persists, operative synovectomy is carried out and at the same time cuff tears may be repaired. Excision of the lateral end of the clavicle may relieve acromioclavicular pain.

In advanced cases, pain and stiffness can be very disabling and may call for either arthroplasty or arthrodesis. Shoulder replacement gives good pain relief and improved function, even though the range of movement remains well below normal. If there is inadequate bone stock for a shoulder replacement, then the shoulder may have to be arthrodesed.

OSTEOARTHRITIS

Glenohumeral osteoarthritis is usually secondary to other fairly obvious disorders: congenital dysplasia, local trauma, long-standing rotator cuff lesions, rheumatoid disease or avascular necrosis of the head of the humerus.

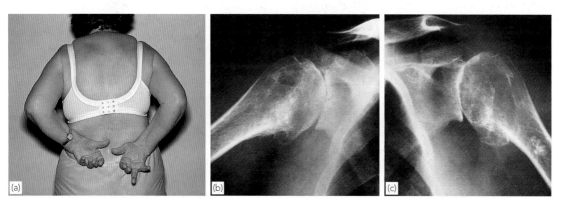

13.18 Osteoarthritis of the shoulder (a) This woman has advanced osteoarthritis of both shoulders. Movements are so restricted that she has difficulty dressing herself and combing her hair. (b,c) X-rays show the severe degree of articular destruction.

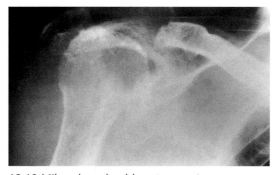

13.19 Milwaukee shoulder The x-ray features are arresting. There is gross destruction of the joint and calcification in the soft tissues around the shoulder.

Clinical features

Patients, usually 50–60 years old, complain of pain; they may give a history of previous shoulder problems. The most typical sign is progressive restriction of shoulder movements.

X-rays show the characteristic features of loss of the articular space, distortion of the joint, subchondral sclerosis and marginal osteophyte formation.

Treatment

Analgesics and anti-inflammatory drugs relieve pain, and exercises may improve mobility. Most patients manage to live with the restrictions imposed by stiffness, provided pain is not severe.

If pain and stiffness become intolerable, joint replacement is justified. It may not improve mobility much, but it does relieve pain.

RAPIDLY DESTRUCTIVE SHOULDER ARTHROPATHY

Occasionally a patient presents with swelling of the shoulder and x-rays show a bizarrely destructive form of arthritis. Similar conditions are encountered in other joints (see page 44). It has been suggested that this is a crystal-induced, rapidly progressive arthropathy; it is sometimes associated with massive tears of the rotator cuff. The name *'Milwaukee shoulder'* was suggested in

an early description of the condition by McCarty, who hailed from the city of that name.

There is no satisfactory treatment. Arthroplasty may relieve pain but will not improve function because the joint is unstable.

DISORDERS OF THE SCAPULA AND CLAVICLE

CONGENITAL ELEVATION OF THE SCAPULA (SPRENGEL'S SHOULDER)

The scapulae normally complete their descent from the neck by the third month of fetal life; occasionally one remains unduly high. The shoulder on the affected side is elevated; the scapula looks and feels abnormally high, smaller than usual and somewhat prominent. Movements are painless, but abduction may be limited. Associated deformities such as fusion of cervical vertebrae, kyphosis or scoliosis may be present.

Treatment

Mild cases are best left untreated. Marked limitation of abduction or severe deformity may necessitate an operation to lower the scapula.

KLIPPEL–FEIL SYNDROME

This rare congenital disorder comprises bilateral failure of scapular descent and fusion of several cervical vertebrae. The neck is unusually short and may be webbed; cervical mobility is restricted. The condition is usually left untreated.

WINGED SCAPULA

In this condition the scapula juts out under the skin, like a small wing. It is due to weakness of the serratus anterior, the muscle which stabilizes the scapula on the thoracic cage. It may cause asymmetry of the shoulders, but it is often not apparent until the patient tries to contract the serratus anterior against resistance (e.g. pushing hard against a wall).

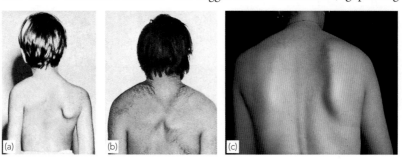

13.20 Scapular disorders
(a) Sprengel shoulder;
(b) Klippel–Feil syndrome;
(c) winged scapula.

Weakness of the serratus anterior may arise from: (1) damage to the long thoracic nerve; (2) injury to the brachial plexus or the fifth, sixth and seventh cervical nerve roots; (3) viral infections of the nerve roots (neuralgic amyotrophy); and (4) certain types of muscular dystrophy.

A less obvious form of scapular instability may be caused by weakness of the trapezius following injury to the spinal accessory nerve.

Treatment

Some of the disorders causing winged scapula are self-limiting and the condition gradually improves. Even if it doesn't, disability is usually slight and is best accepted. However, if function is markedly impaired, the scapula can be stabilized by tendon transfer.

GRATING SCAPULA

This is found in about one-third of normal people; a cause is usually not found but occasionally a tangential x-ray (or better still a CT scan) will show a bone lesion such as an osteochondroma.

ACROMIOCLAVICULAR INSTABILITY

This is a common condition, resulting from dislocation of the acromioclavicular joint and rupture of the ligaments which tether the outer end of the clavicle. The patient may complain of discomfort and weakness during strenuous activities with the arm above shoulder height. On examination there is a fairly obvious bump over the acromioclavicular joint and pressure on the joint may be painful. If the diagnosis is not obvious on plain x-ray, re-examination with the patient standing up and holding a heavy weight (to drag the shoulder downwards) will show the displacement.

Treatment

The condition causes little disability during non-strenuous activities and treatment is therefore unnecessary. However, certain types of work activity may be seriously curtailed and in such cases reconstructive surgery should be considered.

OSTEOARTHRITIS OF THE ACROMIOCLAVICULAR JOINT

Clinical features

Acromioclavicular osteoarthritis is common in old people and usually develops spontaneously. When it occurs in younger individuals it might be due to previous injury or repetitive stress (for example habitually carrying weights on the shoulder or working with pneumatic hammers or drills).

The patient complains of pain over the top of the shoulder, particularly while using the arm above shoulder height. Tenderness and swelling are localized to the acromioclavicular joint.

X-rays show the characteristic features of osteoarthritis.

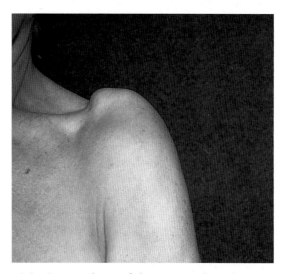

13.21 Osteoarthritis of the acromioclavicular joint Osteophytic thickening of the acromioclavicular joint produces a small (but very tender) bump on top of the left shoulder. Occasionally the joint capsule herniates, producing a large 'cyst' over the acromioclavicular joint.

Treatment

If analgesics and corticosteroid injections are ineffectual, pain may be relieved by excision of the lateral end of the clavicle.

OPERATIONS

ARTHROSCOPY

Arthroscopy is useful for the diagnosis of periarticular and intra-articular disorders, such as rotator cuff disruption and instability. At the same time a biopsy can be taken which may assist in the diagnosis of synovial disorders such as rheumatoid arthritis or pigmented villonodular synovitis.

Arthroscopic surgery is now well established. There has been a transition over the last 20 years from its usage in diagnosis to that of repair and reconstructive procedures. Because it is safer and recovery is quicker, it is the first-line surgical option for subacromial decompression, acromioclavicular joint excisions, debridement of rotator cuff tears and release of frozen shoulder. Arthroscopic repair of anterior shoulder instability produces results comparable to those obtained by open surgery.

ARTHROPLASTY OF THE SHOULDER

Shoulder replacement was initially introduced for the treatment of proximal humeral fractures but technical advances have allowed it to be used for end-stage glenohumeral osteoarthritis and rheumatoid arthritis if non-operative treatment fails. The options are either replacement of just the humeral head or of both the head and the glenoid socket.

Complications

The commonest are loosening of the components, glenohumeral instability, rotator cuff failure, periprosthetic fracture, infection and implant failure. Glenoid fixation remains a challenge; radiographic lucent lines around the glenoid component (usually regarded as a sign of implant loosening) are very common, although not always symptomatic.

Outcome

This depends largely on the indications for surgery. Generally, pain relief is excellent but range of movement is often disappointing.

ARTHRODESIS

Arthrodesis of the glenohumeral joint is now seldom performed, but it is still a useful operation for severe shoulder dysfunction associated with paralysis, uncontrollable instability and failed shoulder replacement. A prerequisite is stable and powerful scapulothoracic movement, because with a fused shoulder 'movement' is achieved entirely by rotation of the scapula on the thorax.

The optimal position is 30 degrees of flexion, 30 degrees of abduction and 30 degrees of internal rotation. The arthrodesis is held by internal fixation with a plate and screws.

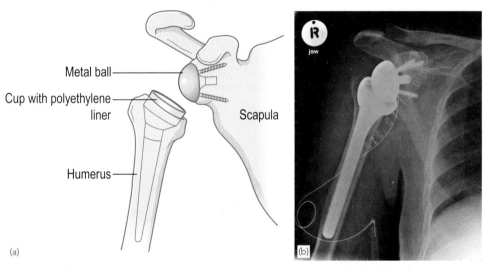

13.22 Shoulder replacement (a) Illustration showing principles of total shoulder replacement.
(b) Postoperative x-ray of this type of implant. Other ball-and-socket configurations are also available.

CHAPTER 14

THE ELBOW

CLINICAL ASSESSMENT

HISTORY

- *Pain* may be felt diffusely on the medial side of the joint (ulnohumeral), the posterolateral side (radiohumeral) or acutely localized to one of the humeral epicondyles ('tennis elbow' on the lateral side and 'golfer's elbow' on the medial side). Pain over the back of the elbow is often due to an olecranon bursitis.
- *Stiffness*, if severe, can be very disabling; the patient may be unable to reach to the mouth (loss of flexion) or the perineum (loss of extension); limited supination makes it difficult to hold something in the palm or to carry large objects.
- *Swelling* may be due to injury or inflammation; a soft lump on the back of the elbow suggests an olecranon bursitis.
- *Deformity* is usually the result of previous trauma: (a) *cubitus varus* due to a malunited supracondylar fracture, or (b) *cubitus valgus* due to an old displaced and malunited fracture of the lateral condyle.
- *Instability* is not uncommon in the late stage of rheumatoid arthritis.
- *Ulnar nerve symptoms* (tingling and numbness in the little and ring fingers, weakness of the hand) may occur in elbow disorders because the nerve is so near the joint.
- *Loss of function* is noticed in grooming activities, carrying and hand work.

EXAMINATION

Both upper limbs must be completely exposed and it is essential to look at the back as well as the

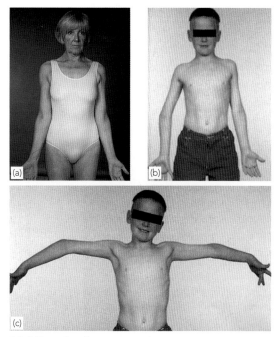

14.1 Examination (a) Note that the elbows are normally held in 5–10 degrees of valgus (the carrying angle). (b) This young boy ended up with slight varus angulation after a supracondylar fracture of the distal humerus. The deformity is much more obvious (c) when he raises his arms (the gun-stock deformity).

front. The neck, shoulders and hands should also be examined.

Look

Looking at the patient from the front, with his or her arms outstretched alongside the body and the palms facing forwards, the elbows are seen to be held in 5–15 degrees of valgus; this is the normal 'carrying angle'. Anything more, especially if unilateral, is regarded as a valgus deformity. Varus deformity is less obvious, but if the patient raises the arms to shoulder height, it is easily seen.

The most common swelling is in the olecranon bursa at the back of the elbow.

Feel

Important bony landmarks are the medial and lateral condyles and the tip of the olecranon. These are palpated to determine whether the joint is correctly positioned.

Superficial structures are examined for warmth and subcutaneous nodules. The joint line (including the radioulnar joint depression) is located and palpated for synovial thickening. Tenderness can usually be localized to a particular structure.

The ulnar nerve is fairly superficial behind the medial condyle and here it can be rolled under the fingers to feel if it is thickened or tapped to find if it is hypersensitive.

Move

Flexion and extension are compared on the two sides. Then, with the elbows tucked into the sides and flexed to a right angle, the radioulnar joints are tested for pronation (palms downwards 0–90 degrees) and supination (palms upwards 0–90 degrees).

General examination

If the symptoms and signs do not point clearly to a local disorder, other parts are examined: the neck (for cervical disc lesions), the shoulder (for cuff lesions) and the hand (for nerve lesions).

X-rays

The position of each bone is noted, then the joint line and space. Next, the individual bones are inspected for evidence of old injury or bone destruction. Finally, loose bodies are sought.

In children, while the epiphyses are still incompletely ossified the anatomy has to be deduced from the shape and position of the emerging secondary ossific centres; the average ages at which they appear can be remembered from the mnemonic CRITOE: Capitulum – 2 years; Radial head – 4 years; Internal epicondyle – 6 years; Trochlea – 8 years; Olecranon – 10 years; External epicondyle – 12 years.

ELBOW DEFORMITIES

CUBITUS VARUS

Varus (or 'gun-stock') deformity is most obvious when the elbows are extended and the arms are elevated (see Figure 14.1(c)). The most common cause is malunion of a supracondylar fracture. The deformity can be corrected by a wedge osteotomy of the lower humerus.

CUBITUS VALGUS

The most common cause is non-union of a fractured lateral condyle; this may give gross deformity and a bony knob on the inner side of the joint. The importance of valgus deformity is the liability for delayed ulnar palsy to develop; years after the causal injury, the patient notices weakness of the hand with numbness and tingling of the ulnar fingers. The deformity itself needs no treatment, but for delayed ulnar palsy the nerve should be transposed to the front of the elbow.

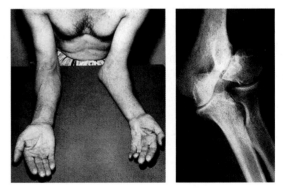

14.2 Cubitus valgus This man's valgus deformity, the sequel to an ununited fracture of the lateral condyle, has resulted in an ulnar nerve palsy.

STIFF ELBOW

A stiff elbow can be a severe impediment. Patients may be unable to reach out to, or bring back from, their environment; others, again, cannot turn the hand palm downwards to pick up something, or palm upwards to lift something. Causes include congenital disorders, trauma and arthritis. If physiotherapy does not help, surgery is needed.

TUBERCULOSIS

Clinical features

Although the disease begins as synovitis or osteomyelitis, tuberculosis of the elbow is rarely seen until arthritis supervenes. The onset is insidious, with a long history of aching and stiffness. The most striking physical sign is the marked wasting. While the disease is active, the joint is held flexed, looks swollen, feels warm and is diffusely tender; movement is considerably limited and accompanied by pain and spasm.

X-ray examination typically shows generalized rarefaction and an apparent increase of joint space because of bone erosion.

Treatment

In addition to antituberculous drugs, the elbow is rested, at first in a splint, but later simply by applying a collar and cuff. Surgical debridement is rarely needed.

RHEUMATOID ARTHRITIS

Clinical features

The elbow is involved in more than 50% of patients with rheumatoid arthritis. Rheumatoid nodules can often be detected over the olecranon. There is pain and tenderness, especially around the head of the radius. Eventually the whole elbow may become swollen and unstable. Often both elbows are affected.

X-rays

Bone erosion, with gradual destruction of the radial head and widening of the trochlear notch of the ulna, is typical of chronic inflammatory arthritis.

Treatment

In addition to general treatment, the elbow should be splinted during periods of active synovitis. For chronic, painful arthritis of the radiohumeral

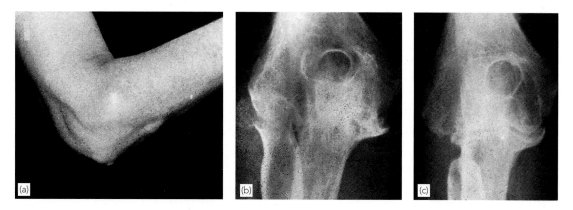

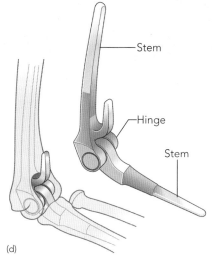

14.3 Rheumatoid arthritis (a) This patient has a painful elbow as well as the typical rheumatoid nodules over the olecranon. (b) His x-rays show deformity of the radial head and marked erosion of the rest of the elbow joint. (c) Excision of the radial head combined with synovectomy relieved the pain. (d) Total elbow arthroplasty: hinged implants.

joint, resection of the radial head and partial synovectomy give reasonably good results. If the entire joint is severely damaged, joint replacement should be considered. The preferred operation is a semi-constrained arthroplasty: stemmed metal implants are cemented into the distal humerus and the proximal ulna; the protruding ends articulate with each other on a polythene bearing. The result is often excellent, at least compared to the preoperative situation. With modern techniques complications such as infection, instability and implant loosening are much less common than in the past.

OSTEOARTHRITIS

The elbow is an uncommon site for osteoarthritis. When it does occur, it may be secondary to trauma. 'Primary' osteoarthritis of the elbow should suggest an underlying disorder such as pyrophosphate arthropathy or congenital dysplasia, but usually occurs spontaneously.

The usual symptoms are pain and stiffness, but in late cases the joint may become unstable. Occasionally ulnar palsy is the presenting feature. The elbow may look and feel enlarged and movements are somewhat limited.

X-rays show diminution of the joint space with subchondral sclerosis and marginal osteophytes; one or more loose bodies may be seen.

Treatment

Osteoarthritis of the elbow rarely requires more than symptomatic treatment; loose bodies, however, should be removed arthroscopically if they cause locking. If stiffness is sufficiently disabling, removal of osteophytes (by either open or arthroscopic surgery) can improve the range of movement. If there are signs of ulnar neuritis, the nerve may have to be transposed to the front of the elbow.

LOOSE BODIES

The commonest cause of a single loose body in the elbow is osteochondritis dissecans of the capitulum. Multiple loose bodies may occur with osteoarthritis or synovial chondromatosis.

The cardinal clinical feature is sudden locking of the elbow. If this is troublesome, the loose bodies can be removed arthroscopically.

OLECRANON BURSITIS

The olecranon bursa sometimes becomes enlarged as a result of pressure or friction. When it is also painful, the cause is more likely to be infection, gout or rheumatoid arthritis.

Gout is suspected if there is a history of previous attacks, if the condition is bilateral, if there are tophi, or if x-ray shows calcification in the bursa. Even then it is not easy to distinguish from acute infection, unless pus is aspirated.

Rheumatoid arthritis causes both swelling and nodularity over the olecranon. In almost all cases this will be associated with a typical symmetrical polyarthritis. In the late stages, erosion of the elbow joint may cause marked instability.

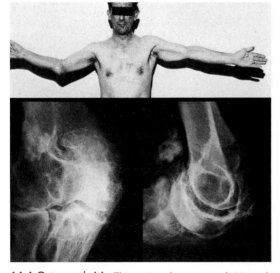

14.4 Osteoarthritis This patient has osteoarthritis and loose bodies in the elbow.

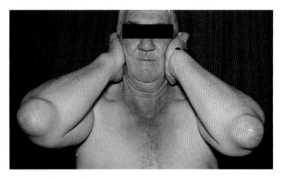

14.5 Olecranon bursitis The enormous red lumps over the points of the elbows are due to swollen olecranon bursae; the patient's ruddy complexion completes the typical picture of gout.

Treatment

The underlying disorder must be treated. Septic bursitis may need local drainage. Occasionally a chronically enlarged bursa has to be excised.

'TENNIS ELBOW' AND 'GOLFER'S ELBOW'

The cause of these common disorders is unknown, but they are seldom due to either tennis or golf. Most cases occur spontaneously as part of a natural degenerative process in the tendon aponeuroses attached to either the lateral or medial humeral epicondyle. Pain is probably due to a vascular repair process similar to that of rotator cuff tendinitis around the shoulder. Often there is a history of occupational stress or unaccustomed activity, such as house painting, carpentry or other activities that involve strenuous wrist movements and forearm muscle contraction.

Clinical features

In 'tennis elbow', pain is felt over the outer side of the elbow, but in severe cases it may radiate widely. It is initiated or aggravated by movements such as pouring out tea, turning a stiff door-handle, shaking hands or lifting with the forearm pronated. The elbow looks normal and flexion and extension are full and painless. Tenderness is localized to a spot just in front of the lateral epicondyle, and pain is reproduced by getting the patient to extend the wrist against resistance, or simply by passively flexing the wrist so as to stretch the common extensors.

In 'golfer's elbow', similar symptoms occur around the medial epicondyle and, owing to involvement of the common tendon of origin of the wrist flexors, pain is reproduced by passive extension of the wrist in supination.

Treatment

Rest, or avoiding the precipitating activity, may allow the lesion to heal. A splint and physiotherapy may help. If pain is severe, the area of maximum tenderness is injected with a mixture of corticosteroid and local anaesthetic.

Persistent pain which fails to respond to conservative measures may call for operative treatment. The affected common tendon on the lateral or medial side of the elbow is detached from its origin at the humeral epicondyle.

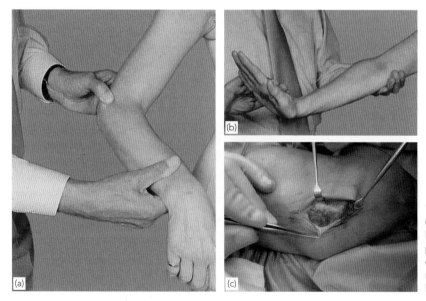

14.6 Tennis elbow
(a) Tenderness over the lateral epicondyle. (b) Pain is provoked by resisted wrist extension. (c) Extensor carpi radialis brevis origin may have to be released.

CHAPTER 15

THE WRIST

CLINICAL ASSESSMENT

HISTORY

- *Pain* may be localized to the radial side (especially in tenovaginitis of the thumb tendons), to the ulnar side (possibly from the radioulnar joint) or to the dorsum (the usual site in disorders of the carpus).
- *Stiffness* is often not noticed until it is severe. Loss of pronation or supination is more readily noticed and may be very disabling.
- *Swelling* may signify involvement of either the joint or the tendon sheaths.
- *Deformity* is a late symptom except after trauma.
- *Loss of function* affects both the wrist and the hand. Firm grip is possible only with a strong, stable, painless wrist that has a reasonable range of movement.

EXAMINATION

Examination of the wrist is not complete without also examining the elbow, forearm and hand. Both upper limbs should be completely exposed.

Look

The skin is inspected for scars. Both wrists and forearms are compared to see if there is any deformity. If there is swelling, note whether it is diffuse or localized to one of the tendon sheaths.

Feel

Undue warmth is noted. Tender areas must be accurately localized and the bony landmarks compared with those of the normal wrist.

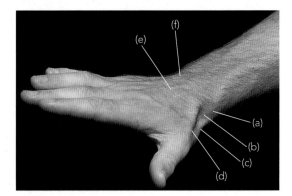

15.1 Tender points at the wrist (a) Tip of the radial styloid process; (b) anatomical snuff-box, bounded on the radial side by (c) the extensor pollicis brevis and on the ulnar side by (d) the extensor pollicis longus; (e) the extensor tendons of the fingers; and (f) the head of the ulna.

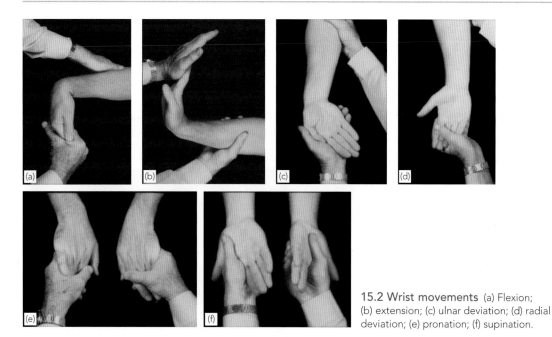

15.2 Wrist movements (a) Flexion; (b) extension; (c) ulnar deviation; (d) radial deviation; (e) pronation; (f) supination.

Move

Passive flexion and extension of the wrist can be measured on each side in turn. To view both sides simultaneously and compare them, ask the patient first to place his or her palms together in a position of prayer, elevating the elbows, then to repeat the manoeuvre with the wrists back-to-back. The normal range for both flexion and extension is 80–90 degrees. Radial deviation and ulnar deviation are measured in the palms-up position; ulnar deviation is normally about 40 degrees and radial deviation only about 15 degrees. Pronation and supination are included in wrist movements, although they depend also on the condition of the elbow and movement between the forearm bones. The normal range is 0–90 degrees in both directions.

Active movements should be tested against resistance; loss of power may be due to pain, tendon rupture or muscle weakness. Grip strength can be gauged by having the patient squeeze the examiner's hand; mechanical instruments allow more accurate assessment.

Imaging

X-rays are routinely obtained; often both wrists must be examined for comparison. Special oblique views are necessary to show up difficult scaphoid fractures.

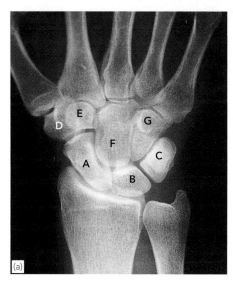

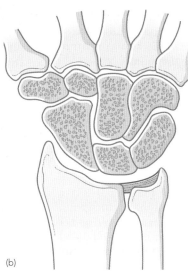

15.3 X-rays (a) Note the shape and position of the bones which make up the wrist: **(A)** scaphoid, **(B)** lunate, **(C)** triquetrum overlain by pisiform, **(D)** trapezium, **(E)** trapezoid, **(F)** capitate, **(G)** hamate. (b) Schematic section showing the carpal articulations and the triangular fibrocartilaginous ligament (coloured green).

191

Note the position of the carpal bones and look for evidence of joint-space narrowing, especially at the carpometacarpal joint of the thumb.

Magnetic resonance imaging (MRI) is useful for demonstrating soft-tissue lesions or the early signs of avascular necrosis in one of the carpal bones.

Arthrography, combined with computed tomography (CT) or MRI, is a sensitive way to diagnose ligament tears.

Arthroscopy

This is the most reliable way of diagnosing tears of the triangular fibrocartilage complex (TFCC). It will also reveal the early changes of osteoarthritis.

WRIST DEFORMITIES

CONGENITAL VARIATIONS

Embryonic abnormalities of the upper limb are likely to affect more than one segment (or indeed the whole) of the limb; therefore, congenital anomalies often appear together in the forearm, wrist and hand. Furthermore, other organs developing during the same period may be affected and thus there may be associated congenital abnormalities.

These are rare conditions; the overall incidence of upper limb anomalies is estimated to be about 1 in 600 live births, but in only a fraction of those affected are the defects severe enough to require corrective surgery. A few of the least unusual deformities affecting the wrist are described here.

Radial dysplasia

The infant is born with the wrist in marked radial deviation, hence the common name *radial club-hand*; one-half of the patients are affected bilaterally. There is absence of the whole or part of the radius, and usually also the thumb.

Treatment in the neonate consists of gentle stretching and splintage. Serious cases can be treated by distraction prior to a tension-free soft-tissue correction which has less effect on growth of the carpus and distal ulna than the older technique of 'centralizing' the carpus over the remaining forearm structures. Prolonged splintage is still required to avoid recurrence of the deformity.

Always examine the elbow: if the joint is stiff, a radially deviated wrist can actually be advantageous, as the child can then get the hand to his or her mouth (for eating) and the perineum (for toilet care). Surgical correction of the wrist in these cases can be disastrous.

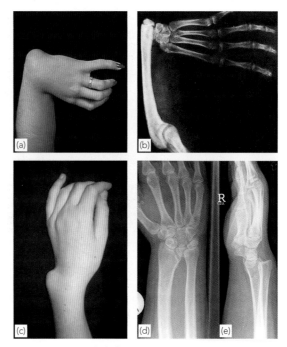

15.4 Congenital deformities (a,b) Radial club-hand. (c–e) Madelung's deformity.

If function deteriorates, centralization of the carpus over the ulna is recommended, preferably before the age of 3 years.

Madelung's deformity

In this deformity the lower radius curves forwards (ventrally), carrying with it the carpus and hand but leaving the distal end of the ulna projecting on the back of the wrist. Although the abnormality is present at birth, the deformity is rarely seen before the age of 10 years, after which it increases until growth is complete. Despite the deformity, function is usually undisturbed.

Treatment may be unnecessary, but if the deformity is severe, the lower end of the ulna can be shortened; this is sometimes combined with osteotomy of the radius.

ACQUIRED DEFORMITY

Physeal injuries can result in malunited fractures or subluxation of the distal radioulnar joint. Osteotomy of the radius or stabilization of the ulna may be needed.

Non-traumatic deformities are seen typically in rheumatoid arthritis and cerebral palsy. These disorders are discussed in Chapters 3 and 10, respectively.

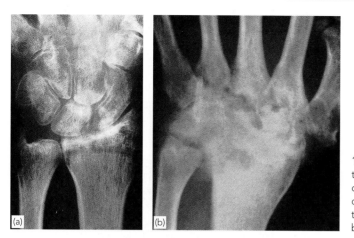

15.5 Tuberculosis (a) Subacute tuberculous arthritis; note the marked osteoporosis in the distal radius and the carpus. (b) A much more advanced case of tuberculous arthritis giving rise to extensive bone destruction.

TUBERCULOSIS

Tuberculous arthritis sometimes occurs at the wrist. Pain and stiffness come on gradually and the hand feels weak. The forearm looks wasted; the wrist is swollen and feels warm. Involvement of the flexor tendon compartment may give rise to a large fluctuant swelling that crosses the wrist into the palm (what used to be called a 'compound palmar ganglion'). Movements are restricted and painful. In a neglected case there may be a sinus.

X-ray examination shows localized osteoporosis and irregularity of the radiocarpal and intercarpal joints, and sometimes bone erosion.

Diagnosis

The condition must be differentiated from rheumatoid arthritis. Bilateral arthritis of the wrist is nearly always rheumatoid in origin; when only one wrist is affected, the signs resemble those of tuberculosis. X-rays and serological tests may help, but sometimes a biopsy is necessary.

Treatment

Antituberculous drugs are given and the wrist is splinted. If an abscess forms, it must be drained. If the wrist is destroyed, systemic treatment should be continued until the disease is quiescent and the wrist is then arthrodesed.

RHEUMATOID ARTHRITIS

Clinical features

After the metacarpophalangeal joints, the wrist is the most common site of rheumatoid arthritis. Pain, swelling and tenderness may at first be localized to the radioulnar joint, or to one of the tendon sheaths. Sooner or later the whole wrist becomes involved and tenderness is much more ill defined. In late cases the wrist is deformed and unstable. Extensor tendons may rupture where they cross the dorsum of the wrist, causing one or more of the fingers to drop into flexion.

X-rays show the characteristic features of osteoporosis and bony erosions. Tell-tale signs are usually more obvious in the metacarpophalangeal joints.

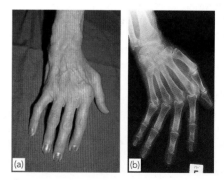

15.6 Rheumatoid arthritis (a) The wrist is deviated radialwards and the fingers ulnarwards; this is the typical zig-zag deformity of established rheumatoid arthritis in the wrist and hand. (b) X-ray of the same patient.

Treatment

Management in the early stage consists of splintage and local injection of corticosteroids, combined with systemic treatment. Persistent synovitis (usually affecting the extensor tendon sheaths) may call for synovectomy and soft-tissue stabilization of the wrist. If the radioulnar joint is involved, synovectomy can be combined with excision of the distal end of the ulnar head. Flexor synovitis may cause median nerve compression (carpal tunnel syndrome), which should be treated by operative release of the flexor retinaculum.

In the late stage, tendon ruptures at the wrist, joint destruction, instability and deformity may require reconstructive surgery, including either arthroplasty or arthrodesis.

OSTEOARTHRITIS OF THE RADIOCARPAL JOINT

Osteoarthritis of the wrist joint proper is unusual except as a sequel to intra-articular injuries of the distal radius or the carpal bones, or avascular necrosis of the lunate (Kienböck's disease). The patient may have forgotten the old injury, but some years later he or she begins to complain of pain, progressive loss of movement and weakness of grip. The appearance is usually normal, but the wrist is tender and movements are restricted and painful.

X-ray features are narrowing of the radiocarpal joint, bone sclerosis and irregularity of one or more of the proximal carpal bones. There may also be signs of the old injury or Kienböck's disease.

Treatment

Rest in a splint is often sufficient treatment. Painful but limited osteoarthritis following a scaphoid fracture can be alleviated by excision of the radial styloid process. Widespread osteoarthritis may require more extensive surgery, including replacement or arthrodesis of the wrist.

OSTEOARTHRITIS OF THE FIRST CARPOMETACARPAL JOINT

Osteoarthritis of the thumb carpometacarpal joint is common in postmenopausal women. The patient complains of pain and swelling around the

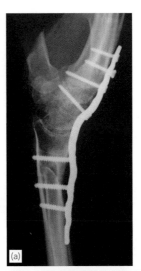

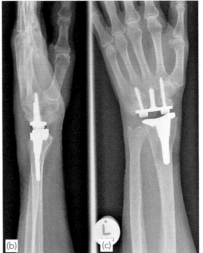

15.7 Osteoarthritis of the wrist Severe symptoms may call for either (a) total wrist fusion or (b,c) total joint replacement.

proximal end of the thumb metacarpal. Careful examination will show that tenderness is sharply localized to the carpometacarpal joint, about 1 cm distal to the radial styloid process. The condition is

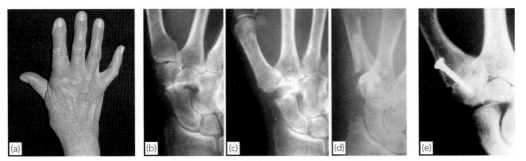

15.8 Osteoarthritis of the first carpometacarpal (CMC) joint (a) Typical deformity: note the swelling over the first CMC joint. (b) X-ray changes. Choice of treatment is between (c) trapeziectomy, (d) replacement arthroplasty and (e) arthrodesis.

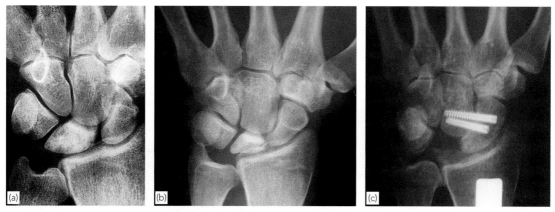

15.9 Kienböck's disease (a) Typical x-ray features of avascular necrosis of the lunate. (b) Late changes – marked distortion of the lunate. (c) Treatment, in this case, was first by osteotomy and shortening of the radius (the plate is still present) and then, when this failed to relieve pain, by lunate excision and scaphocapitate fusion.

often bilateral, and Heberden's nodes of the finger joints are common. In late cases, fixed adduction of the first metacarpal produces a characteristic deformity. *X-ray* examination shows the usual features of joint-space narrowing, sclerosis and osteophyte formation.

Treatment

Local injection of corticosteroid usually relieves pain, and movements may improve. If this fails, operation may be advisable. The surest way of abolishing pain and preserving function is to excise the trapezium. A more sophisticated, but less reliable, option is joint replacement. Joint arthrodesis is difficult and causes stiffness.

KIENBÖCK'S DISEASE

After injury or stress, the lunate bone sometimes develops a patchy avascular necrosis. A predisposing factor may be relative shortening of the ulna (negative ulnar variance), which could result in excessive stress being applied to the lunate where it is squeezed between the distal surface of the (over-long) radius and the second row of carpal bones.

The patient, usually a young adult, complains of ache and stiffness. Tenderness is localized to the centre of the wrist on the dorsum; wrist extension may be limited.

Imaging

The earliest signs of osteonecrosis can be detected only by MRI. Typical x-ray signs are increased density in the lunate and, later, flattening and irregularity of the bone. Ultimately there may be features of osteoarthritis of the wrist.

Treatment

During the early stage, while the shape of the lunate is more or less normal, osteotomy of the distal end of the radius may reduce pressure on the bone and thereby protect it from collapsing. Microsurgical revascularization of the bone is also worth considering if the necessary expertise is available. In late cases, partial wrist arthrodesis or proximal row excision or even joint replacement are considered.

TEARS OF THE TRIANGULAR FIBROCARTILAGE

The TFCC fans out from the base of the ulnar styloid process to the medial edge of the distal radius, acting somewhat like a meniscus in the wrist joint (see Figure 15.3). Chronic pain in the wrist may be related to an old 'sprain' in which a more serious injury to the TFCC was overlooked. In addition to pain, there may be loss of grip strength and clicking on supination of the forearm. The diagnosis can be confirmed by arthroscopy.

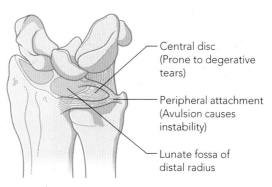

Central disc (Prone to degerative tears)

Peripheral attachment (Avulsion causes instability)

Lunate fossa of distal radius

15.10 Triangular fibrocartilage complex.

Operative treatment may be needed if the symptoms are marked. Peripheral tears can be re-attached by either open or arthroscopic techniques; central tears, in the absence of ulnocarpal impaction (see below) are best managed by arthroscopic debridement to remove the ragged fragments.

ULNOCARPAL IMPACTION AND TFCC DEGENERATION

Chronic degeneration of the TFCC may be associated with a relatively long ulna, impaction of the ulnar head against the ulnar side of the lunate and ulnocarpal arthritis (*the ulnocarpal impaction syndrome*). This may result when an impacted Colles fracture leaves the radius relatively shorter than usual. X-ray examination shows a relatively long ulna ('positive ulnar variance') and in late cases there may be arthritic changes in the ulnolunate articulation.

Treatment starts with simple analgesics, splintage and steroid injections. If the positive ulnar variance is slight (less than 3 mm) arthroscopic excision of the distal dome of the ulnar head may be successful; otherwise the long ulna can be shortened using a special jig and compression plate.

CHRONIC CARPAL INSTABILITY

The wrist functions as a system of intercalated segments (i.e. adjacent congruous bones) stabilized by ligaments and by the scaphoid, which bridges the two rows of carpal bones. Following trauma to the carpus, there may be partial collapse of this structure, a condition which is not always recognized at the time. Some years later, the patient complains of progressive pain and weakness in the wrist.

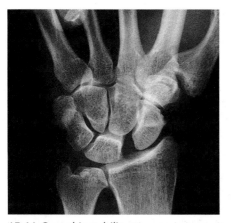

15.11 Carpal instability The scapholunate ligament has ruptured – the X-ray shows a large gap between the two bones and the scaphoid is foreshortened.

Diagnosis

The different types of carpal instability are described on page 392. The most easily spotted example is a rupture of the scapho-lunate ligament, which appears on x-ray as an unusual gap between the scaphoid and lunate and foreshortening of the scaphoid image (Figure 15.11).

Treatment

The best form of treatment is prevention. Acute 'wrist sprains' should be carefully assessed for signs of carpal displacement and instability (see page 392). Carpal displacement must be reduced, the ligament repaired and the bones held in position with Kirschner wires (K-wires).

Patients with chronic instability can often be treated by splintage, analgesics and specific physiotherapy. Occasionally operative treatment is indicated, involving soft-tissue augmentation or partial fusion of the wrist.

TENOSYNOVITIS AND TENOVAGINITIS

The extensor retinaculum contains six compartments which transmit tendons lined with synovium. Tenosynovitis can be caused by unaccustomed movement; sometimes it occurs spontaneously. The resulting synovial inflammation causes secondary thickening of the sheath and stenosis of the compartment, which further compromises the tendon. Early treatment, including rest, anti-inflammatory medication and injection of corticosteroids, may break this vicious circle.

The first dorsal compartment (enclosing abductor pollicis longus and extensor pollicis brevis) and the second dorsal compartment (extensor carpi radialis longus and brevis) are the ones most commonly affected.

DE QUERVAIN'S DISEASE

Tenovaginitis of the first dorsal compartment is usually seen in women between the ages of 30 and 50 years. There may be a history of unaccustomed activity, such as pruning roses, cutting with scissors or wringing out clothes. It is quite common shortly after childbirth.

Clinical features

Pain, and sometimes swelling, is localized to the radial side of the wrist. The tendon sheath feels thick and hard. Tenderness is most acute at the very tip of the radial styloid.

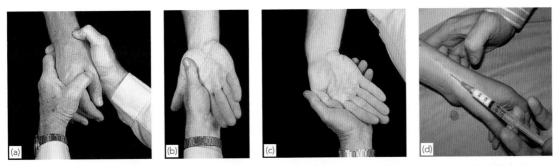

15.12 De Quervain's disease (a) There is point tenderness at the tip of the radial styloid process. (b,c) Finkelstein's test: ulnar deviation with the thumb left free is relatively painless (b), but if the movement is repeated with the thumb held close to the palm (c), the pull on the thumb tendons causes intense pain. (d) Injecting the tendon sheath.

The pathognomonic sign is elicited by *Finkelstein's test*. Hold the patient's hand firmly, keeping the thumb tucked in close to the palm, then turn the wrist sharply towards the ulnar side. A stab of pain over the radial styloid is a positive sign. Repeating the movement with the thumb left free is relatively painless.

Treatment

In early cases, symptoms can be relieved by ultrasound therapy or a corticosteroid injection into the tendon sheath, sometimes combined with splintage of the wrist. Resistant cases need an operation, which consists of slitting the thickened tendon sheath. Care should be taken to prevent injury to the dorsal sensory branches of the radial nerve, which may cause intractable dysaesthesia.

OTHER SITES OF EXTENSOR TENOSYNOVITIS

Tenosynovitis of *extensor carpi radialis brevis* (the most powerful extensor of the wrist) or *extensor carpi ulnaris* may cause pain and point tenderness just medial to the anatomical snuffbox or immediately distal to the head of the ulna,

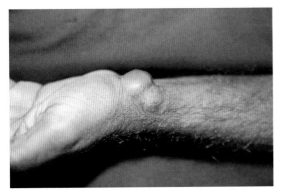

15.13 Volar wrist ganglion

respectively (see Figure 15.1). Splintage and corticosteroid injections are usually effective.

GANGLION

The ubiquitous ganglion is seen most commonly on the back of the wrist. It arises from cystic degeneration in the joint capsule or tendon sheath. The distended cyst contains a glairy fluid.

The patient, often a young adult, presents with a painless lump, usually on the back of the wrist, but sometimes on the front. Occasionally there is a slight ache. The lump is well defined, cystic and not tender. It may be attached to one of the tendons.

The ganglion often disappears after some months, so there should be no haste about treatment. If the lesion continues to be troublesome, it can be aspirated; if it recurs, excision is justified, but the patient should be told that there is a 30% risk of recurrence, even after careful surgery.

CARPAL TUNNEL SYNDROME

This is the commonest and best known of all the nerve entrapment syndromes. In the normal carpal tunnel there is barely room for all the tendons and the median nerve; consequently, any swelling is likely to result in compression and ischaemia of the nerve. Usually the cause eludes detection; the syndrome is, however, common in women at the menopause, in rheumatoid arthritis, in pregnancy and in myxoedema. The usual age group is 40–50 years.

Clinical features

The history is most helpful in making the diagnosis. Pain and paraesthesia occur in the distribution of the median nerve in the hand. Night after night the patient is woken with burning pain, tingling and numbness. Patients tend to seek relief by hanging the arm over the side of the bed or shaking the arm;

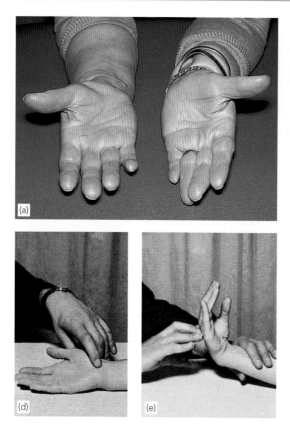

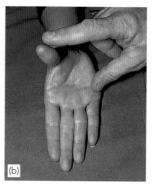

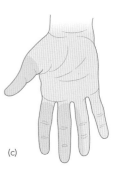

15.14 Median nerve compression (a) In the right hand there is wasting of the thenar eminence. (b) Testing for abductor power shows that it is weaker than that in the normal hand. (c) Area of diminished sensibility. (d) Tapping on the nerve may cause tingling in the hand (Tinel's sign), and holding the wrist flexed for 2 minutes may also produce tingling in the median nerve distribution (e).

however, merely changing the position of the wrist will usually help.

Early on there is little to see, but there are two helpful tests: sensory symptoms can often be reproduced by percussing over the median nerve (*Tinel's sign*) or by holding the wrist fully flexed for a minute (*Phalen's test*). In late cases there is wasting of the thenar muscles, weakness of thumb abduction and sensory dulling in the median nerve territory.

Electrodiagnostic tests, which show slowing of nerve conduction across the wrist, are reserved for those with atypical symptoms.

Radicular symptoms of cervical spondylosis may confuse the diagnosis and may coincide with carpal tunnel syndrome.

Treatment

Light splints that prevent wrist flexion can help those with night pain or with pregnancy-related symptoms. Steroid injection into the carpal canal, likewise, provides temporary relief.

Open surgical division of the transverse carpal ligament usually provides a quick and simple cure; this can usually be done under local anaesthesia. The incision should be kept to the ulnar side of the thenar crease so as to avoid accidental injury to the palmar cutaneous (sensory) and thenar motor branches of the median nerve. Endoscopic carpal tunnel release offers an alternative with slightly quicker postoperative rehabilitation.

CHAPTER 16

THE HAND

CLINICAL ASSESSMENT

The hand is (in more senses than one) the medium of introduction to the outside world. Deformity and loss of function are quickly noticed – and often bitterly resented.

HISTORY

- *Pain* is usually felt in the palm or in the finger joints. A poorly defined ache may be referred from the neck, shoulder or mediastinum.
- *Swelling* may be localized, or may occur in many joints simultaneously. Characteristically, rheumatoid arthritis causes swelling of the proximal joints and osteoarthritis the distal joints.
- *Deformity* can appear suddenly (due to tendon rupture) or slowly (suggesting bone or joint pathology).
- *Loss of function* is particularly troublesome in the hand. The patient may have difficulty handling eating utensils, holding a cup or glass, grasping a doorknob (or a crutch), dressing or (most trying of all) attending to personal hygiene.
- *Sensory symptoms and motor weakness* provide clues to neurological disorders affecting the lower cervical nerve roots and their peripheral extensions.

EXAMINATION

Both upper limbs should be bared for comparison. Examination of the hand needs patience and meticulous attention to detail.

Look

The skin may be scarred, altered in colour, dry or moist, and hairy or smooth. Wasting and deformity, and the presence of any lumps, should be noted; a crimped appearance of the skin in the palm is characteristic of Dupuytren's contracture. The resting posture of the hand and fingers is an important clue to nerve or tendon damage. Swelling may be in the subcutaneous tissue, in a tendon sheath or in a joint – typically the metacarpophalangeal (MCP) joints in rheumatoid arthritis or the interphalangeal (IP) joints in osteoarthritis.

Feel

The temperature and texture of the skin are noted. Swelling or thickening may be in the subcutaneous tissue, a tendon sheath, a joint or one of the bones. If a nodule is felt, the underlying tendon should be moved by flexing the finger to discover if the nodule is attached to that tendon. Tenderness should be accurately localized to one of these structures.

Move

Passive movements should be tested first, to see whether the joints are 'movable' before you ask the patient to move them actively. The range of movement for each digit is recorded, starting with the MCP joints and then going on to the proximal interphalangeal (PIP) and distal interphalangeal (DIP) joints.

Active movements reflect, simultaneously, the state of the joints, the integrity of the tendons and motor nerve function in each digit.

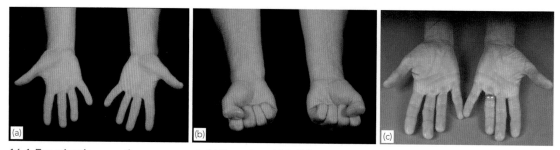

16.1 Examination – active movement (a) Extension. (b) Full flexion. (c) Testing finger abduction. The abducted little fingers are forced against each other; the weaker one will collapse.

Ask the patient to place both hands with palms facing upwards and the fingers extended, then to curl the fingers into full flexion; a 'lagging finger' is immediately obvious.

MCP flexion and IP extension are activated by the intrinsic muscles (lumbricals and interossei). This is tested by asking the patient to extend the fingers with the MCP joints flexed (the 'duckbill' position).

The interossei also motivate finger abduction and adduction (fingers together and then spread widely apart). Active power can be roughly gauged by having the patient abduct the fingers while the examiner presses against the spread-out index and little fingers, trying to force them back to the neutral position. A better way is to ask the patient to spread the fingers of both hands to the maximum; the examiner then grasps the patient's hands, pushes them towards each other and forces the two little fingers against each other; the weaker (non-dominant) side will normally give way first, but if the difference in one or other hand is marked it signifies true abductor weakness, a sign of ulnar nerve or T1 root dysfunction.

Thumb movements (and their nomenclature) are unusual, comprising the combined mobility of both the first carpometacarpal (CMC) and the first MCP joint. With the hand lying flat, palm upwards, five types of movement are recognized:

- Extension (sideways movement in the plane of the palm).
- Abduction (upward movement at right angles to the palm).
- Adduction (pressing against the palm).
- Flexion (sideways movement across the palm).
- Opposition (touching the tips of the fingers).

Weakness of abduction (tested simply by pressing against the abducted thumb of each hand) is a cardinal feature of median nerve dysfunction. In advanced cases there will also be obvious wasting of the thenar eminence.

Pain, deformity and loss of motion at the base of the thumb (the first CMC joint) are common symptoms of osteoarthritis.

Testing for musculotendinous function

Flexor digitorum profundus (FDP) is tested by simply immobilizing the PIP joint and then asking the patient to bend the tip of the finger.

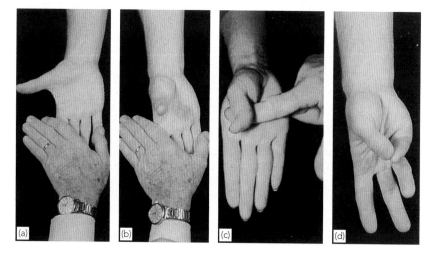

16.2 Thumb movements (a) Hold the patient's hand flat on the table and ask him or her to 'stretch to the side' (extension); (b) 'point to the ceiling' (abduction); (c) 'pinch my finger' (adduction); and (d) 'touch your little finger' (opposition).

Flexor digitorum superficialis is more complicated. The FDP must first be inactivated, otherwise one cannot tell which of the two tendons is flexing the PIP joint. This is done by grasping all the fingers, except the one being examined, and holding them firmly in full extension; because the profundus tendons share a common muscle belly, this manoeuvre automatically prevents *all* the profundus tendons from participating in finger flexion. The patient is then asked to flex the isolated finger which is being examined; this movement must be activated by flexor digitorum superficialis.

There are two exceptions to this rule: first, the little finger sometimes has no independent flexor digitorum superficialis; second, the index finger often has a separate flexor profundus which cannot be inactivated by the usual mass action manoeuvre. Instead, for these two fingers flexor superficialis is tested by asking the patient to pinch hard with the DIP joint in full extension and the PIP joint in full flexion; this position can be maintained only if the superficialis tendon is active and intact.

The *long extensors* are tested by asking the patient to extend the MCP joints. However, inability to do this does not necessarily signify paralysis or tendon rupture: the long extensor tendon may have slipped off the knuckle into the interdigital gutter (a common occurrence in rheumatoid arthritis).

Flexor pollicis longus is tested by immobilizing the thumb MCP joint and asking the patient to bend the single IP joint.

Grip strength

Grip strength is assessed (rather crudely) by asking the patient to squeeze the examiner's fingers; it may be diminished because of muscle weakness, tendon damage, finger stiffness or wrist instability. Strength can be measured more accurately with a mechanical dynamometer. Pinch grip also should be measured.

Neurological assessment

If symptoms such as numbness, tingling or weakness exist – and in all cases of trauma – a full neurological examination of the upper limbs should be carried out, testing power, reflexes and sensation. Further refinement is achieved by testing two-point discrimination, sensitivity to heat and cold, stereognosis and fine pressure (see Chapter 11).

Functional tests

Function can be measured subjectively using patient-completed scales, but objective tests are more reliable. There are several types of grip, which can be tested by giving the patient a variety of tasks to perform: picking up a pin (*precision grip*), holding a sheet of paper (*pinch*), holding a key (*sideways pinch*), holding a pen (*chuck grip*), holding a bag handle (*hook grip*), holding a glass (*span*) and gripping a hammer handle (*power grip*).

Stereognosis is evaluated using Moberg's pick-up test – asking the patient to pick up and identify, with eyes closed, a number of objects from the desk-top; the procedure is timed and the affected hand is compared with the 'good' hand.

Each finger has its special task: the thumb and index finger are used for pinch, but the index finger is also a sensory organ; slight loss of movement matters little but if sensation is abnormal the patient may not want to use the finger at all. The middle finger controls the position of objects in the palm. The ring and little fingers are used essentially for power grip (e.g. wielding a hammer or a wrench); here stiffness is a real handicap.

Dexterity is important in all these functions; it may be lost in any type of nerve lesion – e.g. in a severe carpal tunnel syndrome (median nerve compression) because of the combination of thenar weakness, reduced sensation and diminished stereognosis and proprioception.

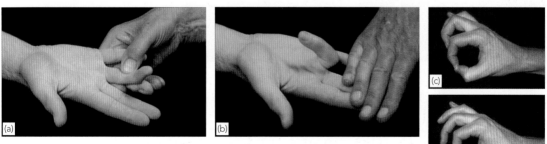
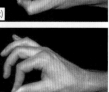

16.3 Testing musculotendinous function (a) Flexor digitorum profundus (FDP) lesser finger. (b) Flexor digitorum superficialis (FDS) lesser fingers. (c) FDP index. (d) FDS index.

CONGENITAL VARIATIONS

The hand and foot are much the most common sites of congenital deformities of the locomotor system; the incidence is about 1:1000 live births. Early recognition is important, and definitive treatment should be timed to fit in with the functional demands of the child. There are seven types of malformation:

- *Failure of formation*: total or partial absence of parts may be transverse ('congenital amputations') or axial (missing rays).
- *Failure of differentiation*: fingers may be partly or wholly joined together (syndactyly). This may be corrected by separating the fingers and repairing the defects with skin grafts.
- *Duplication*: polydactyly (extra digits) is the most common hand malformation. The extra finger should be amputated, if only for cosmetic reasons.
- *Under-growth*: the thumb can be very small or even absent.
- *Over-growth*: a giant finger is unsightly, but attempts at operative reduction are fraught with complications.
- *Constriction bands*: these have the appearance of an elastic band constricting the finger. In the worst cases this may lead to amputation.
- *Generalized malformations*: the hand may be involved in generalized disorders such as Marfan's syndrome ('spider hands') or achondroplasia ('trident hand'). See Chapter 8.

ACQUIRED DEFORMITIES

Deformity may be due to disorders of the skin, subcutaneous tissues, muscles, tendons, joints, bones or neuromuscular function.

SKIN CONTRACTURE

Cuts and burns of the palmar skin are liable to heal with contracture; this may cause puckering of the palm or fixed flexion of the fingers. *Surgical incisions should never cross flexor creases.* Established contractures may require excision of the scar and Z-plasty of the overlying skin.

DUPUYTREN'S CONTRACTURE

This is a nodular hypertrophy and contracture of the palmar aponeurosis. The condition is familial, but there is a higher than usual incidence in people with diabetes and acquired immunodeficiency syndrome (AIDS) and in patients with epilepsy receiving phenytoin therapy. Smoking and heavy alcohol consumption are also risk factors.

Clinical features

The patient – usually a middle-aged man – complains of a nodular thickening in the palm. Gradually this progresses distally to involve the ring or little finger. Pain is unusual. Often both hands are involved, one more than the other. The palm is puckered, nodular and thick. If the subcutaneous cords extend into the fingers, they may produce flexion deformities at the MCP and PIP joints. Sometimes the dorsal knuckle pads are thickened.

Similar nodules may be seen on the soles of the feet (Ledderhose's disease). There is a rare, curious association with fibrosis of the corpus cavernosum (*Peyronie's disease*).

Diagnosis

Dupuytren's contracture must be distinguished from skin contracture (where a previous laceration

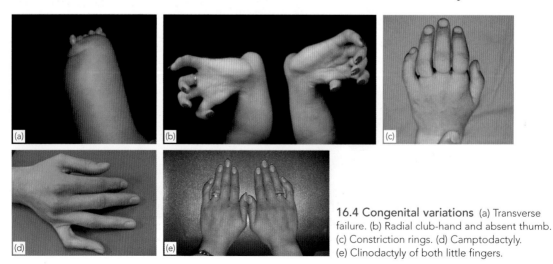

16.4 Congenital variations (a) Transverse failure. (b) Radial club-hand and absent thumb. (c) Constriction rings. (d) Camptodactyly. (e) Clinodactyly of both little fingers.

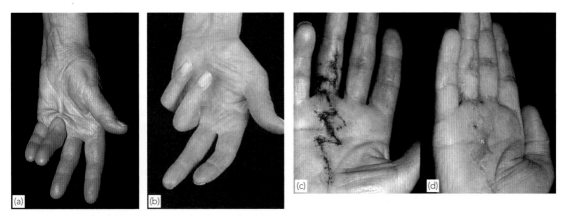

16.5 Dupuytren's disease Contractures at (a) the palmar crease and (b) the proximal interphalangeal joint. (c) Z-plasty shortly after operation and (d) 2 weeks later.

is usually obvious) and tendon contracture (where the 'cord' moves on passive flexion of the finger).

Treatment

If the deformity is static and there is no loss of function, no treatment is needed. If the condition is marked, operative treatment may be called for. The aim is reasonable, not complete, correction; a satisfactory outcome is more predictable at the MCP joint than the PIP joint, but there is still a risk of recurrence or extension. If the disease is extensive, the affected area is approached through a Z-shaped incision that does not cross directly over a skin crease; after carefully freeing the nerves and blood vessels, the thickened part of the fascia is excised. Following operative correction the hand is splinted for a few days and then active movement is encouraged, but night splinting for a few months may reduce recurrence. An alternative to surgery is the injection of a drug, collagenase, to dissolve the cord.

NEUROMUSCULAR DISORDERS

Ulnar 'claw-hand' (intrinsic-minus deformity)

Ulnar nerve lesions characteristically cause hyper-extension at the MCP joints and flexion at the IP joints. This is due to paralysis of the intrinsic muscles which normally activate MCP flexion and IP extension. Thus it is sometimes called an *intrinsic-minus deformity*.

Shortening of intrinsic muscles (intrinsic-plus deformity)

Intrinsic muscle shortening produces flexion at the MCP joints with extension of the IP joints and adduction of the thumb – an *intrinsic-plus deformity*. Anatomically this is the opposite of the intrinsic-minus deformity described above. The

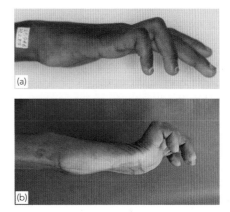

16.6 Ulnar 'claw-hand' (a) *High ulnar nerve paralysis* causing a *partial claw-hand* deformity: the paralysed intrinsic muscles cause the loss of flexion at the MCP joints and loss of extension at the IP joints, but because flexor digitorum profundus (FDP) is also partially paralysed the index and middle fingers are straight. (b) *Low ulnar nerve paralysis* (lower than the innervation of FDP), causing a *total claw-hand* deformity in which all the long flexors are still active.

main causes are muscle scarring or shortening after trauma or infection. Moderate contracture can be treated by releasing the intrinsic muscles where they cross the MCP joints.

Ischaemic contracture of the forearm muscles

This follows circulatory insufficiency due to injuries at or below the elbow (see page 374). There is shortening of the long flexors; the fingers are held in flexion and can be straightened only when the wrist is flexed. Sometimes the picture is complicated by associated damage to the ulnar or median nerve (or both). If disability is marked,

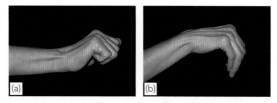

16.7 Contracture of the long flexors (a) When the wrist is extended, the fingers involuntarily curl into tight flexion. (b) When the wrist is flexed, tension on the long flexor muscles is relaxed and the fingers can uncurl to a certain extent.

some improvement may be obtained by releasing the shortened muscles at their origin above the elbow, or else by excising the dead muscles and restoring finger movement with tendon transfers.

TENDON LESIONS

'Mallet' finger

The patient suddenly cannot straighten the terminal joint, but passive movement is normal. This is due to injury at the attachment of the extensor tendon to the terminal phalanx. The DIP joint should be splinted for 8 weeks, with the proximal joint free.

Ruptured extensor pollicis longus

The long thumb extensor may rupture after fraying where it crosses the wrist (e.g. after a Colles' fracture, or in rheumatoid arthritis). Direct repair is unsatisfactory and a tendon transfer, using the extensor indicis, is needed.

Dropped fingers

The patient is unable to hold the fingers in extension at the MCP joints. The cause usually lies not at the MCP joint but at the wrist, where the extensor tendons have ruptured (typically in rheumatoid arthritis). If only one finger is affected, direct repair may be possible; otherwise the distal portion of the tendon can be attached to an adjacent finger extensor.

Boutonnière

This is a flexion deformity of the PIP joint, due to interruption of the central slip of the extensor tendon. The lateral slips separate and the head of the proximal phalanx pops through the gap like a finger through a buttonhole. It is seen after trauma or in rheumatoid disease. Post-traumatic rupture can sometimes be repaired; the chronic deformity in rheumatoid disease usually defies correction.

Swan-neck deformity

This is the reverse of boutonnière: the PIP joint is hyperextended and the DIP joint flexed. It is due to imbalance of extensor versus flexor action in the finger, and is often seen in rheumatoid arthritis. The deformity may be corrected by tendon rebalancing.

'TRIGGER FINGER'

This common condition presents as an intermittent 'deformity', usually of the ring or middle finger, sometimes of the thumb. The patient complains

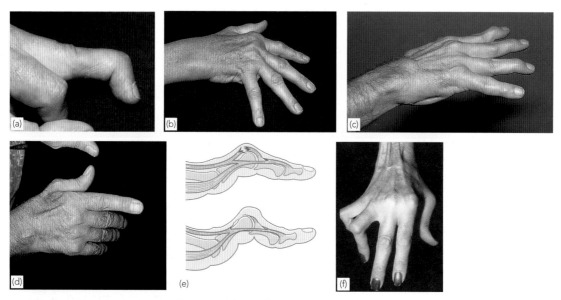

16.8 Deformities due to tendon lesions (a) Mallet finger. (b) Dropped fingers due to extensor tendon ruptures at the wrist. (c) Swan-neck deformities. (d) Rupture of extensor pollicis brevis. (e,f) Boutonnière deformities.

that, when the hand is clenched and then opened, the finger (or thumb) gets stuck in flexion; with a little more effort, it suddenly snaps into full extension. The usual cause is thickening of the fibrous tendon sheath: the flexor tendon becomes temporarily trapped at the entrance to its sheath and then, on forced extension, it passes the constriction with a snap. A similar entrapment may occur due to a bulky tenosynovitis (e.g. in rheumatic disorders). A tender nodule or thickened tendon can usually be felt at the distal palmar crease. The condition is more common in diabetes.

Infantile trigger thumb ('*snapping thumb*') is usually misdiagnosed as a 'dislocating thumb'; sometimes it goes completely undiagnosed and the child grows up with the thumb permanently bent or the distal phalanx under-developed. Feel for the tell-tale thickening on the palmar aspect at the base of the thumb.

Treatment

The condition often improves spontaneously, so there is no urgency about treatment. However, if it persists, or is particularly annoying, it can usually be cured by an injection of corticosteroid carefully placed at the entrance of the tendon sheath.

Refractory cases need operation: the fibrous sheath is incised, allowing the tendon to move freely. In the case of the thumb, take particular care to avoid injuring the digital nerve, which runs close to the sheath.

For children treatment (as above) can be deferred until the child is 3 years old, as spontaneous recovery is quite common.

BONE LESIONS

Malunited fractures may cause metacarpal or phalangeal deformity. Occasionally this needs correction by osteotomy and internal fixation.

ACUTE INFECTIONS OF THE HAND

Infection of the hand is frequently limited to one of several well-defined compartments: under the nailfold (paronychia); the pulp space (whitlow); subcutaneous tissues elsewhere; a tendon sheath; one of the deep fascial spaces or a joint. Almost invariably the cause is a *Staphylococcus* which has been implanted by trivial or unobserved injury.

Pathology

Acute inflammation and suppuration in small closed compartments (e.g. the pulp space or tendon sheath) may cause an increase in pressure to levels at which the local blood supply is threatened. In neglected cases tissue necrosis is an imminent risk. Even if this does not occur, the patient may end up with a stiff and useless hand unless the infection is rapidly brought under control.

Clinical features

Usually there is a history of trauma, but it may have been so trivial as to pass unnoticed. A thorn prick can be as dangerous as a cut. Within a day or two, the finger (or hand) becomes painful and tensely swollen. The patient may feel ill and feverish and the pain becomes throbbing. There is obvious redness and tension in the tissues, and exquisite tenderness over the site of infection. Finger movements may be markedly restricted.

Principles of treatment

Antibiotics

As soon as the diagnosis is made and specimens have been taken for microbiological investigation, antibiotic treatment is started – usually with flucloxacillin and, in severe cases, with fusidic acid or a cephalosporin as well. This may later be changed when bacterial sensitivity is known.

Rest and elevation

In a mild case the hand is rested in a sling. In a severe case the arm is elevated in a roller towel while the patient is kept in hospital under observation. Analgesics are given for pain.

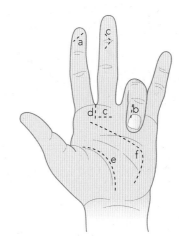

16.9 Incisions for infection The incisions for surgical drainage are illustrated here: (a) pulp space (directly over the abscess); (b) nailfold (it may also be necessary to excise the edge of the nail); (c) tendon sheath (two incisions, one distal and one proximal); (d) web space; (e) thenar space; (f) midpalmar space.

Drainage

If there are signs of an abscess (throbbing pain, marked tenderness and toxaemia), the pus should be drained. A tourniquet and either general or regional block anaesthesia are essential. The incision should be made at the site of maximal tenderness, *but never across a skin crease*. Necrotic tissue is excised and the area thoroughly washed and cleansed. The wound is either left open or lightly sutured and then covered with non-stick dressings. A pus specimen is sent for microbiological investigation.

Splintage

After draining tendon sheath or fascial space infections or if conservative treatment is likely to be prolonged, a removable splint should be applied – *always with the joints in the position of safe immobilization*, that is with the wrist slightly extended, the MCP joints in 70-degrees flexion, the IP joints extended and the thumb in abduction.

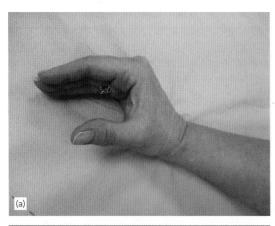

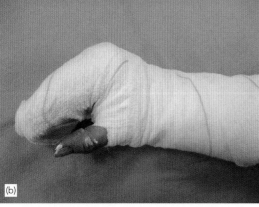

16.10 Position of safe immobilization (a,b) The metacarpophalangeal joints are 70 degrees flexed, the finger joints extended and the thumb abducted. This is the position in which the ligaments are at their longest and splintage is least likely to result in stiffness.

Physiotherapy

Once the acute inflammation subsides, movements are encouraged. Ideally this should be done under the direction of a physiotherapist specialized in 'hand therapy'. The splint is re-applied between exercise sessions.

SPECIFIC TYPES OF INFECTION

Paronychia

Infection under the nailfold is common. The area is swollen, red and tender. At the first sign of infection, antibiotic treatment alone may be effective. If pus is present, it can often be released simply by lifting the nailfold from the nail; otherwise the nailfold must be incised. Occasionally a portion of the nail needs to be removed.

Pulp-space infection (felon)

Pulp-space infection (usually due to a prick or splinter) causes throbbing pain. The fingertip is swollen, red and acutely tender. Antibiotic treatment is started immediately. However, if pus has formed, it must be released through a small incision over the site of maximal tenderness.

Other subcutaneous infections

Anywhere in the hand, a blister or superficial cut may become infected, causing redness, swelling and tenderness. A local collection of pus should be drained through a small incision over the site of maximal tenderness. It is important to exclude a deeper pocket of pus in a nearby tendon sheath or in one of the deep fascial spaces.

Tendon-sheath infection

Suppurative tenosynovitis is uncommon but dangerous. The affected digit is painful and swollen; it is held bent, is very tender and the patient will not move it or permit it to be moved. Unless treatment is swift and effective, there is a risk of tendon necrosis and the patient may end up with a useless finger.

Treatment must be started as soon as the diagnosis is suspected. The hand is splinted and elevated and antibiotics are administered intravenously – initially a broad-spectrum penicillin or a systemic cephalosporin, to be modified if necessary once the organism has been cultured and tested for antibiotic sensitivity. If there is no improvement after 24 hours, surgical drainage is essential. Two incisions are needed, one at the proximal end of the sheath and one at the distal end; using a fine catheter, the sheath is then irrigated with saline or Ringer's lactate solution (always from proximal to

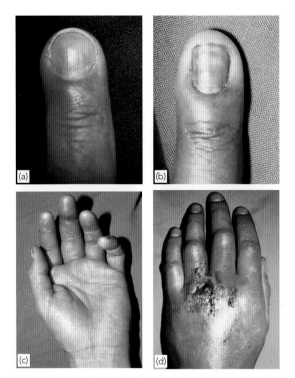

16.11 Types of hand infection (a) Acute nailfold infection (paronychia). (b) Chronic paronychia. (c) Flexor tenosynovitis of the middle finger following a cortisone injection. (d) Septic human bite resulting in acute infection of the fourth metacarpophalangeal joint.

distal). The catheter is left in place for postoperative irrigation during the next 2 days.

Tendon-sheath infection in the thumb or little finger may spread proximally to the synovial bursa. This has to be drained through a further incision just above the wrist.

At the end of the operation, the hand is swathed in absorbent dressings and splinted in the position of safe immobilization (Figure 16.10).

Deep fascial space infection

Infection from a web space or from an infected tendon sheath may spread to either of the deep fascial spaces of the palm. The palm is ballooned, so its normal concavity is lost. There is extensive tenderness and the whole hand is held still.

For drainage, an incision is made directly over the abscess and sinus forceps inserted; if the web space is also infected, it too should be incised. Postoperatively the hand is dressed and splinted as described above.

Joint infection

Any of the joints may be infected, either directly by a penetrating injury on injection, or indirectly from adjacent structures. At the onset, the clinical features may be hard to distinguish from those of acute gout. Joint aspiration will provide the answer.

Intravenous antibiotics are administered and the hand is splinted. If symptoms and signs do not improve within 24 hours, open drainage is needed.

Bites

Animal bites are usually inflicted by cats, dogs or farm animals. Many become infected and, although the common pathogens are staphylococci and streptococci, unusual organisms are also encountered.

Human bites and lacerations sustained during fist-fights are generally thought to be even more prone to infection. A variety of organisms (including anaerobes) are encountered, the commonest being *Staphylococcus aureus*, *Streptococcus* group A and *Eikenella corrodens*. All such wounds should be assumed to be infected. X-rays should be obtained, to exclude a fracture or foreign body.

Treatment should be started immediately. Fresh wounds are carefully examined in the operating theatre and swab samples are taken for bacterial culture and sensitivity. If necessary, the wound should be extended and debrided; search for a fragment of tooth or a divit of articular cartilage from the joint. The hand is then splinted and elevated and antibiotics are given prophylactically until the laboratory results are obtained.

Established infection in bite wounds will need debridement, wash-outs and intravenous antibiotic treatment. The common organisms are all sensitive to broad-spectrum penicillins and cephalosporins. With animal bites one should also consider the possibility of rabies.

Postoperative treatment consists, as usual, of copious wound dressings, splintage in the 'safe' position and encouragement of movement once the infection has resolved. Tendon lacerations can be dealt with when the tissues are completely healed.

RHEUMATOID ARTHRITIS

The hand, more than any other part of the body, is where rheumatoid arthritis displays its story. Early on, there is synovitis of the proximal joints and tendon sheaths; later, joint and tendon erosions prepare the ground for mechanical derangement; in the final stage, joint instability and tendon rupture cause progressive deformity and loss of function.

Clinical features

Pain and stiffness of the fingers are early symptoms; often the wrist also is affected. Examination may show swelling of the MCP and PIP joints; both hands are affected, more or less symmetrically. Joint mobility and grip strength are diminished.

As the disease progresses, deformities begin to appear (and are increasingly difficult to correct). In the late stage one sees the characteristic ulnar deviation of the fingers and subluxation of the MCP joints, often associated with swan-neck or boutonnière deformities. When these abnormalities become fixed, functional loss may be so severe that the patient needs help with washing, dressing and feeding.

X-rays

During the initial stages, x-rays show only soft-tissue swelling and osteoporosis around the joints. Later there is narrowing of the joint spaces and small periarticular erosions appear. In the last stage, articular destruction may be marked, with joint deformity and dislocation.

Treatment

In early cases, treatment is directed at controlling the systemic disease and the local synovitis. In addition to general measures, splints may reduce pain and swelling.

Persistent synovitis may benefit from local injections of methylprednisolone, but sometimes surgical synovectomy is needed.

As the disease progresses, it becomes important to prevent deformity. Uncontrolled synovitis

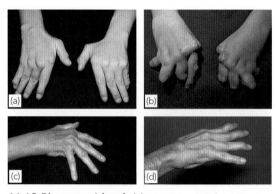

16.12 Rheumatoid arthritis (a) Typical deformities in established rheumatoid arthritis. The proximal joints are the ones most severely affected; there is subluxation of the metacarpophalangeal (MCP) joints and the fingers are deviated ulnarwards. (b) Severe rheumatoid deformities with dislocation of the MCP joints and ulceration of the skin over the knuckles. (c) 'Dropped fingers' due to rupture of extensor tendons where they cross the back of the wrist. (d) Swan-neck deformities of the fingers.

requires synovectomy followed by physiotherapy. Isolated tendon ruptures are repaired or bypassed by appropriate tendon transfers. Joint instability may require stabilization or arthroplasty.

In late cases with established deformities, reconstructive surgery may be needed, but

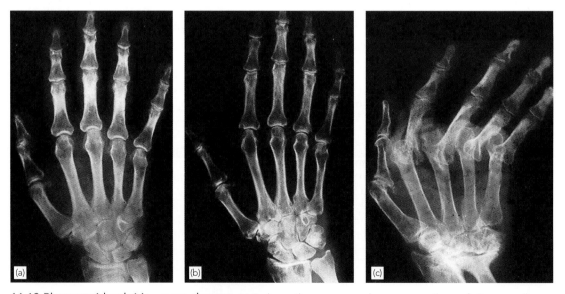

16.13 Rheumatoid arthritis – x-ray changes (a) Early on, the x-rays may show no more than soft-tissue swelling and juxta-articular osteoporosis. (b) A later stage showing characteristic tiny punched-out juxta-articular erosions at the second and third metacarpophalangeal (MCP) joints. The wrist is now also involved. (c) In the most advanced stage, the MCP joints are dislocated and the hand is severely deformed.

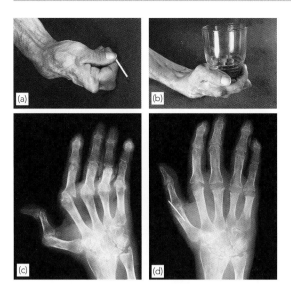

16.14 Rheumatoid arthritis – treatment (a,b) Even with severe deformities, the patient may regain good function. Why interfere if the disease is quiescent and the hand works well? (c,d) If function is markedly restricted, reconstructive surgery has a useful role. X-rays before and after metacarpophalangeal (MCP) joint replacement with Silastic spacers and fusion of the thumb MCP joint.

treatment should be directed at restoring function rather than merely correcting deformity.

OSTEOARTHRITIS

Osteoarthritis of the DIP joints is very common in postmenopausal women and is usually a manifestation of polyarticular osteoarthritis. It often starts with pain in one or two fingers; the distal joints become swollen and tender, the condition usually spreading to all the fingers of both hands. On examination, there is bony thickening around the DIP joints (Heberden's nodes) and some restriction of movement. Not infrequently, some of the PIP joints are involved (Bouchard's nodes)

and the CMC joint of the thumb may show similar changes.

The distinction from rheumatoid arthritis is very important. In both conditions, the finger joints are swollen and stiff. However, whereas rheumatoid arthritis affects the proximal joints (particularly the MCP joints), osteoarthritis affects mainly the terminal IP joints.

Treatment is symptomatic; pain and tenderness gradually subside and the patient is left with painless, knobbly fingers. Occasionally (if pain or deformity is particularly marked), fusion of the DIP joint may be called for. If the PIP joint or the MCP joint are involved they can be replaced.

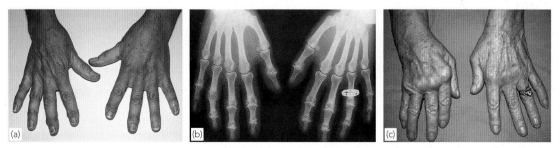

16.15 Osteoarthritis (a,b) Osteoarthritis affects mainly the distal interphalangeal joints. The knobbly joints are called Heberden's nodes. (c) Rheumatoid arthritis can look similar, but here it is mainly the proximal joints that are affected.

CHAPTER 17

THE NECK

CLINICAL ASSESSMENT

HISTORY

The common symptoms of neck disorder are pain and stiffness.

- *Pain* is felt in the neck itself, but it can also be referred to the suprascapular areas, the shoulders or the upper arms. It may start suddenly (as with an acute intervertebral disc prolapse) or gradually (as in chronic disc degeneration). Always ask if it is associated with paraesthesia in the arm or hand, a particularly significant combination.
- *Stiffness* may be either intermittent or continuous. Sometimes it is so severe that the patient can scarcely move his or her head.
- *Deformity* usually appears as a wry neck, due to muscle spasm; think of a disc prolapse or a previously undiagnosed fracture.
- *Numbness, tingling and weakness* in the upper limbs may be due to pressure on a nerve root; weakness in the lower limbs may result from cord compression in the neck.
- *Headache* sometimes emanates from the neck, but if this is the only symptom other causes are more likely.

Always ask about previous neck injuries.

EXAMINATION

The entire upper trunk and both upper limbs should be exposed. Start the examination with the patient standing; neck posture and movements are most easily observed in this position. The shoulders also are examined while the patient is upright. The anterior structures (trachea, thyroid, oesophagus) are best felt with the patient seated and the examiner standing behind the chair. The third part of the examination is carried out with the patient lying down; it is easier (and more reliable) to feel for muscle spasm and point tenderness with the patient lying prone with his or her neck supported over a pillow. Neurological examination is performed with the patient lying supine.

Look

Any deformity is noted. From the back, skin blemishes, scapular abnormalities or muscular asymmetry can be seen. One shoulder may be higher and there may be muscle wasting in the arm or hand.

Feel

The neck and shoulders should be carefully palpated for tender areas, lumps and muscle spasm.

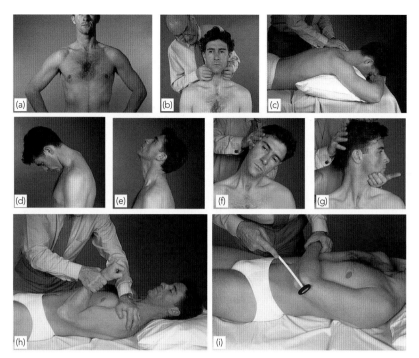

for any deformity or superficial blemish which might suggest a disorder affecting the cervical spine. (b) The front of the neck is felt with the patient seated and the examiner standing behind him. (c) The back of the neck is most easily and reliably felt with the patient lying prone over a pillow; this way muscle spasm is reduced and the neck is relaxed.
(d–g) Movement: flexion ('chin on chest'); extension ('look up at the ceiling'); lateral flexion ('tilt your ear towards your shoulder'); and rotation ('look over your shoulder').
(h,i) Neurological examination is mandatory.

Move

Flexion, extension, lateral flexion and rotation are tested and the range of movements noted. Shoulder movements, likewise, should be recorded.

Spurling's test is helpful. The patient is instructed to rotate the neck to one side with the chin elevated: if this reproduces ipsilateral upper limb pain and paraesthesiae, it would increase the suspicion of a disc prolapse with cervical nerve root compression. Pain may be relieved by having the patient place the arm overhead (the abduction relief sign).

Neurological examination

Neurological examination of the upper limbs is mandatory in all cases; in some the lower limbs also should be examined. Muscle power, reflexes and sensation should be carefully tested; even small degrees of abnormality may be significant.

IMAGING

X-ray examination should include all levels from the base of the occiput to T1. The anteroposterior view should show the regular, undulating outlines of the lateral masses; their symmetry may be disturbed by destructive lesions or fractures. A projection through the mouth is required to show the upper two vertebrae.

When looking at the lateral view, make sure that all seven vertebrae are visible; patients have been

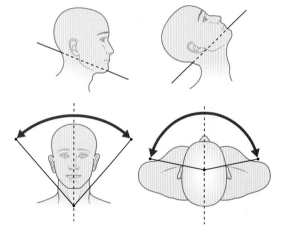

17.2 Normal range of movement Flexion and extension of the neck are best gauged by observing the angle of the occipitomental line – an imaginary line joining the tip of the chin and the occipital protuberance. In full flexion the chin normally touches the chest; in full extension the occipitomental line forms an angle of at least 45 degrees with the horizontal, and over 60 degrees in young people. Lateral flexion is usually achieved up to 45 degrees and rotation to 80 degrees each way.

paralysed, and some have lost their lives, because a fracture–dislocation at C6/7 or C7/T1 was missed. The normal cervical curve shows four parallel lines: one along the anterior surfaces of the vertebral bodies, one along their posterior surfaces, one along the posterior borders of the lateral masses and one along the bases of the spinous processes; any malalignment suggests subluxation. The disc spaces are inspected; loss of disc height and the presence of osteophytic spurs at the margins of adjacent vertebral bodies are features of chronic intervertebral disc degeneration, a common finding in elderly people and not necessarily the cause of neck pain. The posterior interspinous spaces are compared; if one is wider than the rest, this may signify chronic instability of that segment, possibly due to a previously undiagnosed subluxation. Flexion and extension views may be needed to demonstrate instability, though after an acute injury such movements are best avoided!

Computed tomography (CT) and *magnetic resonance imaging (MRI)* are essential for defining the intervertebral discs, the neural structures and the outlines of the spinal canal and intervertebral foramina. Remember, though, that 20% of asymptomatic people show significant abnormalities and the scans must therefore be interpreted alongside the clinical assessment.

DEFORMITIES OF THE NECK

TORTICOLLIS ('WRY NECK', 'SKEW NECK')

In torticollis the chin is twisted upwards and towards one side. It may be either *congenital* or *secondary* to other local disorders.

Infantile (congenital) torticollis

Skew neck is sometimes seen in an infant or very young child. The sternomastoid muscle on one side is fibrous and fails to elongate as the child grows. In some cases a well-defined lump is felt in the muscle during the first few weeks of life, but deformity may not become apparent until the child is 2 or 3 years old. As the neck grows, the contracted sternomastoid tethers the skull on one side, thus twisting the chin towards the opposite side. Secondary facial deformities may occur.

Treatment: if a child has a sternomastoid 'tumour', subsequent deformity may be prevented by gentle, daily manipulation of the neck. Non-operative treatment is successful in most cases, but if the condition persists beyond 1 year operative treatment is required to prevent progressive facial deformity. The contracted muscle is divided (usually at its lower end but sometimes at the upper end or at both ends) and the head is manipulated into the neutral position. After operation, correction is maintained with a temporary orthosis followed by stretching exercises.

Secondary torticollis

Wry neck, due to muscle spasm, may develop as a result of acute disc prolapse (the most common cause in adults), inflamed neck glands, vertebral infection, injuries of the cervical spine or ocular disorders.

VERTEBRAL ANOMALIES

Cervical vertebral anomalies are dealt with in Chapter 8. Odontoid dysplasia is particularly important and the subject warrants repetition in this section.

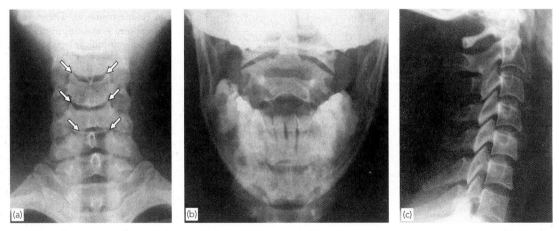

17.3 Imaging – normal x-rays (a) Anteroposterior view – note the smooth, symmetrical outlines and the clear, wide uncovertebral joints (arrows). (b) Open mouth view – to show the odontoid process and atlantoaxial joints. (c) Lateral view – showing all seven cervical vertebrae.

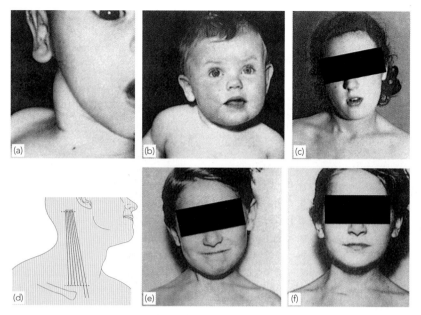

17.4 Torticollis Natural history: (a) sternomastoid tumour in a young baby; (b) early wry neck; (c) deformity with facial hemiatrophy in the adolescent. Surgical treatment: (d) two sites at which the sternomastoid may be divided; (e,f) before and a few months after operation.

ODONTOID ANOMALIES

The odontoid may be absent or hypoplastic, an anomaly that should be suspected (and looked for even if the patient does not complain) in any case of skeletal dysplasia involving the spine. This is especially important in patients undergoing operation; there is a risk that the atlantoaxial joint may subluxate under anaesthesia. Some patients present with pain or torticollis, or neurological complications such as transient paralysis or sphincter disturbances. In the majority of cases the anomaly is discovered by chance in a routine cervical spine x-ray following trauma. Patients with symptoms should have surgical stabilization.

ACUTE INTERVERTEBRAL DISC PROLAPSE

Cervical disc prolapse may be precipitated by local strain or injury, especially sudden unguarded flexion and rotation. It usually occurs immediately above or below the sixth cervical vertebra; in many cases (perhaps in all) there is a predisposing abnormality of the disc with increased nuclear tension.

The disc protrusion may press on the posterior longitudinal ligament, causing neck pain and stiffness as well as pain referred to the upper arm. Even more suggestive are associated symptoms of pain and paraesthesia in one or both arms.

Clinical features

The original attack may occasionally be related to a definite and severe strain. Subsequent attacks may be sudden or gradual in onset, and with trivial cause. The patient may complain of: (1) pain and stiffness of the neck, the pain often radiating to the scapular region and sometimes to the occiput; (2) pain and paraesthesia in one upper limb (rarely both), often radiating to the outer elbow, back of the wrist and to the index and middle fingers. Weakness is rare. Between attacks the patient feels well, although the neck may feel a bit stiff.

The neck may be tilted forwards and sideways. The muscles are tender and movements are restricted. The arms should be examined for neurological signs suggestive of nerve root irritation or compression.

Imaging

X-rays may show narrowing of the disc space. However, the diagnosis should be confirmed by *MRI*, which will show whether the disc protrusion is pressing on the adjacent nerve root.

Differential diagnosis

Acute soft-tissue strain: acute strains of the neck can cause pain and stiffness which may last for weeks or months. The absence of neurological symptoms and signs is significant.

Neuralgic amyotrophy (acute brachial neuritis): pain is sudden and severe, and situated over the shoulder, or the back of the shoulder, rather than in the neck itself. Multiple neurological levels are affected. Look for signs of serratus anterior weakness (winging of the scapula).

213

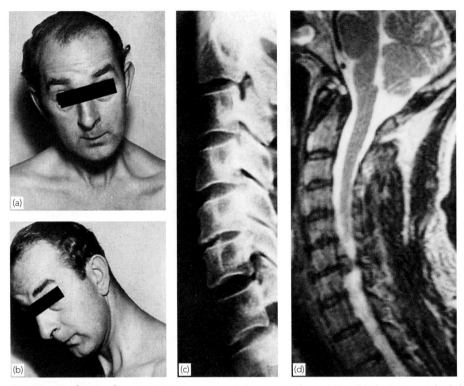

17.5 Acute disc prolapse (a,b) Acute wry neck due to a prolapsed disc. (c) The intervertebral disc space at C5/6 is reduced. (d) MRI in another case showing a large disc prolapse at C6/7.

Cervical spine infections: pain is unrelenting and local spasm severe. X-rays show erosion of the vertebral end-plates.

Cervical tumours: neurological signs are progressive and x-rays or MRI may show bone destruction.

Treatment

Heat and analgesics are soothing but, as with lumbar disc prolapse, there are only three satisfactory ways of treating the prolapse itself:

- Rest: a collar will prevent unguarded movement; it may be made of felt, sponge-rubber or polythene.
- Reduce: traction may enlarge the disc space, permitting the prolapse to subside. The head of the couch is raised and weights (up to 8 kg) are tied to a harness fitting under the chin and occiput. Traction is applied intermittently for no more than 30 minutes at a time.
- Remove: if symptoms are refractory and severe enough, the disc may be removed through an anterior approach; bone grafts are inserted to fuse the affected area and to restore the normal intervertebral height. Nowadays the operation

can also be performed using endoscopic techniques.

CHRONIC DISC DEGENERATION (CERVICAL SPONDYLOSIS)

Intervertebral disc degeneration is common from middle age onwards, even in people who have not been aware of any acute episode in former years. With time, the discs collapse and flatten, and bony spurs appear at the anterior and posterior margins of the vertebral bodies on either side of the affected discs; those that develop posteriorly may encroach upon the intervertebral foramina, causing pressure on the nerve roots. Several levels may be affected and the condition is then usually referred to as '*spondylosis*'. The condition is not always symptomatic, and many people go throughout life without experiencing anything more than slight stiffness.

Clinical features

Troublesome symptoms come on gradually. The patient, usually aged over 40 years, complains of neck pain and stiffness. The pain may radiate widely: to the occiput, the scapular muscles and down one or both arms. Paraesthesia, weakness and clumsiness are occasional symptoms. Typically there are exacerbations of more acute discomfort, and long periods of relative quiescence.

The appearance is usually normal. There may be tenderness in the soft tissues at the back of the neck and above the scapulae; neck movements are limited and painful at the extremes.

Careful neurological examination may show abnormal signs in one or both upper limbs.

Imaging

Typical x-ray features are narrowing of several disc spaces, bony spur formation at the anterior and posterior edges of the vertebral bodies and (in the anteroposterior view) osteoarthritic changes in the tiny uncovertebral joints. Oblique views may show bony encroachment on the intervertebral foramina. MRI will show whether there is nerve root compression.

Differential diagnosis

Other disorders associated with neck or arm pain and sensory symptoms must be excluded. Cervical vertebral spur formation is very common in older people and this can be misleading in patients with other disorders.

Rotator cuff lesions: pain around the shoulder may resemble the referred pain of cervical spondylosis. However, features such as rotator cuff tenderness and restricted shoulder movements should suggest a local problem.

Nerve entrapment syndromes: median or ulnar nerve entrapment may give rise to intermittent symptoms of pain and paraesthesia in the hand. Characteristically the symptoms are worse at night or are related to posture. In doubtful cases, nerve conduction studies and electromyography will help to establish the diagnosis. Remember, though, that the patient may have symptoms from both a peripheral and a central abnormality.

Cervical tumours: with tumours of the vertebrae,

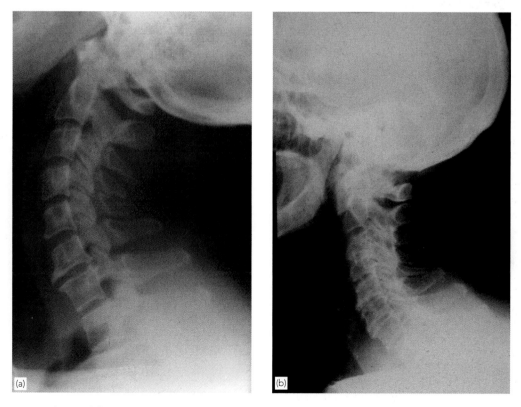

17.6 Cervical spondylosis – x-rays (a) Degenerative features at one level, C6/7. Note the prominent 'osteophytes' at the anterior and posterior borders of these two vertebral bodies. (b) Marked degenerative changes at multiple levels.

spinal cord, nerve roots or lymph nodes the symptoms are unremitting. Imaging studies should reveal the diagnosis.

Treatment

During painful episodes, heat and massage are soothing; some patients benefit from a period in a restraining collar. Physiotherapy is the mainstay of treatment, patients usually being maintained in relative comfort by various measures including exercises, gentle passive manipulation and intermittent traction.

Surgical treatment is indicated if severe symptoms are relieved only by a rigid and irksome support, particularly if there are neurological changes due to nerve root compression.

Foraminotomy

If the main problems are referred pain in the upper limb and/or neurological symptoms and signs, and the MRI shows foraminal narrowing and nerve root compression at one or two levels, foraminotomy (through a posterior approach) may be indicated. Only part of the facet joint is removed so this segment should not become unstable. However, patients should be warned that pre-existing neck pain may not be eliminated.

Anterior discectomy and fusion

This operation is particularly suitable if the problem is primarily one of unrelieved neck pain and stiffness. Through a transverse incision at the front of the neck, the intervertebral disc is removed without disturbing the posteriorly situated neurological structures. After preparation of the intervertebral space, a suitably-shaped autogenous bone graft (usually taken from the iliac crest) is inserted firmly between the adjacent vertebral bodies. An anterior plate is added if there is uncertainty about stability or if several levels are being fused. Operative complications such as injury to the recurrent laryngeal nerve or (worse) the vertebral artery are unusual if sufficient care is exercised. Graft dislodgement and failed fusion are less likely with intervertebral plating.

Intervertebral disc replacement

Disc replacement operations are now being performed in several countries. This has the (theoretical) advantage of removing the offending disc and preserving movement at the affected site. Short-term results appear to be as good as those achieved with anterior spinal fusion, with added benefits of lesser morbidity and shorter hospital stay. However, it is too early to assess the long-term outcome of these procedures.

PYOGENIC INFECTION

Pyogenic infection of the cervical spine is uncommon, and therefore often misdiagnosed in the early stages when antibiotic treatment is most effective. The organism – usually a staphylococcus – reaches the spine via the blood stream. Initially, destructive changes are limited to the intervertebral disc space and the adjacent parts of the vertebral bodies. Later, abscess formation occurs and pus may extend into the spinal canal or into the soft-tissue planes of the neck.

Clinical features

Vertebral infection may occur at any age. The patient complains of pain in the neck, often associated with muscle spasm and stiffness. Neck movements are severely restricted. Systemic symptoms are often mild but blood tests may show a leucocytosis and an elevated erythrocyte sedimentation rate (ESR).

X-rays at first show either no abnormality or only slight narrowing of the disc space; later more obvious signs of bone destruction appear.

Treatment is by antibiotics and rest. The cervical spine is 'immobilized' by traction; once the acute phase subsides, a collar may suffice. Operation is seldom necessary; if there is abscess formation, this will require drainage. As the infection subsides the

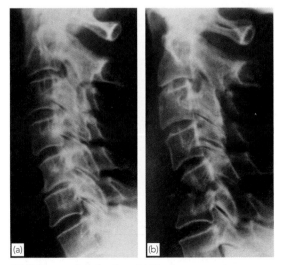

17.7 Pyogenic infection (a) The first x-ray, taken soon after the onset of symptoms, shows narrowing of the C5/6 disc space. (b) Three weeks later there is destruction and collapse of the adjacent vertebral bodies.

intervertebral space is obliterated and the adjacent vertebrae usually fuse.

TUBERCULOSIS

Cervical spine tuberculosis is rare. The organism is blood-borne and the infection localizes in the intervertebral disc and the anterior parts of the adjacent vertebral bodies. As the bone crumbles, the cervical spine collapses into kyphosis. A retropharyngeal abscess forms and points behind the sternomastoid muscle at the side of the neck. In late cases cord damage may cause neurological signs varying from mild weakness to tetraplegia.

Clinical features

The patient – usually a child – complains of neck pain and stiffness. In neglected cases a retropharyngeal abscess may cause difficulty in swallowing or swelling in the posterior triangle of the neck. The neck is extremely tender and all movements are restricted. In late cases there may be obvious kyphosis, a fluctuant abscess in the neck or a retropharyngeal swelling. The limbs should be examined for neurological defects.

X-rays show narrowing of the disc space and erosion of the adjacent vertebral bodies.

Treatment

Treatment is initially by antituberculous drugs and 'immobilization' of the neck in a cervical brace or plaster cast for 6–18 months. Operative debridement of necrotic bone and anterior cervical vertebral fusion with bone grafts may be offered as an alternative to such prolonged immobilization. More urgent indications for operation are: (1) to drain a retropharyngeal abscess; (2) to decompress a threatened spinal cord; or (3) to fuse an unstable spine.

RHEUMATOID ARTHRITIS

The cervical spine is severely affected in 30% of patients with rheumatoid arthritis. Three types of lesion are common: (1) erosion of the atlantoaxial joints and the transverse ligament, with resulting instability; (2) erosion of the atlanto-occipital articulations, allowing the odontoid peg to ride up into the foramen magnum; and (3) erosion of the facet joints in the midcervical region, sometimes ending in fusion but more often leading to subluxation. Considering the amount of atlantoaxial displacement that occurs (often greater than 1 cm), neurological complications are uncommon.

Clinical features

The patient is usually a woman with advanced rheumatoid arthritis. She has neck pain and movements are markedly restricted. Symptoms and signs of root compression may be present

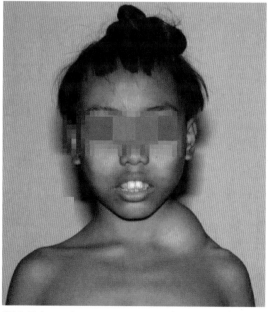

17.8 Tuberculosis This child had been complaining of neck pain and stiffness for several months. When she was brought to the clinic she had a large lump at the side of her neck – a typical tuberculous abscess.

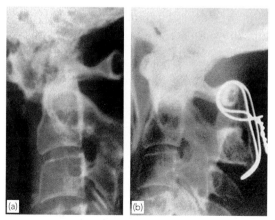

17.9 Rheumatoid arthritis (a) Atlantoaxial subluxation is common; erosion of the joints and the transverse ligament has allowed the atlas to slip forward about 2 cm. (b) Reduction and posterior fusion with wire fixation.

in the upper limbs; less often there are upper motor neuron signs and lower limb weakness due to cord compression. However, there may be symptoms of vertebrobasilar insufficiency, such as vertigo, tinnitus and visual disturbance. Some patients, though completely unaware of any neurological deficit, are found on careful examination to have mild sensory or motor disturbance. Bear in mind that peripheral joint involvement and general debility can mask the signs of myelopathy.

Imaging

X-rays show the features of an erosive arthritis, usually at several levels. Atlantoaxial instability is visible in lateral films taken in flexion and extension; in flexion the anterior arch of the atlas rides forwards, leaving a gap of 5 mm or more between the back of the anterior arch and the odontoid process; on extension the subluxation is reduced. Atlanto-occipital erosion is more difficult to see, but a lateral tomograph shows the relationship of the odontoid to the foramen magnum. Normally the odontoid tip is less than 5 mm above McGregor's line (a line from the posterior edge of the hard palate to the lowest point on the occiput); in erosive arthritis the odontoid tip may be 10–12 mm above this line.

CT and *MRI* are useful for imaging 'difficult' areas such as the atlantoaxial and atlanto-occipital articulations, and for viewing the soft-tissue structures (especially the cord).

Treatment

Despite the startling x-ray appearances, serious neurological complications are uncommon. Pain can usually be relieved by wearing a collar.

The indications for operative stabilization of the cervical spine are: (1) severe and unremitting pain; and (2) neurological signs of root or cord compression. Arthrodesis (usually posterior) is by bone grafting followed by a halo body cast, or by internal fixation (posterior wiring or a rectangular fixator) and bone grafting. Postoperatively a cervical brace is worn for 3 months; however, if instability is marked and operative fixation insecure, a halo jacket may be necessary. In patients with very advanced disease and severe erosive changes, postoperative morbidity and mortality are high.

ANKYLOSING SPONDYLITIS

Ankylosing spondylitis can affect the cervical spine, causing neck pain and stiffness some years after the onset of backache. The neck gradually becomes rigid and kyphotic, although some movement is usually preserved at the atlanto-occipital and atlantoaxial joints.

An unacceptable 'chin-on-chest' deformity, and inability to lift the head high enough to see more than ten paces ahead, are indications for cervical spine osteotomy. The patient should be told that surgery carries a high complication rate.

CHAPTER 18

THE BACK

CLINICAL ASSESSMENT

HISTORY

The usual symptoms of back disorders are pain, stiffness and deformity in the back, and pain, paraesthesia or weakness in the legs. The mode of onset is very important: did it start suddenly (perhaps after lifting) or gradually? Are the symptoms constant, or are there periods of remission? Are they related to any particular posture?

- *Bachache*, either sharp and localized or chronic and diffuse, is the commonest presenting symptom. It is usually felt low down and on either side of the midline, but it may extend into the upper part of the buttock and even into the thighs. If there were no other symptoms it would be difficult to tell whether the pain originated in the intervertebral disc, the nerve root, the vertebral facet joints or the soft-tissue supports at that level of the lumbar spine.
- *Sciatica* is the term originally used to describe intense pain radiating from the buttock into the thigh and calf – more or less following the distribution of the sciatic nerve and therefore suggestive of nerve root compression or irritation. However, Jonas Kellgren (more than 30 years ago) showed that almost any structure in a lumbar spinal segment can, if irritated sufficiently, give rise to *referred pain* radiating into the lower limbs. Unfortunately, with the passage of time, clinicians have taken to describing all types of pain extending from the lumbar region into the lower limb as 'sciatica'. This is at best confusing and at worst a preparation for misdiagnosis! True sciatica, most commonly due to a prolapsed intervertebral disc pressing on a nerve root, is characteristically more intense than referred low back pain, is aggravated by coughing and straining and is often accompanied by symptoms of root pressure such as numbness and paraesthesiae.
- *Stiffness* may be sudden and almost complete (after a disc prolapse) or continuous and predictably worse in the mornings (suggesting arthritis or ankylosing spondylitis).
- *Deformity* is usually noticed by others, but the patient may become aware of shoulder asymmetry or of clothes not fitting well. In disc prolapse, arthritis and ankylosing spondylitis, deformity is usually secondary to, and overshadowed by, pain and stiffness. In structural disorders, such as scoliosis, it may be the only complaint.
- *Numbness or paraesthesia* is felt anywhere in the lower limb, but can usually be mapped fairly accurately over one of the dermatomes. It is

important to ask if it is aggravated by standing upright or walking and relieved by bending forward or sitting down – a classic feature of spinal stenosis.

■ *Other symptoms* important in back disorders are *urethral discharge, diarrhoea* and *sore eyes*; these are features of Reiter's disease, one of the causes of 'reactive' spondylitis.

SIGNS WITH THE PATIENT STANDING

Adequate exposure is essential; patients must strip to their underclothes.

Look

Begin by standing face to face with the patient and note his or her general physique and posture. Then move round and stand behind the patient. Does he or she stand upright or do they lean over to one side? Is the pelvis level or is one leg shorter than the other? Does the spine look straight or curved (*scoliosis*)? Are there scars or other skin markings that may suggest a spinal disorder?

Seen from the side, the thoracic spine normally has a gentle forward curve or *kyphosis*. An unduly prominent kyphotic curve is sometimes called *hyperkyphosis*; if it is sharply angulated, the prominence is called a *kyphos* or *gibbus*.

By contrast, the lumbar spine is normally bent slightly backwards (*lordosis*). In some conditions the lower back may be unusually flat or excessively lordosed.

If the patient consistently stands with one knee bent (even though the legs are equal in length) this suggests nerve root tension on that side; flexing the knee relaxes the sciatic nerve and reduces the pull on the nerve root.

Feel

The spinous processes and the interspinous ligaments are palpated, noting any prominence or a 'step'. Feel for tenderness at each interspinous level.

Move

Flexion: ask the patient to bend forward and try to touch the floor. Even with a stiff back he or she may be able to do this by flexing the hips; so watch the lumbar spine to see if it really moves, or better still, measure the spinal excursion (see Figure 18.2). The mode of flexion is also important; hesitant movements, especially on regaining the upright position, may signify pain or segmental instability.

Extension: ask the patient to lean backwards; with a stiff spine he or she may cheat by bending the knees. The 'wall test' will unmask a disguised loss of extension: standing with the back flush against a wall, the heels, buttocks, shoulders and occiput normally all make contact with the surface.

Lateral flexion: ask the patient to bend first to one side and then to the other; compare the range of movement to right and left.

Rotation: ask the patient to twist the trunk to each side in turn while the pelvis is anchored by the examiner's hands; this is essentially a thoracic movement and should not be limited in lumbosacral disease.

Chest expansion: rib excursion is assessed by measuring the chest circumference in full expiration and then full inspiration; the normal excursion is about 7 cm.

Muscle power: distal muscle power is conveniently tested and compared by asking the patient to stand up on their toes (plantar flexion) and then to rock

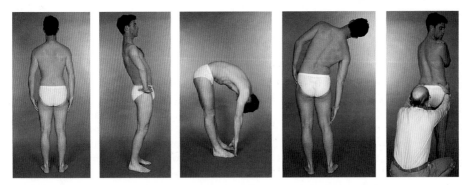

18.1 Examination With the patient standing upright, look at his general posture and note particularly the presence of any asymmetry or frank deformity of the spine. Then ask him to lean backwards (extension), forwards to touch his toes (flexion) and then sideways as far as possible comparing his level of reach on the two sides. Finally, hold the pelvis stable and ask the patient to twist first to one side and then to the other (rotation). Note that rotation occurs almost entirely in the thoracic spine and not in the lumbar spine.

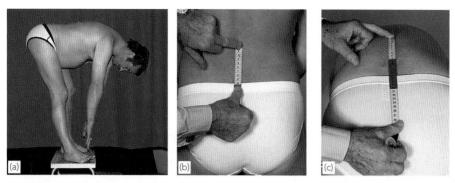

18.2 Measuring the range of flexion Bending down and touching the toes may look like lumbar flexion but this is not always the case. The patient in (a) has ankylosing spondylitis and a rigid lumbar spine, but he is able to reach his toes because he has good flexibility at the hips. Compare his flat back with the rounded back of the model in Fig. 18.1(c). You can measure the lumbar excursion. With the patient upright, select two bony points 10 cm apart and mark the skin (b); as the patient bends forward, the two points should separate by a least a further 5 cm (c).

back on the heels (dorsiflexion); small differences between the two sides are easily spotted.

SIGNS WITH THE PATIENT PRONE

Bony outlines and small lumps can be felt more easily with the patient lying face down.

Deep tenderness is easy to localize, but difficult to ascribe to a particular structure.

Some neurological features are ideally elicited with the patient lying prone. *Hamstring power* is tested by having the patient flex the knee against resistance. The *femoral stretch test* is performed by bending the patient's knee with the hip flat against the couch; a positive sign is pain felt in the front of the thigh and the back, suggesting lumbar root tension.

Popliteal and posterior tibial pulses are conveniently felt in this position.

SIGNS WITH THE PATIENT SUPINE

The patient is observed for pain and stiffness as he or she turns over. Hip and knee mobility are examined before testing for cord or nerve root involvement. Also check the femoral and pedal pulses.

The straight leg raising test: this is the classic test for lumbosacral root tension. With the patient's knee held absolutely straight, the leg is lifted from the couch until the patient experiences pain – not merely in the lower back (which is common and not significant) but also in the buttock, thigh and calf (Lasègue's test). The angle at which this occurs is noted; normally it should be possible to raise the leg to 90 degrees without causing undue discomfort. In a full-blown disc prolapse with nerve root compression, straight-leg raising may be restricted to less than 30 degrees because of severe pain in the sciatic distribution. At the point where the patient experiences discomfort, passive dorsiflexion of the foot may cause an additional stab of pain.

A gentler way of testing straight-leg raising is to ask the patient to raise the leg with the knee straight and rigid – and to stop when he or she feels pain.

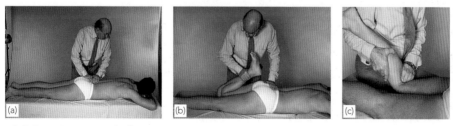

18.3 Examination with the patient prone (a) Feel for tenderness, watching the patient's face for any reaction. (b) Performing the femoral stretch test. You can test for lumbar root sensitivity either by hyperextending the hip or by acutely flexing the knee with the patient lying prone. Note the point at which the patient feels pain and compare the two sides. (c) While the patient is lying prone, take the opportunity to feel the pulses. The popliteal pulse is easily felt if the tissues at the back of the knee are relaxed by slightly flexing the knee.

The *bowstring sign* is even more specific. Raise the patient's leg gently to the point where he or she experiences sciatic pain; now, without reducing the amount of lift, bend the knee so as to relax the sciatic nerve. Buttock pain is immediately relieved; pain may then be re-induced without extending the knee by simply pressing on the lateral popliteal nerve behind the posterolateral side of the knee, to tighten the nerve like a bowstring.

Sometimes straight leg raising on the unaffected side produces pain on the affected side. This 'crossed sciatic tension' is indicative of severe root compression, usually due to a large central disc prolapse, and warns of the risk to the sacral nerve roots that control bladder function (the cauda equina syndrome – one of very few surgical emergencies in spinal disorders).

Neurological examination: a full neurological examination of the lower limbs is essential. An absent ankle jerk on the side with sciatica, combined with paraesthesiae along the lateral border of the foot, suggests compression of the S1 nerve root; normal reflexes combined with paraesthesiae on the dorsum of the foot suggest compression of the L5 nerve root.

General examination: while the patient is lying undressed, a rapid examination is carried out to detect the presence of any suspicious lumps in the breasts, abdomen or genitalia.

IMAGING

X-rays

In the *anteroposterior view* the spine should look perfectly straight and the soft-tissue shadows should outline the normal muscle planes. Curvature (scoliosis) is obvious, and best shown in erect views. Check the outlines of the pedicles, which normally look like oval footprints near the lateral edges of each rectangular vertebral body: a missing or misshapen pedicle could be due to erosion by infection, a neurofibroma or metastatic disease. Individual vertebrae may show asymmetry or collapse. The sacroiliac joints may show erosion or ankylosis, as in tuberculosis (TB) or ankylosing spondylitis, and the hip joints may show features of osteoarthritis, not to be missed in the older patient with backache. Don't forget the soft tissues: bulging of the psoas muscle or loss of the psoas 'shadow' may indicate a paravertebral abscess.

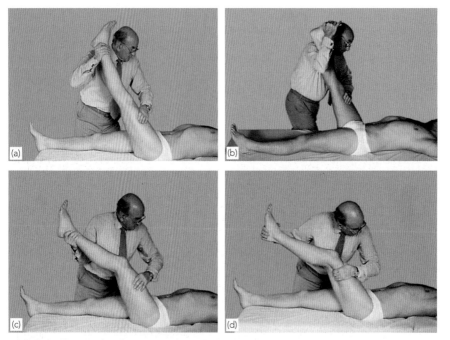

18.4 Sciatic stretch tests (a) Straight-leg raising. The knee is kept absolutely straight while the leg is slowly lifted; note where the patient complains of tightness and pain in the buttock – normally around 80–90 degrees – and compare the two sides. (b) At that point, passive dorsiflexion of the foot causes an added stab of pain. (c) Sciatic tension can also be shown by the bowstring sign. At the point where the patient experiences pain during straight leg raising, relax the tension by bending the knee slightly; the pain should disappear. Then apply firm pressure behind the lateral hamstrings (d); this tightens the common peroneal nerve and the pain recurs with renewed intensity.

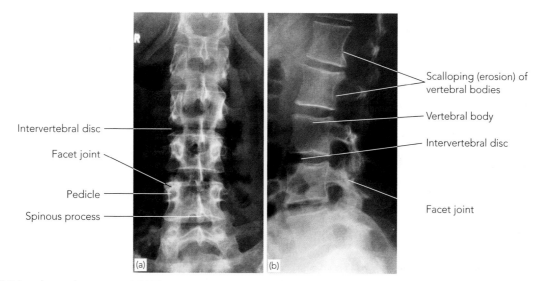

18.5 Lumbar spine x-rays (a,b) The most important normal features are demonstrated in the lower lumbar spine. In this particular case there are also signs of marked posterior vertebral body and facet joint erosions at L1 and L2, features that are strongly suggestive of an expanding neurofibroma.

In the *lateral view* the normal thoracic kyphosis (up to 40 degrees) and lumbar lordosis should be regular and uninterrupted. Anterior shift of an upper segment upon a lower (spondylolisthesis) may be associated with defects of the posterior arch, shown best in oblique views. Vertebral bodies, which should be rectangular, may be wedged or biconcave, deformities typical of osteoporosis or old injury. The intervertebral spaces may be edged by bony spurs (suggesting long-standing disc degeneration) or outlined by fine bony bridges (syndesmophytes – a cardinal feature of ankylosing spondylitis).

Computed tomography (CT)

CT is helpful in the diagnosis of structural bone changes (e.g. a vertebral fracture) and intervertebral disc prolapse. When combined with myelography it gives valuable information about the contents of the spinal canal.

Magnetic resonance imaging (MRI)

MRI has virtually done away with the need for myelography, discography, facet arthrography, and much of CT scanning. The spinal canal and disc spaces are clearly outlined in various planes.

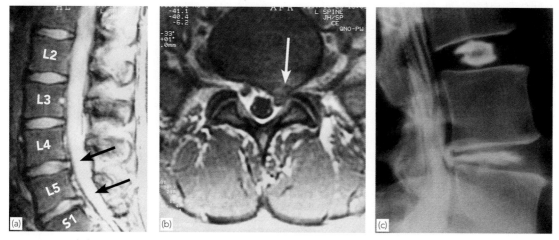

18.6 MRI and discography (a) The lateral T2-weighted MRI shows a small posterior disc bulge (arrow) at L4/5 and a larger protrusion at L5/S1. (b) The axial MRI shows the disc prolapse encroaching on the intervertebral canal and the nerve root on the left side. (c) Discography, showing normal appearance at the upper level and a degenerate disc with prolapse at the level below.

Scans can reveal the physiological state of the disc as regards dehydration, as well as the effect of disc degeneration on bone marrow in adjacent vertebral bodies.

SCOLIOSIS

Scoliosis is an apparent lateral (sideways) curvature of the spine. 'Apparent' because, although lateral curvature does occur, the commonest form of scoliosis is actually a triplanar deformity with lateral, anteroposterior and rotational components. Two broad types of deformity are defined: postural and structural.

POSTURAL SCOLIOSIS

In postural scoliosis the deformity is secondary or compensatory to some condition outside the spine, such as a short leg or a pelvic tilt due to contracture of the hip. When the patient sits (thereby cancelling leg length asymmetry) the curve disappears. Local muscle spasm associated with a prolapsed lumbar disc may also cause a skew back.

STRUCTURAL SCOLIOSIS

In structural scoliosis there is a non-correctable deformity of the affected spinal segment, an essential component of which is vertebral rotation. The spinous processes swing round towards the concavity of the curve and the transverse processes on the convexity rotate posteriorly. In the thoracic

region the ribs on the convex side stand out prominently, producing the rib hump. Secondary (compensatory) curves nearly always develop to counterbalance the primary deformity; they too may later become fixed.

Once established, the deformity is liable to increase throughout the growth period (and sometimes even afterwards).

Most cases have no obvious cause (*idiopathic scoliosis*); other varieties are *congenital* or *osteopathic* (due to bony anomalies), *neuropathic*, *myopathic* (associated with some muscle dystrophies) and a miscellaneous group of *connective-tissue disorders*.

Clinical features

Deformity is usually the presenting symptom: an obvious skew back or a rib hump in thoracic curves, and asymmetrical prominence of one hip in thoracolumbar curves. Balanced curves sometimes pass unnoticed until an adult presents with backache. *Pain* is a rare complaint and should alert the clinician to the possibility of a neural tumour and the need for MRI. *A family history* of scoliosis is not uncommon.

The spine may be obviously deviated from the midline, or this may become apparent only when the patient bends forward. The level and direction of the major curve convexity are noted: e.g. 'right thoracic' means a curve in the thoracic spine and convex to the right; the hip juts out on the concave side and the scapula on the convex. With thoracic scoliosis, rotation causes the rib angles to protrude, thus producing a rib hump on the

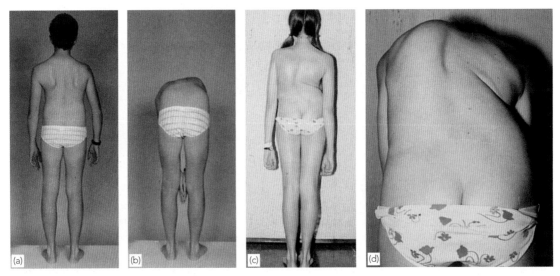

18.7 Structural scoliosis (a) Slight curves are often missed on casual inspection but the deformity becomes apparent when the spine is flexed (b). The young girl in (c) has a much more obvious scoliosis and asymmetry of the hips but what really worries her is the prominent rib hump, seen best when she bends over (d).

convex side of the curve. In balanced deformities the occiput is over the midline; in unbalanced (or decompensated) curves it is not. Side-on posture should also be observed. There may appear to be excessive kyphosis or lordosis.

The diagnostic feature of fixed (as distinct from postural or mobile) scoliosis is that forward bending makes the curve more obvious. Spinal mobility should be assessed and the effect of lateral bending on the curve noted; is there some flexibility in the curve and can it be passively corrected?

Neurological examination is important. Any abnormality suggesting a spinal cord lesion calls for CT and/or MRI.

General examination includes a search for the possible cause and an assessment of cardiopulmonary function (which is reduced in severe curves). Skin pigmentation and congenital anomalies such as sacral dimples or hair tufts are sought.

Imaging

Full-length posteroanterior (PA) and lateral x-rays of the spine and iliac crests must be taken with the patient erect. Structural curves show vertebral rotation: in the PA x-ray, vertebrae towards the apex of the curve appear to be asymmetrical and the spinous processes are deviated towards the concavity.

The upper and lower ends of the curve are identified as the levels where vertebrae start to angle away from the curve. The degree of curvature is measured by drawing lines on the x-ray at the upper border of the uppermost vertebra and the lower border of the lowermost vertebra of the curve; the angle subtended by these lines is the angle of curvature (*Cobb's angle*).

The site of the curve apex should be noted. Right thoracic curves are the commonest, the great majority in girls in adolescent idiopathic scoliosis. The primary structural curve is usually balanced by smaller, compensatory curves above and below. Lateral bending views are taken to assess the degree of curve correctability.

A view of the upper part of the pelvis will show whether the iliac apophysis has fully ossified and fused (*Risser's sign* of skeletal maturity) after which progression of the curve is minimal.

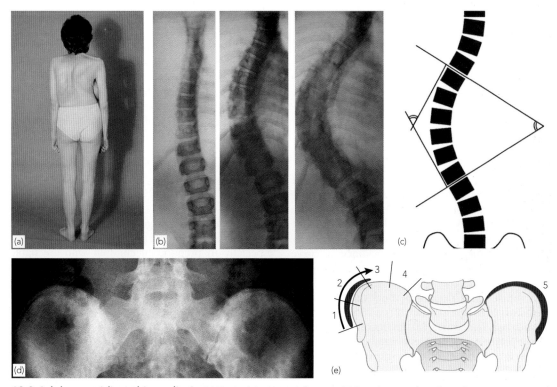

18.8 Adolescent idiopathic scoliosis (a) Typical thoracic deformity. (b) Serial x-rays show how this curve increased over a period of 4 years. (c) The angle of curvature is measured on the x-ray by Cobb's method: lines projected from the top of the uppermost and the bottom of the lowermost vertebral bodies in the primary curve define *Cobb's angle*. An AP view of the pelvis is needed to assess *Risser's sign* (d,e). The iliac apophyses normally ossify progressively from lateral to medial; when fusion is complete, we know that spinal maturity has been reached and further increase in the angle of curvature is negligible.

CT and MRI may be necessary to define a vertebral abnormality or cord compression.

Special investigations

Patients with severe chest deformities should undergo pulmonary function tests. A marked reduction in vital capacity is associated with diminished life expectancy and carries obvious risks for surgery.

Patients with muscular dystrophies or connective tissue disorders require full biochemical and neuromuscular investigation.

Treatment

Prognosis is the key to treatment: the aim is to prevent severe deformity. The younger the child and the higher the curve the worse is the prognosis. Management differs for the different types of scoliosis, which are considered below.

IDIOPATHIC SCOLIOSIS

This group constitutes about 80% of all cases of scoliosis. The deformity is often familial and the population incidence of serious curves (over 30 degrees and therefore needing treatment) is 3 per 1000. The age at onset has been used to define three subgroups: adolescent, juvenile and infantile. A simpler division now in general use is *early-onset* (before puberty) and *late-onset* scoliosis (after puberty).

LATE-ONSET (ADOLESCENT) IDIOPATHIC SCOLIOSIS (AGED 10 YEARS OR OVER)

This is the commonest type, occurring in 90% of cases, mostly in girls. Primary thoracic curves are usually convex to the right, lumbar curves to the left. Progression is not inevitable; most curves of less than 20 degrees either resolve spontaneously or remain unchanged. However, once a curve starts to progress, it usually goes on doing so throughout the remaining growth period (and, to a much lesser degree, beyond that). Reliable predictors of progression are: (1) a very young age; (2) marked curvature; (3) an incomplete Risser sign at presentation. In prepubertal children, rapid progression is liable to occur during the growth spurt.

Treatment

The aims of treatment are: (1) to prevent a mild deformity from becoming severe; (2) to correct an existing deformity that is unacceptable to the patient. A period of preliminary observation may be needed before deciding between conservative and operative treatment. At 4–9-monthly intervals the patient is examined, photographed and x-rayed so that curves can be measured and checked for progression.

Non-operative treatment

If the patient is approaching skeletal maturity and the deformity is acceptable (less than 30 degrees and well balanced), treatment is probably unnecessary unless x-rays show definite progression.

Exercises have no effect on the curve but they do maintain muscle tone and may inspire confidence in a favourable outcome.

Bracing has been used for many years in treating progressive curves of 20–30 degrees. The *Milwaukee brace* consists of a pelvic corset connected by adjustable steel supports to a cervical ring carrying occipital and chin pads; its purpose is to reduce the lumbar lordosis and encourage active stretching and straightening of the thoracic spine. The *Boston brace* is a snug-fitting underarm brace that provides lumbar or low thoracolumbar support. Corrective pads may be added to these devices to apply pressure at a particular site. A well-made brace does not preclude full daily activities, including sport and exercises.

Although bracing is still being used, it is now recognized that it does not actually improve the curve – at best it merely stops it from getting worse. Many orthopaedic surgeons no longer employ this method of treatment, arguing that there is insufficient evidence of its benefits. Their preference now is to wait for the curve to progress to the stage when corrective surgery would be justified.

Operative treatment

The indications for surgery are: (1) curves of more than 30 degrees that are cosmetically unacceptable, especially in prepubertal children who are liable to develop marked progression during the growth spurt; and (2) milder deformity that is deteriorating rapidly. Balanced, double primary curves require operation only if they are greater than 40 degrees and progressing.

The objectives are: (a) to halt progression of the deformity; (b) to straighten the curve (including the rotational component) by some form of instrumentation; and (c) to arthrodese the entire primary curve by bone grafting. Surgical options include:

The Harrington system: in the original system a rod was applied posteriorly along the concave side of the curve; attached to the rod were movable

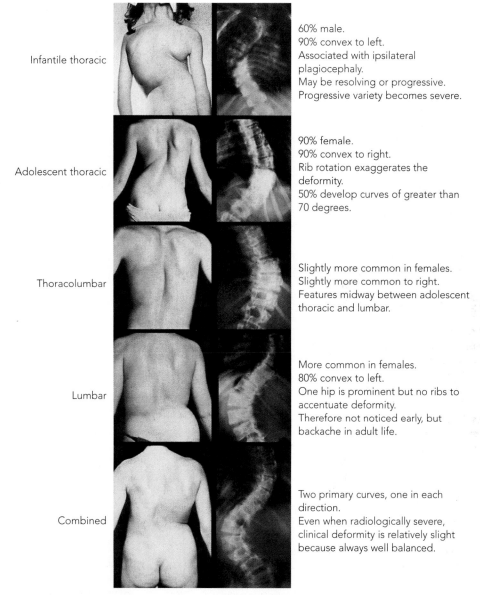

Infantile thoracic

60% male.
90% convex to left.
Associated with ipsilateral plagiocephaly.
May be resolving or progressive.
Progressive variety becomes severe.

Adolescent thoracic

90% female.
90% convex to right.
Rib rotation exaggerates the deformity.
50% develop curves of greater than 70 degrees.

Thoracolumbar

Slightly more common in females.
Slightly more common to right.
Features midway between adolescent thoracic and lumbar.

Lumbar

More common in females.
80% convex to left.
One hip is prominent but no ribs to accentuate deformity.
Therefore not noticed early, but backache in adult life.

Combined

Two primary curves, one in each direction.
Even when radiologically severe, clinical deformity is relatively slight because always well balanced.

18.9 Patterns of idiopathic scoliosis Bracing is used far less than previously because of serious doubts as to its effectiveness beyond natural history.

hooks that were engaged in the uppermost and lowermost vertebrae so as to distract the curve. If the curve is flexible, it will passively correct and bone grafts are then applied to obtain fusion over the length of the curve. A major drawback is that this does not correct the rotational deformity and thus the rib prominence remains virtually unchanged.

Rod and sublaminar wiring (Luque): this is a modification of the Harrington system. Wires are passed under the vertebral laminae at multiple levels and fixed to the rod on the concave side of the curve, thus providing a more controlled and secure fixation. By bending the rod and arranging the mechanism so that the wires pull backwards rather than merely sideways, the rotational component of the deformity can also be substantially improved. However, the sublaminar wires are dangerously close to the dura and the risk of neurological damage is increased.

The Cotrel–Dubousset system: this mechanism combines a pedicle screw 'box' foundation at the

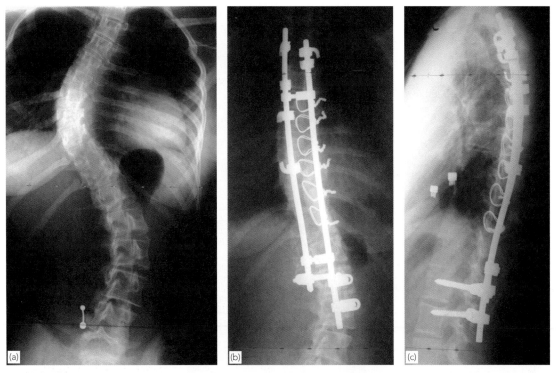

18.10 Scoliosis – posterior instrumentation Idiopathic scoliosis treated by posterior double-rod fixation.

caudal end of the deformity, with multiple hooks placed at various levels to produce either distraction or compression. Using double rods one can distract on the concave and compress on the convex side of the curve. It is claimed that this system can correct the rotational deformity as well. Moreover, it is sufficiently rigid to make postoperative bracing unnecessary.

Anterior instrumentation (Dwyer, Zielke, Kaneda): rigid curves and thoracolumbar curves associated with lumbar lordosis can be corrected by approaching the spine from the front, removing the discs throughout the curve and then applying a compression device along the convex side of the curve. Bone grafts are added to achieve fusion. In some cases combined anterior and posterior instrumentation is necessary. Advantages of this system are: (a) that it provides strong fixation with fewer vertebral segments having to be fused; and (b) that overall shortening of the deformed section (by disc excision and vertebral compression) lessens the risk of cord injury due to spinal distraction.

Warning: whatever method is used, spinal cord function should be monitored during the operation. Ideally this is done by measuring somatosensory and motor evoked potentials during spinal correction. If these facilities are not available,

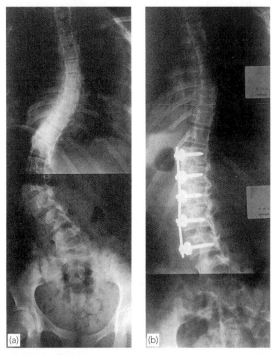

18.11 Scoliosis – anterior instrumentation (a) This 14-year-old girl had a very stiff lumbar curve. It was planned to correct this by two-stage anterior and posterior release and fusion. (b) X-ray taken after the Zielke anterior instrumentation.

the 'wake-up test' is used: anaesthesia is reduced to bring the patient to a semi-awake state and he or she is then instructed to move their feet. If there are signs of cord compromise, the instrumentation is relaxed or removed and re-applied with a lesser degree of correction. Patients have no memory of the wake-up procedure.

Rib hump: none of the instrumentation systems can completely eliminate the rib hump – and it is often this that troubles the patient most of all. If the deformity is marked, it can be reduced significantly by performing a costoplasty, where short sections of rib are excised at multiple levels on the convex side.

Complications of surgery

- *Neurological compromise*: with modern techniques the incidence of permanent paralysis has been reduced to less than 1%.
- Spinal decompensation: over-correction may produce an unbalanced spine. This should be avoided by careful preoperative planning.
- Pseudarthrosis: incomplete fusion occurs in about 2% of cases and may require further operation and grafting.
- *Implant failure*: hooks may cut out and rods may break. If this is associated with a symptomatic pseudarthrosis, revision surgery will be needed.

EARLY-ONSET (JUVENILE) IDIOPATHIC SCOLIOSIS (AGED 4–9 YEARS)

This type is uncommon. The characteristics are similar to those of the adolescent group but the prognosis is worse and surgical correction may be necessary before puberty. However, if the child is very young, a brace may hold the curve stationary until the age of 10 years, when fusion is more likely to succeed.

EARLY-ONSET (INFANTILE) IDIOPATHIC SCOLIOSIS (AGED 3 YEARS OR UNDER)

This is rare, perhaps because most babies nowadays are allowed to sleep prone. Although 90% of infantile curves resolve spontaneously, progressive curves can become very severe and this may, in addition, cause cardiopulmonary dysfunction.

Curves assessed as being potentially progressive should be treated by applying serial elongation–derotation–flexion (EDF) plaster casts under general anaesthesia, until the deformity resolves or until the child is big enough to manage in a brace. From about the age of 4 years onwards, curve progression slows down or ceases and the child

may not need further treatment. If the deformity continues to deteriorate, surgical correction may be required.

OSTEOPATHIC (CONGENITAL) SCOLIOSIS

The commonest bony cause is some type of vertebral anomaly – hemivertebra, wedged vertebra (failure of formation) and fused vertebrae – sometimes combined with absent or fused ribs. There may also be visceral abnormalities (e.g. in the patient with spina bifida). While congenital scoliosis is often mild, some cases progress to severe deformity, particularly those with unilateral fusion of vertebrae. Before any operation is undertaken, advanced imaging is needed to exclude an associated dysraphism, particularly diastematomyelia and cord tethering, which must be dealt with prior to curve correction.

Treatment is more difficult and specialized than that of idiopathic infantile scoliosis. Progressive deformities (usually involving rigid curves) will not respond to bracing alone, and surgical correction carries a significant risk of cord injury. These children should be treated in special units: the approach is to undertake staged resection of the curve apex, followed by instrumentation and spinal fusion. If multiple segments of the spine are involved, surgery may be too hazardous and should probably be withheld.

NEUROPATHIC AND MYOPATHIC SCOLIOSIS

Neuromuscular conditions associated with scoliosis include poliomyelitis, cerebral palsy, syringomyelia, Friedreich's ataxia and the rarer lower motor neuron disorders and muscle dystrophies. The typical paralytic curve is long, convex towards the side with weaker muscles, and at first mobile. In severe cases the greatest problem is loss of stability and balance, which may make even sitting difficult or impossible. *X-ray* with traction applied shows the extent to which the deformity is correctable.

Treatment depends upon the degree of functional disability. Mild curves may require no treatment at all. Moderate curves with spinal stability are managed as for idiopathic scoliosis. Severe curves, associated with pelvic obliquity and loss of sitting balance, can often be managed by fitting a suitable sitting support; if this does not suffice, operative treatment may be indicated. This involves stabilization of the entire paralysed segment by combined anterior and posterior instrumentation and fusion.

SCOLIOSIS AND NEUROFIBROMATOSIS

About one-third of patients with neurofibromatosis develop spinal deformity, the severity of which varies from very mild (and not requiring any form of treatment) to the most marked manifestations accompanied by skin lesions, multiple neurofibromata and bony dystrophy affecting the vertebrae and ribs. The scoliotic curve is typically 'short and sharp'. Other clues to the diagnosis lie in the appearance of the skin lesions and any associated skeletal abnormalities.

Mild cases are treated as for idiopathic scoliosis. More severe deformities will usually need combined anterior and posterior instrumentation and fusion.

KYPHOSIS

Rather confusingly, the term 'kyphosis' is used to describe both the normal (the gentle rounding of the dorsal spine) and the abnormal (excessive dorsal curvature). In the latter sense it signifies a well-recognized deformity which may be progressive; some people prefer the term *hyperkyphosis*.

Postural kyphosis is common ('round back' or 'drooping shoulders') and may be associated with other postural defects such as flat-feet. If treatment is needed, this consists of postural exercises.

Structural kyphosis is fixed and associated with changes in the shape of the vertebrae. It may occur in osteoporosis of the spine (the common round back of elderly people), in ankylosing spondylitis and in Scheuermann's disease (adolescent kyphosis).

A kyphos (or gibbus) is a sharp posterior angulation due to localized collapse or wedging of one or more vertebrae. This may be the result of a congenital anomaly, a fracture (sometimes pathological) or spinal TB.

CONGENITAL KYPHOSIS

Vertebral anomalies leading to kyphosis may be due to failure of formation (Type I), failure of segmentation (Type II) or a combination of these.

Type I is the commonest (and the worst) type. Progressive deformity and posterior displacement of the residual vertebral segment may lead to cord compression. In children younger than 6 years with curves of less than 40 degrees, posterior spinal fusion alone may prevent further progression. Older children or more severe curves may need

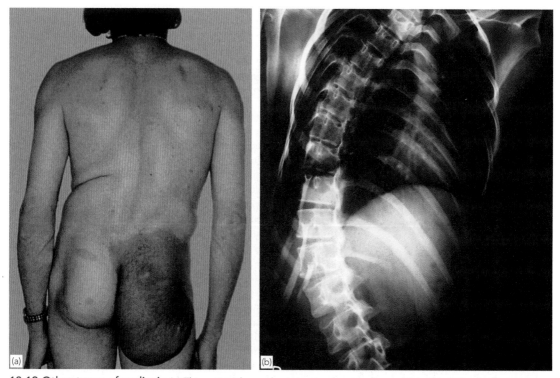

18.12 Other types of scoliosis (a) This patient has a short structural curve plus multiple skin lesions – features suggesting neurofibromatosis. (b) By contrast, the typical postpoliomyelitis 'paralytic' scoliosis shown in this x-ray is characterized by a long C-shaped curve.

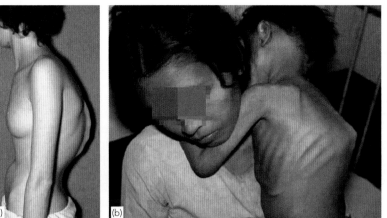

18.13 Kyphosis and kyphos (a) *Kyphosis* – a generalized exaggeration of the normal thoracic 'rounding' of the back, in this case due to Scheuermann's disease. (b) *Kyphos* – a localized spinal angulation, or gibbus, due to collapse of one or two spinal segments (here following tuberculous spondylitis).

combined anterior and posterior fusion, and those with neurological complications will require cord decompression as well.

Type II (failure of segmentation) usually takes the form of an anterior intervertebral bar; as the posterior elements continue to grow, that segment of the spine gradually becomes kyphotic. The risk of neurological compression is much less, but if the curve is progressive a posterior fusion will be needed.

ADOLESCENT KYPHOSIS (SCHEUERMANN'S DISEASE)

This is a 'developmental' disorder in which there is abnormal ossification (and possibly some fragmentation) of the ring epiphyses that appear on the upper and lower surfaces of each vertebral body in the growing spine. As a consequence

these cartilaginous end-plates are weaker than normal and the affected vertebrae in the thoracic spine (which is normally mildly kyphotic) may give way slightly and become wedge shaped. If this happens, the normal *kyphosis* is exaggerated. In the lumbar spine the compressive forces are more evenly distributed and deformity does not occur. Sometimes there may also be small central herniations of disc material into the vertebral body; these are called *Schmorl's nodes*.

Clinical features

Thoracic Scheuermann's disease

The usual form of Scheuermann's disease appears in the midthoracic vertebrae. The condition starts at or shortly after puberty and is more common in boys than in girls. The parents notice that the child, an otherwise fit teenager, is becoming increasingly

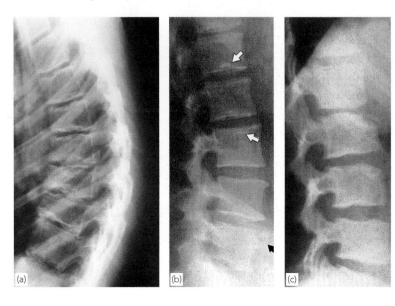

18.14 Scheuermann's disease – x-rays (a) X-rays of the young girl in Figure 18.13(a). (b,c) In lumbar Scheuermann's there is less wedging than in the thoracic region. End-plate fragmentation can be mistaken for a fracture of the vertebral body. Arrows show typical Schmorl's nodes.

'round-shouldered'. The patient may complain of backache and fatigue. Examination reveals a smooth but well-marked thoracic kyphosis (or 'hyperkyphosis') which does not improve with changes in posture.

X-ray features are typical: in the lateral views one can see patchiness or irregularity of the vertebral end-plates and, in some cases, Schmorl's nodes at several intervertebral levels. Later, the vertebral bodies become noticeably wedge shaped.

Treatment depends on the severity of the clinical and x-ray changes. In some cases the early features are so mild that they go unremarked and it is only when, as an adult, the person is x-rayed for some unrelated reason, that the features of an 'old Scheuermann's' are recognized. If there is concern about back pain and/or deformity, an extension brace worn for 1 year or 18 months will often allow a return to normal vertebral growth. If this fails, or if the deformity is already marked when the patient is first seen, operative correction and fusion may be needed.

Thoracolumbar Scheuermann's disease

Thoracolumbar changes may appear together with thoracic kyphosis or may occur on their own. Compared to thoracic Scheuermann's, this condition is less common, tends to occur in late adolescence or early adulthood, does not give rise to local deformity and usually presents as low back pain. X-ray changes are similar to those seen in the thoracic spine, but with little or no vertebral wedging. Patients with low back pain may respond to back-strengthening exercises. Operative treatment is not indicated unless there are associated features of discogenic disease.

PYOGENIC INFECTION

Acute pyogenic infection of the spine is uncommon; elderly, chronically ill and immunodeficient patients are at greatest risk.

Pathology

Staphylococcus aureus is responsible in 50–60% of all cases, but in immunosuppressed patients Gram-negative organisms such as *Escherichia coli* and *Pseudomonas* are the most common. The usual sources of infection are: (1) haematogenous spread from a distant focus of infection; or (2) inoculation during invasive procedures (spinal injections and disc operations).

The infection usually begins in the vertebral end-plates with secondary spread to the disc and adjacent vertebra. It may also spread along the anterior longitudinal ligament or outwards into the paravertebral soft tissues. The spinal canal is rarely involved but when it is (in the form of an epidural abscess) that is a surgical emergency! Despite rapid surgical decompression, the patient is often left with some degree of permanent paralysis.

Clinical features

Localized pain is often intense, unremitting and associated with muscle spasm and restricted movement. There may be point tenderness over the affected vertebra. Enquire about any invasive spinal procedure or a distant infection during the preceding few weeks. Systemic signs such as pyrexia and tachycardia are often present but not marked. In children the diagnosis can be particularly difficult; however, restricted back movement is suspicious.

X-rays may show no change for several weeks. Early signs are loss of disc height, irregularity of the disc space, erosion of the vertebral end-plate and reactive new bone formation. The early loss of disc height distinguishes vertebral osteomyelitis from metastatic disease, where the disc can remain intact despite advanced bone destruction.

Radionuclide scanning will reveal increased activity at the site but this is non-specific.

MRI may show characteristic changes in the vertebral end-plates, intervertebral disc and paravertebral tissues; this investigation is highly sensitive but not specific.

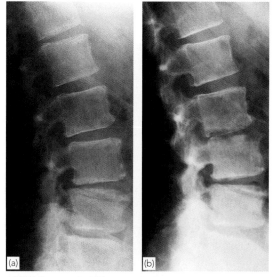

18.15 Pyogenic infection (a) Typical x-ray features of acute vertebral osyeomyelitis. (b) Progressive end-plate erosion after 6 months.

Special investigations

The white cell count, C-reactive protein (CRP) level and erythrocyte sedimentation rate (ESR) are usually elevated, and antistaphylococcal antibodies may be present in high titres. Agglutination tests for *Salmonella* and *Brucella* should be performed, especially in endemic regions and in patients who have recently visited these areas. Blood culture may be positive; however, if it is negative a closed needle biopsy is performed for bacteriological culture and tests for antibiotic sensitivity.

Treatment

Treatment is started on the basis of a clinical diagnosis of infection and includes bed rest, pain relief and intravenous antibiotic administration using a 'best guess' preparation that can be changed once the laboratory results and sensitivities are known.

Intravenous antibiotics are continued for 4–6 weeks; if there is a good response (clinical improvement, a falling CRP and ESR and a normal white cell count), oral antibiotics are then used for a further 6–8 weeks and the patient is mobilized in a spinal brace. The duration of antibiotic treatment depends on the further clinical, haematological and radiological findings.

Operative treatment is seldom needed. The indications for an open biopsy and decompression are: (1) failure to obtain a positive yield from a closed needle biopsy and a poor response to conservative treatment; (2) the presence of neurological signs; (3) the need to drain a soft-tissue abscess. An anterior approach is preferred; necrotic and infected material is removed and, if necessary, the cord is decompressed. If the spine is unstable, internal fixation may be necessary. Postoperatively the spine is supported in a brace until healing occurs.

With prompt and effective treatment the outcome is usually favourable. Spontaneous fusion of infected vertebrae is a common feature of healed staphylococcal osteomyelitis.

DISCITIS

Infection limited to the intervertebral disc is rare and when it does occur it is usually due to direct inoculation following discography, chemonucleolysis or discectomy. The vertebral end-plates are rapidly attacked and the infection then spreads into the vertebral body.

With direct infection there is always a history of some invasive procedure. Acute back pain and muscle spasm following an injection into the disc should never be attributed merely to the irritant effect of the injection. Systemic features are usually mild, but the ESR is elevated.

In children the infection is assumed to be blood-borne. The child complains of back pain, perhaps after a flu-like illness. Back movements are severely limited. X-rays, radioscintigraphy and MRI show the same features as in pyogenic spondylitis.

Prevention is better than cure: following an injection into the disc, a broad-spectrum antibiotic should be administered intravenously. Non-iatrogenic discitis is usually self-limiting.

During the acute stage bed rest and analgesics are essential. If symptoms do not resolve rapidly, a needle biopsy is advisable. Only if there are signs of abscess formation or cord or nerve root pressure is surgical evacuation or decompression indicated. This is rarely necessary.

TUBERCULOSIS

The spine is the most common site of skeletal TB, accounting for 50% of all musculoskeletal TB.

Pathology

Blood-borne infection settles in a vertebral body adjacent to the intervertebral disc. Bone destruction and caseation follow, with infection spreading to the disc space and the adjacent vertebra. A paravertebral abscess may form, and then track along muscle planes to involve the sacroiliac or hip joint, or along the psoas muscle to the inner thigh. The affected vertebral bodies may collapse to form a sharp gibbus (or kyphos). There is a major risk of cord damage due to pressure by the abscess, granulation tissue, sequestra or displaced bone.

With healing, the vertebrae re-calcify and bony fusion may occur between them. Nevertheless, if there has been much angulation, the spine is usually 'unsound', and flares are common. With progressive kyphosis there is again a risk of cord compression.

Clinical features

There is usually a long history of ill health and backache; in late cases a gibbus deformity is the dominant feature. Concurrent pulmonary TB is a feature in most children under 10 years with thoracic spine involvement. Occasionally the patient may present with a cold abscess pointing in the groin, or with paraesthesiae and weakness of the legs. There is local tenderness in the back and spinal movements are restricted. Neurological examination may show motor and/or sensory changes in the lower limbs. As spinal TB is found mostly in the thoracic spine, spastic paraparesis is a common presentation in adults.

In areas where TB is no longer common, the infection may be confined to a single vertebral body, symptoms may be mild and deformity can be slight. It is important to be alert to the possibility of this diagnosis, especially in patients who are human immunodeficiency virus (HIV)-positive.

Imaging

The entire spine should be x-rayed, because vertebrae distant from the obvious site may also be affected. The earliest signs of infection are local osteoporosis of two adjacent vertebrae and narrowing of the intervertebral disc space, with fuzziness of the end-plates. Progressive disease is associated with signs of bone destruction and collapse of adjacent vertebral bodies into each other. Paraspinal soft-tissue shadows may be due either to oedema or a paravertebral abscess. A chest x-ray is essential. With healing, bone density increases, the ragged appearance disappears and paravertebral abscesses may undergo resolution, fibrosis or calcification.

MRI and CT may reveal hidden lesions, paravertebral abscesses, an epidural abscess and cord compression. Myelography is appropriate when these facilities are not available.

Special investigations

The Mantoux test may be positive and in the acute stage the ESR is raised. In patients with no neurological signs a needle biopsy is recommended to confirm the diagnosis by histological and microbiological investigations. If this does not provide a firm diagnosis, tissue should be obtained by open operation. If there are signs of neurological involvement, operative debridement and decompression of the spinal cord will be required. Patients with HIV infection should be referred for appropriate management.

Differential diagnosis

Spinal TB must be distinguished from other causes of vertebral pathology, particularly pyogenic and fungal infections, malignant disease and parasitic infestations such as hydatid disease. Disc space collapse is typical of infection; metastatic lesions may cause vertebral body collapse similar to that seen in TB but the disc space is usually preserved.

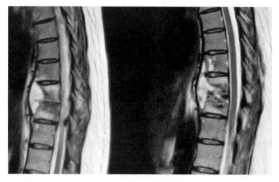

18.17 Spinal tuberculosis – MRI Sagittal MR images of advanced tuberculous infection with abscess formation beneath the anterior longitudinal ligament.

Treatment

The objectives are: (1) to eradicate or arrest the infection; (2) to prevent or correct deformity; and (3) to prevent or treat the major complication – paraplegia.

Ambulant chemotherapy alone is suitable for early or limited disease with no abscess formation or neurological deficit. Rifampicin 600 mg daily plus isoniazid 300 mg daily plus pyrazinamide 2 g daily are given in combination for 6–12 months or until

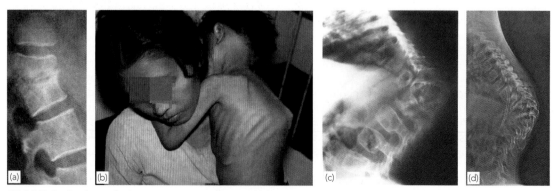

18.16 Spinal tuberculosis (a) Early x-ray changes with loss of disc space. (b) A child with a severe kyphotic deformity. (c,d) X-rays before and after operative debridement and spinal fusion using a rib strut graft.

the x-ray shows resolution of the bone changes, but stopping the pyrazinamide after the first 2 months. (The dosages listed are for adults of average weight.) However, because TB is often a complication of acquired immunodeficiency syndrome (AIDS), resistant mycobacteria are an increasing problem. Ethionamide and streptomycin may have to be substituted for isoniazid.

Continuous bed rest and chemotherapy may be used for more advanced disease when the necessary skills and facilities for radical anterior spinal surgery are not available, or where the technical problems are too daunting – provided there is no abscess that needs to be drained.

Operative treatment is indicated: (1) when there is an abscess that can readily be drained; (2) for advanced disease with marked bone destruction and threatened or actual severe kyphosis; and (3) neurological deficit, including paraparesis, that has not responded to drug therapy. Through an anterior approach, all infected and necrotic material is evacuated or excised and the gap is filled with iliac crest or rib grafts that act as a strut. If several levels are involved, anterior or posterior fixation and fusion may be needed for additional stability. Children who are growing and are seen to be at risk of developing severe kyphosis may need fusion of the posterior elements to minimize the expected deformity. Antituberculous chemotherapy is still necessary, of course.

Pott's paraplegia

Early-onset paresis (usually within 2 years of disease onset) is due to pressure by inflammatory oedema, an abscess, caseous material, granulation tissue or sequestra. The patient presents with lower limb weakness, upper motor neuron signs, sensory dysfunction and incontinence. The diagnosis is confirmed by MRI or myelography. The condition is treated by early anterior decompression and debridement followed by spinal fusion. The prognosis for neurological recovery following surgery is good.

Late-onset paresis is due to direct cord compression from increasing deformity, or (occasionally) vascular insufficiency of the cord. If MRI or myelography reveals direct cord compression, operative removal of necrotic tissue is probably still worthwhile. If there is no actual compression, operation is unlikely to be of use.

AIDS and spinal TB

One of the main reasons for the resurgence of TB, especially in the developing world, is the spread of HIV. Spinal TB, which is an extrapulmonary focus, is AIDS defining. Patients with this condition are prone to developing opportunistic infections and atypical mycobacterial infections.

The tuberculous infection usually involves multiple vertebrae and results in severe deformity. A primary epidural abscess is not uncommon. Decompression and stabilization for neurological deficit are performed through an extrapleural posterolateral approach with instrumentation to minimize pulmonary complications. A primary epidural abscess is drained through a laminectomy.

Postoperatively antituberculous therapy and antiretroviral treatment are commenced. Compliance with treatment and regular monitoring of viral loads and CD4/CD8 counts are essential to ensure a successful outcome.

ANKYLOSING SPONDYLITIS (SPONDYLOARTHROPATHY)

This group of disorders is dealt with in Chapter 3.

INTERVERTEBRAL DISC LESIONS

About one-quarter of the length of the vertebral column is made up of fibrocartilaginous discs that are squeezed between adjacent vertebral bodies, to which they are anchored at the cartilage end-plates. It is the discs that lend limited flexibility to the spine.

In the lumbar region the discs are about 1 cm thick. Their posterior edges lie on the anterior boundary of the spinal canal and posterolaterally they skirt the right and left intervertebral canals close to the nerve roots that exit at successive levels. Little wonder that disc disorders are often accompanied by neurological symptoms.

Structurally the disc consists of a central gel-like portion (proteoglycans in a collagen latticework), called the *nucleus pulposus*, which merges into surrounding lamellae of more fibrous consistency – the *annulus fibrosus*. With ageing there is a gradual loss of proteoglycans and the disc becomes somewhat dehydrated and degenerate. This is thought to be the underlying cause of two important disorders that occur particularly in the lumbar and cervical regions and to a lesser extent in the thoracic spine: intervertebral disc herniation and chronic intervertebral disc degeneration.

INTERVERTEBRAL DISC DEGENERATION

With increasing age, as the lumbar intervertebral discs gradually dry out, the nucleus pulposus changes from a turgid bulb to a brownish,

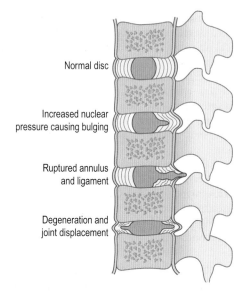

Normal disc

Increased nuclear
pressure causing bulging

Ruptured annulus
and ligament

Degeneration and
joint displacement

18.18 Intervertebral disc prolapse and degeneration Diagrammatic representation of progressive stages in the development of *disc prolapse*. At first there is only bulging of the posterior part of the disc; the annulus fibrosus may go on to rupture and the nucleus pulposus is extruded posteriorly to one or other side. In disc degeneration (lowest figure) the disc becomes desiccated and collapses, causing displacement of the posterior facet joints.

desiccated structure. The annulus fibrosus develops fissures parallel to the vertebral end-plates running mainly posteriorly, and small herniations of nuclear material squeeze into and through the annulus. The discs flatten down and bulge slightly beyond the margins of the vertebral bodies. Where they protrude against the surrounding ligaments, reactive new bone formation produces bony ridges (erroneously called 'osteophytes') and the adjacent vertebral end-plates ossify and become sclerotic. The picture as a whole is referred to as *spondylosis*; it occurs in over 80% of people who live for more than 50 years and, although characteristic changes can be seen on x-ray examination (flattening of the disc 'space' and marginal spur formation), the condition is usually asymptomatic. However, other secondary effects may ensue: slight displacement of the posterior vertebral facet joints, facet joint osteoarthritis and narrowing of the lateral recesses of the spinal canal and the intervertebral foramina. It is then that patients experience the common and ill-defined symptoms of recurrent backache, sometimes with pain radiating towards the buttocks or thighs.

Imaging

X-ray examination typically shows flattening of the 'disc spaces' and spur formation at the borders of the vertebral bodies, often accompanied by characteristic features of osteoarthritis in the small facet joints.

MRI scans may show bulging of one or more discs in both sagittal and axial projections. There may also be subtle changes such as diminished thickness and reduced signal intensity, or small tears and fissures in the disc. Secondary changes, evidently arising from altered loading characteristics of the degenerating disc, can usually be identified in the adjacent vertebral bodies.

Treatment

Asymptomatic lumbar disc degeneration does not necessarily presage the future onset of symptoms and does not need any treatment.

Patients with chronic low-back pain and nothing more than x-ray signs of disc degeneration may benefit from postural and muscle strengthening exercises, as well as some modifications to their daily activities. Their long-term progress is determined mainly by whether they go on to develop any associated features such as facet joint osteoarthritis, degenerative spondylolisthesis or spinal stenosis. In the absence of any such changes, treatment should be conservative.

ACUTE INTERVERTEBRAL DISC HERNIATION

Intervertebral disc herniation or *protrusion* is a bulging of the disc with the outer part of the annulus intact, either directly posteriorly or to one or other side of the posterior longitudinal ligament towards the intervertebral foramen. Acute disc herniation is usually initiated by mechanical stress – a combination of flexion and compression – but even at L4/5 or L5/S1 (where stress is most severe) it is unlikely that a disc would herniate unless there was some prior disturbance of the hydrophilic properties of the nucleus pulposus. If the disc *ruptures*, fibrocartilaginous material may *sequestrate* and lie free in the spinal canal or the intervertebral foramen.

A posterolateral protrusion can compress the nerve root proximal to its point of exit through the intervertebral foramen; a herniation at L4/5 will compress the fifth lumbar nerve root, and a herniation at L5/S1, the first sacral root; a large central herniation or sequestration may cause compression of the cauda equina. A local inflammatory response and oedema may aggravate this situation.

Acute back pain at the onset of disc herniation probably arises from disruption of the outermost layers of the annulus fibrosus and stretching or tearing of the posterior longitudinal ligament. If the disc protrudes to one side, it may irritate the dural covering of the adjacent nerve root causing pain in the buttock, posterior thigh and calf (*sciatica*). Pressure on the nerve root itself causes *paraesthesia* and/or *numbness* in the corresponding dermatome, as well as *weakness* and *depressed reflexes* in the muscles supplied by that nerve root.

Clinical features

The patient is usually a fit young adult, though children and old people can be affected. Typically, while lifting or stooping (or perhaps merely coughing) the patient is seized with back pain and is unable to straighten up. Either then, or a day or two later, pain is felt in the buttock and lower limb (sciatica). Both backache and sciatica are made worse by coughing or straining. Later there may be paraesthesia or numbness in the leg or foot, and occasionally muscle weakness. *Urinary retention – due to compression of the cauda equina – is uncommon but it signals an emergency and may lead to permanent dysfunction of sphincter control if treatment is unduly delayed.*

The patient usually stands with a slight list to one side ('sciatic scoliosis'). All back movements are severely limited, and during forward bending the list may increase.

There is often tenderness in the midline of the low back, and paravertebral muscle spasm. Straight leg raising is limited and painful on the affected side; dorsiflexion of the foot and bowstringing of the lateral popliteal nerve may accentuate the pain. Sometimes raising the unaffected leg causes acute sciatic tension on the painful side ('crossed sciatic tension'). With a prolapse at L3/4 the femoral stretch test may be positive.

Neurological examination may show muscle weakness (and, later, wasting), diminished reflexes and sensory loss corresponding to the affected level. L5 impairment causes weakness of big toe extension and knee flexion, with sensory loss on the outer side of the leg and the dorsum of the foot. S1 impairment causes weak plantarflexion and eversion of the foot, a depressed ankle jerk and sensory loss along the lateral border of the foot. With cauda equina compression, urinary retention is accompanied by loss of sensation over the sacrum.

Imaging

X-rays are essential, not to show the disc space but to exclude bone disease. However, after several attacks the disc space may indeed be flattened. A *myelogram* or radiculogram outlines the disc well, but side-effects are unpleasant.

CT and *MRI* are the best ways of identifying the disc and localizing the lesion. Minor disc bulges are common and unlikely to be the cause of neurological symptoms. See whether the disc herniation is actually abutting against an adjacent nerve root.

Differential diagnosis

The full-blown syndrome is unlikely to be misdiagnosed, but with repeated attacks and with lumbar spondylosis gradually supervening, the features often become atypical. Three groups of disorders must be excluded:

■ *Inflammatory disorders*, such as ankylosing spondylitis, cause severe and more generalized stiffness and typical x-ray changes.

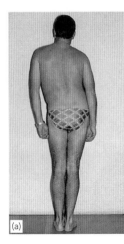
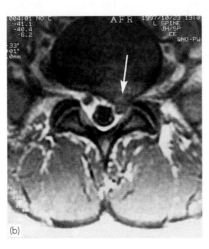

18.19 Prolapsed disc – clinical and MRI (a) This patient presented with acute low back pain and sciatica. He has the characteristic sideways list (or tilt) due to paravertebral muscle spasm. (b) MRI showing the disc prolapse, with posterolateral protrusion towards the intervertebral foramen at L5/S1 (arrow).

- *Vertebral tumours* cause constant pain; x-rays show bone destruction or a pathological fracture.
- *Nerve tumours* may cause sciatica but pain is continuous; CT or MRI may delineate the lesions.

Treatment

There are four elements in the treatment of acute disc herniation: *rest, reduction, removal*, and *rehabilitation*.

Rest: during an acute attack the patient should be kept in bed, with hips and knees slightly flexed. An anti-inflammatory medication is useful.

Reduction: continuous bed rest and traction for 2 weeks may allow the herniation to reduce. If the symptoms and signs do not improve significantly by then, *an epidural injection* of corticosteroid and local anaesthetic may help. If conservative measures fail, then discectomy is the treatment of choice.

Removal: the indications for operative removal of a disc are: (1) a cauda equina compression syndrome which does not clear up within 6 hours of starting bed rest and traction; this is an emergency; (2) persistent pain and severely limited straight leg raising after 2 weeks of conservative treatment; (3) neurological deterioration while under conservative treatment; and (4) frequently recurring attacks. The presence of a herniated disc, and the level, must be confirmed by CT or MRI before operating.

Through a posterior approach between adjacent vertebral laminae, the dural sac is retracted to one side and the bulging disc is exposed. The friable, partially shredded material is removed. This can be done by open operation or by endoscopic surgery (microdiscectomy).

Rehabilitation: after recovery from an acute disc rupture, or disc removal, the patient is taught isometric exercises and how to lie, sit, bend and lift with the least strain. Light work is resumed after 1 month and heavy work after 3 months. At that stage, if recovery is anything but total, the patient should be advised to avoid heavy lifting tasks altogether.

LUMBAR OSTEOARTHRITIS

With advanced degeneration and flattening of the intervertebral disc there is inevitably some displacement of the posterior vertebral facet joints, and this may lead to osteoarthritis at one or several levels. In the worst cases hypertrophic bone formation at the facet joints may cause progressive spinal stenosis.

Clinical features

The patient is usually over 40 years and otherwise fit. He or she may give a history of acute disc rupture followed by recurrent attacks of pain over several years. In many cases, however, disc degeneration gradually progresses without any acute episode of disc herniation, causing chronic backache and a sense of lumbar instability and muscle weakness. Back pain may be intermittent and related to spells of strenuous physical activity, standing or walking a lot, or sitting in one position during a long journey; it is usually relieved by lying down. The patient may also complain of acute incidents of 'locking' or 'giving way' in the back.

Tender areas are often felt in the back and buttocks. Lumbar movements are limited and may be painful at their extremes. A typical feature is difficulty in straightening up from the forward bend position. Neurological examination may show residual signs of an old disc prolapse (e.g. an absent ankle jerk).

In long-standing cases the patient may present with symptoms of spinal stenosis (see below).

Imaging

X-rays show narrowing (flattening) of the intervertebral disc 'spaces', accompanied by osteoarthritic changes in the facet joints.

CT or *MRI* will show whether there is bone encroachment into the spinal canal and/or the intervertebral foramina. These investigations are called for if the patient has symptoms and signs of nerve root entrapment or spinal stenosis.

Treatment

If symptoms are not severe, conservative measures are encouraged for as long as possible. These consist of instruction in modified activities, physiotherapeutic exercises, manipulation during acute episodes and, if necessary, the wearing of a lumbar corset.

The use of a walking stick sometimes relieves tension on the paravertebral muscles and this can ease the backache. Advice about posture, avoiding obesity and carrying weights is helpful. If these measures, conscientiously applied, cannot control pain, spinal fusion may have to be considered.

Chronic back pain can be psychologically debilitating; counselling and support are often welcomed by the patient.

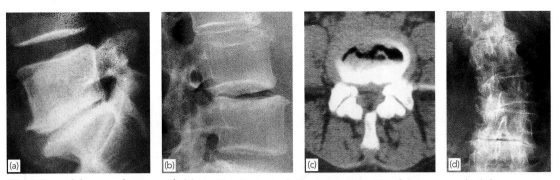

18.20 Spondylosis and osteoarthritis (a,b) Typical x-ray features are narrowing of the intervertebral disc space and marginal spur formation. (c) CT showing a 'vacuum sign' in the disc area and hypertrophic osteoarthritis of the facet joints. (d) In advanced cases several levels are involved and there may be deformity of the spine.

SPONDYLOLISTHESIS

'Spondylolisthesis' means vertebral displacement. Normal laminae and facets constitute a locking mechanism which prevents each vertebra from moving forwards on the one below. Forward shift (or slip) occurs only when this mechanism fails. Listhesis (slippage) is nearly always between L4 and L5, or between L5 and the sacrum. This usually happens for one of the following reasons:

- Dysplasia of the lumbosacral facet joints (20% of cases).
- Separation or stress fracture (lysis) through the neural arch (the pars interarticularis), allowing the anterior part of the vertebra to slip forward upon the one below (50% of cases).
- Osteoarthritic degeneration of the facet joints, causing them to lose their normal stability. This usually occurs at L4/5 (25% of cases).
- Destructive conditions such as fracture, TB and neoplasia (5% of cases).

Clinical features

Dysplastic spondylolisthesis is seen in children. It is usually painless but the mother may notice the unduly protruding abdomen. There may be an associated scoliosis.

Lytic spondylolisthesis is the commonest variety. It occurs in adults and intermittent backache is the usual presenting symptom. Pain may be initiated or exacerbated by exercise or strain. On examination the buttocks look curiously flat, the sacrum appears to extend to the waist and transverse loin creases may be prominent. A 'step' can often be felt when the fingers are run down the spine. Movements are usually normal in younger patients but may be restricted in older people.

Degenerative spondylolisthesis usually occurs in patients over 40 years with long-standing backache due to facet joint arthritis. Sometimes the presenting symptom is spinal 'claudication' due to narrowing of the spinal canal (see under *spinal stenosis*).

Imaging

X-rays show the forward shift of the upper part of the spinal column on the stable vertebra below; elongation of the arch or defective facets may be seen. The gap in the pars interarticularis is more easily seen in oblique x-ray views, and best of all in CT scans.

Treatment

Conservative treatment, similar to that for other types of back pain, is suitable for most patients.

Operative treatment is indicated: (1) if the symptoms are disabling and interfere significantly with work and recreational activities; (2) if the upper vertebra has slipped forwards over more than 50% of the vertebral body below; and (3) if neurological compression is significant.

For children, posterior intertransverse fusion in situ is almost always successful; if neurological signs appear, decompression can be carried out later. For adults, either posterior or anterior fusion is suitable. However, in the 'degenerative' group, where neurological symptoms predominate, decompression without fusion may suffice.

SPINAL STENOSIS

One of the long-term consequences of disc degeneration and osteoarthritis is narrowing of the spinal canal due to hypertrophy at the posterior disc margin and the facet joints. This is more likely if the canal was always small, or if a spondylolisthesis decreases its anteroposterior diameter. Spinal stenosis is also common in people with congenital vertebral dysplasia (e.g. in those with achondroplasia).

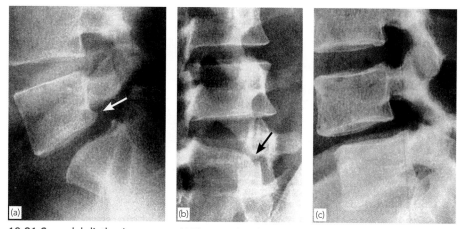

18.21 Spondylolisthesis – x-rays (a) There is a break in the pars interarticularis of L5, allowing the anterior part of the vertebra to slip forwards. In this case the gap is easily seen in the lateral x-ray, but usually it is better seen in the oblique view (b). In degenerative spondylolisthesis there is no break in the pars – the degenerate disc and eroded facet joints permit one vertebra to slide forwards on the other (c).

Clinical features

Typically, a patient with backache complains of aching and/or numbness and paraesthesia in the thighs, legs or feet. The symptoms come on after standing upright or walking for 5–10 minutes and are consistently relieved by sitting or squatting with the spine somewhat flexed (hence the term 'spinal claudication').

Examination, especially after getting the patient to reproduce the symptoms by walking, may show neurological defects in the lower limbs. *Always check the upper limbs for signs of polyneuropathy and the lower limbs for evidence of peripheral vascular disease.*

Nerve conduction studies and electromyography are helpful in establishing the diagnosis and severity of neurological change.

Symptoms are sometimes unilateral, suggesting an asymmetrical stenosis or intervertebral root canal stenosis. The distribution of pain and sensory abnormality will indicate which levels are affected.

Imaging

Lateral view x-rays may show degenerative spondylolisthesis or advanced disc degeneration and osteoarthritis. Measurement of the spinal canal may be carried out on plain films, but more reliable information is obtained from CT and MRI.

Treatment

Conservative measures, including instruction in spinal posture, may suffice. Localized symptoms due to root canal stenosis often respond to injection of a long-acting local anaesthetic and corticosteriod

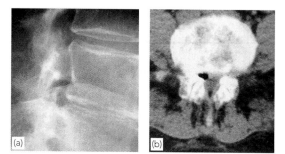

18.22 Spinal stenosis (a) A lateral x-ray shows marked narrowing of the spinal canal, but the CT scan (b) provides even more convincing evidence.

injection, which can be repeated two or three times at 3- or 6-monthly intervals.

If these measures fail to provide sufficient relief, operative decompression will be needed. However, patients must be warned that the operation will not improve their backache. If there are clear-cut signs of spinal instability, segmental fusion may also be needed.

THE BACKACHE PROBLEM

Backache is such a frequent cause of disability that it has become almost a disease in itself. Careful history taking and examination will uncover one of five patterns.

Transient backache following muscular activity

This suggests a simple back strain that will respond to a short period of rest followed by gradually increasing exercise. People with thoracic kyphosis (of whatever origin), or fixed flexion of the hip, are particularly prone to back strain because they tend to compensate for the deformity by holding the lumbosacral spine in hyperlordosis.

Sudden, acute pain and sciatica

In young people (those under the age of 20 years) it is important to exclude *infection* and *spondylolisthesis*; both produce recognizable x-ray changes. Patients aged 20–40 years are more likely to have an *acute disc prolapse*: diagnostic features are a history of a lifting strain, unequivocal sciatic tension and neurological symptoms and signs. Elderly patients may have osteoporotic *compression fractures*, but *metastatic disease* and *myeloma* must be excluded.

Intermittent low back pain after exertion

Patients of almost any age may complain of recurrent backache following exertion or lifting activities and this is relieved by rest. Features of disc prolapse are absent but there may be a history of acute sciatica in the past. In early cases x-rays usually show no abnormality; later there may be signs of *lumbar spondylosis* in those over 50 years and *osteoarthritis* of the facet joints is common. These patients need painstaking examination to determine whether those features are incidental or are likely to account for the patient's symptoms. Disorders such as *ankylosing spondylitis*, *chronic infection* and *myelomatosis* must be excluded by appropriate imaging and blood investigations.

Back pain plus pseudoclaudication

These patients are usually aged over 50 years and may give a history of previous, longstanding back trouble. The diagnosis of *spinal stenosis* should be confirmed by CT and/or MRI.

Severe and constant pain localized to a particular site

This suggests local bone pathology, such as *a compression fracture*, *Paget's disease*, *a tumour* or *infection*. Spinal osteoporosis in middle-aged men is pathological and calls for a full battery of tests to exclude primary disorders such as *myelomatosis*, *metastases*, *gonadal insufficiency*, *alcoholism* or *corticosteroid usage*.

'CHRONIC BACKACHE SYNDROME'

Patients with chronic backache may despair of finding a cure and they often develop affective and psychosomatic ailments that subsequently become the chief focus of attention. This 'illness behaviour' is self-perpetuating and may become accompanied by *'non-organic' physical signs* such as extreme tenderness, pain elicited by pressing vertically on the spine or passively rotating the entire trunk, variations in response to tests for straight-leg raising or muscle power, sensory and/or motor abnormalities that do not fit the known anatomical and physiological patterns and over-determined behaviour during physical examination (trembling, sweating, hyperventilating, inability to move, a tendency to fall and exaggerated withdrawal) – usually accompanied by loud groaning and exclamations of discomfort. Patients with these features are unlikely to respond favourably to surgery and they may require prolonged support and management in a special pain clinic – but only after every effort has been made to exclude organic pathology.

THE HIP

CLINICAL ASSESSMENT

HISTORY

- *Pain* arising in the hip joint is felt in the groin, down the front of the thigh and, sometimes, in the knee; occasionally knee pain is the only symptom! Pain at the back of the hip is seldom from the joint; it usually derives from the lumbar spine.
- *Limp* is the next most common symptom. It may be a way of coping with pain, or it may be due to a change in limb length, weakness of the hip abductors or joint instability. Walking distance may be curtailed; or, reluctantly, the patient starts using a walking stick.
- *Stiffness and deformity* are late symptoms, and tend to be well compensated for by pelvic mobility.

SIGNS WITH THE PATIENT UPRIGHT

Start by standing face to face with the patient and note his or her *general build* and the symmetry of the lower limbs.

While in this position, it is convenient to perform *Trendelenburg's test* for postural stability when the patient stands on one leg. Normally, in one-legged stance, the person's body moves over the standing leg and the pelvis is hitched upwards on the unsupported side. However, if the weightbearing hip is unstable, the pelvis will *drop* on the unsupported side, showing a positive Trendelenburg sign. If the difference between the two hips is marked, you can detect this abnormality by simply looking at the patient's stance. However, small differences are not so obvious. In the classical Trendelenburg test the examiner stands behind the patient, who is asked to stand first on one leg and then on the other: see if the buttock-line drops on the side opposite to the weightbearing hip – which would denote a positive Trendelenburg sign on the weightbearing side.

The causes of a positive Trendelenburg sign are: (1) pain on weightbearing; (2) weakness of the hip abductors; (3) shortening of the femoral neck; and (4) dislocation or subluxation of the hip.

Now ask the patient to walk, and observe each phase of the gait. The commonest abnormalities are:

- A short-leg limp – a regular, even dip on the short side.
- An antalgic gait – the patient moves quickly off the painful side.
- A Trendelenburg lurch – a variant of Trendelenburg's sign.

While the patient is upright, take the opportunity to examine the spine for deformity or limitation of movement.

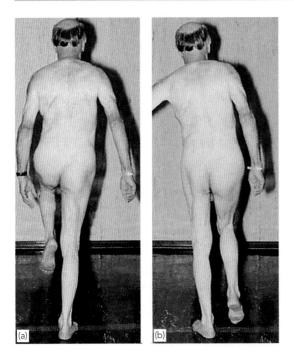

19.1 Examination – Trendelenburg's sign Look carefully at how the patient walks and stands. If the hips are completely normal the pelvis remains level even when the patient stands on one leg. (a) This man has osteoarthritis of the left hip. Standing on his right leg he is well supported by his right hip, the pelvis is level or, if anything, tilted towards the right and the left buttock fold is higher than the right. (b) Standing on his left leg is more difficult. His left hip cannot support him properly, the pelvis tilts towards the right and the right buttock fold drops below the left. The Trendelenburg test is positive for the left side (i.e. abnormal).

SIGNS WITH THE PATIENT LYING DOWN

Look

Make sure that the patient is lying comfortably with the pelvis horizontal (both anterior superior iliac spines at the same level) and the legs placed symmetrically. Check to see if the medial malleoli are at the same level, or if one leg is shorter than the other. Better still, measure the distance from the anterior superior iliac spine to the medial malleolus on each side.

Be alert to the possibility that limb length discrepancy may be *apparent* but not *real*. This occurs when the pelvis is tilted and one limb is hitched upwards. Almost invariably this is due to an uncorrectable deformity in the hip: with fixed adduction on one side, the limbs would tend to be crossed; when the legs are placed side by side the pelvis has to tilt upwards on the affected side, giving the impression of a shortened limb. The exact opposite occurs when there is fixed abduction, and the limb seems to be longer on the affected side.

If there is real shortening on one side, it is usually possible to establish where the fault lies. With the knees flexed and the heels together, it can be seen whether the discrepancy is below or above the knee. If it is above, the next question is whether the abnormality lies above the greater trochanter. The thumbs are pressed firmly against the anterior superior iliac spines and the middle fingers grope for the tops of the greater trochanters; any elevation of the trochanter on one side is readily felt.

Feel

Bone contours are felt when levelling the pelvis and judging the height of the greater trochanters. Tenderness may be elicited in and around the joint. The surface marking of the femoral head is halfway between the anterior superior iliac spine and the pubic tubercle.

Move

The assessment of hip movements is difficult because any limitation can easily be obscured by movement of the pelvis. Thus, even a gross limitation of extension, causing *a fixed flexion deformity*, can be completely masked simply by arching the back into excessive lordosis. Fortunately it can be just as easily unmasked by performing Thomas' test: both hips are flexed simultaneously to their limit, thus completely obliterating the lumbar lordosis; holding the 'sound' hip firmly in this position (and thus keeping the pelvis still), the other limb is lowered gently; with any flexion deformity the knee will not rest on the couch. Meanwhile the full range of *flexion* will also have been noted; the normal range is about 130 degrees.

Similarly, when testing abduction the pelvis must be prevented from tilting sideways. This is achieved by placing the 'sound' hip (the hip

243

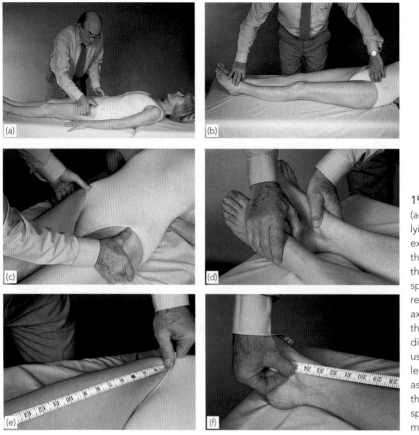

19.2 Measurement
(a–c) Make sure the patient is lying straight on the examination couch and that the pelvis is absolutely level – the anterior superior iliac spines at the same level in relation to the longitudinal axis of the body. Then check the medial malleoli (d); discrepancy in leg length will usually be obvious. (e,f) Leg length is most accurately assessed by measuring from the anterior superior iliac spine to the tip of the medial malleolus on each side.

opposite to the one being examined) in full abduction and keeping it there, thus fixing the pelvis in the coronal plane. A hand is placed on one iliac crest to detect the slightest movement of the pelvis. Then after checking that the anterior superior iliac spines are level, the affected joint is moved gently into abduction. The normal range is about 45 degrees. Adduction is tested by crossing the one limb over the other; the pelvis must be watched and felt to determine the point at which it starts to tilt. The normal range of adduction is about 30 degrees.

To test *rotation* both legs, lifted slightly off the couch by the ankles, are rotated first internally then externally; the patellae are watched to estimate the amount of rotation. Rotation-in-flexion is tested with the hip and knee each flexed 90 degrees.

Abnormal movement, i.e. movement greatly in excess of the norm, or the ability to elicit 'telescoping' by alternately pulling and pushing the limb in its long axis, suggests either instability or an established pseudoarthrosis of the hip.

IMAGING

The minimum required is an anteroposterior *x-ray* view of the pelvis showing both hips, and a lateral view of each hip separately. The two sides can be compared: any difference in the size, shape or position of the femoral heads is important. With a normal hip *Shenton's line*, which follows the inferior border of the femoral neck to the inferior border of the pubic ramus, looks continuous; any interruption in the line suggests an abnormal position of the femoral head. Narrowing of the joint 'space' is a sign of articular cartilage loss, a feature of both inflammatory and non-inflammatory arthritis. Increased radiographic density in the femoral head is associated with avascular necrosis; however, the early changes of femoral head necrosis can be detected only on *magnetic resonance imaging (MRI)*.

Ultrasonography is useful for detecting an intra-articular effusion. This is also the ideal method for demonstrating neonatal hip dysplasia; x-rays are unable to display an image of the cartilaginous femoral head and acetabulum.

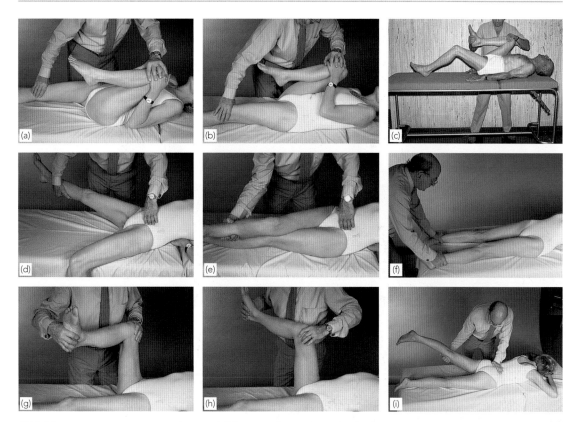

19.3 Movement (a) Forcing one hip into full flexion will straighten out the lumbar spine; the other hip should still be capable of full extension in this position. (b) Now the position is reversed. The right hip is held in full flexion; (c) if the hip cannot straighten out completely, this is referred to as a fixed flexion deformity. (d) Testing for abduction. The pelvis is kept level by placing the opposite leg over the edge of the examination couch with that hip also in abduction (the examiner's left hand checks the position of the anterior spines) before abducting the target hip. (e) Testing for adduction. (f) External and internal rotation are assessed (f) first with the hips in full extension and then (g,h) in 90 degrees of flexion. (i) Testing for extension.

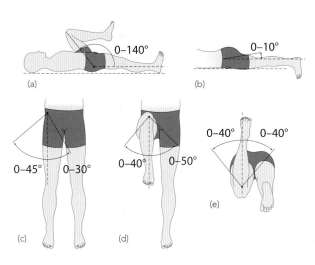

19.4 Normal range of movements (a) The hip should flex until the thigh meets the abdomen, but (b) it can extend only a few degrees. (c) Abduction is usually greater than adduction. The relative amounts of internal and external rotation may vary according to whether the hip is in (d) flexion or (e) extension.

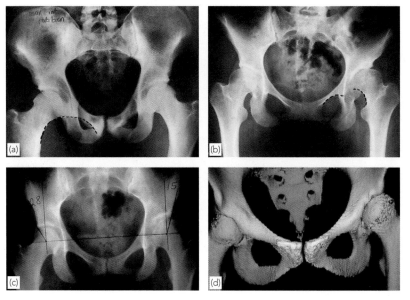

19.5 Imaging
(a) Anteroposterior x-ray of normal hips showing Shenton's line. (b) X-ray of a patient with secondary osteoarthritis of the left hip due to congenital subluxation. The joint 'space' is narrowed and Shenton's line is broken. (c,d) X-ray and three-dimensional CT showing how shallow the acetabula are, especially on the left side.

ARTHROSCOPY

Arthroscopy of the hip is used mainly for the diagnosis of conditions that are not detectable by imaging techniques and for operative procedures such as the repair of a torn or detached acetabular labrum.

Table 19.1 The diagnostic calendar (age of onset as a guide to probable diagnosis)

Age of onset (years)	Probable diagnosis
Neonatal	Developmental dysplasia
0–5	Infections
5–10	Perthes' disease
10–20	Slipped epiphysis
Adult	Arthritis

DEVELOPMENTAL DYSPLASIA OF THE HIP

Developmental dysplasia of the hip (DDH), comprises a spectrum of disorders: an unusually shallow acetabulum without actual displacement of the joint; a shallow acetabulum with subluxation (partial displacement) of the femoral head; or frank dislocation during the neonatal period. Whether the instability comes first and then affects acetabular development because of imperfect seating of the femoral head, or is the result of a primary acetabular dysplasia, is still not known for sure. Both mechanisms might be important.

The reported incidence of neonatal hip instability in Northern Europe is 5–20 per 1000 live births; however, most of these hips stabilize spontaneously, and on re-examination 3 weeks after birth the incidence is only 1 or 2 per 1000 infants. Among the Inuit people of Northern Canada and the Sami people of Finland the incidence is much higher; among African peoples the incidence is considerably lower.

Girls are much more commonly affected than boys (a ratio of about 7:1), and the left hip more often than the right; in 1 in 5 cases the condition is bilateral.

Aetiology and pathogenesis

Genetic factors must be important, for DDH tends to run in families and even in entire populations. Two heritable features which could predispose to hip instability are generalized joint laxity and shallow acetabula.

Hormonal changes in late pregnancy may aggravate ligamentous laxity in the infant. This could account for the rarity of hip instability in premature babies.

Intrauterine malposition, especially a breech position with extended legs, would favour dislocation.

Postnatal factors play a part in maintaining any tendency to instability. This may account for the unusually high incidence of DDH in Inuit and

Sami peoples, who swaddle their babies and carry them with hips and knees fully extended; compare the rarity of DDH in African peoples, who carry their babies astride their backs with hips abducted.

Pathology

The acetabulum is unusually shallow (shaped like a saucer instead of a cup) and its roof slopes too steeply; the femoral head slides out posteriorly and then rides upwards. The capsule is stretched and the ligamentum teres becomes elongated and hypertrophied. Superiorly the acetabular labrum and its capsular edge may be pushed into the socket by the dislocated femoral head; this fibrocartilaginous limbus may obstruct any attempt at closed reduction of the femoral head. Maturation of the acetabulum and femoral epiphysis is retarded and the femoral neck is unduly anteverted.

Clinical features

The ideal, still unrealized, is to diagnose every case at birth. For this reason, every newborn child should be examined for signs of hip instability. Where there is a family history of congenital dislocation, and with breech presentations, extra care is taken and the infant may have to be examined more than once.

Neonatal diagnosis

There are several ways of testing for instability. In *Ortolani's test*, the baby's thighs are held with the thumbs medially and the fingers resting on the greater trochanters; the hips are flexed to 90 degrees and gently abducted. Normally there is smooth abduction to almost 90 degrees. In congenital dislocation the movement is usually impeded, but if pressure is applied to the greater trochanter there is a soft 'clunk' as the dislocation

reduces, and then the hip abducts fully (the 'jerk of entry'). If abduction stops half-way and there is no jerk of entry, there may be an irreducible dislocation.

Barlow's test is performed in a similar manner, but here the examiner's thumb is placed in the groin and, by grasping the upper thigh, an attempt is made to lever the femoral head in and out of the acetabulum during abduction and adduction. If the femoral head is normally in the reduced position, but can be made to slip out of the socket and back in again, the hip is classed as 'dislocatable' (i.e. unstable).

Every hip with signs of instability – however slight – should be examined by *ultrasonography*. This provides a dynamic assessment of the shape of the cartilaginous socket and the position of the femoral head.

Late features

Ideally all children should be examined again at 6 months, 12 months and 18 months of age, so as to be sure that late-appearing signs of DDH are not missed. Occasionally dislocation does not occur until several months after birth.

An observant parent may spot asymmetry, a clicking hip, or difficulty in applying the napkin (diaper) because of limited abduction.

With unilateral dislocation the skin creases look asymmetrical and the leg is slightly short; with bilateral dislocation there is an abnormally wide perineal gap. Abduction is restricted and a thumb in the groin may feel that the femoral head is 'missing'.

Late walking is not a marked feature, but if the child is not walking by 18 months, or if there is hint of a limp or a waddle, dislocation must be excluded.

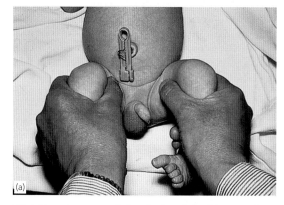
(a)

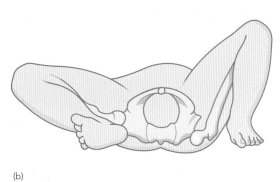
(b)

19.6 Developmental dysplasia of the hip – early signs (a) Position of the hands for performing Ortolani's test. (b) Showing why abduction is limited if the hip is dislocated.

Imaging

Ultrasonography has replaced radiography for imaging hips in the newborn. The acetabulum and femoral head can, with practice, be displayed with static and dynamic ultrasound. Sequential assessment allows monitoring of the hip during an initial period of splintage.

X-ray examination is helpful after the first 6 months. The bony part of the acetabular roof slopes upwards abnormally and the socket is unusually shallow. The ossific centre of the femoral head is under-developed, and from its position it may be apparent that the head is displaced upwards and outwards. Though the bones are incompletely ossified (and therefore difficult to place in x-ray images), the relationship of the femoral head to the acetabular socket can be assessed by studying various geometric projections on the x-ray images (see Figure 19.7).

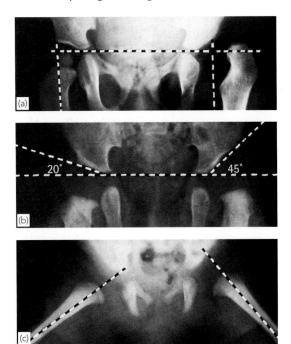

19.7 Developmental dysplasia of the hip – x-rays
(a) The left hip is dislocated, the femoral head is under-developed and the acetabular roof slopes upwards much more steeply than on the right side. In this case the features are very obvious but lesser changes can be gauged by geometrical tests. The epiphysis should lie medial to a vertical line which defines the outer edge of the acetabulum (Perkins' line) and below a horizontal line which passes through the triradiate cartilages (Hilgenreiner's line). (b) The acetabular roof angle should not exceed 30 degrees. (c) Von Rosen's lines: with the hips abducted 45 degrees, the femoral shafts should point into the acetabula. In each case the left side is shown to be abnormal.

Management

Untreated congenital dislocation leads to progressive deformity and disability. With bilateral involvement, because the changes are symmetrical, disability is, for some years, less marked. Children in whom treatment is started only after the first year of life probably have no more than a 50% chance of remaining free of trouble in later life.

Children under 6 months

Every newborn child with signs of hip instability – however slight – should ideally be examined by ultrasonography. If this shows any abnormality, the infant is placed in a splint with the hips flexed and abducted and is recalled for re-examination – in the splint – at 2 weeks and at 6 weeks. By then it should be possible to assess whether the hip is reduced and stable, reduced but unstable (dislocatable by Barlow's test), subluxated or dislocated.

If the scan shows that the hip is reduced and has a normal cartilaginous outline, no treatment is required but the child is kept under observation for 3–6 months.

In the presence of acetabular dysplasia or persistent hip instability, splintage in flexion and abduction is maintained and ultrasound scanning is repeated at intervals until stability and normal anatomy are restored or a decision is made to abandon splintage in favour of more aggressive treatment.

If ultrasound is not available, the simplest policy is to regard all infants with a high-risk background or a positive Ortolani or Barlow test, as 'suspect' and to nurse them in double napkins or an abduction pillow for the first 6 weeks. At that stage they are re-examined: those with stable hips are left free but kept under observation for at least 6 months; those with persistent instability are treated by more formal abduction splintage (see below) until the hip is stable and x-ray shows that the acetabular roof is developing satisfactorily (usually 3–6 months). If the hip fails to locate, splintage should be abandoned in favour of closed or operative reduction at a later date.

Splintage calls for careful attention. It is crucial to ensure that the hip is properly reduced before it is splinted; this can be checked by ultrasound. The object is to hold the hips about 100 degrees flexed and somewhat abducted. Extreme positions are avoided and the joints should be allowed some movement in the splint. Von Rosen's splint is an H-shaped malleable appliance that is easy to apply. The Pavlik harness is more difficult to apply but gives the child more freedom while still maintaining

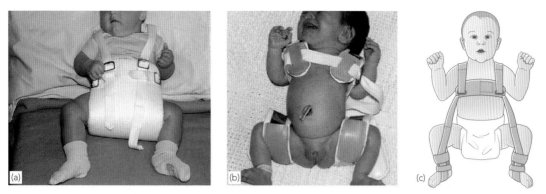

19.8 Developmental dysplasia of the hip – early treatment Three types of abduction splint: (a) pillow type; (b) Von Rosen splint; (c) Pavlik harness.

position. Whatever method is adopted, follow-up is continued until the child is walking.

Persistent dislocation: 6–18 months

If, after early treatment, the hip is still incompletely reduced, or if the child presents late with a 'missed' dislocation, the hip must be reduced (if necessary by operation) and held reduced until acetabular development is satisfactory.

Closed reduction by manipulation under anaesthesia carries a high risk of femoral head necrosis; to minimize this risk, reduction should be gradual: traction is applied to both legs, preferably on a vertical frame, and abduction is gradually increased until, by 3 weeks, the legs are widely separated. This manoeuvre alone (aided if necessary by adductor tenotomy) may achieve stable, concentric reduction. Arthrography will show whether the femoral head is fully seated in the acetabulum.

Splintage is still important. When concentric reduction has been achieved, the hips (both) are held in a spica cast at 60 degrees of flexion, 40 degrees of abduction and 20 degrees of internal rotation. After 6 weeks the spica is changed and the stability of the hip(s) assessed under anaesthesia. Provided the position and stability are satisfactory, the spica is retained for a further 6 weeks. Following plaster removal the hip is either left unsplinted or managed in a removable abduction splint which is retained for up to 6 months, depending on radiological evidence of satisfactory acetabular development.

Open reduction is needed if, at any stage, concentric reduction has not been achieved. The psoas tendon is divided, obstructing tissues (redundant capsule and thickened ligamentum teres) are removed and the hip is reduced. It is usually stable in 60 degrees of flexion, 40 degrees of abduction and 20 degrees of internal rotation. A spica cast is applied and the hip is splinted as described above. If stability can be achieved only by markedly internally rotating the hip, a corrective subtrochanteric osteotomy of the femur is carried out, either at the time of open reduction or 6 weeks later. In young children this usually gives a good result.

Persistent dislocation: 18 months–4 years

In the older child, closed reduction carries an even greater risk of causing avascular necrosis of the femoral head, due to tightness of the soft tissues. The preferred approach is to proceed straight to arthrography and open reduction. An arthrogram will show whether there is an in-turned limbus or any marked degree of acetabular dysplasia.

Through an anterolateral approach the joint capsule is opened, all soft tissues blocking reduction are removed and the femoral head is seated in the acetabulum. Often a de-rotation femoral osteotomy (held by a plate and screws) will be needed; at the same time a 1 cm segment can be removed from the proximal femur to lessen pressure on the reduced hip. Some type of acetabular osteotomy may also be required to ensure concentric reduction.

After operation the child should be placed in a hip spica cast with the hip in about 90 degrees of flexion and about 60 degrees of abduction; this is maintained for 3 months and thereafter unsupported movements are encouraged. Intermittent clinical and radiological surveillance should be continued until the child reaches skeletal maturity.

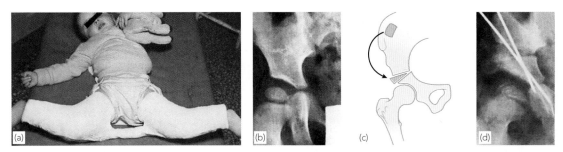

19.9 Developmental dysplasia of the hip – later treatment (a) Reduced open but stable only in medial rotation. If the femoral head remains poorly covered (b) this can be treated by innominate osteotomy (c,d).

After the age of 4 years

For unilateral dislocation, operative reduction is still feasible, at least up to the age of 8–10 years; as in the former group, it may be necessary to combine this with corrective osteotomies of the femur and/or pelvis.

In older children, the force needed for reduction may damage the hip and cause avascular necrosis, so it may be better to leave well alone and wait until pain and abnormal function call for further reconstructive surgery.

With bilateral dislocation the deformity is symmetrical and therefore less noticeable. The risk of operative intervention is also greater because failure on one or other side results in asymmetrical deformity. Therefore, most surgeons avoid operation unless pain or deformity is unusually severe. The untreated patient has a waddling gait through life and may be surprisingly uncomplaining. However, if disability becomes severe, reconstructive surgery may be justified.

Persistent dislocation in adulthood

Adults who appear to have managed quite well for many years may present in their 30s or 40s with increasing discomfort due to an unreduced congenital dislocation. Walking becomes more and more tiring and backache is common. With bilateral dislocation, the loss of abduction may hamper sexual intercourse in women.

Disability may be severe enough to justify *total joint replacement*. The operation is difficult and should be undertaken only by those with experience of hip reconstructive surgery. The femoral head is seated above a shallow acetabulum. A new socket should be fashioned at the normal anatomical site and it may have to be augmented by building up the roof of the socket with bone grafts. It is often difficult to bring the femoral head down to the level of the socket without risking damage to the sciatic nerve; if necessary, a small segment of femoral bone can be removed to allow a safe fit.

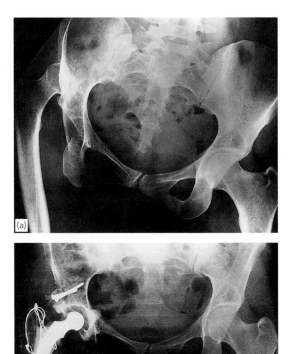

19.10 Untreated developmental dysplasia of the hip (a) This patient, aged 35 years, had a short leg, a severe limp and back pain. (b) Hip replacement restored her to near normality.

ACETABULAR DYSPLASIA AND SUBLUXATION OF THE HIP

Acetabular dysplasia may be genetically determined or may follow incomplete reduction of a congenital dislocation, damage to the lateral acetabular epiphysis or maldevelopment of the femoral head. The socket is unusually shallow, the roof is sloping and there is deficient coverage of the femoral head; in some cases the hip subluxates. Faulty load transmission in the lateral part of the joint may lead to secondary osteoarthritis in later life.

Clinical features

During infancy, limited abduction of the hip is suspicious and ultrasonography may reveal a deficient acetabulum.

In children the condition is usually asymptomatic and discovered only when the pelvis is x-rayed for some other reason. Sometimes, however, the hip is painful – especially after strenuous activity – and the child may develop a limp. If there is subluxation the Trendelenburg sign is positive, leg length may be asymmetrical and movement – particularly abduction in flexion – is restricted.

Adolescents and young adults may complain of pain over the lateral side of the hip, probably due to muscle fatigue and/or increased bone stress in the lateral part of the acetabulum. Some experience episodes of sharp pain in the groin, possibly the result of a labral tear or detachment. However, the majority go through life without experiencing really intrusive symptoms.

Older adults (those in their 40s) may present with features of secondary osteoarthritis. In Southern Europe dysplasia of the hip is a common cause of symptomatic osteoarthritis.

Imaging

X-rays should be taken lying and standing (the latter may show minor degrees of incongruity). The acetabulum looks shallow, the roof is sloping and the femoral head is uncovered. Lesser degrees of dysplasia are revealed by measuring the depth of the socket and the relationship between the centre of the femoral head and the edge of the acetabulum – Wiberg's centre–edge (CE) angle, which should

be no less than 30 degrees. If the femoral head is displaced, Shenton's line will be broken.

Computed tomography (CT) and *MRI* are helpful if operative treatment is being considered. Three-dimensional CT reconstruction is particularly useful in providing an accurate picture of the anatomy.

Treatment

Infants with subluxation are treated as for dislocation: the hip is splinted in abduction until the acetabular roof looks normal.

Children and adolescents, provided the hip is reducible and congruent, often manage with no more than muscle strengthening exercises. If symptoms persist, they may need an operation to improve the acetabular roof, either a lateral shelf procedure or a pelvic osteotomy to re-orientate the position of the acetabular roof; these operations can, if necessary, be combined with a varus osteotomy of the proximal femur.

Adults with pain, weakness, instability and subluxation of the hip are candidates for periacetabular osteotomy or three-dimensional re-orientation of the entire hip (see Figure 19.12).

Patients with secondary osteoarthritis may need total hip replacement.

ACQUIRED DISLOCATION OF THE HIP

Dislocation occurring after the first year of life is usually due to one of three causes: *pyogenic arthritis*, *muscle imbalance* or *trauma*.

Dislocation following sepsis

Pyogenic infection of the joint, whether primary or secondary to osteomyelitis of the femoral neck, carries a serious risk of enzymatic 'digestion' of the articular cartilage. In the past, septic arthritis in early childhood (when the epiphysis is still mainly

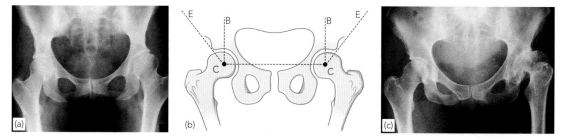

19.11 Acetabular dysplasia (a) X-ray showing a dysplastic left acetabulum. The socket is shallow and the roof sloping, leaving much of the femoral head uncovered. (b) Method of measuring Wiberg's centre–edge angle. (c) Left untreated, this sometimes progresses to severe osteoarthritis.

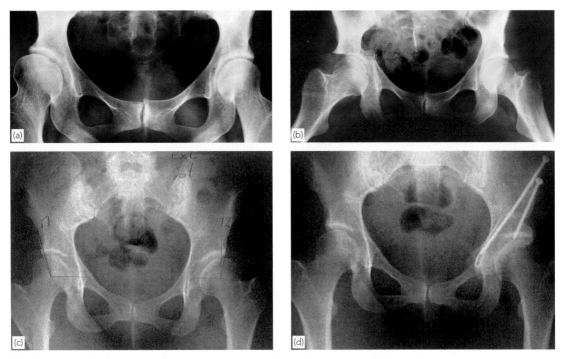

19.12 Acetabular reconstruction (a) Acetabular dysplasia of the right hip. (b) X-ray after innominate osteotomy (Chiari operation). (c) Bilateral acetabular dysplasia, worse on the left side. (d) X-ray after left side periacetabular osteotomy and outward rotation of the socket to cover the loadbearing part of the femoral head.

cartilaginous) often resulted in partial or complete dissolution of the femoral head and dislocation of the hip – a so-called Tom Smith dislocation.

On *x-ray* the femoral head appears to be completely absent; however, part of it often survives, although it is too osteoporotic to be seen.

Treatment is by traction, followed, if necessary, by open reduction. In the absence of a femoral head, the greater trochanter can be placed in the acetabulum; varus osteotomy of the upper femur helps to achieve a measure of stability. Further reconstructive surgery will almost certainly be needed in later life.

Dislocation due to muscle imbalance

Unbalanced paralysis in childhood may result in the hip abductors being weaker than the adductors. This is seen in *cerebral palsy*, in *myelomeningocele* and after *poliomyelitis* (see Chapter 10). The greater trochanter fails to develop properly, the femoral neck becomes valgus and the hip may subluxate or dislocate. Treatment is similar to that of very late congenital dislocation, but in addition some muscle re-balancing operation is essential.

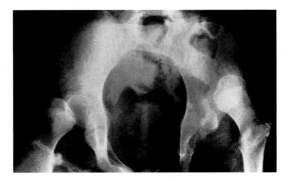

19.13 Acquired dislocation of the hip Muscle imbalance in a child with spina bifida has led to bilateral hip dislocation.

Traumatic dislocation

Occasionally dislocation of the hip is missed while attention is focused on some more distal (and more obvious) injury. Reduction is essential, if necessary by open operation; even if avascular necrosis or hip stiffness supervenes, a hip in the anatomical position presents an easier prospect for reconstructive surgery than one that remains persistently dislocated.

PROTRUSIO ACETABULI

In this condition the socket is too deep and bulges into the cavity of the pelvis. The 'primary' form shows a slight familial tendency. It affects females much more often than males and develops soon after puberty; at this stage there are usually no symptoms although movements are limited.

X-rays show the sunken acetabulum, with the inner wall bulging beyond the iliopectineal line. Secondary osteoarthritis may develop in later life, but until then the condition does not require treatment.

Protrusio may occur in later life secondary to bone 'softening' disorders, such as osteomalacia or Paget's disease, and in long-standing cases of rheumatoid arthritis.

Treatment is indicated only if pain is severe or movements are markedly restricted. This calls for total joint replacement.

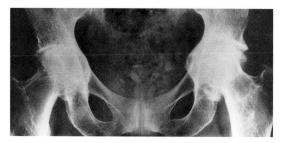

19.14 Protrusio acetabuli X-ray examination of the pelvis shows the typical bulging of the inner wall of the acetabulum on each side. The condition has been present since adolescence and has resulted in osteoarthritis.

COXA VARA

The normal femoral neck–shaft angle is 160 degrees at birth, decreasing to 125 degrees in adult life. An angle of less than 120 degrees is called *coxa vara*. The deformity may be either congenital or acquired.

Congenital coxa vara

This is a rare disorder of infancy and early childhood. It is due to a defect of endochondral ossification in the medial part of the femoral neck. When the child starts to crawl or stand, the femoral neck bends or develops a stress fracture; with continued weightbearing it collapses increasingly into varus. Sometimes there is also shortening or bowing of the femoral shaft. The condition is bilateral in about one-third of cases.

The abnormality is usually diagnosed when the child starts to walk. The leg is short and the thigh may be bowed. *X-ray* shows that the physeal line is too vertical; typically, in the infant, there is a separate triangular fragment of bone in the inferior portion of the metaphysis (Fairbank's triangle).

With bilateral coxa vara the patient may not be seen until he or she presents as a young adult with osteoarthritis.

If shortening is progressive, the deformity should be corrected by a subtrochanteric valgus osteotomy. Varus does not recur, but there may be some permanent shortening.

Acquired coxa vara

Coxa vara can develop at any age if the bone at the femoral neck gives way. This is seen in certain of the osteochondral dystrophies, in rickets, in fibrous dysplasia, following severe grades of epiphysiolysis (slipped femoral epiphysis) and in adult osteomalacia. Malunited or ununited femoral neck fractures also may result in varus deformity of the femoral neck.

Often no treatment is required, but if the condition is troublesome it can be improved by corrective intertochanteric or subtrochanteric osteotomy.

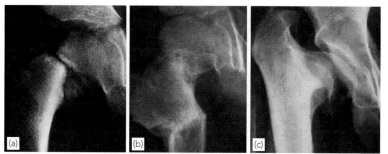

19.15 Infantile coxa vara (a) Typical x-ray features before displacement of the femoral neck. The physis is too vertical and there is a large triangular fragment of bone on the undersurface of the femoral neck. (b) Abduction osteotomy in a young patient with established coxa vara. (c) Untreated coxa vara.

FEMORAL ANTEVERSION (IN-TOE GAIT)

The commonest cause of in-toe gait is excessive anteversion of the femoral neck, so that internal rotation of the hip is increased and external rotation diminished. The gait may look clumsy, but is no bar to athletic prowess and usually improves with growth. These children often sit on the floor in the so-called 'television position' (with the knees facing each other); they should be encouraged to adopt the 'Buddha position' (knees turned outwards).

Correction by osteotomy is feasible, but rarely indicated, and certainly not before the age of 8 years.

PERTHES' DISEASE

Perthes' disease is a disorder of childhood characterized by necrosis of the femoral head. Although the incidence is only 1 in 10,000, it should always be considered in the differential diagnosis of hip pain in young children. Patients are usually 4–10 years old and often show delayed skeletal maturity; boys are affected four times as often as girls.

Pathogenesis

Up to the age of 4 months, the femoral head is supplied by: (1) metaphyseal vessels which penetrate the growth disc; (2) lateral epiphyseal vessels running in the retinacula; and (3) scanty vessels in the ligamentum teres. The metaphyseal supply gradually declines until, by the age of 4 years, it has virtually disappeared; by the age of 7, however, the vessels in the ligamentum teres have developed. Between 4 and 7 years of age the femoral head may depend for its blood supply almost entirely on the lateral epiphyseal vessels whose situation in the retinacula makes them susceptible to stretching and to pressure from an effusion. The precipitating cause is probably an effusion into the hip joint following either trauma, of which there is a history in over one-half of the cases, or a non-specific synovitis.

Pathology

The pathological process takes 2–4 years to complete, passing through three stages.

- *Stage 1: bone death*: following one or more episodes of ischaemia, part of the bony femoral head dies; it still looks normal on plain x-ray but it stops enlarging.
- *Stage 2: revascularization and repair*: new blood vessels enter the necrotic area and new bone is laid down on the dead trabeculae, producing the appearance of increased density on the x-ray. Some of the necrotic parts are resorbed

and replaced by fibrous tissue, producing the x-ray appearance of epiphyseal 'fragmentation'. If only part of the epiphysis is involved and the repair process is rapid, the bony architecture may be completely restored.

- *Stage 3: distortion and re-modelling*: if a large part of the bony epiphysis is damaged, or the repair process is slow, the epiphysis may collapse and subsequent growth at the head and neck will be distorted. Sometimes the epiphysis ends up flattened ('*coxa plana*') but enlarged ('*coxa magna*') and the femoral head is incompletely covered by the acetabulum.

Clinical features

The patient – usually a boy of 4–8 years – complains of pain and starts to limp. Symptoms may continue for weeks or recur intermittently. Clinically, the hip looks deceptively normal, although there may be a little wasting. Early on, the joint is 'irritable', so all movements are diminished and their extremes painful. Often the child is not seen till later, when most movements are full; but abduction is nearly always limited and usually internal rotation also.

X-rays

Even before x-ray changes appear, the ischaemic area can sometimes be demonstrated as a 'void' on radionuclide scanning. A subtle early change is widening of the radiographic joint 'space'. The classic feature of increased radiographic density in the bony epiphysis appears somewhat later. Flattening, false 'fragmentation' and lateral displacement of the epiphysis follow, with rarefaction and broadening of the metaphysis. The picture varies with the age of the child, the extent of ischaemia and the stage of the disease.

Various prognostic grading systems are employed, based mainly on x-ray appearances. Common to all of these systems is the importance of the structural integrity of the superolateral (principal loadbearing) part of the femoral head. The one described by Herring is recommended here (Herring JA: *Journal of Bone and Joint Surgery* **76A**:448–458,1994). In the anteroposterior x-ray, the femoral head is divided into three 'pillars' by lines at the medial and lateral edges of the central 'sequestrum'. **Group A** comprises those with normal height of the lateral pillar. **Group B** are patients with partial collapse (but still more than 50% height) of the lateral pillar; those under 9 years of age usually have a good outcome but older children are likely to develop flattening of the femoral head. **Group C** cases show more severe collapse of the lateral pillar (less than 50%

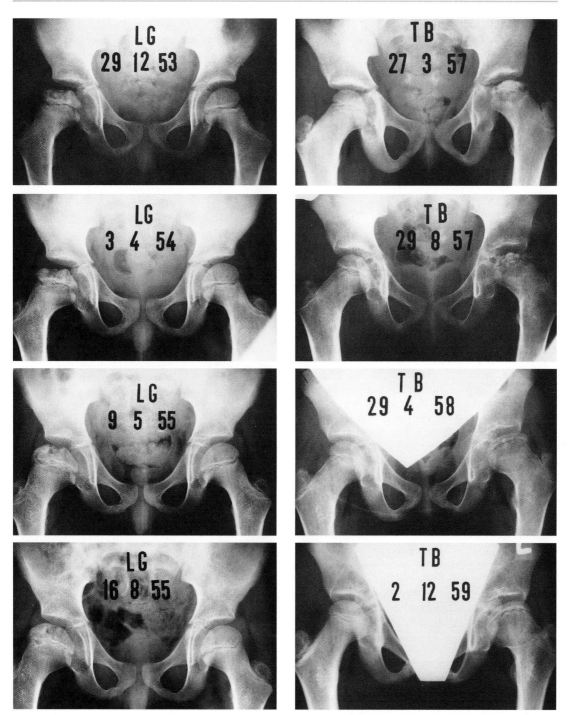

19.16 Perthes' disease – prognostic classification The Herring classification is based on the severity of structural disintegration of the lateral pillar of the femoral epiphysis. Column 1 shows the changes in a boy with moderately severe Perthes' disease of the right hip. Although the central part of the epiphyseal ossific centre seems to be 'fragmented', the lateral part of the epiphysis is intact throughout the natural progress of the disease. This is a favourable feature and serial x-rays show how the femoral head has gradually re-formed. Column 2 shows progressive changes in another young boy with severe Perthes' disease of the left hip. The epiphysis is widely involved from the outset, 'fragmentation' extends to the most lateral portion of the epiphysis and there is progressive flattening of the epiphysis resulting in permanent distortion of the femoral head.

of normal height); these usually end up with significant distortion of the femoral head.

Differential diagnosis

The commonest cause of hip pain in children is a non-specific transient synovitis – the so-called *irritable hip*. Ultrasound may show a joint effusion, but the x-rays are always normal. Symptoms last for 1–2 weeks and clear up completely. The child should be kept in bed until pain disappears and the effusion resolves.

General management

As long as the hip is painful the child should be in bed, with severe symptoms sometimes requiring a period of skin traction applied to the affected leg. Once pain has subsided, which usually takes about 3 weeks, movement is encouraged.

The clinical and radiographic features are then reassessed and the bone age is determined from x-rays of the wrist. The choice of further management is between: (a) symptomatic treatment; and (b) containment.

Symptomatic treatment means renewed pain control (if necessary), gentle exercise to maintain movement and regular reassessment. During asymptomatic periods the child is allowed out and about but sport and strenuous activities are avoided.

Containment means taking active steps to seat the femoral head congruently and as fully as possible in the acetabular socket, so that it may retain its sphericity and not become displaced during the period of healing and re-modelling. This is achieved (a) by holding the hips widely abducted in a plaster cast or in a removable brace for at least 1 year (ambulation, though awkward, is just possible) or (b) by operation, either a varus osteotomy of the femur or an innominate osteotomy of the pelvis, or both.

Operative reconstruction provides better containment and earlier mobilization, but there is no convincing evidence of improvement in the natural history of the disorder or (in particular) the likelihood of needing an arthroplasty in later life.

Guidelines to treatment

There is no general agreement on the 'correct' course of treatment for all cases. Decisions are based on an assessment of the age of the patient, the clinical features, the stage of the disease and the prognostic x-ray classification.

Children under 6 years

No specific form of treatment has much influence on the outcome. Symptomatic treatment, including activity modification, is appropriate.

Children aged 6–8 years

Here the bone age is more important than the chronological age:

- Bone age at or below 6 years:
  - Lateral pillar group A and B – symptomatic treatment.
  - Lateral pillar group C – abduction brace.
- Bone age over 6 years:
  - Lateral pillar group A and B – brace or varus osteotomy.
  - Lateral pillar group C – outcome probably unaffected by treatment, but some would operate.

Children 9 years and older

Except in very mild cases (which are rare), operative containment is the treatment of choice.

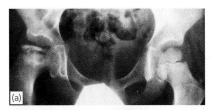
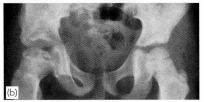

19.17 Perthes' disease – operative treatment
(a) The x-ray shows advanced Perthes' changes and lateral displacement of the right femoral head.
(b) Following an innominate osteotomy the femoral head is much better 'contained' and, although not normal, is developing reasonably well.

SLIPPED UPPER FEMORAL EPIPHYSIS

Displacement of the proximal femoral epiphysis – also known as *epiphysiolysis* – is uncommon and virtually confined to children going through the pubertal growth spurt. Boys are affected more often than girls. If one side slips there is a 30% risk of the other side slipping as well.

Aetiology

A slipped epiphysis is, to all intents and purposes, an insufficiency fracture through the hypertrophic zone of the cartilaginous growth plate. Trauma may be the precipitating cause, but often there is also an underlying abnormality. The disorder seems to occur in children who are unusually tall or obese and have delayed gonadal development. Perhaps this means that in these children there is an imbalance between pituitary growth hormone (which stimulates bone growth) and gonadal hormone (which promotes stable physeal fusion). Thus, during the pubertal growth spurt the relatively immature physis might be too weak to resist the stress imposed by the increased body weight.

Pathology

Following physeal disruption the femoral shaft rolls into external rotation and the femoral neck is displaced forwards while the epiphysis remains seated in the acetabulum. If the slip is severe, the anterior retinacular vessels are torn. However, at the back of the femoral neck the periosteum is lifted from the bone with the vessels intact; this may be the main – or the only – source of blood supply to the femoral head, and damage to these vessels by manipulation or operation may result in avascular necrosis.

Physeal disruption leads to premature fusion of the epiphysis – usually within 2 years of the onset of symptoms. This is accompanied by considerable bone modelling and, although there may be a permanent external rotation deformity and apparent coxa vara, adaptive changes often ensure good joint function even without treatment.

Clinical features

The patient – usually a boy of 14 or 15 years – presents with pain in the groin, the anterior part of the thigh or the knee (referred pain); he may also limp. The onset may be sudden and in 30% there

is a history of trauma (*an 'acute slip'*). However, in the majority symptoms are protracted (*a 'chronic slip'*), or else a long period of pain may culminate in a sudden climax following minor trauma (*an 'acute-on-chronic slip'*). Two-thirds of the patients are overweight and sexually under-developed, or unusually tall and thin.

On examination the leg is externally rotated and is 1 or 2 cm short. Characteristically there is limitation of abduction and medial (internal) rotation. Following an acute slip, the hip is irritable and all movements are accompanied by pain.

> ⚠ Beware the 'fat boy' with pain in or just above the knee! Look also at the hip.

X-rays

Even when slipping is trivial, changes can be detected. In the anteroposterior view the epiphyseal plate seems to be too wide and too 'woolly'. A line drawn along the superior surface of the femoral neck remains superior to the head instead of passing through it (*Trethowan's sign*). In the lateral view the femoral epiphysis is tilted backwards; small degrees of tilt can be detected by measuring the angle between the epiphyseal base and the femoral neck (see Figure 19.19).

Complications

Slipping at the opposite hip occurs in one-third of cases – sometimes while the patient is in bed. Forewarned is forearmed: always check the opposite side by x-ray. At the least sign of abnormality the epiphysis should be pinned.

Avascular necrosis is the most serious complication. It is seen only after a slip has been reduced or pinned, and is presumably due to the remaining leash of vessels being damaged.

Coxa vara deformity may result if the displacement is not reduced and the epiphysis fuses in its deformed position. The patient limps but the condition is usually painless. Osteotomy may be needed to correct the deformity and in the hope of preventing secondary osteoarthritis.

Secondary osteoarthritis is a likely sequel if displacement has not been reduced, and inevitable if there has been avascular necrosis.

Treatment

Closed reduction of the 'slip' is dangerous and should not be attempted.

- *Minor displacement*: displacement of less than one-third the width of the epiphysis is treated by accepting the position and fixing the epiphysis

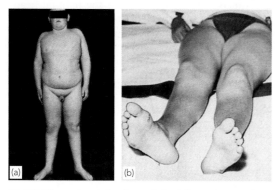

19.18 Slipped epiphysis – clinical features (a) This boy complained only of pain in his right knee. His build is unmistakable and the resting posture of his right lower limb tends towards external rotation (b). On examination, abduction and internal rotation were restricted.

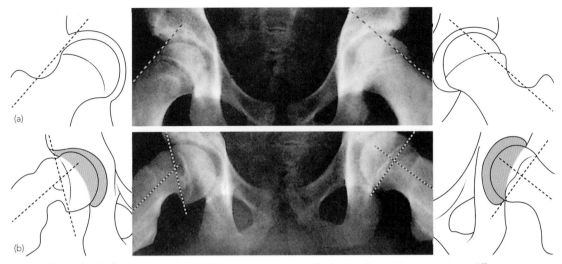

19.19 Slipped epiphysis – x-rays Careful x-ray examination is the key to diagnosis; even minute differences between the two sides may be important. In the anteroposterior view (a) Trethowan's line passes just above the femoral head on the right but cuts through the superior part of the femoral head on the left (normal) side. The lateral view (b) is diagnostically more reliable; even minor degrees of slip can be shown by drawing lines through the base of the epiphysis and up the middle of the femoral neck – if the angle indicated is less than 90 degrees, the epiphysis has slipped posteriorly.

with two thin threaded pins or screws. This is always done under x-ray control.

- *Moderate displacement*: displacements of one-third to one-half the epiphyseal width can often be treated by pinning alone. With further growth the proximal femur may be re-modelled to an acceptable degree; if this does not happen the residual deformity can be corrected later by an osteotomy lower down.
- *Severe displacement*: if the displacement is more than one-half the epiphyseal width, corrective surgery will be needed. In skilled hands this can be achieved by exposing the slip, removing a small piece of the femoral neck in order to permit replacement of the epiphysis, and pinning. A safer method is to fix the epiphysis in the displaced position and follow this some

while later with a compensatory osteotomy lower down. The femur is divided just below the greater trochanter; the distal fragment is re-positioned and fixed in valgus, flexion and medial rotation.

PYOGENIC ARTHRITIS

Pyogenic arthritis of the hip is usually seen in children under 2 years of age. The organism (usually a staphylococcus) reaches the joint either directly from a distant focus or by local spread from osteomyelitis of the femur. Unless the infection is rapidly aborted the femoral head, which is largely cartilaginous at this age, is liable to be destroyed by the proteolytic enzymes of bacteria and pus.

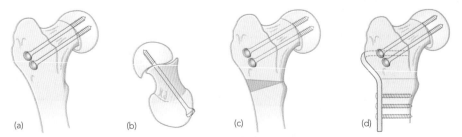

19.20 Slipped epiphysis - treatment (a,b) In this case slipping was minimal so no reduction was attempted, but further slipping was prevented by pinning the epiphysis in that position. (c,d) In more severe degrees of slip, the epiphysis should be fixed without attempting reduction and then, at a later stage, a complex compensatory osteotomy (d) can be performed to restore the normal position of the limb.

Clinical features

The child is ill and in pain, but it is often difficult to tell exactly where the pain is! The affected limb may be held absolutely still and all attempts at moving the hip are resisted. With care and patience it may be possible to localize a point of maximum tenderness over the hip; the diagnosis is confirmed by aspirating pus from the joint.

In neonates the most common presenting feature is a total lack of movement in the affected limb (*pseudoparalysis*). Local signs of inflammation are usually absent and blood tests are often normal.

During the acute stage of bone infection *x-rays* may show slight lateral displacement of the femoral head, suggesting the presence of a joint effusion. Ultrasound scans also will help to reveal a joint effusion. In children the epiphysis may become necrotic and later appear unusually dense or 'fragmented' on x-ray. In adults the defining feature is rapidly progressive erosion of the articular surfaces.

Treatment

Antibiotics should be given as soon as the diagnosis is reasonably certain, but not before obtaining a sample of joint fluid (or pus) for microbiological investigation and testing for antibiotic sensitivity. The joint is aspirated under general anaesthesia and, if pus is withdrawn, arthrotomy is advisable; antibiotics are instilled locally and the wound is closed without drainage. The hip is kept on traction or splinted in abduction until all evidence of disease activity has disappeared.

TUBERCULOSIS

The disease may start as a synovitis, or as an osteomyelitis in one of the adjacent bones. Once arthritis develops, destruction is rapid and may result in pathological dislocation. Healing usually leaves a fibrous ankylosis with considerable limb shortening and deformity.

Clinical features

Pain in the hip is the usual presenting symptom, though in late, neglected cases a cold abscess may point in the thigh or buttock. The patient walks with a limp; muscle wasting may be obvious and joint movements are limited and painful.

X-rays

The first x-ray change is general rarefaction of bone around the hip, a sign of inflammatory joint disease. In a child, the femoral epiphysis may be enlarged, again suggestive of chronic synovitis. Later changes are erosion and eventually destruction of the articular surfaces on both sides of the joint. The resemblance to rheumatoid arthritis is liable to lead to misdiagnosis in areas where tuberculosis is uncommon. A more unusual radiographic feature is the appearance of a bone abscess in the femoral neck or the greater trochanter.

Complications

Early disease may heal leaving a normal or almost normal hip. However, if the joint is destroyed the usual result is an unsound fibrous ankylosis. The leg is scarred and thin, and shortening is likely to be severe.

Treatment

If the disease is caught early, antituberculous chemotherapy should result in healing. During the acute phase the joint may need to be splinted in

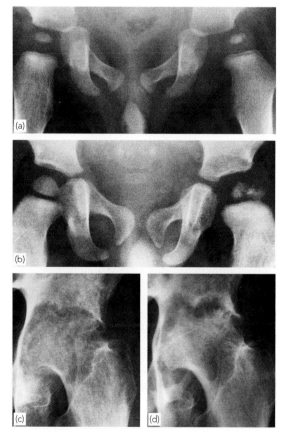

19.21 Pyogenic arthritis (a,b) In an infant. The left hip is distended and the head is drifting out of the socket. Six months later the epiphysis appears to be necrotic. (c,d) Rapid bone destruction in an adult over a period of 3 weeks!

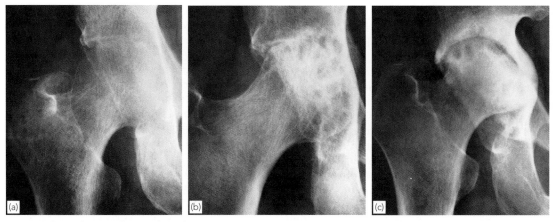

19.22 Tuberculous arthritis of the hip Serial x-rays showing (a) rarefaction of the bones on either side of the joint and loss of articular cartilage; (b) further joint erosion and abscesses in the femoral head; (c) healing after antituberculous drug treatment. If movement is restricted and painful, hip replacement can now be considered.

abduction or held in traction until the symptoms subside. An abscess in the femoral neck is best evacuated; if the joint infection does not settle, a surgical 'debridement' should be considered. After the disease subsides, the patient is allowed up and movement is encouraged, but chemotherapy should be continued for several months (see Chapter 2).

If the joint has been destroyed, *arthrodesis* may become necessary, but usually not before the age of 14 years. In older patients with residual pain and deformity, if the disease has clearly been inactive for a long time, *total joint replacement* is feasible and often successful; with antituberculous drugs, which are essential, the chance of recurrence is small.

THE IRRITABLE HIP

This condition – most probably due to a non-specific, short-lived synovitis with an effusion in the hip joint – is the most common cause of an acute limp and/or hip pain in children; it has a reported frequency of 14 per 1000. It usually occurs in 3–8 year olds, with boys affected twice as often as girls. The exact cause is unknown.

Clinical features

Typically the child presents with pain around the hip and a limp, often intermittent and following activity. The cardinal sign is restriction of all movements with pain at the extremes of the range in all directions. The diagnosis is based primarily on the clinical features; laboratory investigations are normal and x-rays show nothing more than slight widening of the medial joint space. This is caused by the effusion which allows the femoral head to sublux slightly; it may be confirmed by ultrasonography.

Characteristically, symptoms last for 1 or 2 weeks and then subside spontaneously; hence the synonym '*transient synovitis*'. The child may experience more than one episode, with an interval of months between attacks of pain.

Differential diagnosis

The condition is important largely because it resembles a number of serious disorders which have to be excluded:

- *Perthes' disease* is the main worry. Acute symptoms usually last longer than 2 weeks, and later the x-ray features are unmistakable.
- *Slipped epiphysis* may present as an 'irritable hip'. Initially the x-ray looks normal but if the age and general build are suggestive, or if the symptoms persist, the x-ray should be repeated.
- *Septic arthritis* and *tuberculous synovitis* should always be borne in mind. The early symptoms and signs are sometimes misleading, but blood tests will be abnormal and x-ray changes will inevitably appear.
- *Juvenile chronic arthritis* and *ankylosing spondylitis* may start with synovitis of one hip and it may take months before other joints are affected. Look for systemic features and a raised erythrocyte sedimentation rate (ESR). In doubtful cases, synovial biopsy may be helpful.

Treatment

Treatment involves bed rest, reduced activity and observation, which may be supervised at home or in hospital. Most children recover within a few days and any deterioration in signs or symptoms requires urgent reassessment.

Ultrasonography is repeated at intervals and weightbearing is allowed only when the symptoms disappear and the effusion resolves.

RHEUMATOID ARTHRITIS

The hip joint is frequently affected in rheumatoid arthritis. The hallmark of the disease is progressive bone destruction on both sides of the joint without any reactive osteophyte formation.

Clinical features

Usually the patient already has rheumatoid disease affecting many joints. Pain in the groin comes on insidiously; limp, though common, may be ascribed to pre-existing arthritis of the foot or knee. With advancing disease the patient has difficulty getting into or out of a chair, and even movement in bed may be painful.

Wasting of the buttock and thigh is often marked, and the limb is usually held in external rotation and fixed flexion. All movements are restricted and painful.

X-rays

During the early stages there is osteoporosis and diminution of the joint space; later, the acetabulum and femoral head are eroded. In the worst cases (and especially in patients on corticosteroids) there is gross bone destruction and the floor of the acetabulum may be perforated.

Treatment

If the disease can be arrested by general treatment (as described in Chapter 3), hip deterioration may be slowed down. But once cartilage and bone are eroded, no treatment will influence the progression

to joint destruction. Total joint replacement is then the best answer; it relieves pain and restores a useful range of movement. This is advocated even in younger patients, because the polyarthritis so limits activity that the implants are not unduly stressed. *Care should be taken to avoid perforation or fracture of the osteoporotic bone.*

OSTEOARTHRITIS

Osteoarthritis (OA) is the commonest non-traumatic disorder of the hip in middle and late age. Usually no specific 'cause' is identified but in younger patients (those under the age of 40 years) OA may appear as a sequel to childhood and adolescent disorders such as acetabular dysplasia, coxa vara, Perthes' disease or slipped femoral epiphysis, all of which may result in malcongruence between the acetabular socket and the femoral head.

A less obvious precursor – femoroacetabular impingement with scuffing of the acetabular labrum and the articular cartilage at the edge of the acetabulum – is now also recognized as a cause of hip OA. These are subtle changes which can easily be overlooked; special x-ray projections and magnetic resonance arthrography are needed to confirm the diagnosis.

In older patients secondary OA may appear in the aftermath of rheumatoid arthritis, avascular necrosis or Paget's disease.

Pathology

The articular cartilage becomes soft and fibrillated while the underlying bone shows cyst formation and sclerosis. These changes are most marked in the area of maximal loading (chiefly the top of the joint); at the margins of the joint there are the characteristic osteophytes. Synovial hypertrophy and capsular fibrosis may account for joint stiffness.

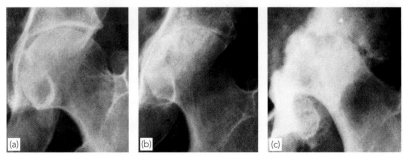

19.23 Rheumatoid arthritis Three stages in the development of rheumatoid arthritis: (a) loss of joint space; (b) erosion of the bone after cartilage has disappeared; (c) perforation of the acetabular floor – such marked destruction is more likely to occur if the patient is being treated with corticosteroids.

Clinical features

Pain is felt in the groin but may radiate to the knee. Typically it occurs after periods of activity but later it is more constant and sometimes disturbs sleep. Stiffness at first is noticed chiefly after rest; later it increases progressively until putting on socks and shoes becomes difficult. Limp is often noticed early and, if the hip is adducted, the patient may think the leg is getting shorter.

The patient is usually fit and over 50 years, but secondary osteoarthritis can occur at 30 or even 20 years. There may be an obvious limp and, except in early cases, a positive Trendelenburg sign. The affected leg usually lies in external rotation and adduction, so it appears short; there is nearly always some fixed flexion, although this may only be revealed by Thomas' test. Muscle wasting is detectable but rarely severe. Deep pressure may elicit tenderness, and the greater trochanter is situated somewhat high and posterior. Movements, though often painless within a limited range, are restricted.

X-rays

The earliest sign is a decreased joint space (loss of articular cartilage), usually maximal in the superior weightbearing region but sometimes affecting the entire joint. Later signs are subarticular sclerosis, cyst formation and osteophytes at the edges of the joint. There may also be tell-tale signs of previous abnormalities dating back to childhood or adolescence.

Treatment

Analgesics and anti-inflammatory drugs are helpful, and warmth is soothing. The patient is encouraged to use a walking stick (held in the opposite hand) and to try to preserve movement and stability by performing exercises within the range of comfort. Joint manipulation sometimes relieves pain for long periods.

Patients should be advised on ways of changing their lifestyle so as reduce impact loading on the affected hip: e.g. cutting down on uphill walking, climbing up and down stairs, carrying heavy weights or even sitting in one position for very long periods. Functional aids will help with daily activities such as bathing and dressing. Of course none of these measures will restore damaged cartilage, but they will lessen the patient's symptoms.

Operative treatment: details of operative treatment can be found in Chapter 12. The indications for surgery are relentlessly intrusive pain, a progressive decrease in joint movements and walking ability, increasing difficulty with activities of daily living and x-ray signs of progressive joint deterioration.

The procedure of choice will usually be *total joint replacement*, especially if the patient is over 50 years of age and unlikely to stress the hip excessively during their remaining lifetime. In experienced hands the results are usually very good over a period of 15–20 years, but the patient should be warned that failures do occur and may necessitate revision of the arthroplasty.

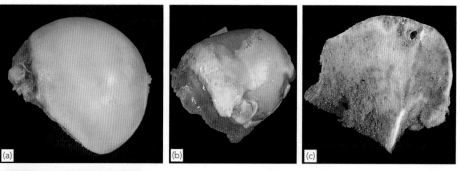

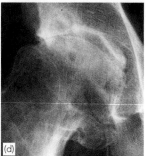

19.24 Osteoarthritis (a,b) Pathology – loss of articular cartilage over the dome of the femoral head and osteophyte formation around the periphery. Subarticular cysts are seen in the coronal section (c). These features are well demonstrated in the x-ray (d).

For younger patients, who will probably need at least one revision during their remaining lifetime, other procedures are worth considering. If the hip is dysplastic and a significant area of articular cartilage still preserved, a *re-positioning intertrochanteric osteotomy* may buy 5–10 years of satisfactory function, by which time a total hip replacement may be more suitable.

In recent years *osteochondroplasty* has gained attention following the recognition of femoro-acetabular impingement as a cause of early acetabular cartilage damage (see below).

Arthrodesis of the hip is a practical solution for very young adults with marked destruction of a single joint, and particularly when the conditions for advanced reconstructive surgery are not available. If well executed, the operation guarantees freedom from pain and permanent stability, though it has the disadvantages of restricted mobility and a significant incidence of later backache.

FEMOROACETABULAR IMPINGEMENT

In recent years it has been recognized that some cases of so-called primary OA of the hip may be caused by minimal deformities of the femoral head or acetabular socket – specifically, by initial damage to the articular cartilage due to impingement of the femoral head against the edges of the acetabular socket (femoroacetabular impingement, or FAI). The two main types of FAI are described as *pincer* and *cam*.

In *pincer impingement* there is over-coverage of the femoral head by the anterior edge of the acetabulum, either due to excessive depth or retroversion of the acetabular socket or at a localized site by a protruding acetabular osteophyte. In this case the hard acetabular margin abuts against the femoral head during movement, causing degeneration of the acetabular labrum and the adjacent articular cartilage.

In *cam impingement* the 'deformity' is at the femoral head/neck junction: an unusual degree of bony thickening causes jamming of the femoral neck against the front of the acetabulum and abrasion of the articular cartilage (and possibly also damage to the acetabular labrum).

In most cases both types of FAH co-exist, though the cam type predominates. Initially the anterosuperior part of the joint is affected but in the long term this may progress to full-blown OA.

Clinical features

Patients are usually fit adults in their 30s or 40s whose main complaint is pain in the groin, particularly after strenuous activity. The women tend to develop pincer lesions; the men are often strongly built athletes or sportsmen and usually present with cam lesions. Hip movements may be restricted and sometimes provoke pain in the hip.

Specialized imaging techniques, including magnetic resonance arthrography, are required to reveal these unusual disorders.

Treatment

Physiotherapy and pain-relieving medication may be helpful, but in addition strenuous physical activity will have to be curtailed.

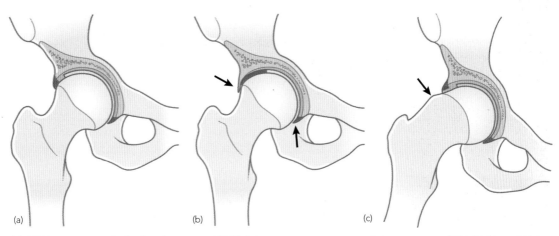

19.25 Femoroacetabular impingement (FAI) Schematic representation of the two types of FAI. (a) Normal hip. (b) Pincer type FAI. (c) Cam type FAI.

If clinical and imaging examinations reveal unequivocal signs of FAI, operative osteochondroplasty should be considered. This involves shaving back the protuberant bone at the anterosuperior part of the femoral neck in cam lesions, and/or removal of acetabular bone excrescences in pincer lesions, as well as debridement of damaged cartilage and labral tissue. Short- to midterm results are reputed to be good, but longer follow-up studies are awaited to indicate whether this is a worthwhile approach to treatment.

THE KNEE

CLINICAL ASSESSMENT

HISTORY

■ *Pain* is the most common symptom. In inflammatory or degenerative disorders it is usually diffuse – gradual in onset with osteoarthritis but typically sudden and severe with gout or infection. In mechanical disorders (especially after injury) it is usually localized: think of a torn meniscus or ligament; it helps if the patient can point to the painful spot.

■ *Swelling*, too, may be diffuse or localized. When diffuse, it is suggestive of fluid within the joint or synovial thickening. If there was an injury, ask whether the swelling appeared immediately (suggesting a haemarthrosis) or gradually (typical of a torn meniscus). Chronic diffuse swelling is characteristic of arthritis or synovitis. Intermittent swelling suggests an old meniscal tear or a loose body.

  ● A soft, well-defined, localized swelling either in front of or behind the knee may be due to an inflamed bursa.

  ● A firm, fixed swelling along the lateral joint line is typical of a meniscal cyst; a loose body in the joint is also firm but it tends to move around on pressure.

  ● A bony hard swelling at the distal end of the femur or the proximal end of the tibia is more sinister: x-ray examination may reveal a tumour.

■ *Stiffness* is also a common complaint. Ask whether it fluctuates and when it feels worse or better. Early morning stiffness suggests an inflammatory disorder; stiffness after periods of inactivity is typical of osteoarthritis.

■ *'Locking'* is different from stiffness. The joint is not really 'locked' in the sense that it cannot move at all. One minute it moves perfectly well and the next it can still flex as before but it cannot extend fully; something has got jammed between the articular surfaces (usually a torn meniscus or a loose body). *'Unlocking'* is even more suggestive: the obstructing object has shifted and the joint can now move freely again.

■ Do not be misled by 'pseudolocking', when movement is suddenly stopped by pain or the fear of impending pain.

■ *Deformity*, especially if it is of recent onset, is quickly noticed. It may be unilateral or bilateral: *valgus* or *varus*, *fixed flexion* or *hyperextension*. Knock-knees and bandy-legs are common in children and usually correct spontaneously as the child grows.

■ *Giving way* can be due to muscle weakness, but more often it is caused by a mechanical disorder such as a torn meniscus or a faulty patellar extensor mechanism.

■ *Loss of function* manifests as difficulty in standing up from a low chair, a progressively diminishing walking distance, inability to run and difficulty going up and down steps.

> ⚠ **Pain in the knee**
> Check the hip as well – it could be referred pain.

SIGNS WITH THE PATIENT STANDING

Uncover the lower limbs from groin to toe and position the patient with both feet pointing forward and slightly apart. Getting the patient to stand upright unmasks deformities better than with the patient lying down. Look at the overall shape and alignment of the limb: is there an asymmetry; are the muscles wasted; do the limbs appear to be bow-legged (genu varum) or knock-kneed (genu valgum)? Remember it is often easier to pick up subtle changes of alignment looking from behind the patient than from the front.

Then ask the patient to walk. Is there a limp and, if so, is it because the knee does not move freely as it swings through or because it does not straighten well when planted on the ground? Is there an irregular rhythm with the patient trying to diminish weightbearing on one or other side?

If the history suggests a possible meniscal injury, the *Thessaly test* is useful. The patient is instructed to stand with the affected knee flexed to 20 degrees and the foot placed flat on the ground, taking his or her full weight on that leg (the examiner can support the patient for balance). The patient is then asked to twist his or her body first to one side and then to the other three times (thus exerting a rotational force in the knee with each turn), while still keeping the knee flexed at 20 degrees. Patients with meniscal tears experience medial or lateral joint line pain and may feel that the knee is locking.

SIGNS WITH THE PATIENT SITTING

With the patient sitting on the edge of the examination couch look at the position of the patella: is it seated centrally or is it shifted to one side? Does it appear higher (*patella alta*) or lower (*patella baja / infera*) than usual? Ask the patient to straighten each knee in turn. Note the movement of the patella. Does it glide upwards in a smooth manner or does it momentarily veer sideways (maltracking or patellar instability)?

SIGNS WITH THE PATIENT LYING SUPINE

Always compare the two sides; subtle differences are easier to detect by comparing the abnormal with the normal side.

Look

Is there any asymmetry? Are there tell-tale scars from previous injuries or operations? Is there muscle wasting? Always confirm the visual impression by measuring the girth of the thigh at a fixed point above each knee. Is there swelling and is it diffuse or localized? Is there bruising that may help localize the injury?

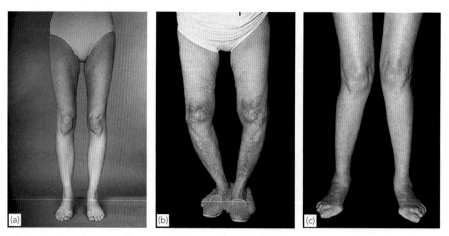

20.1 Examination standing (a) Look at the general shape and posture, first from in front and then from behind. Normally the knees are in slight valgus. (b) Varus deformity (osteoarthritis). (c) Valgus deformity (rheumatoid arthritis).

Feel

Run the back of your hand down each limb from the thigh and across the knee. Does the knee feel warmer on one side, suggesting inflammation? Now bend the patient's knee to about 70 degrees and sit on the edge of the couch facing the knee. Feel the bony contours around the joint, the attachments of ligaments and tendons, and the joint line. Note where there is tenderness.

Synovial thickening is best diagnosed as follows. Grasp the patella between the thumb and middle finger and try to lift it off the femoral groove: normally it can be gripped quite firmly but if the synovium is thickened, your fingers simply slip off the edges of the patella.

The patellofemoral joint can be felt only at its medial and lateral edges. Straighten the patient's knee and push the patella first towards the medial and then towards the lateral side, feeling with the fingers of your other hand for tenderness along the undersurface of the bone. Rubbing the patella against the femoral trochlea may also elicit pain. A more sensitive test is to press gently against the proximal edge of the patella and ask the patient to contract the quadriceps muscles: as the patella is dragged forcefully along the front of the femur the patient may wince with pain – a feature that is often encountered in patellofemoral chondromalacia or osteoarthritis.

Move

Ask the patient to bend and straighten the knee fully. Note the range of movement. Repeat the motion while placing a hand over the front of the knee; *crepitus* is felt as a grating sensation between the patella and femur – a sign of patellofemoral degeneration. Finally check if passively moving the knee alters the range.

The patellar apprehension test is a useful way of detecting unstable patellar movement. While passively flexing the patient's knee slowly, use your thumb to press the patella laterally: if the patient becomes increasingly anxious and resistant to further movement, it suggests that he or she has

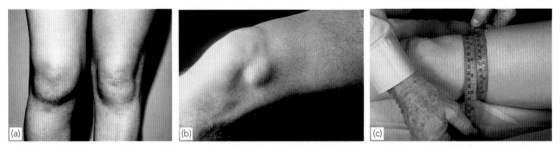

20.2 Examination with the patient supine Swelling may involve either the whole joint, as in (a), a patient with synovitis of the right knee, or may be due to a localized lesion, as in (b), a patient with a large loose body slipping around in the joint. Quadriceps wasting is common in all types of joint derangement; it can be accurately assessed by (c) measuring the thigh girth at a fixed distance above the joint line of each knee and comparing the two sides.

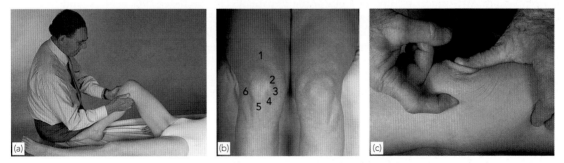

20.3 Feeling for tenderness (a) This is the best position for eliciting tenderness around the knee. (b) Landmarks are: 1, quadriceps tendon; 2, edge of patella; 3, medial collateral ligament; 4, the joint line; 5, lateral collateral ligament; 6, patellar ligament. (c) By pushing the patella to one or other side of the midline one can feel under its edge.

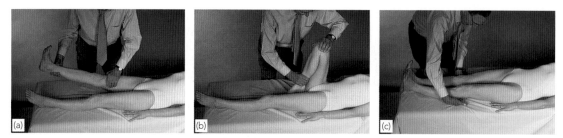

20.4 Movement The knee should move from full extension (a) through a range of 150 degrees to full flexion (b). Small degrees of flexion deformity (loss of full extension) can be detected by placing the hands under the knees while the patient forces the legs down on the couch (c); if your hand can be extracted more easily on one side than the other, this indicates loss of the final few degrees of complete extension.

either experienced a previous patellar dislocation of subluxation or fears an impending subluxation because of patellar instability.

Tests for intra-articular fluid

Cross-fluctuation

This test is applicable only if there is a sizable joint effusion. The left hand is used to compress and empty the suprapatellar pouch while the right hand straddles the front of the joint below the patella; by squeezing with each hand alternately, a fluid impulse is transmitted across the joint.

The patellar tap

The suprapatellar pouch is compressed with the left hand to squeeze any fluid from the pouch into the joint. With the other hand the patella is then tapped sharply backwards onto the femoral condyles. In a positive test the patella can be felt striking the femur and bouncing off again (a type of ballottement).

The bulge test

This is a useful method of testing when there is very little fluid in the joint, though it takes some practice to get it right! After squeezing any fluid out of the suprapatellar pouch, the medial compartment is emptied by pressing on the medial aspect of the joint; that hand is then lifted away and the lateral side is sharply compressed – a distinct ripple is seen on the flattened medial surface as fluid is shunted across.

The juxtapatellar hollow

If both knees are bent gradually and observed from below, a hollow appears lateral to the patellar ligament and disappears on further flexion; if there is fluid in the joint, this hollow fills quickly and disappears at a lesser angle of flexion, or it may not be seen at all.

Tests for ligamentous stability

Collateral ligaments

The medial and lateral ligaments are tested by stressing the knee into valgus and varus: this is best done by tucking the patient's foot under your arm and holding the extended knee firmly with one hand on each side of the joint; the leg is then angulated alternately towards abduction and adduction. The test is performed at full extension and again at 30 degrees of flexion. There is normally some mediolateral movement at 30 degrees, but if this is excessive (compared to the normal side) it suggests a torn or stretched collateral ligament. Sideways movement in full extension is always abnormal; this may be due either to torn or stretched ligaments and capsule, or to loss of articular cartilage or bone on one side of the knee which allows the affected compartment to collapse.

Cruciate ligaments

Routine examination for cruciate ligament stability involves testing for abnormal gliding movements in the anteroposterior (sagittal) plane. With the patient's knees flexed 90 degrees and the feet resting on the couch, the upper tibia is inspected from the side; if its upper end has dropped back, or can be gently pushed back, this indicates a tear of the posterior cruciate ligament (the 'sag sign'). With the knee in the same position, the foot is anchored by the examiner sitting on it (provided this does not cause pain); then, using both hands, the upper end of the tibia is grasped firmly and rocked backwards and forwards to see if there is any anteroposterior glide (the 'drawer test'). Excessive anterior movement (a positive anterior drawer sign) denotes anterior cruciate laxity; excessive posterior movement (a positive posterior drawer sign) signifies posterior cruciate laxity.

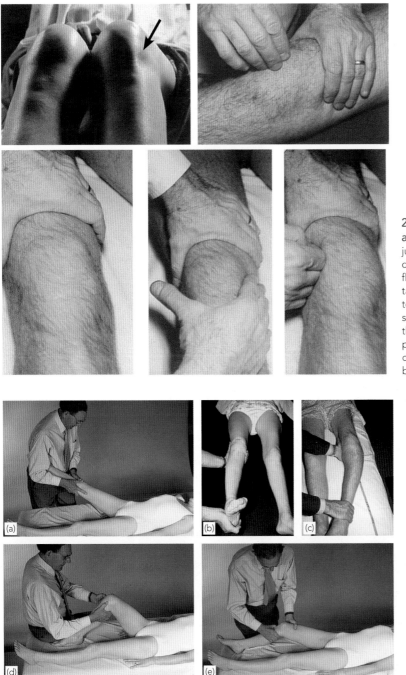

20.5 Testing for intra-articular fluid (a) The juxtapatellar hollow, which disappears in flexion if there is fluid in the knee. (b) Patellar tap test. (c–e) Doing the bulge test: compress the suprapatellar pouch (c); empty the medial compartment (d); push fluid back from the lateral compartment and watch for the bulge on the medial side (e).

20.6 Testing for instability There are two ways of testing the collateral ligaments (side-to-side stability): (a) by gripping the foot close to your body and guiding the knee alternately towards valgus and varus; (b) by gripping the femoral condyles (provided your hand is big enough) and then forcing the leg alternately into valgus and varus. (c) In this case there was gross instability on the lateral side, allowing the knee to be pulled into marked varus. Cruciate ligament instability can be assessed by either the drawer test (d) or the Lachman test (e) as described in the text.

More sensitive is the *Lachman test*, but this is difficult if the patient has big thighs (or the examiner has small hands). The patient's knee is flexed 20 degrees; with one hand grasping the lower thigh and the other the upper part of the leg, the joint surfaces are shifted backwards and forwards upon each other. If the knee is stable, there should be no gliding.

Rotatory instability

If multiple ligaments and the capsule are torn, the knee can become unstable to rotatory forces.

Special clinical tests have been developed to detect these abnormalities; the best known is the *pivot shift test*. The patient lies supine with the lower limb completely relaxed. The examiner lifts the leg with the knee held in full extension and the tibia internally rotated. This produces a position of slight rotational subluxation if the lateral collateral, anterior cruciate and part of the posterolateral capsule are torn (see Chapter 32). A valgus force is then applied to the lateral side of the joint as the knee is flexed; a sudden posterior movement of the tibia is seen and felt as the joint is fully re-located. The test is sometimes quite painful.

SIGNS WITH THE PATIENT LYING PRONE

Scars or lumps in the popliteal fossa are noted. If there is a swelling, is it in the midline (most likely a bulging capsule) or to one side (possibly a bursa)? The soft tissues are carefully palpated. If there is a lump, where does it originate? Does it pulsate? Can it be emptied into the joint?

The joint line is located about a finger's breadth below the flexion crease. A *semimembranous bursa* is usually just above the joint line, a *Baker's cyst* below it.

Apley's test (also called the *grinding* test) is sometimes helpful. The knee is flexed to 90 degrees and rotated while a compression force is applied; this may reproduce symptoms if a meniscus is torn. Rotation is then repeated while the leg is pulled upwards with the surgeon's knee holding the thigh flat on the couch; this, *the distraction test*, produces increased pain only if there is ligament damage.

Table 20.1

Three causes of:

Acute swelling	**Chronic swelling**
Synovitis	Rheumatoid arthritis
Haemarthrosis	Osteoarthritis
Septic arthritis	Tuberculosis

Giving way

Torn meniscus
Torn ligaments
Unstable patella

IMAGING

X-rays

Anteroposterior and lateral views are routine; it is often useful also to obtain tangential ('skyline') patellofemoral views and intercondylar (or tunnel) views. The skyline view gives additional information on how the patella lies within the femoral groove and may reveal poor tracking of this sesamoid bone; the tunnel view reveals the articular portions of the medial and lateral femoral condyles where osteoarticular lesions (osteochondritis dissecans) may exist.

The anteroposterior view should always be taken with the patient standing: unless the femorotibial compartment is loaded, narrowing of the articular space may be missed.

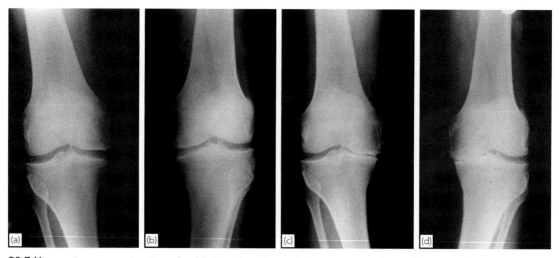

20.7 X-rays Anteroposterior views should always be taken with the patient standing. (a,b) Images obtained with the patient lying on the x-ray couch show only slight narrowing of the medial joint space on each side; but with weightbearing (c,d) it is clear that the changes are much more marked than at first thought.

Magnetic resonance imaging (MRI)

MRI has evolved to become the standard imaging method for diagnosing and grading the severity of many intra-articular and extra-articular problems. It is able to detect meniscal tears, ligament and capsular injuries, osteoarticular fractures and both benign and malignant tumours.

ARTHROSCOPY

Arthroscopy is useful: (1) to establish or refine the accuracy of diagnosis (e.g. biopsies can be taken); (2) to help in deciding a treatment strategy or to plan the operative approach; (3) to record the progress of a knee disorder; and (4) to perform certain operative procedures, particularly for meniscal tears and ligament reconstructions. Arthroscopy is not a substitute for clinical examination and imaging; a detailed history, meticulous assessment of the physical signs and careful scrutiny of imaging are indispensable preliminaries and remain the sheet anchor of diagnosis.

SWELLINGS AROUND THE KNEE

A common complaint is of swelling – either of the entire joint or asymmetrically on one or other aspect of the joint. The following conditions should be considered.

ACUTE SWELLING OF THE ENTIRE JOINT

Traumatic synovitis

Any moderately severe injury (including a torn or trapped meniscus or a torn cruciate ligament) can precipitate a reactive synovitis, but typically the swelling appears only after several hours.

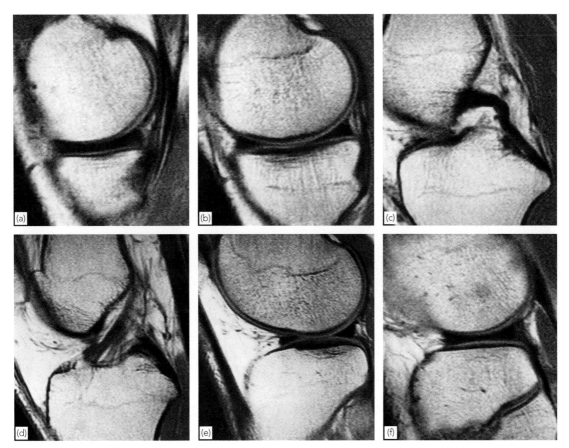

20.8 MRI A series of sagittal T1-weighted images proceeding from medial to lateral show the normal appearances of: (a,b) the medial meniscus; (c) the posterior cruciate ligament; (d) the somewhat fan-shaped anterior cruciate ligament; and (e,f) the lateral meniscus.

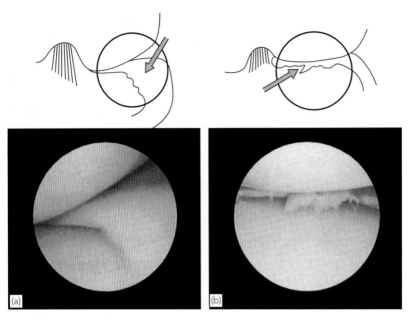

20.9 Arthroscopy
Arthroscopic images of the interior of the right knee from the lateral side, showing (a) a normal medial meniscus and (b) a torn medial meniscus.

Post-traumatic haemarthrosis

Tense swelling immediately after injury means blood in the joint. The knee is painful and it feels warm, tense and tender. Movements are restricted. X-rays are essential to see if there is a fracture; if there is not, then suspect a tear of the anterior cruciate ligament.

Non-traumatic haemarthrosis

In patients with clotting disorders, the knee is a common site for acute bleeds. If the appropriate clotting factor is available, the joint should be aspirated and splinted. Bleeds can also occur from tears to vascular lesions in the knee (e.g. pigmented villonodular synovitis).

Acute septic arthritis

The joint is swollen, painful and inflamed; this may be accompanied with systemic features such as malaise, pyrexia, a high temperature and elevation of the white cell count, erythrocyte sedimentation rate (ESR) and C-reactive protein. Aspiration reveals pus in the joint; fluid should be sent for microbiological investigation, including anaerobic culture. *This should always be done before starting antibiotic treatment.* The organism is usually *Staphylococcus aureus*, but in adults gonococcal infection is almost as common. Treatment consists of intravenous antibiotics and drainage of the joint.

Aseptic inflammatory arthritis

Acute swelling without a history of trauma or signs of infection suggests gout or pseudogout. The joint may be inflamed and very tender. Aspiration will provide fluid which may look like pus but is sterile; microscopy (using polarized light) reveals the characteristic crystals. Treatment with anti-inflammatory drugs is usually effective.

Another cause of acute inflammatory synovitis is Reiter's disease (see page 36). Always enquire about symptoms due to urogenital or bowel infection. If *Chlamydia* are isolated, treatment should include a prolonged course of tetracycline.

CHRONIC SWELLING OF THE ENTIRE JOINT

Non-infective arthritis

The commonest causes of chronic swelling are *osteoarthritis* and *rheumatoid arthritis*. Other signs, such as deformity, loss of movement or instability, may be present and x-ray examination will usually show characteristic features.

Chronic infective arthritis

The most important condition to exclude is *tuberculosis*, of which there has been a resurgence of cases in the last two decades. Typically, the knee is swollen and the thigh muscles are wasted. Further details are given on page 279.

Other synovial disorders

Unusual conditions such as *synovial chondromatosis* and *pigmented villonodular synovitis* (PVNS) should not be forgotten. In synovial chondromatosis there are multiple, pearly cartilaginous loose bodies enveloped in synovial folds. PVNS is a type of synovial tumour which causes erosion and excavation of the articular surfaces; at operation the synovium is seen to be swollen, often covered in villi and golden-brown in colour – the effect of haemosiderin deposition. Rare disorders such as these are usually diagnosed only by careful imaging studies and arthroscopy. Treatment involves operative removal of pathological tissue. Not surprisingly, there is a considerable recurrence rate and some patients may even require joint replacement.

SWELLINGS IN FRONT OF THE KNEE

Prepatellar bursitis

This fluctuant swelling is confined to the front of the patella and the joint itself is normal. It is an uninfected bursitis due to constant friction between skin and bone. As such, it is seen mainly in carpet layers, paving workers, floor cleaners and miners who do not use protective knee pads. Treatment consists of firm bandaging, and kneeling is avoided; occasionally aspiration is needed. In chronic cases the lump is best excised.

Infrapatellar bursitis

The swelling is below the patella and superficial to the patellar ligament, being more distally placed than prepatellar bursitis. Treatment is similar to that for prepatellar bursitis.

SWELLINGS AT THE BACK OF THE KNEE

Semimembranosus bursa

The bursa between the semimembranosus and the medial head of gastrocnemius may become enlarged in children or adults. It presents usually as a painless lump behind the knee, slightly to the medial side of the midline and is most conspicuous with the knee straight. The lump is fluctuant and transilluminates. The knee joint is normal. A waiting policy, even if the lump causes an ache, is wise as it usually disappears with time.

Popliteal 'cyst'

Bulging of the posterior capsule and synovial herniation may produce a swelling in the

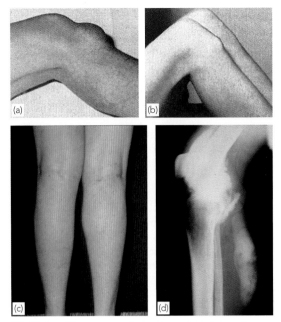

20.10 Swellings around the knee (a) Infrapatellar bursitis. (b) Osgood–Schlatter's disease (see also Figure 20.26). (c) Swelling in the right popliteal fossa and upper calf, due to a large joint effusion. In this case the joint capsule ruptured and synovial fluid trickled into the popliteal space, as revealed in the arthrogram (d).

popliteal fossa. It is usually caused by rheumatoid or osteoarthritis, but it is still often called a 'Baker's cyst' (even though Baker's original description probably referred to an association with tuberculous arthritis). Occasionally the 'cyst' ruptures and the synovial contents spill into the muscle planes causing pain and swelling in the calf – a combination which can easily be mistaken for deep vein thrombosis. The swelling may diminish following aspiration and injection of hydrocortisone; excision is not advised, because recurrence is common unless the underlying condition is treated.

Popliteal aneurysm

Before plunging a knife into a popliteal swelling, make sure that the 'lump' is not an aneurysm! If there is any doubt, use a fine needle to aspirate the 'cyst'.

SWELLINGS AT THE SIDE OF THE JOINT

Meniscal cyst

This presents as a small, tense swelling, usually on the lateral side at or just below the joint line.

273

Sometimes it is so tense that it can easily be mistaken for a bony lump. It is usually tender on pressure (see also page 277).

Calcification of the collateral ligament

An acutely painful swelling may suddenly appear, usually on the medial side of the joint. It is rubbery in consistency and acutely tender. Operative decompression will confirm the diagnosis (the calcific material is extruded like toothpaste) and provide immediate relief.

Bony swellings

Bony lumps (exostosis or bone tumours) arising in the metaphyses of the distal femur or proximal tibia may cause visible and palpable swelling on any aspect close to the joint. The diagnosis is revealed by x-ray examination and, if necessary, biopsy.

DEFORMITIES OF THE KNEE

PHYSIOLOGICAL BOW-LEGS AND KNOCK-KNEES

Bow-legs in babies and knock-knees in 4 year olds are so common that they are considered to be stages of normal development. Bilateral bow-legged appearance can be recorded by measuring the distance between the knees with the child standing and the heels touching; it should be less than 6 cm. Similarly, knock-knee can be estimated by measuring the distance between the medial malleoli when the knees are touching with the patellae facing forwards; it is usually less than 8 cm. In the occasional case where, by the age of 10 years, the deformity is still marked (i.e. the intercondylar distance is more than 6 cm or the intermalleolar distance more than 8 cm), operative correction can be offered. This is done by inserting a staple or small plate on the side of the physis (the convex side of the deformity) that needs growth restriction (*hemi-epiphyseodesis*). When the deformity has been corrected, the staple or plate is removed.

PATHOLOGICAL BOW-LEGS AND KNOCK-KNEES IN CHILDREN

A unilateral deformity is likely to be pathological, as is a severe bilateral deformity (by the measures cited above). Unilateral deformities are usually caused by eccentric growth from the physis of the distal femur or proximal tibia; this may result from rickets, injury, infection, or an inherent growth disorder. The clinical deformity is usually progressive. Operative correction by osteotomy should be deferred until near the end of growth lest the deformity recur with further growth.

Blount's disease is a progressive bow-legged deformity due to abnormal growth of the posteromedial part of the proximal tibia. It tends to affect children of black African descent more frequently than others. Typically, and in the adolescent variety, the child is overweight and walks with an outward thrust at the knee. On x-ray, the proximal tibial epiphysis is flattened medially and the adjacent metaphysis is beak shaped. Spontaneous resolution is rare. Hemi-epiphyseodesis may not always work and correction by osteotomy is usually needed.

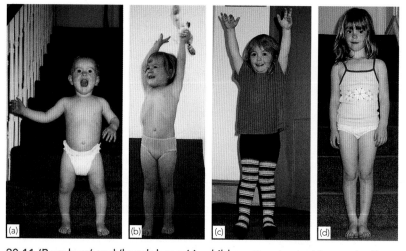

20.11 'Bow-legs' and 'knock-knees' in children Two sisters with natural self-correcting 'deformities' of the knees. (a,b) Tamzin at 1½ and 2½ years; (c,d) Jessy at 3 and 4½ years.

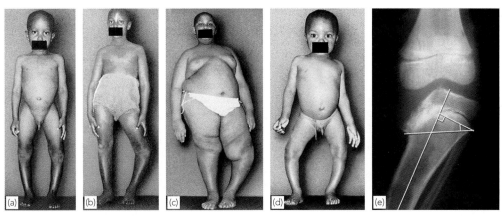

20.12 Pathological bow-legs (a) Child with healed rickets. (b) Growth deformity following a fracture through the proximal tibial physis. (c) This deformity was due to a 'slipped' tibial epiphysis in a child with an endocrine disorder. (d,e) Blount's disease in a young boy who developed progressive 'bow-legs' from the time he started walking. X-rays showed the typical distortion of the tibial epiphysis. The deformity can be accurately assessed by measuring the metaphyseodiaphyseal angle: a line is drawn perpendicular to the long axis of the tibia and another across the metaphyseal flare as shown on the x-ray; the acute angle formed by these two lines should normally not exceed 11 degrees.

PATHOLOGICAL BOW-LEGS AND KNOCK-KNEES IN ADULTS

Angular deformities are common in adults (usually bow-legs in men and knock-knees in women). While this may be a sequel to a childhood problem, the deformity usually arises from an asymmetrical cartilage or bone loss on one side of the joint, e.g. in osteoarthritis, rheumatoid arthritis, subchondral fractures or Paget's disease. Provided the joint is stable, a corrective osteotomy may be all that is required. However, a unilateral ligament injury may also cause an unstable valgus or varus deformity; this will call for ligament reconstruction. In some cases partial or total joint replacement will be needed.

LESIONS OF THE MENISCI

MENISCAL TEARS

The menisci have three important roles:

- Improving articular congruency and stability.
- Controlling the complex rolling and gliding actions of the joint.
- Distributing load during weightbearing.

These functions are compromised if the menisci are torn or removed. The medial meniscus is less mobile than the lateral and, consequently, more liable to tearing when subjected to abnormal stresses. Grinding forces split the fibres of the

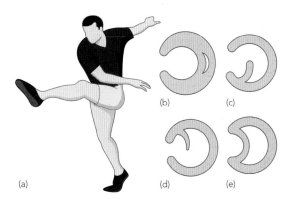

20.13 Torn medial meniscus (a) The meniscus is usually torn by a twisting force with the knee bent and taking weight; the initial split (b) may extend anteriorly (c), posteriorly (d) or both ways to create a 'bucket-handle' tear (e).

meniscus (which are arranged circumferentially). If the separated fragment remains attached at the front and back, the lesion is called a *bucket-handle tear*. The torn portion sometimes displaces towards the centre of the joint and, if jammed between femur and tibia, it can block the knee extending fully ('locking'). If the tear emerges at the free edge of the meniscus, it leaves a tongue based anteriorly (an *anterior horn tear*) or posteriorly (a *posterior horn tear*).

Horizontal tears are usually 'degenerative' or due to repetitive minor trauma. Some are associated with meniscal cysts (see below). Some tears, if peripheral (outer third), can heal after suture but others, closer to the centre of the joint, do not heal because they are avascular.

Clinical features

The patient is usually a young person who sustains a twisting injury to the knee. Pain is often severe and further activity is avoided. Occasionally the knee is 'locked' in partial flexion. Almost invariably swelling appears a few hours later, or perhaps the following day.

With rest the initial symptoms subside, only to recur periodically after trivial twists or strains. Sometimes the knee gives way spontaneously and this is again followed by pain and swelling.

It is important to remember that in patients aged over 40 years the initial injury may be unremarkable and the main complaint is of recurrent 'giving way' or 'locking'.

'Locking' (the sudden inability to extend the knee fully) suggests a bucket-handle tear. The patient sometimes learns to 'unlock' the knee by bending it fully or by twisting it from side to side.

On examination the joint may be held slightly flexed and there is often an effusion. In late presentations, the quadriceps will be wasted. Tenderness is localized to the joint line, in the vast majority of cases on the medial side. Flexion is usually full but extension is often slightly limited.

Between attacks of pain and effusion there is a disconcerting paucity of signs, but special tests may alert one to the diagnosis.

McMurray's test is based on the fact that a loose meniscal tag can sometimes be trapped between the articular surfaces and then induced to snap free with a palpable and audible click. The knee is flexed as far as possible; one hand steadies the joint and the other rotates the leg medially and laterally while the knee is slowly extended. The test is repeated several times, with the knee stressed in valgus or varus, the examiner all the time feeling and listening for the click. A positive test is helpful but not pathognomonic and a negative test does not exclude a tear. This classic way of diagnosing a torn meniscus is seldom used now that the diagnosis can be made by MRI; however, advanced imaging is not always available and the clinical test has not been altogether discarded.

In *Apley's grinding test* the meniscus is forcibly compressed and the leg is rotated from side to side between the articular surfaces; a painful response signifies the likelihood of a torn or degenerate meniscus.

The *Thessaly test* is based on a dynamic reproduction of load transmission in the knee joint under normal or trauma conditions. With the affected knee flexed to 20 degrees and the foot placed flat on the ground, the patient is told to put full weight on that leg while being supported by the examiner (for balance). The patient is then instructed to twist his or her body to one side and then to the other three times; with each turn, a rotational force is exerted on the knee. Patients with meniscal tears experience medial or lateral joint line pain and may have a sense of the knee 'locking'.

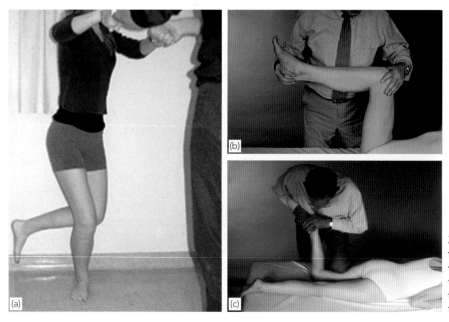

20.14 Meniscal tears (special tests) (a) Thessaly test. (b) McMurray's test. (c) The grinding test.

Imaging

Plain x-rays are normal but MRI is a reliable method for confirming the diagnosis, and may even reveal tears that are missed by arthroscopy.

Arthroscopy

Arthroscopy has the advantage that, if a lesion is identified, it can be treated at the same time (see Figure 20.9). You have to be certain, though, that the lesion which you see is the one causing the patient's symptoms!

Treatment

In the past, meniscal tears were treated by open operation. Nowadays arthroscopic surgery is preferable. For peripheral tears, operative repair is feasible. In other cases, the displaced portion should be cleanly excised. Postoperative physiotherapy is an important part of the treatment.

MENISCAL CYSTS

A meniscal cyst can be likened to a ganglion, inasmuch as it contains gelatinous fluid and is surrounded by fibrous tissue, but in reality it is distinct. It is probably traumatic in origin, arising from either a small horizontal tear or repeated squashing of the peripheral part of the meniscus.

The patient presents with pain and a small lump can be seen and felt, usually on the lateral side of the joint; it may feel surprisingly firm (or tense), particularly when the knee is extended.

If the symptoms are sufficiently troublesome, the cyst can be decompressed or removed arthoscopically; any meniscal lesion can be dealt with at the same time.

OSTEOCHONDRITIS DISSECANS

A small, well-demarcated, avascular fragment of bone and overlying cartilage sometimes separates from one of the femoral condyles and later appears as a loose body in the joint. The most likely cause is trauma, either a single impact with the edge of the patella or repeated contact with an adjacent tibial ridge. The incidence appears to be increasing and this may parallel growing participation of adolescents in competitive sport. Over 80% of

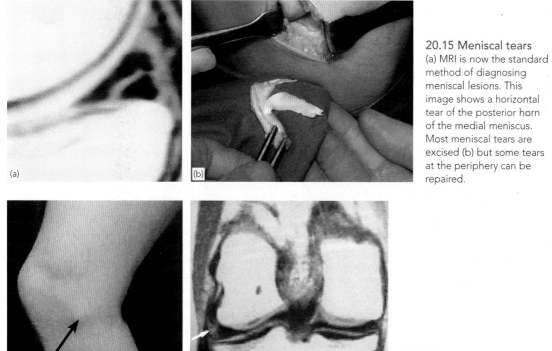

20.15 Meniscal tears
(a) MRI is now the standard method of diagnosing meniscal lesions. This image shows a horizontal tear of the posterior horn of the medial meniscus. Most meniscal tears are excised (b) but some tears at the periphery can be repaired.

20.16 Meniscal cyst
(a) Typical appearance of a small, firm swelling at or just below the joint line. (b) MRI showing the cyst arising from the edge of the meniscus (arrow).

lesions occur on the lateral part of the medial femoral condyle and lesions are bilateral in 25% of cases.

Clinical features

The patient, usually a male aged 15–20 years, presents with intermittent ache or swelling. Later, there are attacks of giving way and the knee feels unreliable. From time to time the knee may 'lock'.

The quadriceps muscle is wasted and the joint may be slightly swollen; there is usually a small effusion. Two signs which are almost diagnostic are: (a) tenderness localized to one femoral condyle; and (b) Wilson's sign: if the knee is flexed to 90 degrees, rotated medially and then gradually straightened, pain is felt; if the test is repeated with the knee rotated laterally, the patient feels no pain.

Imaging

Plain x-rays, especially intercondylar (tunnel) views, may show a line of demarcation around a lesion, usually in the lateral part of the medial femoral condyle. Once the fragment has become detached, the empty hollow may be seen – and possibly a loose body elsewhere in the joint. *Radionuclide scans* show increased activity around the lesion, and *MRI* consistently shows an area of low signal intensity in the T1-weighted images.

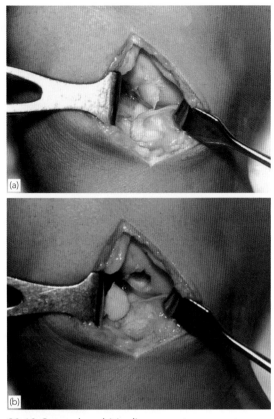

20.18 Osteochondritis dissecans Intraoperative pictures showing the articular lesion (a) and the defect left after removal of the osteochondral fragment (b).

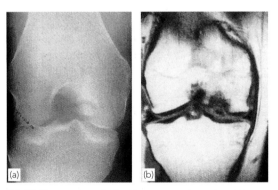

20.17 Osteochondritis dissecans – imaging The lesion is best seen in the 'tunnel view', usually along the lateral side of the medial femoral condyle (a). Here the osteochondral fragment has remained in place but sometimes it appears as a separate body elsewhere in the joint. (b) MRI provides confirmatory evidence.

Treatment

In the earliest stage, when the cartilage is intact and the lesion 'stable', no treatment is needed but activities are curtailed for 6–12 months. Small lesions often heal spontaneously.

If the fragment is 'unstable' – i.e. surrounded by a clear boundary with sclerosis of the underlying bone, or showing MRI features of separation, or even detached – treatment will depend on the size of the lesion. A small or ill-fitting fragment should be removed by arthroscopy and the base drilled; the bed will eventually be covered by fibrocartilage. A large fragment (more than 1 cm in diameter) or one that can be shaped to fill the crater should be fixed in situ with pins or Herbert screws. After any of the above operations the knee is held in a cast for 6 weeks; thereafter, movement is encouraged but weightbearing is deferred until x-rays show signs of healing.

In recent years attempts have been made to fill the condylar defect by cartilage transplantation. This should still be regarded as an experimental procedure.

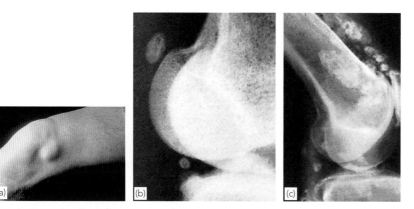

20.19 Loose bodies (a) This loose body slipped away from the fingers when touched; the term 'joint mouse' seems appropriate. (b) Which is the loose body here? Not the large one (which is a normal fabella), but the small lower one opposite the joint line. (c) Multiple loose bodies are seen in synovial chrondromatosis, a rare disorder of cartilage metaplasia in the synovium.

LOOSE BODIES

The knee joint offers a relatively capacious haven for loose bodies. These may be produced by: (1) injury (a chip of bone or cartilage); (2) osteochondritis dissecans (which may produce one or two fragments); (3) osteoarthritis (pieces of cartilage or osteophyte); (4) Charcot's disease (large osteocartilaginous bodies, separated by repeated trauma in a joint that has lost protective sensation); and (5) synovial chondromatosis (cartilage metaplasia in the synovium, sometimes producing hundreds of loose bodies).

Clinical features

The patient may be symptomless, or may complain of sudden locking without injury. The joint gets stuck in a position which varies from one attack to another. Sometimes the locking is only momentary and usually the patient can wriggle the knee until it suddenly unlocks. The patient may be aware of something 'popping in and out of the joint'. Sometimes, especially after the first attack, the knee swells up, due to synovitis.

In some cases there is evidence of an underlying cause. A pedunculated loose body may be felt; one that is truly loose tends to slip away during palpation (aptly named a 'joint mouse'). X-ray will usually confirm the diagnosis; most loose bodies are radio-opaque and the examination also shows an underlying joint abnormality.

A loose body causing symptoms should be removed, unless the joint is severely osteoarthritic. This can usually be done with the aid of arthroscopy.

TUBERCULOSIS

Tuberculosis of the knee may appear at any age, but it is more common in children than in adults.

Clinical features

Pain and limp are early symptoms, or the child may present with a swollen joint and a low-grade fever. The thigh muscles are wasted, thus accentuating the joint swelling. The knee feels warm and there is synovial thickening. Movements are restricted and often painful. The Mantoux test is often positive,

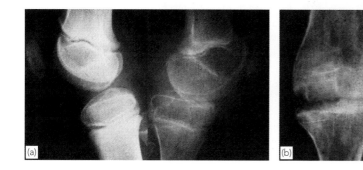

20.20 Tuberculosis – x-rays (a) Lateral views of the two knees. On one side the bones are porotic and the epiphyses enlarged, features suggestive of a severe inflammatory synovitis. (b) Later the articular surfaces are eroded.

the ESR may be increased and the peripheral blood film shows an increase in lymphocytes.

X-rays

Common features are periarticular osteoporosis and, in children, enlargement of the bony epiphyses. Joint space narrowing and progressive erosion of the articular surfaces are late signs.

Diagnosis

During the early stages the condition may resemble monarticular rheumatoid synovitis, or juvenile chronic arthritis. A synovial biopsy may be necessary to establish the diagnosis.

Treatment

Antituberculous chemotherapy should be given for 12–18 months (see page 26).

During the phase of active synovitis the knee is rested in a bed-splint, but exercised intermittently for short spells to prevent ankylosis. If the condition settles and x-rays show that the joint surfaces are intact, movements can be increased and the patient is allowed to start walking. However, if the synovitis does not settle within a few weeks, then surgical debridement will be needed.

In the healing stage the patient can get about wearing a weight-relieving caliper. If the articular cartilage is intact, weightbearing is slowly resumed but the patient should still be kept under observation to detect any recurrence. If the articular surfaces have been destroyed, immobilization is continued until the joint stiffens.

In the aftermath, if the joint is painful, arthrodesis is recommended; in adults this can be done as soon as the disease is inactive, but in children the operation is deferred until growth ceases. In some cases, once it is certain that the disease is quiescent, joint replacement may be feasible.

RHEUMATOID ARTHRITIS

Occasionally, rheumatoid arthritis starts in the knee as a chronic monarticular synovitis. Sooner or later, however, other joints become involved.

Clinical features

During the early stage the patient complains of pain and chronic swelling. There may be a large effusion and wasting of the thigh muscles, features that are common to other types of inflammatory monarthritis such as Reiter's disease and tuberculous synovitis.

With advancing articular erosion the joint becomes unstable, muscle wasting increases and there is some restriction of movement. X-rays may show loss of joint space and marginal erosions; the condition is easily distinguishable from osteoarthritis by the complete absence of osteophytes.

In the late stage the joint becomes increasingly deformed and painful; in some patients there is only a jog of painful movement. X-rays reveal the bone destruction characteristic of advanced disease.

Treatment

In addition to general treatment with anti-inflammatory and disease-modifying drugs, local splintage and injection of triamcinolone will usually reduce the synovitis. A more prolonged effect may be obtained by injecting radiocolloids such as yttrium-90 (^{90}Y).

Synovectomy is indicated if other measures fail to control the synovitis; this can be done very effectively by arthroscopy.

If deformity is marked but the joint is stable, a femoral or tibial osteotomy may improve function and relieve pain. However, once bone destruction is present and the joint is unstable, total joint replacement is advised.

20.21 Rheumatoid arthritis (a) Patient with rheumatoid arthritis showing the typical valgus deformity of the knee; the feet and toes also are affected. (b,c) X-rays showing progressive erosive arthritis resulting in joint destruction and deformity.

OSTEOARTHRITIS

The knee is one of the commonest sites for osteoarthritis. Often there is a predisposing factor: injury to the articular surface, a torn meniscus and ligamentous instability or pre-existing deformity of the knee. However, in many cases no obvious cause can be found, and here the condition is often bilateral and has a strong association with Heberden's nodes.

Cartilage breakdown usually starts in an area of excessive loading. Thus, with long-standing varus the changes are most marked in the medial compartment. The characteristic features of cartilage fibrillation, sclerosis of the subchondral bone and peripheral osteophyte formation are usually present.

Clinical features

Patients are usually over 50 years old; they tend to be overweight and may have long-standing bow-leg deformity.

Pain is the leading symptom, worse after use, or (if the patellofemoral joint is affected) on stairs. After rest, the joint feels stiff and it hurts to 'get going' after sitting for any length of time. Swelling is common, and giving way or locking may occur.

On examination there may be an obvious deformity (usually varus) or the scar of a previous operation. The quadriceps muscle is usually wasted.

Except during an exacerbation, there is little fluid and no warmth; nor is the synovial membrane thickened. Movement is somewhat limited and is often accompanied by patellofemoral crepitus.

X-rays

An anteroposterior x-ray must be obtained with the patient standing and bearing weight; only in

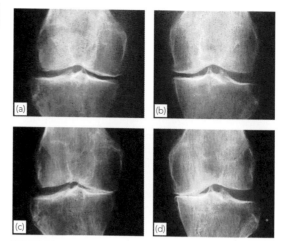

20.23 Knee x-rays *Always ask for weightbearing views.* X-rays taken with this patient lying down (a,b) suggest only minor cartilage loss on the medial side of each knee. Weightbearing views (c,d) show the true position; there is severe loss of articular cartilage in the medial compartment of both knees.

this way can small degrees of articular cartilage thinning be revealed. The tibiofemoral joint space is diminished (often only in one compartment) and there is subchondral sclerosis. Osteophytes and subchondral cysts are usually present and sometimes there is soft-tissue calcification in the suprapatellar region or in the joint itself (chrondrocalcinosis).

Treatment

If symptoms are not severe, treatment is conservative. Analgesics can be prescribed for pain. Local measures include quadriceps exercises and the application of warmth (e.g. radiant heat or shortwave diathermy). Joint loading is lessened by using a walking stick.

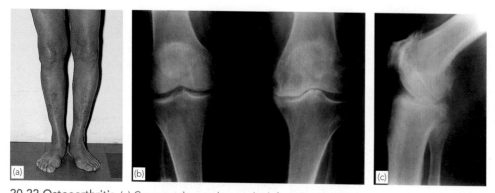

20.22 Osteoarthritis (a) Compare the two knees: the left one rests in slight varus on weightbearing. The x-ray (b) shows loss of 'joint space' (articular cartilage), subchondral sclerosis and peripheral osteophytes – typical of OA – on the medial side of the knee. (c) Sometimes it is the patellofemoral joint that is mainly affected.

The indications for operative treatment are persistent pain unresponsive to conservative treatment, progressive deformity and instability.

Arthroscopic washouts, with trimming of meniscal fragments and osteophytes, may give temporary relief; this is a useful measure when there are contraindications to reconstructive surgery.

Realignment osteotomy (typically an upper tibial valgus osteotomy for medial compartment disease in a young patient) is often successful in relieving symptoms and staving off the need for 'end-stage' surgery.

Replacement arthroplasty is indicated in older patients with progressive joint destruction. This is usually a 'resurfacing' knee replacement; with modern techniques and meticulous attention to anatomical alignment of the knee, the results are excellent.

PATELLOFEMORAL DISORDERS

RECURRENT DISLOCATION OF THE PATELLA

Acute dislocation of the patella is dealt with on page 446. In about 15% of cases (mostly children) the first episode is followed by recurrent dislocation or subluxation after minimal stress. This is due, in some measure, to disruption or stretching of the ligamentous structures which normally stabilize the extensor mechanism. However, in a significant proportion of cases there is no history of an acute strain and the initial episode is thought to have occurred 'spontaneously'. It is now recognized that in all cases of recurrent dislocation, but particularly in the latter group, one or more *predisposing factors* are often present: (1) generalized ligamentous laxity; (2) under-development of the lateral femoral condyle and flattening of the intercondylar groove; (3) maldevelopment of the patella (which may be unusually small or seated too high); (4) valgus deformity of the knee; (5) external tibial torsion; or (6) a primary muscle defect.

Repeated dislocation damages the contiguous articular surfaces of the patella and femoral condyle; this may result in further flattening of the condyle, so facilitating further dislocations.

Dislocation is almost always towards the lateral side; medial dislocation is seen only in rare iatrogenic cases following over-zealous lateral release or medial transposition of the patellar tendon.

Clinical features

Girls are affected more commonly than boys and the condition is often bilateral. The main (or only) complaint is that from time to time the knee suddenly gives way and the patient falls; this may be accompanied by pain and sometimes the knee gets stuck in flexion.

Although the patella always dislocates laterally, the patient may think it has displaced medially because the uncovered medial femoral condyle stands out prominently.

If the knee is seen while the patella is dislocated, the diagnosis is obvious. There is usually tenderness on the medial side of the joint. Later the joint becomes swollen, and aspiration may reveal a blood-stained effusion.

Between attacks clinical signs are sparse; however, the *apprehension test* is positive (see page 267).

Treatment

If the patella is still dislocated, it is pushed back into place while the knee is gently extended. A plaster cylinder or splint is applied and retained for 2–3 weeks; isometric quadriceps strengthening exercises are encouraged and the patient is allowed to walk with the aid of crutches. Exercises should be continued for at least 3 months, concentrating on strengthening the vastus medialis muscle.

If recurrences are few and far between, conservative treatment may suffice; as the child grows older the patellar mechanism tends to stabilize. However, about 15% of children with patellar instability suffer repeated and distressing episodes of dislocation and for these patients surgical reconstruction is indicated.

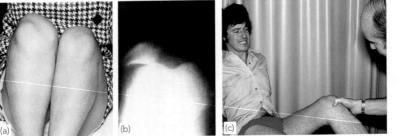

20.24 Patellofemoral instability This young girl presented with recurrent subluxation of the right patella. (a,b) The knee looks abnormal and the x-ray shows the patella riding on top of the lateral femoral condyle. (c) Performing the *apprehension test* – watch the patient's face.

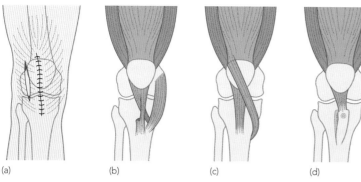

20.25 Patellar instability – operative treatment
Several methods are employed. (a) Lateral release and vastus medialis tethering. (b) Transposition of lateral half of patellar ligament towards the medial side (Roux–Goldthwait). (c) Medial tethering by using semi-tendinosus tendon. (d) Medial transposition of patellar ligament insertion (Elmslie–Trillat).

The principles of operative treatment are: (a) to repair or strengthen the medial patellofemoral ligaments; and (b) to re-align the extensor mechanism so as to produce a mechanically more favourable angle of pull. Some methods are illustrated in Figure 20.25.

CHONDROMALACIA OF THE PATELLA

The common term *'chondromalacia patellae'* has, by long usage, been accepted to designate a condition affecting adolescents and young adults who present with a dominant symptom of anterior knee pain, supposedly due to 'softening' of the patellar articular cartilage. We suggest that a more apt name would be *patellofemoral overload*.

The basic disorder is probably repetitive mechanical overload of the patellofemoral joint due to either: (1) malcongruence of the patellofemoral surfaces because of some abnormal shape of the patella or intercondylar groove; or (2) malalignment of the extensor mechanism, or relative weakness of the vastus medialis, which causes the patella to tilt, or subluxate, or bear more heavily on one facet than the other during flexion and extension of the knee.

Clinical features

The patient, often a teenage girl or an athletic young adult, complains of pain over the front of the knee or 'under the knee-cap'. Symptoms are aggravated by activity or climbing stairs, or when standing up after prolonged sitting. The quadriceps may be wasted and there may be a small effusion.

Patellofemoral pain is elicited by pressing the patella against the femur and asking the patient to contract the quadriceps – first with central pressure, then compressing the medial facet and then the lateral. If, in addition, the apprehension test is positive, this suggests actual previous subluxation or dislocation.

Imaging

X-ray examination should include skyline views of the patella, which may show abnormal tilting or subluxation, and a lateral view with the knee partly flexed to see if the patella is riding high or is unusually small.

The most accurate way of showing and measuring patellofemoral malposition is by *computed tomography (CT)* or *MRI*, with the knees in full extension and varying degrees of flexion.

Arthroscopy

The findings at arthroscopy are usually of mild fibrillation and softening of the articular cartilage on the undersurface of the patella. Arthroscopy is also useful in excluding other causes of anterior knee pain (see Table 20.2).

Table 20.2 Causes of anterior knee pain

Referred from hip

Patellofemoral disorders:
    Patellar instability
    Patellofemoral overload
    Osteochondral injury
    Patellofemoral osteoarthritis

Knee joint disorders:
    Osteochondritis dissecans
    Loose body in the joint
    Synovial chondromatosis
    Plica syndrome

Periarticular disorders:
    Patellar tendinitis
    Patellar ligament strain
    Bursitis
    Osgood–Schlatter's disease

Treatment

In the vast majority of cases the patient will be helped by adjustment of stressful activities and physiotherapy, combined with reassurance that most patients recover. Exercises are directed specifically at strengthening the medial quadriceps so as to counterbalance the tendency to lateral tilting or subluxation of the patella.

If symptoms persist, surgery can be considered – lateral release, or lateral release combined with one of the re-alignment procedures illustrated in Figure 20.25 if there is any sign of patellar instability. Arthroscopic shaving of fibrillated cartilage is sometimes performed, but its efficacy is questionable.

Patients should be reassured that chondromalacia does not inevitably lead to patellofemoral osteoarthritis in later life.

TIBIAL TUBERCLE 'APOPHYSITIS'

This condition (also called *Osgood–Schlatter's disease*) is characterized by pain and swelling of the tibial tubercle. It is a fairly common complaint among adolescents, particularly those engaged in strenuous sports. It is, in fact, a traction injury of the incompletely fused apophysis into which part the patellar ligament is inserted.

On examination the tibial tuberosity is unusually prominent and tender. Sometimes active extension of the knee against resistance also is painful. *X-rays* show displacement or 'fragmentation' of the tibial apophysis.

Spontaneous recovery is usual, but it takes time. During this period activities such as football, cycling, strenuous walking and hill-climbing should be restricted.

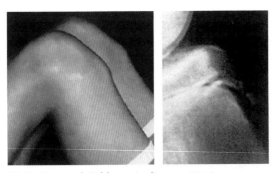

20.26 Osgood–Schlatter's disease This boy complained of a painful bump below the knee. X-ray shows the traction injury of the tibial apophysis.

CHRONIC LIGAMENTOUS INSTABILITY

The knee is a complex hinge which depends heavily on its ligaments for mediolateral, anteroposterior and rotational stability. Ligament injuries, from minor strains through partial ruptures to complete tears, are common in sportsmen, athletes and dancers. Whatever the nature of the acute injury, the victim may be left with chronic instability of the knee – a sense of the joint wanting to give way, or actually giving way, during weightbearing activity.

There are basically three types of tibiofemoral instability: sideways tilt (varus or valgus), excessive glide (forwards or backwards) and unstable rotation. Some patients develop a combination of abnormal movements.

Clinical features

The patient complains of the knee feeling insecure and giving way (or threatening to give way) during weightbearing activities; sometimes this is accompanied by pain. With collateral ligament instability the knee tends to wobble to one side. With anterolateral rotatory instability (due to an old anterior cruciate ligament injury) the knee gives way as the patient pivots on the affected side. In the less common posterior cruciate insufficiency, symptoms are mild and may be felt only on climbing stairs.

The joint looks normal apart from slight wasting; there is rarely tenderness but abnormal movement in one or more directions can usually be demonstrated by performing the appropriate tests (see page 268). Comparison with the normal knee is essential. A useful routine is to observe gait and knee posture in standing and walking, then to examine for hyperextension, then for increased tilting into varus or valgus (at both 0 and 30 degrees of knee flexion), followed by the drawer tests and the more specific Lachman test. Special tests can also be performed for rotational instability.

X-rays may show suspicious signs: avulsion of a small bone fragment at the ligament insertion point, or old ossification in the ligament. However, *MRI* is more useful and can reliably diagnose both ligament and meniscal injuries.

Arthroscopy may be needed to exclude other abnormalities in the joint.

Treatment

Most patients with chronic symptoms – especially those with previous isolated collateral ligament strains – have reasonably good function and will not require an operation. The first approach should always be a well-supervised exercise programme. Some patients will accept the use of a knee brace for specific activities that are known to cause trouble.

The *indications for operation* are: (a) intolerable symptoms of giving way; these are usually patients with severe anterior cruciate insufficiency or combined injuries causing rotatory instability; (b) unacceptably reduced function in patients with specialized occupations (e.g. professional sportspersons); (c) the presence of an associated internal injury such as a torn meniscus or an avulsion fracture of the tibial spine; and (d) symptomatic ligament injuries in adolescents. The operation, in principle, consists of ligament reconstruction or replacement with an autologous graft or an allograft. This is followed by a long period of intensive physiotherapy.

PATELLAR TENDINOPATHY

A patellar ligament strain or partial rupture may lead to a traction 'tendinitis' causing repeated episodes of pain and local tenderness – usually close to its attachment at the lower pole of the patella. If persistent, it may lead to calcification within the ligament. The condition is fairly common in adolescent athletes and has acquired the eponym *Sinding-Larsen–Johansson syndrome*. It usually resolves spontaneously; if it does not, the painful area is carefully removed keeping the major part of the ligament in continuity.

CHAPTER 21

THE ANKLE AND FOOT

CLINICAL ASSESSMENT

HISTORY

The most common presenting symptoms are pain, deformity, swelling and giving way. It is helpful to know whether the symptoms are constant or provoked by standing or walking, or by shoe pressure.

- *Pain* over a bony prominence or a joint is probably due to a local disorder: shoe pressure upon a local deformity, arthritis, tendinitis or – in the younger patient – an 'apophysitis' (inflammation over the point where a tendon inserts). Pain across the entire forefoot (*metatarsalgia*) is less specific and is often associated with uneven loading and muscle fatigue. Always ask whether it started after some unusual activity; metatarsal stress fractures occur even in physically fit athletes, ballet dancers and soldiers on route marches.
- *Swelling* can be diffuse and bilateral, or localized. Swelling over the medial side of the first metatarsal head (a bunion) is common in older women. Bilateral swelling may be due to dependent oedema.

- *Deformity* may be in the ankle, the foot or the toes. Parents often worry about their children who are 'flat-footed' or 'pigeon-toed'. Elderly patients may complain chiefly of having difficulty fitting shoes.
- *'Giving way'* may be due to pain or instability at the ankle or subtalar joint.
- *Corns and callosities* (thickened, often tender, plaques of skin on the toes or the soles of the feet) are a frequent cause for complaints. They are usually produced by localized pressure and friction – perhaps simply from ill-fitting shoes.
- *Numbness and paraesthesia* may be felt in a circumscribed field served by a single nerve, or more generally in all the toes and both feet suggesting a peripheral neuropathy.

SIGNS WITH THE PATIENT STANDING AND WALKING

See that the patient's lower limbs are exposed from the knees down, and examine them first from the front and then again from behind. Normally the heels are in slight valgus while standing and inverted when on tiptoes; the degree of diversion should be equal on the two sides, showing that the subtalar joints are mobile and the tibialis posterior muscles functioning.

Deformities such as flat-foot, cavus (high-arched) foot, hallux valgus and crooked toes are noted. Corns over the proximal toe joints and callosities on the soles are common in older people.

Ask the patient to walk. Note whether the gait is smooth or halting and whether the feet move through the walking cycle symmetrically. Concentrate on the sequence of movements that make up the walking cycle. It begins with heel-strike, then moves into stance, then push-off and finally swing-through before making the next heel-strike. Gait may be disturbed by pain, muscle weakness, deformity or stiffness. A fixed equinus deformity results in the heel failing to strike the ground at the beginning of the walking cycle; sometimes the patient forces heel contact by hyperextending the knee. If the ankle dorsiflexors are weak, the forefoot may strike the ground prematurely, causing a 'slap'; this is called foot-

drop (or drop-foot). In some cases, during swing-through the leg is lifted higher than usual so that the foot can clear the ground; this is known as a high-stepping gait.

SIGNS WITH THE PATIENT SITTING OR LYING

Each foot is examined in turn, so that the findings can be compared.

Look

Holding the heel square, the dorsum, sides and plantar aspects are inspected. Callosities (on the plantar aspect) or corns (on the dorsum) indicate where there is high pressure or friction. Look for swelling over joints or tendon sheaths.

Feel

Pain and tenderness localize well to the affected structures because the foot and ankle are not

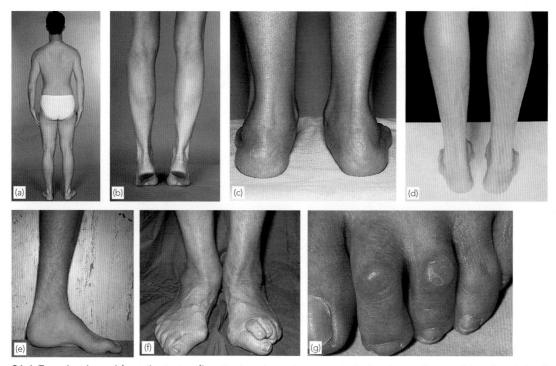

21.1 Examination with patient standing Look at the patient as a whole, first from in front and then from behind. (a,b) The heels are normally in slight valgus and should invert equally when a patient stands on tiptoes. (c) This patient has flat-feet (pes planovalgus), while the patient in (d) has the opposite deformity, varus heels and an abnormally high longitudinal arch – pes cavus (e). From the front you can again notice (f) the dropped longitudinal arch in the patient with pes planovalgus, as well as the typical deformities of bilateral hallux valgus and over-riding toes. (g) Corns on the top of the toes are common.

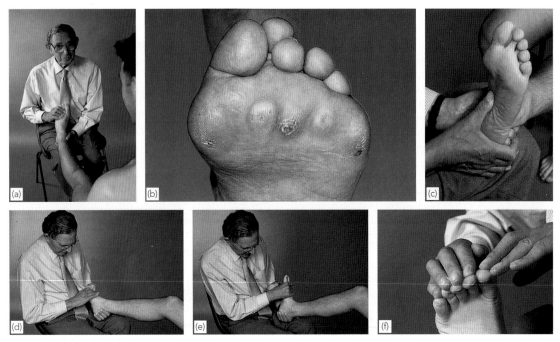

21.2 Examination with patient sitting (a) The patient is seated with his foot on the examiner's lap. Keep an eye on the patient's face as well as the foot. (b) Look for skin lesions and deformities, especially of the toes; don't forget the sole where callosities go together with toe deformities. (c) Feel for tenderness over every joint and along the tendons and ligaments. Then test for movements in the ankle and the toes (d–f).

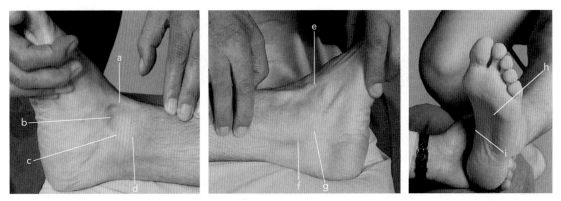

21.3 Foot – surface anatomy Medial aspect. (a, tendon of tibialis anterior, b, medial malleolus, c, tendon of tibialis posterior, d, sulcus behind medial malleolus, e, extensor tendons of toes, f, lateral malleolus, g, peroneal tendons curving behind the lateral malleolus, h, anterior metatarsal arch, i, medial longitudinal arch.)

shielded by thick muscle layers. Feel along the bony prominences, joint lines and tendon sheaths. Feel also for pulses (about 1 in 6 individuals does not have a dorsalis pedis pulse) and check the sensation and skin temperature.

Move

Check each joint in turn for both active and passive movements. Muscle power can be tested at the same time.

Ankle joint

With the heel grasped in the left hand and the midfoot in the right, the ranges of plantarflexion and dorsiflexion are estimated.

Subtalar joint

When assessing inversion and eversion, make sure that the ankle is fully plantigrade (at a right-angle to the leg); this prevents the ankle tilting to one or other side.

Midtarsal joint

The heel is held still with one hand while the other moves the tarsus up and down and from side to side.

Toes

The metatarsophalangeal (MTP) and interphalangeal (IP) joints are tested separately. Extension (dorsiflexion) of the great toe at the MTP joint should normally exceed 70 degrees and flexion 10 degrees.

Tests for stability

Ankle stability should be tested in both coronal and sagittal planes, always comparing the two sides. The ankle is held in 10 degrees of plantarflexion and the joint stressed into valgus and then varus. Anteroposterior stability is assessed by performing an anterior 'drawer test': with the ankle held in 10 degrees of plantarflexion, the distal tibia is gripped with one hand while the other grasps the heel and tries to shift the hindfoot forwards and backwards. Patients with recent ligament injury may have to be examined under anaesthesia. The same tests can be performed under x-ray and the positions of the two ankles measured and compared (see below).

GENERAL EXAMINATION

If there are any symptoms or signs of vascular or neurological impairment, or if multiple joints are affected, a more general examination is essential.

IMAGING

The standard views of the ankle are anteroposterior (AP), mortise (an AP view with the ankle internally rotated 15–20 degrees) and lateral. *Standing views* reveal changes in joint alignment and joint space not usually seen in the standard views. The subtalar joint can be seen best through medial and lateral oblique projections. *Stress x-rays* complement the clinical tests for ankle stability; if stress manoeuvres are painful they can be carried out under general anaesthesia. Both ankles should be examined for comparison. *Computed tomography (CT) scans* are important in assessing fractures and for congenital bony coalitions. *Radio-isotope scanning* is excellent for localizing areas of abnormal blood flow or bone re-modelling activity, signs that suggest the presence of covert infection.

Magnetic resonance imaging (MRI) and *ultrasound* are used to demonstrate soft-tissue problems, such as tendon and ligament injuries. They can be used to diagnose joint effusions and bone infections as well.

GLOSSARY OF FOOT POSTURES

- *Plantigrade* is the normal neutral position of the foot – i.e. when the patient stands the sole is at right angles to the leg.
- *Talipes equinus* refers to the shape of a horse's foot – i.e. the hindfoot is fixed in plantarflexion (pointing downwards).
- *Plantaris* looks similar, but the ankle is neutral and only the forefoot is plantarflexed.
- *Equinovarus* describes a foot that points both downwards and inwards.
- *Calcaneus* is fixed dorsiflexion at the ankle. A dorsiflexion deformity in the midfoot produces a *rocker-bottom foot*.

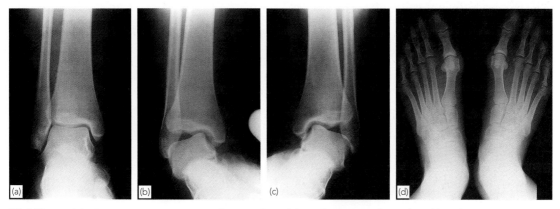

21.4 X-rays (a) AP view in a young woman who complained that, after twisting her right ankle, it kept giving way in high-heeled shoes. The x-ray looks normal; the articular cartilage width (the 'joint space') is the same at all aspects of the joint. The inversion stress view (b) shows that the talus tilts excessively; always x-ray both ankles for comparison and in this case the left ankle (c) does the same! She has generalized joint hypermobility, not a torn lateral ligament. (d) X-rays of the feet should be taken with the feet flat on the ground.

- *The longitudinal arch* forms the medial border of the foot. Even when weightbearing the medial border normally forms a slight arch.
- *The anterior or transverse arch* is formed by the arrangement of the slightly splayed metatarsals in the forefoot.
- *Pes planovalgus (flat-foot)* describes a flattened longitudinal arch. A dropped metatarsal arch is called *anterior flat-foot*.
- *Pes cavus* is a foot with an excessively high arch.
- *Hallux valgus* means lateral deviation of the big toe.
- *Hammer toe* aptly describes a flexion deformity of the proximal IP joint of one of the lesser toes.
- *Claw-toes* denotes curled flexion of all the toes.

CONGENITAL TALIPES EQUINOVARUS (IDIOPATHIC CLUB-FOOT)

In this deformity the foot is curved downwards and inwards – the ankle in equinus, the heel in varus, and the forefoot adducted, flexed and supinated. The skin and soft tissues of the calf and the medial side of the foot are short and under-developed. If the condition is not corrected early, secondary growth changes occur in the bones and these are permanent. Even with treatment the foot is liable to be short and the calf may remain thin.

The deformity is relatively common, with an incidence of 1–3 per 1000 births. Boys are affected twice as often as girls and it occurs bilaterally in nearly one-half of the cases. A family history increases the risk by 20–30 times.

The cause is unknown. There are theories, and some evidence in support, of a chromosomal defect, arrested development in utero, or an embryonic event such as a vascular injury. The abnormal distribution of types 1 and 2 muscle fibres in the affected leg and alteration of electromyography and nerve conduction velocities suggest a neuromuscular basis but the true cause remains unknown.

Similar deformities are seen in some infants with myelomeningocele and arthrogryposis.

Clinical features

The deformity is usually obvious at birth; the foot is both turned and twisted inwards so that the sole faces posteromedially. The heel is usually small and high, and deep creases appear posteriorly and medially. In a normal baby the foot can be dorsiflexed and everted until the toes almost touch the front of the leg. In club-foot this manoeuvre meets with varying degrees of resistance and in severe cases the deformity is fixed.

The infant must always be examined for associated disorders such as congenital hip dislocation and spina bifida.

X-rays

In the newborn x-rays are unhelpful: the tarsal bones are incompletely ossified and the anatomy is therefore difficult to define. However, in older infants the shape and position of the tarsal ossific centres assist in assessing progress after treatment.

Imaging

Plain x-rays are not helpful in the young infant; there are problems positioning the foot reliably and the ossified nuclei of the foot bones are not all present. In older children, some estimate of the severity of the deformity is obtained from the talocalcaneal angle in the AP and lateral views. Perhaps the most important imaging in a new-born child with club-feet is an ultrasound of the hips to ensure they are not dislocated!

Treatment

The aim of treatment is to produce and maintain a plantigrade, supple foot that will function well. The favoured method is the one popularized by Ponseti.

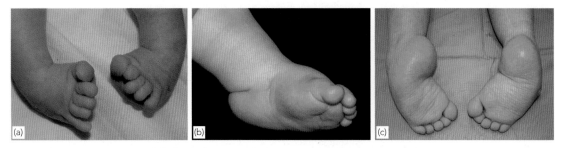

21.5 Talipes equinovarus (club-foot) (a) The sole of the foot often faces posteromedially. There are creases across the back and medially (b) and, in severe cases, across the sole of the foot (c).

Treatment should begin early, preferably within a few days of birth. This consists of repeated manipulation and adhesive strapping or application of plaster of Paris casts which will maintain the correction. If adhesive strapping is used, parents are taught how to do the manipulation and they can then carry out gentle stretches on a regular basis with the strapping still in place. Treatment is supervised by a physiotherapist who alters the strapping as correction is gradually obtained. Plaster of Paris casting requires serial changes and manipulations in a clinic setting. Sometimes percutaneous tenotomy of the Achilles tendon is needed to complete the correction. After correction has been achieved a strict regime of splintage in de-rotation boots is followed until the child is 3 years old.

This method has a high success rate but a second bout of manipulation and casting may be needed when the child is older. Relapse is most likely to occur in children with neuromuscular disorders.

Operative treatment

Resistant cases will need surgery. The objectives are: (a) the complete release of joint tethers (capsular and ligamentous contractures and fibrotic bands); and (b) lengthening of tendons so that the foot can be positioned normally without undue tension. After operative correction the foot is immobilized in its corrected position in a plaster cast. Kirschner wires (K-wires) are sometimes inserted across the talonavicular and subtalar joints to augment the hold. The wires and cast are removed at 6–8 weeks, after which a customized orthosis is used to maintain the correction.

In exceptional circumstances, a more radical approach is needed: the Ilizarov type of external fixation with tensioned wires permits gradual repositioning of the foot and ankle (see page 155).

Late presenters often have severe deformities with secondary bony changes, and the relapsed club-foot is further complicated by scarring from previous surgery. A deformed, stiff and painful foot in an adolescent is best salvaged by corrective osteotomies and fusions.

METATARSUS ADDUCTUS

Metatarsus adductus varies from a slightly curved forefoot to something resembling a mild

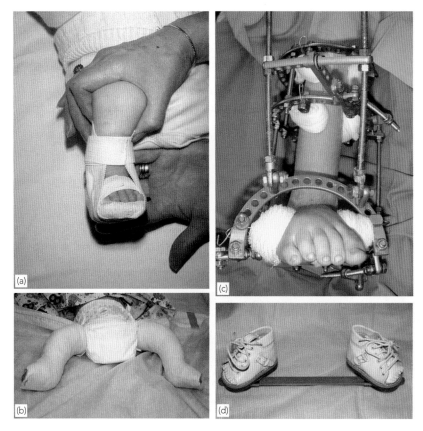

21.6 Congenital talipes equinovarus – treatment First-line treatment is non-operative. This may be by manipulation and strapping (a) or serial casting (b). If insufficient correction is achieved, a formal open release may be needed. (c) Severe relapses need more radical forms of treatment such as the Ilizarov fixator. After successful correction of deformity, relapses may be prevented by using Dennis Browne boots (d).

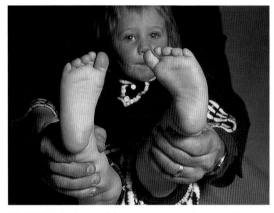

21.7 Metatarsus adductus In contrast to club-foot, the deformity here is limited to the forefoot.

club-foot. The important difference is that in metatarsus adductus the deformity occurs across the tarsometatarsal joints whereas in the club-foot the adduction tends to happen at the midfoot (talonavicular joint).

The majority (90%) either improve spontaneously or can be managed non-operatively using serial corrective casts followed by straight-last shoes. Serial casts work well and may need to be supplemented, for the more resistant forms, by a release of the abductor hallucis muscle.

FLAT-FOOT (PES PLANOVALGUS)

The term 'flat-foot' applies when the apex of the longitudinal arch has collapsed and the medial border of the foot is in contact (or nearly in contact) with the ground; the heel becomes valgus and the foot pronates at the midfoot. The appearance of flat-foot can be normal and without symptoms (the arch is not formed until 4–6 years of age and about 15% of the population have supple asymptomatic flat-feet) but some conditions are characterized by flat-feet that are stiff and painful.

CONGENITAL VERTICAL TALUS (CONGENITAL CONVEX PES VALGUS)

This is a severe neonatal form in which the arch is sometimes reversed leading to a 'rocker-bottom' appearance. This is due to a plantar dislocation of the head of the talus from the navicular, giving the appearance of a 'vertical' talus on the lateral x-ray. The condition is aptly called congenital vertical talus. Unlike the usual flexible forms of flat-foot, passive correction is not possible. The diagnosis can be confirmed by obtaining a lateral x-ray with the foot plantarflexed: in a flexible flat-foot when the ankle is plantarflexed, the talus is seen to line up with the first metatarsal, whereas it does not do so with a vertical talus.

Treatment involves manipulation, serial casting and (in resistant cases) open surgery.

FLAT-FOOT IN CHILDREN AND ADOLESCENTS

Flat-foot is a common complaint among children and teenagers; or rather their parents – the children themselves usually don't seem to mind! When weightbearing, the foot is turned outwards, the medial border of the foot is in contact (or nearly in contact) with the ground and the heel becomes valgus (*pes planovalgus*).

Two forms of the condition are encountered: flexible (by far the most common) and rigid. *Mobile (or 'flexible') flat-foot* often appears in toddlers as a normal stage in development, and it usually disappears after a few years when medial arch development is complete. *Stiff (or 'rigid') flat-foot* which cannot be corrected passively should alert the examiner to an underlying abnormality: tarsal coalition (often a bar of bone connecting the calcaneum to the talus or the navicular); an inflammatory joint condition; or a neurological disorder.

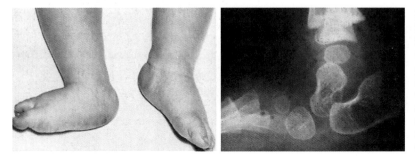

21.8 Congenital vertical talus This infant's right foot is in marked valgus and has a rocker-bottom shape. The deformity is rigid and cannot be corrected. X-ray shows the vertical talus pointing downwards towards the sole and the other tarsal bones rotated around the head of the talus.

Clinical assessment

In the common *flexible flat-foot* there are usually no symptoms but the parents notice that the feet are flat or that the shoes wear badly.

The deformity becomes noticeable when the youngster stands. The first test is to ask him or her to go up on their toes: if the heels invert and the medial arches form up, it is probably a flexible (or mobile) deformity. This can be checked by performing the *jack test (also called the great toe extension test)*: with the child seated, feet planted firmly on the floor, the examiner firmly dorsiflexes the great toe; the medial arch should re-appear while the heel adopts a more neutral position and the tibia rotates externally.

Go on to examine the foot with the child sitting or lying. Feel for localized tenderness and test the range of movement in the ankle, the subtalar and midtarsal joints. A tight Achilles tendon may induce a *compensatory flat-foot* deformity.

Teenagers sometimes present with a *painful, rigid flat-foot*. On examination the peroneal and extensor tendons appear to be in spasm (the condition is sometimes called *spasmodic flat-foot*). These patients should be further investigated for the presence of some underlying condition: a tarsal coalition, an inflammatory arthritis or a neuromuscular disorder; in many cases, however, no specific cause is identified.

The clinical assessment is completed by a general examination for joint hypermobility and signs of any other associated condition.

Imaging

X-rays are unnecessary for asymptomatic, flexible flat-feet. For painful or stiff flat-feet, standing AP,

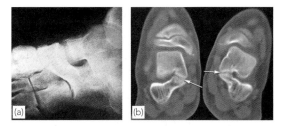

21.10 Tarsal coalition (a) X-ray appearance of a calcaneonavicular bar. (b) CT image showing incompletely ossified talocalcaneal bars bilaterally (arrows).

lateral and oblique views may help to identify underlying disorders. CT scanning is the most reliable way of demonstrating tarsal coalitions.

Treatment

Children with flexible flat-feet seldom require treatment; parents should be reassured and told that the 'deformity' will probably correct itself in time; even if it does not fully correct, function is unlikely to be impaired. However, medial arch supports or heel cups may help but the feet remain flat. In exceptional cases symptomatic mobile flat-

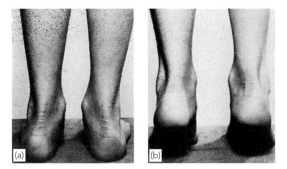

21.9 Flat-feet (a) Standing with the feet flat on the floor, the medial arches are seen to have dropped and the heels are in valgus; but is it flexible or rigid? (b) When the patient goes up on his toes, the medial arches are restored, indicating that these are 'mobile' (flexible) flat feet. If this does not occur, look carefully for a tarsal coalition.

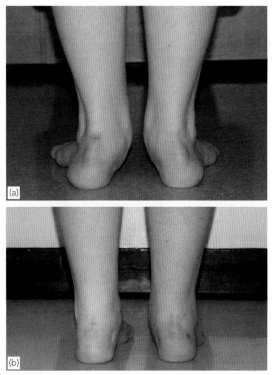

21.11 Flat-feet – operative correction Occasionally surgical correction is justified, as in this patient: (a) before operation; (b) after.

feet can be improved by surgery, e.g. lengthening the lateral side of the foot through an osteotomy in the front of the calcaneum and inserting a wedge of bone graft, or by inserting a titanium implant in the sinus tarsi which elevates the neck of talus and restores the arch.

Where the condition is obviously due to a neuromuscular disorder such as poliomyelitis, splintage or operative correction and muscle rebalancing may be needed.

Painful spasmodic flat-foot can be temporarily relieved by rest in a cast or a splint. Tarsal coalitions can be excised successfully as long as they are not larger than 50% of the joint area.

FLAT-FOOT IN ADULTS

When an adult presents with symptomatic flat-feet, the first thing to ask is whether they have always had flat-feet or whether it is of recent onset. Constitutional flat-feet which have been more or less asymptomatic for many years may start causing nagging pain after a change in daily activities (e.g. taking on work which requires a lot of standing and walking). More recent deformities may be due to an underlying disorder such as rheumatoid arthritis or generalized muscular weakness.

Where there is no underlying abnormality, little can be done apart from giving advice about sensible footwear and arch supports.

Patients with painful, rigid flat-feet may require more robust splintage (and, of course, treatment for any generalized condition such a rheumatoid arthritis).

Unilateral flat-foot should make one think of tibialis posterior synovitis or rupture. Women in later midlife are predominantly affected. Onset is usually insidious, affecting one foot much more than the other. There may be identifiable systemic factors such as obesity, diabetes, corticosteroid medication or past surgery. Aching is felt in the line of the tendon and, as the tendon stretches out, the foot drifts into planovalgus, producing the typical acquired flat-foot deformity. If the tendon ruptures, the ache or pain will often improve, temporarily, but the foot deformity then worsens. Treatment should start before the tendon ruptures. Rest, anti-inflammatory medication, support from an insole, and ultrasound-guided steroid injections into the tendon sheath may be considered. Failure to improve may call for surgery: the tendon sheath can be decompressed and the synovium excised; the calcaneum may be osteotomized to shift the axis of weightbearing more medially, so protecting the tendon. A ruptured tendon can sometimes be reconstructed with a tendon graft. As a last resort a triple arthrodesis of the subtalar, talonavicular and calcaneocuboid joints may be needed to correct or prevent a worsening deformity.

PES CAVUS

In pes cavus the foot is highly arched and the toes are drawn up into a 'clawed' position, forcing the metatarsal heads down into the sole. Often the heel is inverted and the soft tissues in the sole are tight. In the forefoot, under the prominent metatarsal heads, callosities may appear.

The close resemblance to deformities seen in neurological disorders, where the intrinsic muscles are weak or paralysed, suggests that all forms of pes cavus are due to some type of muscle imbalance.

Clinical features

The condition often becomes noticeable by the age of 8–10 years, before there are any symptoms. As a rule both feet are affected and in some cases there is a past history of a spinal disorder.

The overall deformity is usually obvious. At first the position is mobile and the deformity can be

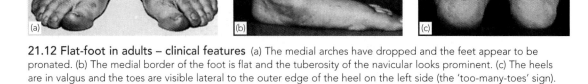

21.12 Flat-foot in adults – clinical features (a) The medial arches have dropped and the feet appear to be pronated. (b) The medial border of the foot is flat and the tuberosity of the navicular looks prominent. (c) The heels are in valgus and the toes are visible lateral to the outer edge of the heel on the left side (the 'too-many-toes' sign).

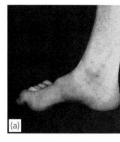
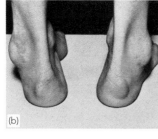
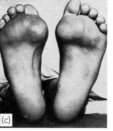

21.13 Pes cavus and claw-toes (a) Typical appearance of 'idiopathic' pes cavus. Note the high arch and claw-toes. (b) This is associated with varus heels. (c) Look for callosities under the metatarsal heads.

corrected passively by pressure under the metatarsal heads; as the forefoot lifts, the toes flatten out automatically. Later the deformities become fixed with the toes hyperextended at the MTP joints and flexed at the IP joints. Pain may then be felt under the metatarsal heads or over the toes where shoe pressure is most marked; callosities appear at the same sites. Walking tolerance is usually reduced.

The Coleman block test is used to check if the deformity is reversible. The patient is helped to stand with the heel and lateral part of the foot resting on a 1 inch (2 cm) block and the medial part of the forefoot and great toe dipping over the edge of the block to touch the floor. If, in this position, the heel varus corrects then mobility of the subtalar joint is demonstrated.

Neurological examination is important, to identify causal disorders such as hereditary motor and sensory neuropathies and spinal cord abnormalities (tethered cord syndrome, syringomyelia). Poliomyelitis is also a significant cause in some parts of the world.

Imaging

Lateral weightbearing x-rays of the foot will reveal the components of the high arch (see Figure 21.14). MRI scans of the entire spine are important to rule out any structural problem in the spinal cord.

Treatment

Often no treatment is required; apart from the difficulty of fitting shoes, the patient has no complaints. Patients with significant discomfort may benefit from fitting custom-made shoes with moulded supports, but this does not alter the deformity or influence its progression.

If symptoms persist and the deformities are still passively correctable, a tendon re-balancing operation may be worthwhile: the long toe flexors are released and transplanted into the extensor expansions to pull the toes straight. Unfortunately even this may offer only temporary relief.

A painful foot with fixed deformities presents a more difficult problem. The aim of surgery is to

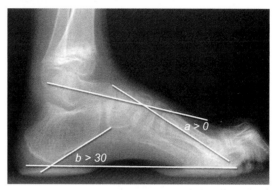

21.14 Pes cavus – weightbearing x-rays
Weightbearing films are essential for showing the components of foot deformities. In standing lateral views, some measurements are helpful in describing the type of high-arched foot: a, the axes of the talus and first metatarsal are parallel in normal feet but cross each other in a plantaris deformity (Meary's angle); b, the calcaneal pitch is greater than 30 degrees in calcaneus deformities.

provide a pain-free, plantigrade, supple but stable foot. This could involve release of contractures, corrective osteotomies and tendon transfers. In principle, the deformity should be corrected before tendon transfers can address the muscle imbalance around the foot.

If recurrence follows corrective surgery, arthrodesis to maintain a functional and stable foot is needed; this is usually an arthrodesis of the talonavicular, calcaneocuboid and subtalar joints – the triple arthrodesis. For the clawed toes, interphalangeal joint fusions may be necessary.

If an underlying neurological cause is identified, this too must be addressed.

HALLUX VALGUS

Hallux valgus is the commonest of the foot deformities (and probably of all musculoskeletal deformities). In people who have never worn shoes the big toe is in line with the first metatarsal, retaining the slightly fan-shaped appearance of the

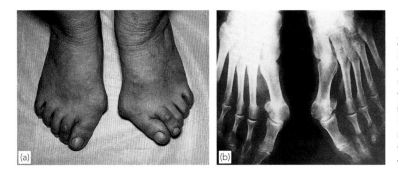

21.15 Hallux valgus This 58-year-old woman (a) complained of painful bunions and corns, unsightly feet and difficulties with fitting shoes. (b) Standing x-rays showed the abnormal first intermetatarsal angulation and the marked valgus angulation at the first metatarsophalangeal joint – worse in the left foot than the right.

forefoot. In people who habitually wear shoes the hallux assumes a valgus position; but only if the angulation is excessive is it referred to as 'hallux valgus'.

Splaying of the forefoot, with varus angulation of the first metatarsal, predisposes to lateral angulation of the big toe in people who wear shoes. This *metatarsus primus varus* may be congenital, or it may result from loss of muscle tone in the forefoot in elderly people. Hallux valgus is also common in rheumatoid arthritis.

The elements of the deformity are lateral deviation and rotation of the hallux, together with a prominence of the medial side of the head of the first metatarsal (a *bunion*); there may also be an overlying bursa and thickened soft tissue. Lateral deviation of the hallux may lead to overcrowding of the lateral toes and sometimes over-riding.

Clinical features

Hallux valgus is most common in women between 50 and 70 years, and is usually bilateral. An important sub-group, with a strong familial tendency, appears during late adolescence.

Often there are no symptoms apart from the deformity. Pain, if present, may be due to: (1) shoe pressure on a large or an inflamed bunion; (2) splaying of the forefoot and muscle strain (metatarsalgia); (3) associated deformities of the lesser toes; or (4) secondary osteoarthritis of the first metatarsophalangeal joint.

X-rays

Standing views will show the degree of metatarsal adduction and hallux angulation (see Figure 21.15). Normally the first intermetatarsal angle is less than 9 degrees and the toe valgus angle at the MTP joint less than 15 degrees. Any greater degree of angulation should be regarded as abnormal. Three types of deformity can be identified (see Figure 21.16):

- MTP joint normally centred but articular surfaces, though congruent, are tilted towards valgus.
- Articular surfaces are not congruent, the phalangeal surface being tilted towards valgus.
- MTP joint both incongruent and slightly subluxated.

Type 1 is a stable joint and any deformity is likely to progress very slowly or not at all. Type 2 is somewhat unstable and likely to progress. Type 3 is even more unstable and almost certain to progress.

Treatment

Adolescents and young adults
Deformity is usually the only 'symptom', but the patient is anxious to prevent it becoming more

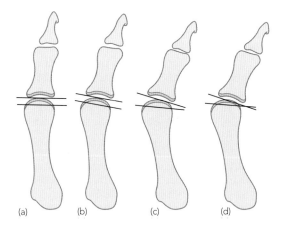

21.16 Type of hallux valgus (a) In *normal feet* the articular surfaces are parallel and centred upon each other. In *congruent hallux valgus* (b) the lines across the articular surfaces are still parallel and the joint is centred, but the articular surfaces are set more obliquely to the long axes of their respective bones. In (c), the *deviated type of hallux valgus*, the lines are not parallel and the articular surfaces are not congruent. In *the subluxated type* (d) the surfaces are neither parallel nor centred.

severe and painful. Conservative treatment is justified as a first measure (operative correction carries a 20–40% recurrence rate in this age group). The patient is encouraged to wear shoes with deep toe-boxes, soft uppers and low heels.

If the deformity is mild (less than 25 degrees at the MTP joint), it can be corrected by either a soft-tissue rebalancing operation or by a metatarsal osteotomy. If the x-ray shows a *congruent* articulation, the deformity is largely bony and therefore amenable to correction by a distal metatarsal osteotomy. If the MTP articulation is *incongruent* the deformity is in the joint and soft-tissue realignment is indicated: tight structures on the lateral side (adductor hallucis, transverse metatarsal ligament, and lateral joint capsule) are released, the prominent bone on the medial side of the metatarsal head is pared down, and the capsule on the medial side is tightened by reefing.

In moderate and severe deformities the hallux valgus angle may be greater than 30 degrees and intermetatarsal angle wider than 15 degrees. If the MTP joint is *congruent*, a distal osteotomy combined with a corrective osteotomy of the base of the proximal phalanx is recommended. For greater deformities, if the joint is subluxed, a soft-tissue adjustment is needed as well as a metatarsal osteotomy to reduce the wide intermetatarsal angle.

Adults

Surgical treatment is more readily offered to older patients. This usually takes the form of excision of the bunion, metatarsal osteotomy and soft-tissue rebalancing. However, if the metatarsophalangeal joint is frankly osteoarthritic, arthrodesis of the joint may be a better option.

Hallux valgus in aged patients with limited mobility is best treated by shoe modifications. The classic Keller's operation (excision of the proximal third of the proximal phalanx, as well as the bunion prominence) has fallen into disuse because of the high rate of recurrent deformity and complications such as loss of control over great toe movement and recurrent metatarsalgia.

HALLUX RIGIDUS

'Rigidity' of the first MTP joint may be due to local trauma or osteochrondritis dissecans of the first metatarsal head, but in older people it is usually caused by long-standing joint disorders such as gout, pseudogout or osteoarthritis. In contrast to hallux valgus, men and women are affected with equal frequency. Clinical problems are due to the fact that, because the big toe cannot extend (dorsiflex), push-off at the end of the stance phase of gait becomes painful and clumsy.

Clinical features

Pain on walking, especially on slopes or rough ground, is the predominant symptom. The hallux is straight and the MTP joint feels knobbly; a tender 'bunion' on the dorsum of the MTP joint (actually a large osteophyte) is characteristic.

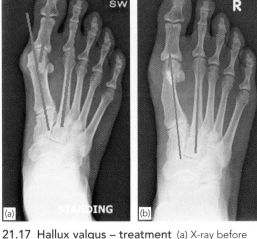

21.17 Hallux valgus – treatment (a) X-ray before operation. (b) X-ray after distal osteotomy. Both the intermetatarsal angle and the metatarsophalangeal valgus angle have been corrected.

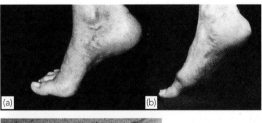

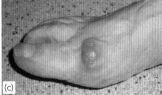

21.18 Hallux rigidus (a) In normal walking, at push-off the big toe dorsiflexes (extends) considerably. With rigidus (b), dorsiflexion is limited and this makes walking difficult. Osteoarthritis in the first metatarsophalangeal joint produces a dorsal bunion (c), in contrast to the medial bunion of hallux valgus.

Extension (dorsiflexion) of the toe is restricted and painful; plantarflexion is also limited, but less so.

X-ray changes are those of osteoarthritis; the joint space is narrowed, there is bone sclerosis and, often, large osteophytes at the joint margins. In younger patients, there may be squaring of the metatarsal head indicating a previous osteochondritis dissecans.

Treatment

A rocker-soled shoe may abolish pain by allowing the foot to 'roll' without the necessity for dorsiflexion at the MTP joint. If walking is painful despite this type of shoe adjustment, an operation is advised. For young patients the best procedure is a simple extension osteotomy of the proximal phalanx, to mimic dorsiflexion at the IP joint. In older patients, where the extent of the disease is limited, simply removing the osteophyte and a little of the metatarsal head dorsally (cheilectomy) might be effective and this can be combined with an extension osteotomy in the proximal phalanx to alter loadbearing. If the joint is more arthritic, then a fusion offers a good chance of returning the patient to function and walking comfortably without a limp.

DEFORMITIES OF THE LESSER TOES

Common deformities of the lesser digits are hammer-toe, claw-toe, mallet-toe and overlapping-toe.

HAMMER TOE

'Hammer-toe' is an isolated flexion deformity of the proximal IP joint of one of the lesser toes –

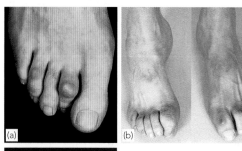

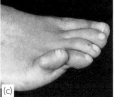

21.19 Disorders of the lesser toes (a) Hammer-toe deformity. (b) Claw-toes (weakness of the intrinsic muscles and cavus feet). (c) Overlapping-fifth toe.

usually the second or third. The distal IP joint and the MTP joint are pulled into hyperextension. Shoe pressure may produce a painful corn on the dorsally projecting proximal IP (PIP) 'knuckle'.

Operative correction is indicated for pain or for difficulty with shoes. The toe is shortened and straightened by excising the PIP joint and performing a fusion.

CLAW-TOE

In this deformity all the toes are affected to greater or lesser degree. The MTP joints are hyperextended and the IP joints are flexed. This suggests that the intrinsic muscles are relatively weak and it is not surprising that the deformity is seen in neurological disorders (e.g. peroneal muscular atrophy, poliomyelitis and peripheral neuropathies) and in rheumatoid arthritis. Often, however, no cause is found. The condition may also be associated with pes cavus.

Clinical features

The patient complains of pain in the forefoot and under the metatarsal heads. Usually the condition is bilateral and walking may be severely restricted.

At first the joints are mobile and can be passively corrected; later the deformities become fixed and the metatarsophalangeal joints subluxed or dislocated. Painful corns and callosities develop and in the most severe cases the skin ulcerates at the pressure sites.

Treatment

So long as the toes can be passively straightened the patient may obtain relief by wearing a metatarsal support (pressure under the metatarsal necks will straighten the mobile joints). If this fails to relieve discomfort, 'dynamic' correction is achieved by transferring the long toe flexors to the extensors. The operation, at one stroke, removes a powerful IP flexor and converts it to a MTP flexor and IP extensor.

When the deformity is fixed, it may either be accepted and accommodated by special footwear, or treated by IP arthrodesis combined with tendon transfers.

If the great toe is clawed, an IP arthrodesis combined with a transfer of extensor hallucis longus through the neck of the first metatarsal (in order to elevate it) works well – the *Jones procedure*.

Excision arthroplasty is also an option if the joint is destroyed (e.g. by rheumatoid disease). The base of the proximal phalanx is removed and the space filled with the extensor tendon sutured to the flexor.

MALLET-TOE

In mallet-toe it is the distal IP joint that is flexed. The toenail or the tip of the toe presses into the shoe, resulting in a painful callosity. If conservative treatment (chiropody and padding) does not help, operation is indicated. The distal IP joint is exposed, the articular surfaces excised and the toe straightened; flexor tenotomy may be needed. A thin K-wire is inserted across the joint and left in position for 6 weeks to hold the joint until fusion is achieved.

OVERLAPPING-TOE

This is often seen when a markedly valgus big toe forces the adjacent second toe to find room for itself by riding up on top of the hallux. The overlapping-toe may fall back into position once the hallux valgus is corrected, but sometimes surgical correction is needed.

Overlapping-fifth toe is a congenital anomaly. If it is sufficiently bothersome, the toe may be straightened by performing a dorsal V/Y-plasty together with transfer of the flexor to the extensor tendon. The toe has to be held in the corrected position with tape or a K-wire for 6 weeks while the soft tissues heal.

RHEUMATOID ARTHRITIS

The ankle and foot are affected almost as often as the wrist and hand. Early on there is synovitis of the joints as well as of the sheathed tendons (usually the peronei and tibialis posterior). As the disease progresses, joint erosion and tendon dysfunction prepare the ground for increasingly severe deformities.

FOREFOOT

Pain and swelling of the MTP joints are among the earliest features of rheumatoid arthritis. Tenderness is at first localized to the MTP joints; later the entire forefoot is painful on pressing or squeezing. There is increasing weakness of the intrinsic muscles and, with joint destruction, the characteristic deformities appear: a flattened anterior arch, hallux valgus, claw-toes and prominence of the metatarsal heads in the sole (patients say it feels like walking on pebbles).

Subcutaneous nodules, corns and callosities are common and may ulcerate. In the worst cases the toes are dislocated, inflamed, ulcerated and useless.

X-rays show osteoporosis and periarticular erosion at the MTP joints. Curiously – in contrast to the situation in the hand – the smaller digits (fourth and fifth toes) are affected first.

Treatment

During the stage of synovitis, corticosteroid injections and attention to footwear, including modifications to accommodate the toe deformities, may relieve symptoms. Synovectomy of the MTP joints may slow disease progression.

Once deformity is advanced, treatment is that of the claw-toes and hallux valgus. An effective operation is excision arthroplasty of the MTP joints of lesser toes in order to relieve pressure in the sole and to correct the toe deformities. For the hallux, an MTP fusion is preferred.

ANKLE AND HINDFOOT

The earliest symptoms are pain and swelling around the ankle. Walking becomes increasingly difficult and, later, deformities appear. On examination, swelling and tenderness are usually localized to the back of the medial malleolus (tenosynovitis of tibialis posterior) or the lateral malleolus (tenosynovitis of the peronei). Less often there is swelling of the ankle joint and its movements are restricted. Inversion and eversion may be painful and limited.

In the late stages the tibialis posterior may rupture (all too often this is missed), or become

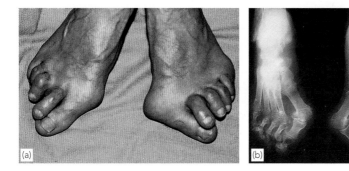

21.20 Rheumatoid arthritis (a,b) Forefoot deformities are like those in non-rheumatoid feet but more severe.

ineffectual; with progressive erosion of the tarsal joints the foot gradually drifts into severe valgus.

X-rays show osteoporosis and, later, erosion of the tarsal and ankle joints. Soft-tissue swelling may be marked.

Treatment

In the stage of synovitis, splintage is helpful (to allow inflammation to subside and to prevent deformity) while waiting for systemic treatment to control the disease. Initially, tendon sheaths and joints may be injected with methylprednisolone, but this should not be repeated more than two or three times. A lightweight below-knee orthosis will restore stability and may be worn almost indefinitely.

If the synovitis does not subside, operative synovectomy may help. Although tendon replacement is technically feasible, progressive joint erosion will ultimately counteract any improvement this might achieve. In the very late stage, arthrodesis of the ankle and tarsal joints can still restore modest function and abolish pain. Arthroplasty for rheumatoid disease of the ankle is becoming popular and can yield good results.

OSTEOARTHRITIS

Osteoarthritis (OA) of the ankle is almost always secondary to some underlying disorder: a malunited fracture, recurrent instability, osteochondritis dissecans of the talus, avascular necrosis of the talus or repeated bleeding with haemophilia. Sometimes the ankle is involved in generalized OA and crystal arthropathy.

Clinical features

The presentation is usually with pain and stiffness localized to the ankle, particularly when first standing up from rest. Patients often indicate the site of pain as being transversely across the front of the ankle. The ankle is usually swollen, with palpable anterior osteophytes and tenderness along the anterior joint line. Dorsiflexion (extension) and plantarflexion at the ankle are restricted and the gait is often antalgic. The foot may be turned outwards in the stance phase, to compensate for the loss of ankle movement.

X-rays show the typical features of OA: joint space narrowing, subchondral sclerosis and osteophyte formation. The predisposing disorder is almost always easily detected.

Treatment

Painful exacerbations can be managed with analgesics or anti-inflammatory medication. Offloading the joint can be achieved with the use of a walking stick; weight loss might be appropriate. Arthrodesis is a good solution for a painful stiff joint although arthroplasty of the ankle may have a place in the low-demand individual.

GOUT

Swelling, redness, heat and exquisite tenderness of the MTP joint of the big toe ('podagra') is the epitome of gout (see also Chapter 4). The ankle joint, or one of the lesser toes, may be similarly affected – especially following a minor injury. The condition may closely resemble septic arthritis, but the systemic features of infection are absent. The serum uric acid level may be raised.

Chronic tophaceous gout is not uncommon. Lumpy tophi may appear around any of the joints. The diagnosis is suggested by the characteristic x-ray features and confirmed by identifying the typical crystals in the tophus.

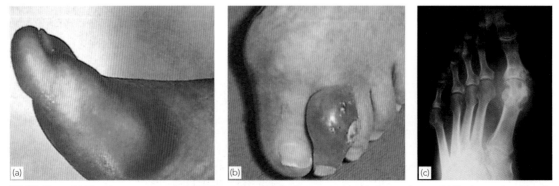

21.21 Gout (a) The classic picture: acute inflammation of the first metatarsophalangeal joint. (b) Tophaceous gout of the second toe. (c) X-ray of the first metatarsophalangeal joint; the large excavations are occupied by crystalline tophi.

Treatment

Treatment with anti-inflammatory drugs will abort the acute attack of gout; until the pain subsides the foot should be rested and protected from injury.

Painful or ulcerating tophi may require local curettage of the bone lesions.

TUBERCULOUS ARTHRITIS

Tuberculous infection of the ankle joint begins as a synovitis or as an osteomyelitis; because walking is painful, the patient may present before true arthritis supervenes. The ankle is swollen and the calf markedly wasted; the skin feels warm and movements are restricted. Sinus formation occurs early.

X-rays show regional osteoporosis, sometimes a bone abscess and, with late disease, narrowing and irregularity of the joint space.

Treatment

In addition to general treatment (Chapter 2) a removable splint is used to rest the foot in neutral position.

If the disease is arrested early, the patient is allowed up non-weightbearing in a calliper, gradually taking more and more weight and then discarding the calliper altogether.

In the long term stiffness is inevitable and, if this is accompanied by pain, arthrodesis is the best treatment.

THE DIABETIC FOOT

The complications of long-standing diabetes mellitus often appear in the foot, causing chronic disability. About 40% of non-trauma related amputations in British hospitals are for complications of diabetes. Factors affecting the foot are: (1) a predisposition to peripheral vascular disease; (2) damage to peripheral nerves; (3) reduced resistance to infection; (4) osteoporosis.

Peripheral vascular disease: the patient may complain of intermittent claudication or ischaemic changes and there may be ulceration or, worse still, gangrene in the foot.

Peripheral neuropathy: early on, patients may complain of symmetrical numbness and paraesthesia, but they are usually unaware of the systemic abnormality. Motor loss may lead to claw-toes with high arches and this, in turn, may predispose to plantar ulceration. Neuropathic joint disease (Charcot joints), occurs in less than 1% of diabetic patients, yet diabetes is the commonest cause of a neuropathic joint in Europe and North America. The midtarsal joints are the most commonly affected, followed by the MTP and ankle joints. A minor provocative incident, such as a twisting injury or a fracture, leads to a painless progressive collapse of the joint. X-rays show destruction of the joint.

Infection: uncontrolled diabetes reduces immunity and, in combination with peripheral neuropathy and ischaemia, increases the risk of infection after minor trauma.

Osteoporosis: loss of bone density in diabetes may be severe enough to result in insufficiency fractures around the ankle or in the metatarsals.

Management

Prevention of foot-related complications of diabetes is through:

- Regular attendance at a diabetic clinic.
- Full compliance with the medication.
- Checks for early signs of vascular or neurological abnormality.
- Taking heed of advice on foot care and footwear.
- A high level of skin hygiene.
- Use of adaptive and supportive orthoses if there is deformity or joint instability.

Diabetic foot clinics are a multi-disciplinary effort of physician, surgeon, podiatrist and orthotist. Regular examination for early signs of neuropathy should include the use of Semmes–Weinstein hairs (for testing skin sensibility) and a biothesiometer (for testing vibration sense). Peripheral vascular examination is enhanced by using a Doppler ultrasound probe.

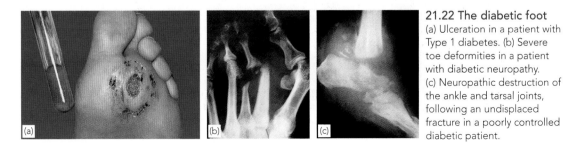

21.22 The diabetic foot
(a) Ulceration in a patient with Type 1 diabetes. (b) Severe toe deformities in a patient with diabetic neuropathy. (c) Neuropathic destruction of the ankle and tarsal joints, following an undisplaced fracture in a poorly controlled diabetic patient.

The presence of ulcers calls for differentiation between vascular, neuropathic or combined causes. Ischaemic changes need the attention of a vascular surgeon who can advise on ways of improving the local blood supply. Neuropathic ulcers require total contact casts followed by custom-made shoes with total contact insoles to avoid recurrence.

Neuropathic joint disease is a major challenge. Arthrodesis has a very poor union rate; 'containment' of the problem in a weight-relieving orthosis may be the best option.

Careful attention is needed for signs of gangrene. Dry gangrene of the toe can be left to demarcate before amputation; wet gangrene and infection may call for immediate amputation.

DISORDERS OF THE TENDO ACHILLIS

ACHILLES TENDINITIS

Athletes, joggers and hikers often develop pain and swelling around the tendo Achillis, due to local irritation of the tendon sheath or the paratenon. Function is inhibited because of pain in the heel-cord, especially at pushoff. The condition may come on gradually or rapidly following a change in sporting activity.

The tendon feels thickened and tender in the watershed area about 4 cm above its insertion. An ultrasound scan may be helpful in confirming the diagnosis. If the onset is very sudden, suspect tendon rupture.

Treatment

Advice on rest, ice, compression and elevation (RICE) and the use of an non-steroidal anti-inflammatory drug (oral or topical) are helpful. When symptoms improve, stretching exercises and muscle strengthening are introduced. A removable in-shoe heel-raise might be helpful. Operative treatment is seldom necessary. Injection with

corticosteroids should only be performed under ultrasound guidance.

ACHILLES TENDON RUPTURE

Rupture probably occurs only if the tendon is degenerate. Consequently most patients are over 40 years old. While pushing off (running or jumping), the calf muscle contracts; but the contraction is resisted by body weight and the tendon ruptures. The patient feels as if he or she has been struck just above the heel, and is unable rise up on tiptoes.

Soon after the tear occurs, a gap can be seen and felt about 5 cm above the insertion of the tendon. Plantarflexion of the foot is weak and is not accompanied by tautening of the tendon. Where doubt exists, *Simmonds' test* is helpful: with the patient prone, the calf is squeezed; if the tendon is intact the foot is seen to plantarflex involuntarily; if the tendon is ruptured the foot remains still. *Ultrasound scans* can be used to confirm the diagnosis.

Treatment

If the patient is seen early, the ends of the tendon may approximate when the foot is passively plantarflexed. If so, a plaster cast or special boot is applied with the foot in equinus and is worn for 8 weeks; thereafter, a shoe with a raised heel is worn for a further 6 weeks. It is usually safe to commence physiotherapy at 4–6 weeks.

Operative repair is probably more reliable, but immobilization in equinus for 8 weeks and a heel raise for a further 6 weeks are still needed.

THE PAINFUL ANKLE

Except after trauma or in rheumatoid arthritis, persistent pain around the ankle usually originates in one of the periarticular structures or in the talus rather than the joint itself. Conditions to be looked for are chronic ligamentous instability, tenosynovitis of the tibialis posterior or peroneal

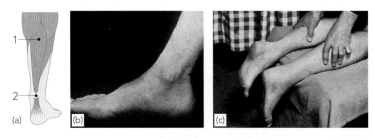

21.23 Rupture of tendo Achillis (a) The soleus may tear at its musculotendinous junction (1), but the tendo Achillis itself ruptures about 5 cm above its insertion (2). (b) There is a visible and palpable depression at the site of rupture just above the heel. (c) Simmonds' test: both calves are being squeezed but only the left foot plantarflexes – the right tendon is ruptured.

tendons, rupture of the tibialis posterior tendon, osteochondritis dissecans of the dome of the talus or avascular necrosis of the talus.

Tenosynovitis

Tenderness and swelling are localized to the affected tendon, and pain is aggravated by active movement – inversion or eversion against resistence. Local injection of corticosteroid usually helps.

Rupture of tibialis posteror tendon

Pain starts quite suddenly and sometimes the patient gives a history of having felt the tendon snap. The heel is in valgus during weightbearing; the area around the medial malleolus is tender and active inversion of the ankle is both painful and weak.

In physically active patients, operative repair or tendon transfer using the tendon of flexor digitorum longus is worthwhile. For poorly mobile patients, or indeed anyone who is prepared to put up with the inconvenience of an orthosis, splintage may be adequate.

Osteochondritis dissecans of the talus

Unexplained pain and slight limitation of movement in the ankle of a young person may be due to a small osteochondral fracture of the dome of the talus. Tangential x-rays will usually show the tiny fragment. MRI is also helpful and the lesion may be visualized directly by arthroscopy. If the articular surface is intact, it is sufficient simply to restrict activities. If the fragment has separated, it may have to be removed.

Avascular necrosis of the talus

The talus is one of the preferred sites of 'idiopathic' necrosis. The causes are the same as for necrosis at other more common sites such as the femoral head (see Chapter 6). If pain is marked, arthrodesis of the ankle may be needed.

Chronic instability of the ankle

This subject is dealt with on page 289.

THE PAINFUL FOOT

Pain may be felt predominantly in the heel, the midfoot or the forefoot. Common causes are: (1) mechanical pressure (which is more likely if the foot is deformed); (2) joint inflammation or stiffness; (3) a localized bone lesion; (4) peripheral ischaemia; or (5) muscular strain – usually secondary to some other abnormality.

PAINFUL HEEL

Traction 'apophysitis' (Sever's disease)

This condition usually occurs in young boys. It is not a 'disease', but a mild traction injury. Pain and tenderness are localized to the tendo Achillis insertion. The x-ray may show increased density or irregularity of the apophysis, but often the painless heel looks similar. The heel of the shoe should be raised a little and strenuous activities restricted for a few weeks.

Calcaneal bursitis

Older girls and young women often complain of painful bumps on the backs of their heels. The posterolateral portion of the calcaneum is prominent and shoe friction causes a bursitis. Treatment should be conservative – attention to footwear (open-back shoes are best) and padding of the heel. If symptoms warrant it, removal of the calcaneal prominence may help.

Plantar fasciitis

Pain under the ball of the heel, or slightly forwards of this, is a fairly common complaint in people (mainly men) aged 30–60 years. It is worse on weightbearing and there is marked tenderness along the distal edge

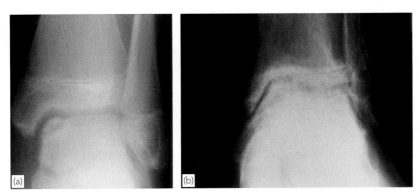

21.24 Osteochrondritis dissecans and osteonecrosis
(a) 'Osteochondritis dissecans' (more correctly, a small osteoarticular fracture) at the common site, the anteromedial part of the articular surface of the talus. (b) More extensive osteonecrosis can lead to secondary osteoarthritis of the ankle.

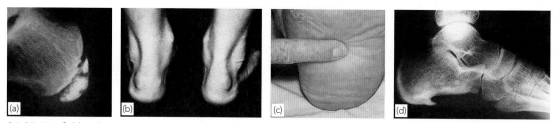

21.25 Painful heel (a) Sever's disease – the apophysis is dense and fragmented. (b) Bilateral 'heel bumps'. (c) The usual site of tenderness in plantar fasciitis. (d) X-ray in patients with plantar fasciitis often shows what looks like a spur on the undersurface of the calcaneum. In reality this is a two-dimensional view of a small ridge corresponding to the attachment of the plantar fascia. It is doubtful whether the 'spur' is responsible for the pain and local tenderness.

of the heel contact area. A lateral x-ray of this site often shows a bone 'spur' extending distally on the undersurface of the calcaneum; this is an associated – not a causative – feature.

Plantar fasciitis is sometimes encountered in patients with inflammatory disorders such as gout, ankylosing spondylitis and Reiter's disease.

Treatment is conservative: anti-inflammatory drugs or local injection of corticosteroids, and a pad under the heel to off-load the painful area. The condition can take 18–36 months or longer to resolve but it is generally self-limiting.

Bone lesions

Calcaneal lesions such as infection, tumours and Paget's disease can give rise to unremitting pain in the heel. The diagnosis is usually obvious on x-ray examination.

PAIN OVER THE MIDFOOT

In children, pain in the midtarsal region is unusual: two possible causes are *Köhler's disease* ('osteochondritis' – flattening and increased density on x-ray of the navicular) or a bony coalition across the midtarsal joints. In both a period of observation is wise; in Kohler's disease spontaneous resolution is likely and not all bony coalitions will need removal.

In adults, especially if the arch is high, a ridge of bone sometimes develops on the adjacent dorsal surfaces of the medial cuneiform and the first metatarsal (the '*overbone*'). A lump can be seen and it feels hard; it may become tender if the shoe presses on it. If shoe adjustment fails to provide relief the lump may be bevelled off.

PAIN IN THE FOREFOOT

Any foot abnormality which results in faulty weight distribution may cause nagging pain in the forefoot – *metatarsalgia*. It is therefore a common

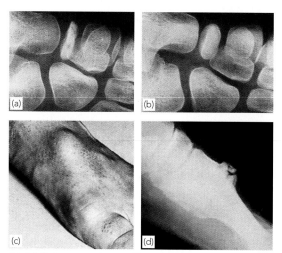

21.26 Pain over the midfoot (a) Köhler's disease compared with (b) the normal foot. (c,d) The bump on the dorsum of the foot due to osteoarthritis of the first cuneiform–metatarsal joint.

complaint in patients with hallux valgus, claw-toes, pes cavus or flat-foot. However, there are several specific disorders which cause localized pain in the forefoot.

Sesamoiditis

Pain and tenderness directly under the first metatarsal head, typically aggravated by walking or passive dorsiflexion of the great toe, may be due to sesamoiditis. Symptoms usually arise from irritation or inflammation of the peritendinous tissues around the sesamoids.

Treatment consists of reduced weightbearing and a pressure pad in the shoe. In resistant cases, a local injection of methylprednisolone and local anaesthetic often helps.

Freiberg's disease

'Osteochondritis' (or 'osteochondrosis') of a metatarsal head is actually a type of traumatic

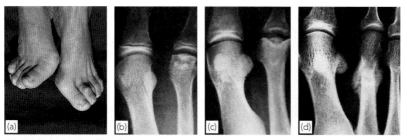

21.27 Pain in the forefoot (a) Long-standing deformities such as dropped anterior arches, hallux valgus, hammer-toe, curly-toes and overlapping-toes (all of which are present in this patient) can cause metatarsalgia. Localized pain and tenderness suggest a more specific cause. (b,c) Stages in the development of Freiberg's disease. (d) Periosteal new bone formation along the shaft of the second metatarsal, the classical sign of a stress fracture.

osteonecrosis of the subarticular bone. It usually affects the second metatarsal head (rarely the third) in young adults. There is pain over the MTP joint and a bony lump (the enlarged metatarsal head) is palpable and tender. *X-rays* show the head to be flattened and wide, the neck thick and the joint space apparently increased.

A walking plaster or moulded sandal will help to reduce pressure on the metatarsal head. If symptoms persist, synovectomy, debridement and trimming of the metatarsal head (cheilectomy) should be considered. Pain relief is usually good and the range of dorsiflexion is improved.

Stress fracture

Stress fractures of the second and third metatarsal bones are seen in young adults after unaccustomed activity. The affected metatarsal shaft feels thick and tender. The x-ray appearance is at first normal, but later shows fusiform callus around a fine transverse fracture. Similar fractures sometimes occur in elderly, osteoporotic patients who (for one reason or another) change their pattern of walking and weightbearing.

Treatment is either unnecessary or consists simply of rest and reassurance.

Interdigital nerve compression (Morton's metatarsalgia)

The patient, usually a woman of around 50 years, complains of pain in the forefoot ('as if walking on a pebble in the shoe') with radiation to the toes. Tenderness is localized to one of the intermetatarsal spaces – usually the third – and pressure just proximal to the interdigital web may elicit both the pain and a tingling sensation distally. Squeezing the metatarsal heads together may produce a painful click (Mulder's click).

This is essentially an entrapment or compression syndrome affecting one of the digital nerves, but secondary thickening of the nerve creates the impression of a 'neuroma'.

If symptoms do not respond to the use of protective padding and wearing wider shoes, a steroid injection into the interspace will provide lasting relief in about 50% of cases. If this too fails, nerve compression can usually be relieved by operative division of the tight transverse intermetatarsal ligament. Intractable cases may need excision of the 'neuroma'.

TOENAIL DISORDERS

The toenail of the hallux may be ingrown, overgrown or undergrown.

Ingrown toenail

The nail burrows into the nail groove; this ulcerates and its wall grows over the nail, so the term 'embedded toenail' would be better. The patient is taught to cut the nail square, to insert pledgets of wool under the ingrowing edges and always to keep the feet clean and dry. If these measures fail, the portion of germinal matrix which is responsible for the 'ingrow' should be ablated, either by operative excision or by chemical ablation with phenol. Rarely is it necessary to remove the entire nail or completely ablate the nail bed.

Over-grown toenail (onychogryposis)

Sometimes the nail, for no apparent reason, becomes unusually hard, thick and curved. A chiropodist can make the patient comfortable, but occasionally the nail may need complete excision.

Subungual bone growth

In this condition the nail is gradually lifted from its bed by an 'exostosis' growing on the dorsum of the terminal phalanx. X-ray examination shows the bony protuberance. The 'exostosis' should be removed, but recurrence is not uncommon.

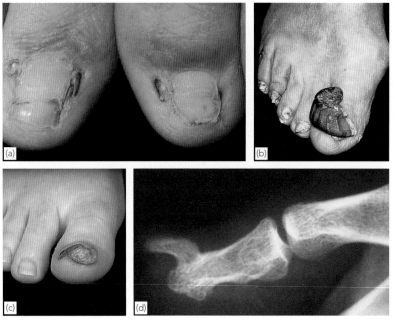

21.28 Toenail disorders
(a) In-grown toenails. (b) Over-grown toenail (onychogryposis). (c,d) Exostosis from the distal phalanx, pushing the toenail up.

SKIN LESIONS

Typical skin lesions are illustrated in Figure 21.29.

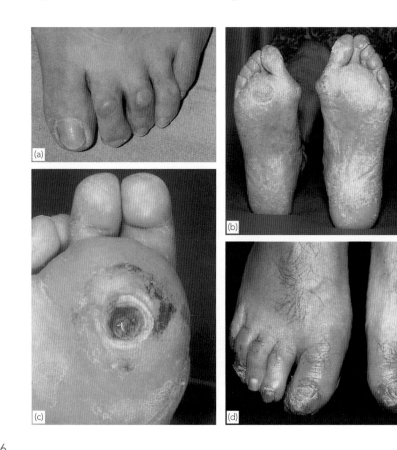

21.29 Skin lesions (a) Corns. (b) Planter callosities in a patient with claw-toes and a 'dropped' anterior metatarsal arch. (c) A typical pressure ulcer in a patient with long-standing diabetic neuropathy. (d) Keratoderma blenorrhagica, a complication of Reiter's disease.

PART 3

FRACTURES AND JOINT INJURIES

THE MANAGEMENT OF MAJOR INJURIES

Throughout the developed world trauma is the commonest cause of death in people under the age of 40 years, with the largest proportion resulting from road accidents. For every death, three victims suffer permanent disability, causing personal tragedy and a drain on a nation's healthcare economy.

These deaths follow a trimodal pattern: 50% of patients die on scene from unsurvivable injuries; 30% survive but die between 1 and 3 hours after injury; the remaining 20% die from complications during the 6 weeks after injury. The second peak in the death rate is due mostly to hypoxia and loss of blood with hypovolaemic shock; these are potentially preventable and hence this period has been called '*the golden hour*'. The third peak is due largely to multi-system failure and sepsis needing high levels of intensive care, but is reducible by early and effective management.

The management of severe injuries proceeds in well-defined stages:

- Emergency treatment immediately after the accident.
- Resuscitation and evaluation in the hospital accident department.
- Early treatment of life-threatening injuries.
- Treatment of potentially life-threatening injuries.
- Long-term rehabilitation.

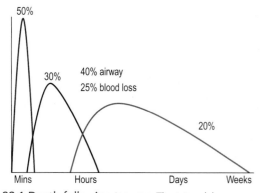

22.1 Death following trauma The trimodal distribution of mortality following severe trauma.

MANAGEMENT AT THE SCENE OF THE ACCIDENT

IMMEDIATE ACTIONS AND TRIAGE

Trauma scenes are hazardous, and personal safety is essential. Medical teams should be provided with personal protective equipment (PPE).

Make contact with emergency service commanders and, if there are multiple casualties, identify priorities by *triage*. This is a sorting system based on the injured person's ability to walk, breathe and maintain a pulse, followed by a scored, physiological assessment placing the individual in one of the following categories:

- Priority 1 Immediate
- Priority 2 Urgent
- Priority 3 Delayed
- Priority 4 Dead

ASSESSMENT AND INITIAL MANAGEMENT

The nature of the incident and pattern of vehicle damage help in predicting the likely injuries. Early recognition is based on a rapid and systematic questioning and examination of the casualty.

Access to an entrapped person may be limited, but an immediate examination can be made of the *airway*, *breathing* and *circulation* – the 'ABC' of trauma assessment, which guides immediate management, extrication and transfer.

Management

Life-threatening injuries in the ABC categories are treated first; the exception to this is *catastrophic external haemorrhage*, in which situation bleeding is controlled first and then the ABC system is followed. Furthermore, *at all times the cervical spine must be immobilized*, in case there is some vertebral injury. Control pain, if necessary.

Airway: casualties with airway obstruction can succumb within minutes. Open the airway by pulling the jaw forward, *but do not extend the neck*, and remove all visible foreign bodies. Use airway devices if the casualty's airway remains obstructed. Intubation following rapid sequence induction of anaesthesia is the gold standard, but this should be performed by an Emergency Medicine doctor trained in anaesthesiology. If intubation fails, a surgical airway will be required.

Breathing: administer high-flow oxygen with a non-rebreathing reservoir mask; support ventilation with a bag–valve–mask (BVM) assembly, and ventilate intubated casualties.

Examine the chest for signs of a *tension pneumothorax* which will need immediate decompression using a large-bore intravenous cannula inserted through the second intercostal space in the midclavicular line, to be followed by thoracostomies if the patient is intubated. Cover open chest wounds with an occlusive, three-sided dressing.

Circulation: control haemorrhage and site intravenous (IV) or intraosseous (IO) cannulas. Limit IV fluids in haemorrhagic shock; titrate Hartmann's in 250 mL boluses to maintain a radial pulse only. Consider bilateral thoracostomies and clamshell thoracotomy if post-traumatic cardiac arrest occurs.

An extended system (ABCDE) would also include

Disability (assess the neurological status using the Glasgow Coma Score [GCS], and note the pupil size) and check the *Environmental situation* (keep the patient exposed but ensure that normothermia is maintained).

Extrication and immobilization

Managing an entrapped casualty is difficult and extrication becomes a priority. Protect the spine using manual immobilization, cervical collars and rigid immobilization devices. Analgesia may be required. Splint limb fractures and dislocations (use femoral traction splints for midshaft femur fractures if the pelvic ring is intact) and stabilize pelvic fractures with compression devices.

Transfer to hospital

Delayed or prolonged transfer to hospital is associated with poor outcomes, but *the ABCs must be addressed before transferring the patient*. The destination hospital should be matched to injury severity, and a 'trauma call' made.

Maintain the casualty's oxygen saturations above 95%, and end-tidal carbon dioxide ($EtCO_2$) at a low normal level (4.0–4.5 kPa) if ventilated. Control haemorrhage and continue IV Hartmann's to maintain a radial pulse.

On-scene priorities
■ Stay safe.
■ Obtain access.
■ Protect the cervical spine.
■ Free the airway.
■ Ensure ventilation.
■ Arrest haemorrhage.
■ Combat shock.
■ Control pain.
■ Splint fractures.
■ Transfer to hospital.

MANAGEMENT IN HOSPITAL

After reaching the hospital, the following factors are important:

- Organization and trauma teams.
- Assessment and management. *The ATLS concept*.
- Initial management.
- Definitive care.

ORGANIZATION AND TRAUMA TEAMS

'Get the right patient to the right hospital in the right amount of time' (Trunkey). Hospitals in the UK are categorized as Levels I–III, with Level I being a centre capable of managing the most serious casualties.

Casualty patients need rapid assessment and resuscitation to avoid their dying during the 'golden hour'. Crucial for this requirement is *a multi-disciplinary team led by a doctor with advanced trauma skills.*

THE ATLS CONCEPT

ATLS® (Advanced Trauma Life Support) is central to the internationally recognized training programme for the management of major injuries. The programme teaches a two-stage initial assessment and management followed by transfer to definitive care. This calls for a *primary survey and simultaneous resuscitation* (rapid assessment and treatment of life-threatening injuries) followed by a *secondary survey* (head-to-toe re-evaluation to identify all other injuries).

Specialist skills such as anaesthesia are employed in addition to core basic ATLS® skills. The following facilities should also be available: electrocardiographic (ECG) monitoring; pulse oximetry (arterial oxygen saturation); EtCO$_2$; arterial blood gas measurements (ABGs); urethral catheters; nasogastric tubes; x-rays (chest and pelvis); Focussed Assessment Sonography for Trauma (FAST); computed tomography (CT).

PRIMARY SURVEY AND RESUSCITATION

Airway obstruction kills in minutes. In degrees of urgency it is followed by respiratory failure,

circulatory failure and expanding intracranial mass lesions. Hence the development of the 'ABC' sequence, the goal of which is to preserve perfusion of the brain with oxygenated blood:

- A Airway with cervical spine protection.
- B Breathing.
- C Circulation with haemorrhage control.
- D Disability or neurological status.
- E Exposure and Environment.

Throughout, the cervical spine must be protected until a vertebral injury has been excluded. This is achieved by manual in-line immobilization or triple immobilization with a cervical collar, head supports and strapping. *Never extend the neck until a cervical spine injury has been excluded.*

A – Airway

The sound of an obstructed airway (stridor) is unmistakable. Support the airway, suction secretions and blood and place oropharyngeal or nasopharyngeal airways. Further options are the laryngeal mask airway, tracheal intubation or operative provision of an airway (cricothyrotomy). The airway must be checked frequently throughout the resuscitation phase; one that appears initially to be safe may not remain so.

B – Breathing

If, despite a clear airway, ventilation is inadequate the chest should be carefully examined for pneumothorax or a flail thoracic segment. *Tension pneumothorax* is a life-threatening complication and should be treated by immediate decompression (see pages 309, 314). *Sucking chest wounds* must be covered and a *flail chest* may require endotracheal intubation and positive pressure ventilation. The BVM is a hand-held device that manually supplies positive pressure ventilation.

It is essential to give all severely injured patients supplemental oxygen and to take a blood sample for measurement of the arterial oxygen tension (PaO_2) and carbon dioxide tension ($PaCO_2$).

C – Circulation with haemorrhage control

Assess for bleeding and shock and control external haemorrhage. Site IV or IO cannulas, and draw samples for diagnostic tests and cross-matching. If blood is available, initially treat shock with 2 L of warmed Hartmann's. Use FAST to identify body cavity haemorrhage.

D – Disability (level of consciousness)

Assess neurological status using the GCS. Consider intoxication but assume a lowered GCS

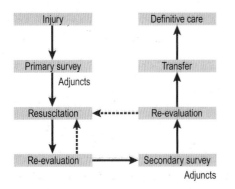

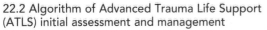

22.2 Algorithm of Advanced Trauma Life Support (ATLS) initial assessment and management

is secondary to a cerebral injury until proved otherwise. Examine pupils for equality.

E – Exposure and environment

Remove clothing and 'log-roll' the patient to examine the entire body. Maintain normothermia and warm fluids and ventilated gases.

Table 22.1 Glasgow Coma Score

Response	Score
Eye opening:	
Spontaneous	4
On command	3
On pain	2
Nil	1
Best motor response:	
Obeys	6
Localizes pain	5
Normal flexor	4
Abnormal flexor	3
Extensor	2
Nil	1
Verbal response:	
Orientated	5
Confused	4
Words	3
Sounds	2
Nil	1

SECONDARY SURVEY

Once the patient has been resuscitated a 'head-to-toe survey' is carried out. The back can be examined by gently 'log-rolling' the patient onto their side.

Take a history if possible and establish whether trauma was subsequent to a medical collapse, and whether the patient is receiving long-term treatment.

Examination

- *Head and face*: examine for contusions, lacerations and fractures, and examine eyes and ears for bleeding. Re-assess the GCS. The presence of facial or head injuries should raise suspicions about concomitant brain injury.
- *Neck*: examine for a step in the cervical spine indicative of fracture/dislocation, and contusions over the anterior neck indicative of laryngeal damage.

- *Chest*: inspect and auscultate to identify a pneumothorax. Palpate to detect fractured ribs, sternum, and subcutaneous emphysema and percuss to reveal a tension pneumothorax and haemothorax.
- *Abdomen*: examine for contusions and wounds; auscultate and palpate. Don't forget the perineum, rectum and vagina.
- *Pelvis*: check for unequal leg length and local tenderness.
- *Limbs*: examine for swelling, contusions, deformity, tenderness and pallor. Feel the pulses.
- *Neurological assessment*: examine for lateralizing signs, loss of sensation and motor power, and abnormality of reflexes. Document levels of sensory loss.

Imaging

CT scanning is now the method of choice for patients with acute major trauma; it should be obtained at the earliest opportunity. Modern CT scanners can provide high definition images within minutes whilst the patient is returned to the emergency department for continuing resuscitation.

X-rays of the chest, pelvis, spine and limbs are obtained as indicated or if the patient is not stable enough for CT.

FAST has replaced peritoneal lavage for detecting intraperitoneal fluid or blood.

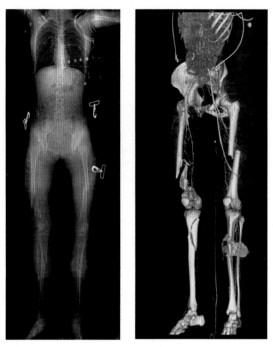

22.3 Imaging CT scanning is the imaging mode of choice. Multiple injuries are rapidly displayed.

GENERAL CARE

Pain management

Pain can be controlled in several ways, depending on the type of trauma:

- *Intravenous analgesia* – titrate morphine against response and administer an antiemetic.
- *Inhalational analgesia* – Entonox is good for short-term use but is contraindicated in patients with untreated pneumothorax.
- *Nerve blocks* – discuss this with the orthopaedic surgeon to avoid masking possible compartment syndrome.

Re-evaluation

The vital signs should be checked repeatedly to assess the response to treatment. The patient should not leave the Emergency Department until his or her condition is stable, unless it is to be taken directly to the operating theatre for the control of haemorrhage or some other surgical emergency.

Intrahospital and interhospital transfer

Transfer is indicated when the patient's needs exceed local resources. Careful planning is essential as monitoring and resuscitation are difficult during transfer.

DEFINITIVE CARE

Specialist care may be required to manage specific injuries identified during the initial assessment and investigation.

AIRWAY AND CERVICAL SPINE

Until the airway is secured and protected, the cervical spine should be stabilized by manual in-line immobilization as a cervical collar makes intubation difficult. Once the airway is securely protected, *triple immobilization with a stiff collar, head blocks and tape should be used until an unstable injury is excluded.*

Awareness

Head injury is the most common cause of airway compromise. As consciousness and muscle tone decrease, the pharynx and tongue obstruct the glottis.

Maxillofacial trauma can disrupt facial bones and this, with tissue swelling and bleeding, may obstruct the pharynx. These patients may need to sit up to open the airway.

Neck trauma causes haemorrhage and swelling, distorting and obstructing the airway. Tracheal intubation can be impossible and surgical alternatives are likely to be difficult.

Laryngeal trauma, heralded by hoarseness and coughing of bright red blood, may cause surgical emphysema and sudden airway obstruction.

Inhalational burns result in rapid swelling and airway obstruction, requiring early and expert intubation.

Recognition

Examine for signs of airway obstruction:

Look:
- Agitation, aggression, anxiety.
- Depressed level of consciousness.
- Cyanosis.
- Sweating.
- Use of accessory muscles of ventilation (tracheal tug and intercostal recession).

Listen:
- Noisy breathing.
- Stridor.
- Hoarse voice.
- Faint or absent sounds of breathing.

Feel:
- Reduced passage of air through mouth and nose.

Management

- *Chin lift*: lift the mandible forwards with fingertips.
- *Jaw thrust*: pull the mandible up and forwards, combined with BVM ventilation. Effective with small jaws, thick necks and in edentulous patients.
- *Oropharyngeal (OP) airway*: slide the airway above the tongue until the flange rests on the teeth. Use only in obtunded patients with absent gag reflexes.
- *Nasopharyngeal (NP) airway*: insert along the floor of the nasal cavity, with caution if a basal skull fracture is suspected.
- *Oropharyngeal suction*: clear secretions and blood.
- *Laryngeal mask airway (LMA)*: insert the LMA over the tongue into the oropharynx and inflate the cuff. This is effective, and requires less training than tracheal intubation. However, it does not protect the airway so it should be replaced with a tracheal tube.
- *Tracheal intubation*: orotracheal intubation is the preferred method for securing and protecting the airway, but it is a difficult procedure in un-anaesthetized casualties.
- *Needle cricothyroidotomy*: this is the insertion of a thin cannula through the cricothyroid membrane into the trachea to allow jet insufflation of the lungs with oxygen; it is used

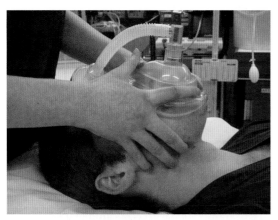

22.4 Jaw thrust with oxygen mask

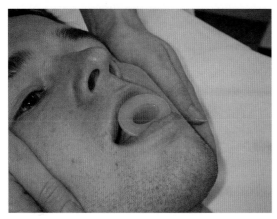

22.5 Oropharyngeal airway – correct position

in 'can't intubate, can't ventilate' situations. Oxygenation is achievable, but ventilation limited. Complications are misplacement, surgical emphysema and barotrauma. It should only be attempted if intubation has failed.

■ *Surgical cricothyroidotomy*: when orotracheal intubation fails, a tracheal tube can be inserted through the cricothyroid membrane into the trachea, thus enabling oxygenation and full ventilation. Complications include haemorrhage, damage to laryngeal structures, false passage formation, misplacement of the tracheal tube, surgical emphysema and barotrauma.

BREATHING AND CHEST INJURIES

Awareness

Only 10% of blunt chest injuries and 20% of penetrating injuries require thoracotomy. Non-surgical management involves supportive treatment and the insertion of chest drains.

Six immediately life-threatening injuries are recognized and managed during the primary survey, and eight potentially life-threatening injuries are sought during the secondary survey (see below).

Recognition

If, despite a clear airway, ventilation is inadequate the chest and surrounding areas should be carefully examined for signs of respiratory dysfunction.

Look:
■ Tachypnoea, laboured breathing and paradoxical respiration.
■ Cyanosis.
■ Plethora and petechiae.
■ Unequal chest inflation.
■ Bruising and contusions.
■ Penetrating chest injuries.
■ Distended neck veins.

Listen:
■ Absent breath sounds.
■ Noisy breathing/crepitations/stridor/wheeze.
■ Reduced air entry unilaterally.

Feel:
■ Tracheal deviation.
■ Tenderness.
■ Crepitus/instability.
■ Surgical emphysema.

Chest x-rays may be performed if the patient is not stable enough for CT. Severely injured patients are given supplemental oxygen and a blood sample is taken for measurement of the PaO_2 and $PaCO_2$.

Management of *immediately* life-threatening chest injuries

Administer high-flow oxygen and ventilate the lungs if breathing is absent or inadequate. Intubated trauma patients must be ventilated.

Tension pneumothorax

Air builds up under pressure in the pleural cavity, leading to collapse of the lung and shift of the mediastinum away from the affected side, obstructing venous return to the heart. This results in hypoxia and loss of cardiac output, and ultimately, pulseless electrical activity (PEA) cardiac arrest.

Diagnosis should be clinical, not radiological: absent breath sounds (*on* the side of the pneumothorax); hyper-resonance (*on* the side of the pneumothorax); deviated trachea (*away* from the side of the tension pneumothorax); surgical emphysema (chest and neck).

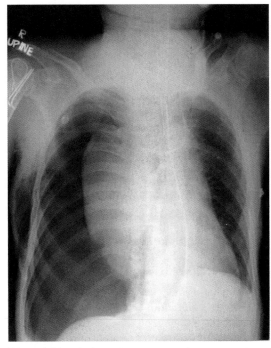

22.6 Right-sided tension pneumothorax

Immediately decompress the tension pneumothorax by inserting a large-bore cannula into the pleural cavity of the affected side, through the second intercostal space, in the midclavicular line. Follow with a wide-bore chest drain, or thoracostomies in an intubated and ventilated patient.

Open pneumothorax

An open wound in the chest wall will result in a simple pneumothorax. With a large defect, air is drawn into the pleural cavity rather than the lung, leading to hypoxia and hypercarbia. A flap valve effect can lead to a tension pneumothorax.

Apply an occlusive dressing, sealed on three sides, leaving the fourth side open to prevent tensioning.

Massive haemothorax

Up to 1500 mL (one-third of the blood volume) can rapidly accumulate in the chest following blunt or penetrating chest injury, leading to hypoxia and shock. Massive bleeds are more likely to require surgical repair and pulmonary lobectomy.

Diagnostic signs are hypoxia, reduced chest expansion, absent breath sounds, dullness to chest percussion, and hypovolaemic shock.

Treat by inserting a chest drain, correcting hypovolaemia and transfusing blood. If more than 1500 mL of blood is drained initially, or bleeding

continues at >200 mL/hour or the patient remains haemodynamically unstable, surgical referral and thoracotomy are indicated.

Cardiac tamponade

This is accumulation of blood within the pericardium resulting in a loss of cardiac output leading to PEA cardiac arrest. Is is more common with penetrating trauma between the nipple lines or scapulae.

Diagnostic signs are distended neck veins, muffled heart sounds, or a fall in arterial blood pressure/paradoxical pulse. Investigate by FAST, CT or transoesophageal echocardiogram.

Manage with clamshell thoracotomy and pericardiotomy. Immediate surgical repair of the myocardium may be required.

Flail chest

Multiple rib fractures damage the structural integrity of the chest wall; as the patient inspires, the flail segment is sucked in (paradoxical respiration). The injury causes a lung contusion resulting in hypoxia, further compromised by pain.

Diagnostic signs are: pain, tenderness and crepitus; fractured ribs on chest x-ray and hypoxia on estimating ABGs.

Manage initially with oxygen and analgesia. Patients may require early intubation and IV fluid restriction. Fractured ribs or costochondral disruption rarely requires surgical stabilization.

Disruption of tracheobronchial tree

Disruption of the tracheobronchial tree can result in a bronchopleural fistula, causing air to leak into the pleura and preventing inflation of the lung, even with a chest drain in situ.

Signs are persistent pneumothorax, pneumomediastinum, pneumopericardium, surgical emphysema and air below the deep fascia of the neck.

Selective endobronchial intubation of the opposite lung may be required.

Management of *potentially* life-threatening chest injuries

Simple pneumothorax

This results from air entering the pleural cavity, causing collapse of the lung and hypoxia. No mediastinal shift develops, and cardiac output is maintained. The cause is usually a lung laceration.

Diagnostic signs are absence or reduction of breath sounds and absent lung markings on chest x-ray. A simple pneumothorax can develop into a tension pneumothorax, precipitated by intubation and ventilation, use of nitrous oxide and air transport.

A chest drain should be inserted. This carries the potential complication of visceral damage, and trochars should not be used. Make a horizontal skin incision in the fifth intercostal space, above the sixth rib, just anterior to the midaxillary line; then bluntly dissect down to and through the pleura with forceps. A finger sweep will confirm entry into the empty pleura, and the chest tube can be introduced with forceps and connected to a valve or underwater drain.

Haemothorax

Smaller haemothoraces are normally self-limiting, and rarely require operative intervention. The only diagnostic sign is dullness to percussion, and this is not very reliable. A supine chest x-ray may show opacification, but may not reveal moderate amounts of blood. FAST or CT is more reliable.

Treatment is placement of a large-calibre basal chest drain. If drainage continues at more than 200 mL/hour, thoracotomy should be considered.

Pulmonary contusion

This is the commonest potentially life-threatening chest injury. Hypoxia is dependent on the extent of the contusion and pain. 50% of patients will develop bilateral acute respiratory distress syndrome (ARDS).

Pulmonary contusion may not be associated with obvious rib fractures, particularly in the young. The initial chest x-ray may not reveal the extent of the contusion, which can develop over 48 hours, and diagnosis depends on the mechanism of injury and hypoxia. The condition is managed supportively with oxygen administration and ventilation.

Tracheobronchial tree injury

This is a rare injury. Diagnostic signs are haemoptysis, surgical emphysema and persistent pneumothorax. CT may be diagnostic, but bronchoscopy may be required.

Treat initially with one or more large chest drains with or without a high-volume, low-pressure pump. Persistent bronchopleural fistulae may require operative intervention.

Blunt cardiac injury

This follows a direct blow to the anterior chest wall, associated with a fractured sternum. Myocardial contusion, chamber rupture and valvular disruption can result in hypotension, dysrhythmias and ventricular fibrillation.

Manage supportively and monitor for 24 hours when risk of dysrhythmia diminishes.

Aortic disruption

This occurs mostly in the proximal thoracic aorta. Specific clinical signs and symptoms are often absent, and the mechanism of injury should provoke suspicion. Chest x-ray shows a widened mediastinum with loss of the aortic knuckle and deviation of the trachea to the right, and CT is highly specific.

Manage supportively, and control blood pressure. Once the injury is confirmed, surgical repair is required.

Diaphragmatic injury

This is associated with blunt and penetrating trauma to the abdomen. Rupture is more common on the left, and rarely found in isolation, being associated with other chest, abdominal and pelvic injuries. Diaphragmatic ruptures associated with penetrating trauma result in a smaller tear.

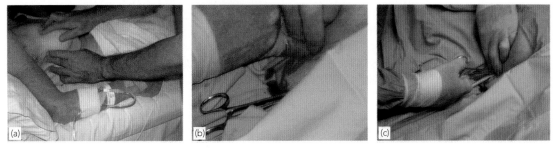

22.7 Chest drain insertion sequence (a) Identify entry point at the fifth intercostal space, just anterior to the midaxillary line. (b) Insert gloved finger through incision into chest cavity; sweep to ensure cavity is empty and the incision is above the diaphragm. (c) Introduce appropriately sized throacostomy tube through incision into chest cavity and attach the tube to an underwater drain. *X-ray to check lung re-inflation.*

Signs and symptoms can be subtle. Chest x-ray may show an elevated but indistinct hemidiaphragm, requiring CT.

Manage supportively, and consider chest drain insertion. Definitive treatment is surgical.

Mediastinal traversing wounds

Penetrating objects that cross the mediastinum may damage the lungs and mediastinal structures. The diagnosis is made by examination of the chest and trauma imaging. The significant finding is an entrance wound in one hemithorax and an exit wound or radiologically visible missile in the other.

Haemodynamically unstable patients should be assumed to have a haemothorax, tension pneumothorax or cardiac tamponade until proved otherwise.

Manage with bilateral chest drains. Stable patients should undergo extensive investigation with ultrasound, CT, angiography, oesophagoscopy and bronchoscopy as indicated, and early consultation with a cardiothoracic surgeon.

CIRCULATION – SHOCK

Shock is circulatory failure and inadequate perfusion of tissues with oxygenated blood, which leads to organ damage and death from multi-organ failure. Management comes after attention to the airway and breathing – unless there is catastrophic external bleeding for which control of the bleeding takes precedence.

Awareness

There are five types of shock:

- *Vasoconstrictive*:
  - Hypovolaemic.
  - Cardiogenic.
- *Vasodilative*:
  - Septic.
  - Neurogenic.
  - Anaphylactic.

Hypovolaemic shock, secondary to haemorrhage, is the most common. As the circulating blood volume decreases, compensatory mechanisms maintain systolic blood pressure up to around 30% blood loss in a fit patient. Above this, compensation increasingly fails until coma is followed by death at around 50% blood loss.

Cardiogenic shock occurs in trauma patients who have suffered a myocardial infarction, or direct myocardial injury.

Neurogenic shock is seen in high spinal cord transections.

Septic shock and *anaphylactic shock* are unusual in acute trauma.

Recognition

Diagnosis depends on a rapid assessment of the patient and assessment of vital signs; blood pressure and pulse alone are not adequate.

The patient becomes apathetic and thirsty; breathing is shallow and rapid; the lips and skin are pale and the extremities feel cold and clammy. As compensation fails, the pulse becomes rapid and feeble, the blood pressure drops and the patient may become confused. Eventually renal function is impaired and urinary output falls.

If it is difficult to measure the blood pressure reliably and repeatedly, continuous intra-arterial pressure monitoring should be instituted. Manual sphygmomanometry with a cuff and stethoscope is considerably more accurate than automated non-invasive blood pressure machines.

Hypovolaemic shock unresponsive to treatment is commonly due to bleeding into body cavities or potential spaces and can be identified by FAST or CT. Remember the epigram: '*Count bleeding onto the floor and four more*' (chest; abdomen; pelvis/retroperitoneum; long bones).

Management

Control bleeding: several methods are available; the choice depends upon the severity of blood

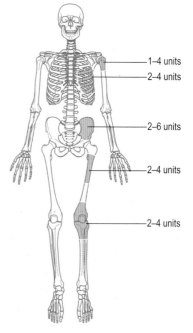

22.8 Severe injuries – blood loss in closed fractures The patient loses more blood than you think.

- 1–4 units
- 2–4 units
- 2–6 units
- 2–4 units
- 2–4 units

loss. Consider elevation and direct pressure; use of tourniquets; wound packing with haemostatic dressings; circumferential pressure dressings; intravenous administration of tranexamic acid (an antifibrinolytic agent). At all times maintain normothermia.

Secure vascular access: venous cannulation is usually appropriate. Site two large-bore cannulas. Central venous cannulation is associated with dangerous complications and should be avoided unless performed by an expert. Femoral vein cannulation is an option.

IO cannulation has superseded cut-down. Cannulae can be inserted through bone cortex into the marrow cavity of the tibia or the humeral head using an EZ-IO® driver and needle set.

Administer intravascular fluids: if blood is immediately available, or haemorrhage controlled, give 2 L of warmed Hartmann's (20 mL/kg in children) followed by transfusion. If bleeding is persistent and blood unavailable, give fluids in 250 mL boluses, titrated against a palpable radial pulse; this minimizes dilutional anaemia and increased bleeding as the blood pressure is restored. There is little evidence to support the use of colloids, and the role of hypertonic solutions has yet to be determined.

Titrate fluids against response, gauged by blood pressure, pulse rate, peripheral perfusion, central venous pressure (CVP) and measurement of metabolic acidosis.

Monitor the response to a fluid challenge. Rapid responders respond quickly and remain stable; transient responders respond and then deteriorate, causing significant on-going shock; non-responders show minimal or no response – suspect exsanguinating haemorrhage or other pathology, e.g. a tension pneumothorax.

Transfuse blood and blood products: transfuse blood, fresh frozen plasma and platelets in a ratio of 1:1:1 to maintain the haemoglobin above 10 g/dL. Regularly check haemoglobin, platelet count and clotting times. Consider giving clotting factors as advised by a haematologist.

The underlying cause of shock should be established and treated alongside resuscitative measures.

HEAD INJURIES

Most head injuries result from a blow that causes either direct damage or intracerebral movement due to rapid acceleration or deceleration. Damage may consist of: (1) minor contusion causing transient loss of consciousness or amnesia; (2) severe contusion or laceration, due either to direct injury or to shearing forces; (3) localized intracranial bleeding; (4) fractures of the skull; (5) diffuse oedema and a rise in intracranial pressure. High-velocity penetrating injuries (e.g. gunshot wounds) also cause diffuse and severe brain damage as the pressure wave moves across the brain.

The primary brain injury occurs at the time of the initial trauma from sudden distortion and shearing of brain tissue. Swelling and raised intracerebral pressure (ICP) are compounded by hypoxia, hypercarbia and hypotension. Extradural, subdural and intracerebral bleeding may contribute further to the rise in ICP. If the ICP is sustained above 20 mmHg, permanent brain damage can result; this is *the secondary brain injury*, which accounts for a significant number of fatalities.

When pressure compensation reaches its limit, the ICP rises exponentially causing uncal herniation with pupillary dilatation on the side of the injury. Ultimately, the cerebellum herniates through the foramen magnum, leading to brainstem death.

Prompt management of the ABCs helps to prevent these secondary changes.

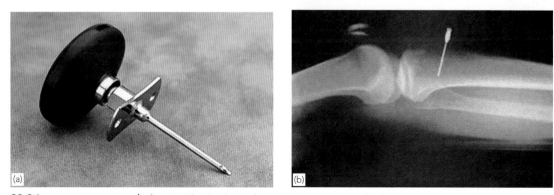

22.9 Intraosseous cannulation (a) The Cook paediatric intraosseous needle. (b) Intraosseous needle in place in the medial proximal tibia.

Awareness

In the UK, head injuries account for more than 50% of trauma deaths, following road traffic crashes, assaults and falls. These injuries can be classified into three groups based on the GCS:

- Mild:
  - GCS 13–15 (80% of cases).
  - 55% have mild disability at 1 year.
- Moderate:
  - GCS 9–12 (10% of cases).
  - 63% have significant disability at 1 year.
- Severe:
  - GCS 3–8 (10% of cases).
  - 85% have significant disability at 1 year.

Recognition

During the primary survey, assess the airway, cervical spine, breathing and circulation and *commence resuscitation before neurological assessment in order to limit the secondary brain injury.* Assess the GCS; examine the pupils for equality, diameter and response to light. With increased intracranial pressure and tentorial herniation, compression of the third nerve results in dilatation of the pupil and a failure to react to light.

Re-assess thoroughly during the secondary survey; look for lateralizing signs and motor and sensory deficits. Diagnostic signs of a basal skull fracture are otorhinorrhoea (cerebrospinal fluid [CSF] leakage from ear or nose), periorbital haematomas ('raccoon eyes'), subconjunctival haemorrhage without a posterior margin and retromastoid bruising (Battle's sign).

Open wounds should be gently explored with a gloved finger to exclude underlying skull fractures.

Patients suffering a severe head injury require an urgent CT. Specific indications include a drop

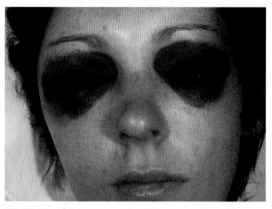

22.10 Head injury Periorbital haematomas ('racoon eyes') suggest the presence of a basal skull fracture.

in GCS, suspected skull fracture, seizures, focal neurological signs, vomiting and amnesia.

Management

Most head injuries are fairly trivial and require no more than careful examination and reassurance. The indications for admission to hospital for observation and reassessment are any of the following: (1) a diminished level of consciousness; (2) a history of transient loss of consciousness or amnesia; (3) a skull fracture; and (4) abnormal neurological signs.

In patients who appear to be comatose, drowsy, restless or merely confused it may be difficult to distinguish the effects of a head injury from those of hypoglycaemia, alcohol or drugs. All such patients, as well as those whose cerebral dysfunction may be due to shock or hypoxia, should be graded on the GCS and kept under observation until the diagnosis is clear. If there is any chance that the patient has suffered an intracranial bleed, a CT scan is urgent.

Concussion

Following a blow, there is a transient loss of consciousness, often associated with amnesia. However brief the period of unconsciousness, the skull should be x-rayed. If the patient was unconscious for only a few minutes and is now fully conscious, and a skull fracture has been excluded, they can be allowed to go home in the care of a responsible adult who will look after them for the next 48 hours. If this cannot be arranged, then they should be admitted for observation. Those with either a skull fracture or an impaired level of consciousness will also need a CT scan.

Scalp wounds

Scalp wounds (after thorough cleaning) can be sutured, provided there is no underlying depressed fracture.

Fractures

A linear fracture may be quite harmless, but a CT should be obtained to exclude intracranial damage or haematoma. If there is a CSF leak (otorrhoea or rhinorrhoea) the patient is given prophylactic benzyl penicillin. A depressed fracture requires exploration, elevation and clearance of damaged tissue.

Extradural haematoma

The classic scenario is of a patient who has a head injury but seems to be perfectly well, is allowed to go home and then rapidly becomes unconscious. There may be a minor fracture which causes bleeding and cerebral compression. Look for a fixed dilated pupil on the affected side. CT shows

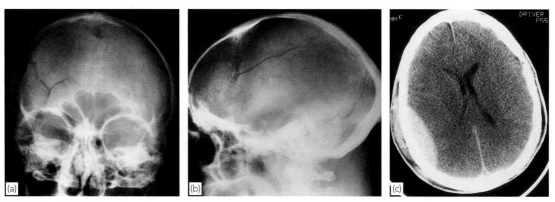

22.11 Head injuries – imaging (a,b) X-rays showing a fracture of the parietal bone. (c) The CT scan shows an extradural haematoma with distortion of the lateral ventricle on that side.

an extradural haematoma and a shift of the brain. This requires urgent treatment: burr holes and evacuation of the haematoma; if necessary, the middle meningeal artery is ligated.

Severe brain contusion

Patients with severe head injuries (a GCS score of 8 or less) require early intubation and ventilation with management on an intensive care unit (ICU) until recovery or brain death. Operative treatment may be required. The main indication for craniotomy is the development of an intracranial haematoma.

ABDOMINAL INJURIES

The immediately life-threatening injury is bleeding into the abdominal cavity.

Head injury: management

- Ensure exemplary oxygenation, normocapnia and normotension.
- *For mild head injury* (GCS 13–15): admission, monitoring and observation.
- CT and referral if deterioration is observed.
- *For moderate head injury* (GCS 9–12): CT and referral to neurosurgeon.
- *For severe head injury* (GCS 3–8): resuscitation, anaesthesia (rapid sequence induction) and intubation.
- Control of vascular filling pressures and CVP monitoring, and maintenance of arterial normotension.
- Early CT and referral to neurosurgeon; IV mannitol 0.5 mg/kg if advised.
- Urgent transfer to a specialist unit.

Awareness

Blunt abdominal trauma is a cause of avoidable death but is difficult to detect. Visceral rupture and laceration cause internal bleeding.

Penetrating injuries between the nipples and the perineum produce unpredictable damage, e.g. from tumbling and fragmenting bullet fragments. High-velocity rounds transfer kinetic energy to the viscera, causing cavitation and tissue destruction despite deceptively small entrance wounds. Look carefully for stab wounds; they may also be very small but they can penetrate deeply and damage several structures.

Recognition

During the primary survey inspect the abdomen for wounds, abrasions and contusions. Examine flanks, posterior abdomen, back, perineum and genitalia, and perform rectal examination. FAST has supplanted diagnostic peritoneal lavage. Early CT is indicated, but a shocked patient may need urgent transfer to surgery.

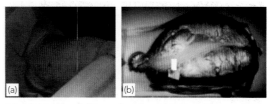

22.12 High velocity gun-shot injury (a) Entry wound. (b) Tissue cavitation.

Management

Control external bleeding and manage shock. If unresponsive, administer further fluid and transfuse blood. Pass a gastric tube and a urinary catheter unless signs of urethral injury are present.

Bleeding into the abdomen is an indication for

immediate laparotomy. The patient will require supportive critical care, and may require ventilation on an ICU.

MUSCULOSKELETAL INJURIES

In the absence of catastrophic bleeding, musculoskeletal injuries are not immediately life threatening, but they may be limb threatening, however.

PELVIC FRACTURES

Bleeding into the pelvis and retroperitoneum can result in non-responsive shock. Potential causes are road accidents, falls from a height or crush injuries.

The injury may be suspected during the primary survey as a cause of circulatory failure. Diagnostic signs are pelvic ring tenderness, leg shortening, swelling and bruising of the lower abdomen, the thighs, the perineum, the scrotum or vulva. Look for blood at urethral meatus. Obtain an anteroposterior (AP) x-ray and/or CT if the patient is stable.

Management

Treat shock. Position a pelvic compression device such as the SAM Sling™ around the pelvis at the level of the greater trochanters, and tighten as indicated. Once in place, do not remove this until surgical intervention is available. Developments in interventional radiology have enabled embolization to be used to control haemorrhage from a fractured pelvis.

SPINAL INJURIES

Indirect injuries are the most common, typically the result of falls or vehicular accidents. *Direct injuries*

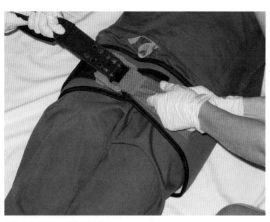

22.13 SAM Sling™ Ratcheted compression belt in use.

are usually associated with firearms and knives. There is an association of cervical spinal damage with all injuries above the clavicles, and 5% of head-injured patients have an associated spinal injury; 10% of those with a cervical spine fracture have a second, non-contiguous spinal fracture.

A high spinal transection will cause vasodilatory, neurogenic shock. Diagnostic signs are hypotension, low diastolic blood pressure, widened pulse pressure, bradycardia and warm, well-perfused extremities.

Spinal injuries are usually recognized during the secondary survey. Be careful to maintain immobilization throughout the examination; log-roll the patient to examine the vertebral column from neck to sacrum. Perform a rectal examination to assess anal tone, and identify loss of somatic sensory and motor function.

If the casualty is conscious, has no neck pain, has no distracting painful injury, is not intoxicated and has not received any analgesia, the cervical spine can be examined and a fracture clinically excluded to enable immobilization to be dispensed with. Obtain x-ray and/or CT during the secondary survey.

Management

In high spinal transections, the patient's respiratory function may be compromised, leading to ventilatory failure. This may require rapid sequence induction and ventilation by an experienced anaesthetist.

Neurogenic shock may need circulatory support with vasoconstrictors and chronotropes.

Spinal fractures and neurological deficit are managed by immobilization and referral to a spinal surgeon.

LONG-BONE INJURIES

Musculoskeletal injuries occur in 85% of patients sustaining blunt trauma. Although not immediately life threatening, they present a potential threat to life and threaten the integrity and survival of the limb. Crush injuries can lead to compartment syndrome, myoglobin release and renal failure.

Examine the patient from head to toe in all planes. Examine limbs but do not specifically elicit crepitus. Assess peripheral circulation and neurological status. Confirm the presence of pulses with Doppler ultrasound. Obtain x-rays as soon as the patient is stable.

Management

Control catastrophic haemorrhage. Reduce fractures and dislocations and splint in the anatomical position with the aid of procedural sedation (e.g. ketamine 0.5–1 mg/kg IV).

BURNS

Risk is highest in the 18–35 year age group; serious burns occur most frequently in children under 5 years. The mortality is 4% in burns centres, with a higher death rate in patients over 65 years.

Thermal burns

The threat to life arises through compromise of the airway, breathing and circulation.

Inhalation of super-heated gases and toxic smoke causes inhalational burns, smoke intoxication and carbon monoxide poisoning. Direct thermal injury is usually limited to the upper airway and can result in rapid airway obstruction. Smoke inhalation initiates an inflammatory reaction in the bronchioles, leading to bronchospasm, oedema and respiratory failure.

Carbon monoxide poisoning causes cerebral hypoxia and coma, due to the tight binding of carbon monoxide to the haemoglobin, forming carboxyhaemoglobin. Hydrogen cyanide can also be present, leading to profound tissue hypoxia.

Depth of burn is classified according to the degree and extent of tissue damage.

Burns are diagnosed during the primary survey, to determine immediately life-threatening airway injuries, respiratory failure, shock and coma. Blood carboxyhaemoglobin levels are assayed to quantify carbon monoxide poisoning. Diagnostic signs are facial burns, singed nasal hair, soot in the mouth or nose, hoarseness, carbonaceous sputum, expiratory wheezing and stridor.

Assess depth of the burn and the extent as a percentage of body surface area (BSA) using the 'rule of nines'. The palmar surface of the patient's hand,

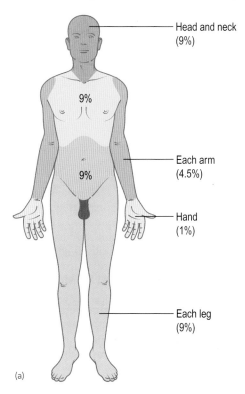

Head and neck (9%)

9%

9%

Each arm (4.5%)

Hand (1%)

Each leg (9%)

(a)

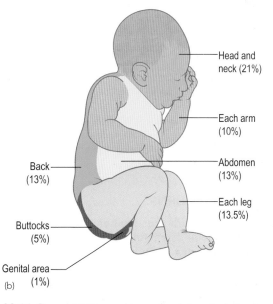

Head and neck (21%)

Each arm (10%)

Back (13%)

Abdomen (13%)

Each leg (13.5%)

Buttocks (5%)

Genital area (1%)

(b)

22.14 Burns (a) Extent of burns in adults – the 'rule of nines'. (*Note that the back of the thorax and the back of the lower torso each carry another 9%; the back of each arm carries another 4.5% and the back of each leg carries another 9%*). (b) Burn extents in infants differ markedly from those in adults.

Depth of burn		
■ *First degree:*	Epidermal	– reddening and pain without blistering.
■ *Second degree:*	Dermal	– superficial or deep partial-thickness with pain, blistering and variable skin damage.
■ *Third degree:*	Full thickness	– painless, charred, leathery with skin destruction.
■ *Fourth degree:*	Subcutaneous	– deep tissue destruction.

including the fingers, represents approximately 1% of the BSA. The values are different in infants since they have a disproportionately larger head and smaller lower limb surface areas.

Management

Secure the airway with anaesthetic support, and optimize oxygenation and ventilation. Temporarily relieve stridor with high-flow helium and oxygen (heliox).

Carboxyhaemoglobin levels may indicate the need for hyperbaric therapy and ventilation with 100% oxygen. Circumferential neck and chest burns may need to be incised to allow effective breathing and ventilation.

Support the circulation with warmed IV Hartmann's in partial and full-thickness burns patients with signs of shock, or a burn greater than 20% BSA. Calculate the volume and rate of fluid administration from the time of the burn according to the Parkland formula (Table 22.2).

Dress wounds with loose, clean, dry dressings, plastic sandwich wrap, specialized gel dressings or saline-moistened dressings. Patients with circumferential, deep burns of the limbs may develop eschars with compromise of the distal circulation requiring surgical escharotomy. Opioid analgesia will be required for partial-thickness burns in addition to cooling and dressing.

Involve a burns specialist for all patients with severe or unusual burns.

CHEMICAL BURNS

These occur with skin exposure to strong alkalis and acids. Full development is slower than that in thermal injury, so the true extent can initially be under-estimated.

Determine the chemical involved and its concentration. *Alkali burns* are often full-thickness and look pale, leathery and slippery. *Acid burns* are frequently partial-thickness and result in erythema and erosion.

Management

Minimize irreversible damage and maximize salvage of reversible damage. If dry powder is present, brush it off before irrigating with tap water. Do not use neutralizing agents. Make an urgent referral to a burns unit.

ELECTRICAL BURNS

These are caused by contact between an electrical source and earth. Severe electrical skin burns are associated with high-voltage shocks, whereas domestic, low-voltage shocks may cause death from ventricular fibrillation without superficial burning. Electrical muscle damage can result in rhabdomyolysis and renal failure.

The airway may be obstructed if the victim is unconscious and prolonged apnoea may follow paralysis of the respiratory muscles. The heart may arrest in ventricular fibrillation or asystole. Examine the entry and exit points, as the extent of underlying muscle damage may not be apparent.

Management

The immediate priority is personal safety. Secure the airway, protect the cervical spine and oxygenate and ventilate the casualty. Gain vascular access and administer fluids if the casualty is shocked or burnt more than 20% BSA. If cardiac arrest occurs, institute advanced life support (ALS). Monitor the heart for arrhythmias.

Tissue damage may need surgical debridement, and compartment syndrome may develop, requiring fasciotomies. Site a urinary catheter and test urine for myoglobinuria; treat with IV fluids and mannitol.

Consult early with burns and critical care specialists.

COLD INJURY AND BURNS

Cold injury can be systemic (hypothermia) or localized (tissue damage).

Hypothermia is a core temperature of below 35°C (95°F). Systemic effects depend on the degree of heat loss: as the core temperature

---

Table 22.2 Intravenous fluid requirements in partial- and full-thickness burn patients

ADULTS

Hartmann's or Ringer's lactate:

4 mL × weight (kg) × % BSA over initial 24 hours

Half over first 8 hours from the time of burn (other half over subsequent 16 hours)

CHILDREN

Hartmann's or Ringer's lactate:

3 mL × weight (kg) × % BSA over initial 24 hours plus maintenance

Half over first 8 hours from the time of burn (other half over subsequent 16 hours)

drops, conscious level deteriorates and the airway obstructs as coma ensues. Respiratory and cardiac functions deteriorate until respiratory and cardiac arrest result.

Localized cold injury is seen in three forms: frostnip; frostbite; and non-freezing injury.

Frostnip is reversible on warming.

Frostbite causes freezing and tissue damage; four degrees are recognized:

- First-degree frostbite: hyperaemia and oedema without skin necrosis.
- Second-degree frostbite: vesicle formation with partial-thickness skin necrosis.
- Third-degree frostbite: full-thickness and subcutaneous tissue necrosis, with haemorrhagic vesicle formation.
- Fourth-degree frostbite: deep necrosis, including muscle and bone.

Non-freezing injury presents as trench or immersion foot, with microvascular endothelial damage, stasis and vascular occlusion.

At the primary survey the patient is cold to the touch, looks grey and is peripherally cyanosed. A temperature probe will gauge the degree of hypothermia.

During the secondary survey local injuries are assessed. The affected part of the body initially appears hard, cold, white and anaesthetic.

Management

Hypothermia is treated by securing the airway, optimizing oxygenation and ventilation and treating shock with warmed IV fluids.

Re-warming depends on the degree of hypothermia: for mild and moderate hypothermia use passive and active external re-warming; for severe hypothermia and hypothermic cardiac arrest, active internal (core) re-warming including cardiopulmonary bypass, is needed.

Localized cold injury is managed by removing wet clothing, elevating and dressing the extremities. Rapid re-warming is the most effective therapy for frostbite. Surgical debridement may be required.

CRUSH SYNDROME

This is seen when a limb is compressed for extended periods, e.g. following entrapment in a vehicle or rubble. The crushed limb is under-perfused and myonecrosis follows, leading to the release of toxic metabolites when the limb is freed and so generating a re-perfusion injury. Reactive oxygen metabolites create further tissue injury. Membrane damage and capillary fluid re-absorption failure

result in swelling that may lead to a compartment syndrome, thus creating more tissue damage from escalating ischaemia. Tissue necrosis also causes systemic problems such as renal failure from free myoglobin, which is precipitated in the renal glomeruli. Myonecrosis may cause a metabolic acidosis with hyperkalaemia and hypocalcaemia.

Clinical features and treatment

The compromised limb is pulseless and becomes red, swollen and blistered; sensation and muscle power may be lost.

The most important measure is prevention. From an intensive care perspective a high urine flow is encouraged with alkalization of the urine with sodium bicarbonate; this prevents myoglobin precipitating in the renal tubules. If oliguria or renal failure occurs, then renal haemofiltration will be needed.

If a compartment syndrome develops, and is confirmed by pressure measurements, then a fasciotomy is indicated. Excision of dead muscle must be radical to avoid sepsis. Similarly, if there is an open wound then this should be managed aggressively. If there is no open wound and the compartment pressures are not high, then the risk of infection is probably lower if early surgery is avoided.

MULTIPLE ORGAN FAILURE

Multiple organ failure, or dysfunction syndrome (MODS), is the clinical manifestation of a severe systemic inflammatory reaction, following a triggering event such as trauma, infection, or inflammation. It develops in 5–15% of patients requiring ICU admission; it is now the commonest cause of long stays in surgical ICUs and the most frequent cause of death.

In its classical form (following severe sepsis) it manifests with pulmonary features of ARDS and is most likely to occur in elderly patients with poor health. Its pathogenesis is still unclear but it appears to be a disorder of the host defence system, involving an unregulated and exaggerated immune response which results in an excessive release of inflammatory mediators. It is these mediators that produce widespread microvascular damage leading to organ failure.

MODS usually progresses through four clinical phases: *shock* (hypoperfusion) – *active resuscitation* – *stable hypermetabolism* (systemic inflammatory response) – *organ failure*.

In the majority of critically ill patients who develop MODS the lungs are the first organs to fail; the other organs following in a sequential fashion. Dysfunction ranges from minor changes to massive alterations in pulmonary physiology – the hallmark of ARDS. Over a period of a few days the picture may change from pulmonary congestion to diffuse alveolar destruction. The early changes are reversible, but once diffuse alveolar damage occurs there is usually an inexorable progression to severe hypoxaemia. In the worst cases this is followed by multiple organ failure and death.

Clinical features

After a variable period following injury with hypovolaemic shock, the patient develops mild dyspnoea. Even before this, if blood gases are measured they may show a diminished PaO_2. These changes are common after long-bone fractures, and 'fat embolism' is often suspected.

By the second or third day the clinical features are more obvious: the patient is restless, with an increased pulse rate, oliguria, mild cyanosis and signs of respiratory distress. X-rays may now show diffuse pulmonary infiltrates. Special lung function tests are required to show the full extent of the condition.

In the most severe cases, by about 10 days postinjury, pulmonary deterioration is followed by liver failure and renal failure. The changes are irreversible and the outcome is fatal.

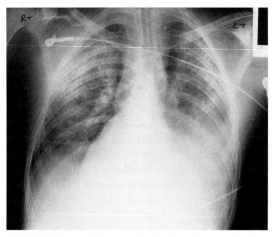

22.15 Adult respiratory distress syndrome X-ray showing diffuse pulmonary infiltrates in both lungs.

Treatment

The most important aspect of management is the early and effective treatment of shock. There is also evidence that – especially in patients with multiple injuries – measures such as the early stabilization of fractures, early excision of necrotic tissue, prompt treatment of infection and expert attention to nutritional requirements will reduce the incidence of pulmonary dysfunction and organ failure.

The treatment of established ARDS is supportive and aims to minimize further lung damage until recovery occurs, whilst optimizing oxygen delivery to the tissues. This requires highly specialized methods of artificial ventilation and continuous cardiopulmonary assessment in an intensive care facility.

THE FAT EMBOLISM SYNDROME

Circulating fat globules larger than 10 µm in diameter occur in most adults after closed fractures of long bones, and histological traces of fat can be found in the lungs and other internal organs. A small percentage of these patients develop clinical features similar to those of ARDS; this was recognized as the *fat embolism syndrome* long before ARDS entered the medical literature. Whether the fat embolism syndrome is an expression of the same condition or whether it is an entirely separate entity is still uncertain.

The source of the fat emboli is probably the bone marrow, and the condition is more common in patients with multiple fractures.

Clinical features

Early warning signs of fat embolism (usually within 72 hours of injury) are a slight rise of temperature and pulse rate. In more pronounced cases there is breathlessness and mild mental confusion or restlessness. Pathognomonic signs are petechiae on the trunk, axillae and in the conjunctival folds and retinae. In more severe cases there may be respiratory distress and coma, due to both brain emboli and hypoxia from involvement of the lungs. The features at this stage are essentially those of ARDS.

There is no infallible test for fat embolism; however, urinalysis may show fat globules in the urine and the blood PaO_2 should always be monitored; values below 8 kPa (60 mmHg or less) within the first 72 hours of any major injury must be regarded as suspicious. A chest x-ray may show classical changes in the lungs.

Management

Management of severe fat embolism is supportive. Symptoms can be reduced with the use of supplemental high inspired oxygen concentrations immediately after injury. Prompt stabilization of long-bone fractures also appears to reduce the likelihood of fat embolism occurring; this also allows the patient to be nursed in the sitting position, which optimizes the ventilation–perfusion match in the lungs. Intramedullary nailing is not thought to increase the risk of developing the syndrome.

CHAPTER 23

FRACTURES AND JOINT INJURIES

A fracture is a break in the structural continuity of bone. It may be no more than a crack, a crumpling or a splintering of the cortex; more often the break is complete and the bone fragments are displaced. If the overlying skin remains intact it is a *closed* (or *simple*) *fracture*; if the skin or one of the body cavities is breached it is an *open* (or *compound*) *fracture*, liable to contamination and infection.

Inevitably the surrounding soft tissues are involved as well. Changes range from local oedema and inflammatory reactions to severe soft-tissue damage and vascular impairment. Some of the most troublesome complications of fractures arise in joints which themselves appeared not to have been injured at the time.

When the joint itself is injured this may take the form of strained ligaments, *subluxation*, *dislocation* or *fracture–dislocation* (a combination of bone and joint injury).

PATHOLOGY OF FRACTURES

Bone is relatively brittle, yet it has sufficient strength and resilience to withstand the normal stresses of everyday activities. Fractures result from: (1) a single highly stressful, traumatic incident; (2) repetitive stress of normal degree persisting to the point of mechanical fatigue; or (3) normal stress acting on abnormally weakened bone (a so-called 'pathological' fracture).

CAUSES OF FRACTURES

Fractures due to sudden trauma

Most fractures are caused by sudden and excessive force, which may be direct or indirect. With direct force the bone breaks at the point of impact and the surrounding soft tissues are also damaged. With *indirect force* the bone breaks at a distance from where the force is applied: a common example is a fracture of the femoral neck due to a blow on the bended knee; soft-tissue damage at the fracture site is not inevitable.

Stress or fatigue fractures

Cracks can occur in normal bone, as in metal and other materials, due to repetitive stress. This is most often seen in the tibia or fibula or the metatarsals, especially in athletes, dancers and army recruits who go on long route marches.

Pathological fractures

Fractures may occur even with normal stresses if the bone has been weakened by a change in its structure (e.g. in osteoporosis, osteogenesis imperfecta or Paget's disease) or through a lytic lesion (e.g. a bone cyst or a metastasis).

TYPES OF FRACTURE

Fractures vary greatly in appearance but for practical purposes they can be divided into a few well-defined groups.

Complete fractures

The bone is completely broken into two or more fragments. The fracture pattern helps to tell how the fracture occurred and how it is likely to behave after reduction. If the fracture is *transverse*, the fragments usually remain in place after reduction; if it is *oblique* or *spiral*, they tend to slip and re-displace even if the bone is splinted. In an *impacted fracture* the fragments are jammed tightly together and the fracture line is indistinct. Double fractures in a long-bone diaphysis, leaving an isolated segment between the breaks, is called a *segmental fracture*. A *comminuted fracture* is one in which there are multiple fragments; because there is poor interlocking of the fragments, these fractures are inevitably unstable.

Incomplete fractures

Here the bone is incompletely divided and the periosteum remains in continuity. In a *greenstick fracture* the bone is buckled or bent (like snapping a green twig); this is seen in children, whose bones are more springy than those of adults. Reduction is usually easy and healing is quick. *Stress fractures* also may be incomplete, with the break initially appearing in only one part of the cortex; nevertheless, they take just as long to heal as complete fractures. *Compression fractures* occur when cancellous bone is crumpled. This is seen most typically in the vertebral bodies.

Physeal fractures

Fractures through the growing physis are a special case. Damage to the cartilaginous growth plate may give rise to progressive deformity out of all proportion to the apparent severity of the injury.

FRACTURE DISPLACEMENT

After a complete fracture the fragments usually become displaced, partly by the force of the injury, partly by gravity and partly by the pull of muscles attached to them. Displacement is usually described in terms of translation, alignment, rotation and altered length.

- *Translation (shift)*: the fragments may be shifted sideways, backwards or forwards in relation to each other, such that the fracture surfaces lose contact. The fracture will usually unite even if apposition is imperfect, and sometimes even if the bone ends lie side by side with the fracture surfaces making no contact at all (Figure 23.1(b)).
- *Alignment (angulation)*: the fragments may be tilted or angulated in relation to each other. If malalignment is marked the bend in the limb may be obvious; small degrees of malalignment are detected only by x-ray (Figure 23.1(d)).
- *Rotation (twist)*: long-bone fragments may be rotated in relation to each other; the bone looks straight but the limb ends up with a torsional deformity.
- *Length*: the fragments may be distracted and separated, or they may overlap, due to muscle spasm, causing shortening of the bone.

SOFT-TISSUE DAMAGE

Low-energy (low-velocity) fractures cause only moderate soft-tissue damage; the classic example is a closed spiral fracture. *High-energy (high-velocity)* fractures cause severe damage; examples are segmental and comminuted fractures, no matter whether open or closed. The state of the enveloping

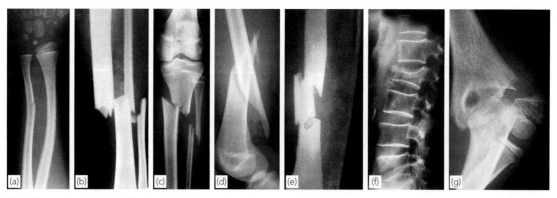

23.1 Common types of fracture (a) Incomplete ('greenstick') fracture of the ulna; (b) displaced transverse fracture; (c) oblique fracture; (d) spiral fracture, due to a twisting force – a typical low-energy fracture; (e) segmental fracture – a typical high-energy injury; (f) compression fracture, typically of an osteoporotic lumbar vertebra; and (g) avulsion fracture – in this case of the lateral condyle of the humerus, due to severe traction on the lateral ligaments of the elbow.

soft tissues has a significant effect on fracture healing. A full description of the fracture should therefore include comment on the soft tissues.

FRACTURE HEALING

Fractures heal by two different methods: with callus or without.

Healing by callus

The process of fracture repair varies according to the type of bone involved and the amount of movement at the fracture site. In a tubular bone, and in the absence of rigid fixation, 'natural' healing proceeds in five stages:

- *Tissue destruction and haematoma formation*: vessels are torn and a haematoma forms around and within the fracture. Bone at the fracture surfaces, deprived of a blood supply, dies back for a millimetre or two.
- *Inflammation and cellular proliferation*: within 8 hours of the fracture there is an acute inflammatory reaction with proliferation of mesenchymal stem cells under the periosteum and within the breached medullary canal. The fragment ends become surrounded by cellular tissue, which bridges the fracture site. The clotted haematoma is slowly absorbed and fine new capillaries grow into the area.
- *Callus formation*: the proliferating cells are potentially chrondrogenic and osteogenic; given the right conditions, they will start forming bone and, in some cases, also cartilage. The cell population also includes osteoclasts (probably derived from the new blood vessels) which begin to mop up dead bone. The thick cellular mass, with its islands of immature bone and cartilage, forms the *callus* (or splint) on the periosteal and endosteal surfaces. As the immature bone (or 'woven' bone) becomes more densely mineralized, movement at the fracture site decreases progressively and the fracture 'unites'. The entire process is driven by inductive proteins, which include fibroblast growth factors, transforming growth factors and bone morphogenetic protein.

- *Consolidation*: with continuing osteoclastic and osteoblastic activity the woven bone is transformed into lamellar bone. The system is now rigid enough to allow osteoclasts to burrow through the debris at the fracture line, and close behind them osteoblasts fill in the remaining gaps between the fragments with new bone. This is a slow process and it may be several months before the bone is strong enough to carry normal loads.
- *Re-modelling*: over time this natural 'weld' is re-shaped by a continuous process of alternating bone resorption and formation. Thicker lamellae are laid down where the stresses are high; unwanted buttresses are carved away; the medullary cavity is re-formed. Eventually, and especially in children, the bone reassumes something like its normal shape.

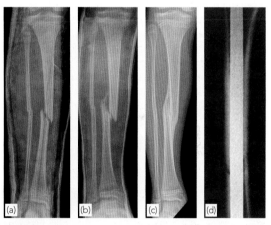

23.3 Fracture healing – x-rays (a–c) X-rays showing fracture healing by callus. (d) Healing with rigid internal fixation (intramedullary nail fitted snugly). In this case no callus is visible on x-ray.

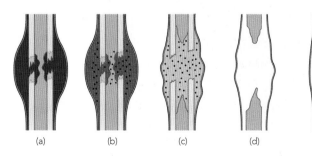

23.2 Fracture healing Five stages of healing. (a) *Haematoma*: tissue damage and bleeding at the fracture site: The bone ends die back for a few millimetres.
(b) *Inflammatory reaction*: inflammatory cells appear in the haematoma. (c) *Callus*: the cell population changes to osteoblasts and osteoclasts; dead bone is mopped up and woven bone appears in the fracture callus.
(d) *Consolidation*: woven bone is replaced by lamellar bone; the fracture has united.
(e) *Re-modelling*: the newly formed bone is re-modelled to resemble the normal structure.

Healing by direct union

Callus is the response to movement at the fracture site. It serves to stabilize the fragments as rapidly as possible – a necessary precondition for bridging by bone. If the fracture site is absolutely immobile (e.g. an impacted fracture in cancellous bone, or a fracture rigidly immobilized by internal fixation) there is no need for callus; instead, new bone formation occurs directly between the fragments. Gaps at the fracture surfaces are invaded by new capillaries and bone-forming cells growing in from the edges. Where the crevices are very narrow (less than 200 μm) osteogenesis produces lamellar bone; wider gaps are filled first by woven bone which is then re-modelled to lamellar bone (gap healing).

Healing by callus, though less direct, ensures mechanical strength while the bone ends heal. With rigid metal fixation, on the other hand, the absence of callus means that there is a long period during which the bone depends entirely upon the metal implant for its integrity. Moreover, the implant diverts stress away from the bone, which may become osteoporotic and not recover fully until the metal is removed.

Union, consolidation and re-modelling

Repair of a fracture is a continuous process and there are no specific events signifying a moment of 'union' or 'consolidation'.

Fracture union is considered to have occurred when the ensheathing callus is calcified. But this is still incomplete repair: though the bone moves in one piece, attempted angulation is still painful and x-ray examination shows that the fracture line is still visible. Repair is incomplete and it is unsafe to subject the unprotected bone to stress.

Consolidation defines the stage in which the callus becomes ossified. Clinically the fracture site is no longer tender, the bone feels rigid, attempted angulation is painless and x-rays show that the fracture line is almost obliterated by crossing trabeculae. Yet, although unprotected function is now safe, there may still be further re-modelling at the fracture site in response to loadbearing; only after the restoration of normal bone density is the process of repair complete.

Delayed union and non-union

Delayed union is when a fracture takes unusually long to heal. The rate of repair depends upon the *type of bone* involved (cancellous bone heals faster than cortical bone), the *type of fracture* (a transverse fracture takes longer than a spiral fracture), the state of the *blood supply* (poor circulation means slow healing), the patient's *general constitution* (healthy bone heals faster) and the patient's *age* (healing is almost twice as fast in children as in adults).

23.4 Fractures that fail to unite Some causes of non-union. (a,b) Excessive movement at the fracture site. Callus forms but the fracture gap cannot be bridged; this is shown more clearly in (b) the CT scan (hypertrophic non-union). (c) Too large a gap between the fracture ends with no attempt at healing (atrophic non-union). (d) Infection. (e) Abnormal bone, as in this case of congenital pseudarthrosis of the tibia.

Non-union is when a fracture fails altogether to unite. Causes are:

- Severe damage to soft tissues, rendering them non-viable (or nearly so).
- Distraction and separation of the fragments.
- Interposition of soft tissues between the fragments.
- Excessive movement at the fracture site.
- Poor local blood supply.
- Abnormal bone.
- Infection.

In such cases cell proliferation is predominantly fibroblastic; the fracture gap is filled by fibrous tissue and the bone fragments remain mobile, eventually creating a false joint or *pseudarthrosis*. In some cases callus formation starts off quite well; the fragment ends become thickened and even splayed, suggesting that periosteal new bone formation is florid but bridging of the fracture gap is prevented (*hypertrophic non-union*). Union is still possible provided the bone fragments are apposed and held immobile. In other cases, bone formation peters out altogether and what one sees on x-ray are the tapered ends of the fracture fragments with no sign of attempted bridging (*atrophic non-union*); the fragments will never unite unless they are immobilized and helped along with bone grafts.

Delayed union and non-union are discussed in more detail in Chapter 25.

CLINICAL FEATURES

History

There is usually a history of *injury*, followed by *inability to use the injured limb*. But beware! The fracture is not always at the site of the injury: a blow to the knee can obviously fracture the patella or the femoral condyles, but it may also fracture the shaft of the femur or even the acetabulum. The patient's age and the mechanism of injury are important. If a fracture occurs with trivial trauma, suspect a pathological lesion. *Pain, bruising* and *swelling* are common symptoms, but they do not distinguish a fracture from a soft-tissue injury. *Deformity* is much more suggestive. Remember also that some children with greenstick fractures and elderly people with impacted fractures of the femoral neck may experience little or no pain or loss of function.

Always enquire about symptoms of *associated injuries*: numbness or loss of movement, skin pallor or cyanosis, blood in the urine, abdominal pain, difficulty with breathing or transient loss of consciousness. A common mistake is to get distracted by the main injury, particularly if it is severe.

Once the acute emergency has been dealt with, ask about *previous injuries* or *any other musculoskeletal abnormality* that might cause confusion when the x-ray is seen. Finally, a *general medical history* is important, in preparation for anaesthesia or operation.

Examination

Unless it is obvious from the history that the patient has sustained a purely local injury, *priority must be given to dealing with the general effects of trauma* (see Chapter 22).

Injured tissues must be handled gently. To try and elicit crepitus or abnormal movement is unnecessarily painful; in any case, x-ray diagnosis is more reliable. Nevertheless, a systematic approach is essential, or damage to arteries, nerves, ligaments and viscera may be overlooked:

- Examine the most obviously injured part.
- Check for arterial damage.
- Test for nerve injury.
- Look for injuries of local soft tissues and viscera.
- Look for injuries in distant parts.

Look

Swelling, bruising and deformity may be obvious, but the important point is whether the skin is intact; even the smallest wound which communicates with the fracture makes it an 'open' injury and therefore vulnerable to infection. Check also whether the skin is stretched over a projecting fragment of bone; this needs special protection to prevent a closed fracture from turning into an open one.

Note also the posture of the distal extremity and the colour of the skin (for tell-tale signs of nerve or vessel damage).

Feel

The injured part is gently palpated for localized tenderness. Some fractures would be missed if not specifically looked for; e.g. the classical sign of a fractured scaphoid is tenderness in the anatomical snuffbox. The common and characteristic associated injuries also should be felt for even if the patient does not complain of them: e.g. an isolated fracture of the ulna may be associated with a dislocated head of radius. In high-energy injuries always examine the spine and pelvis. Vascular and peripheral nerve abnormalities should be tested for, both before and after treatment. If for any reason this cannot be done, it should be documented as such to avoid the assumption that nerve and vascular functions were intact after the injury.

Move

Crepitus and abnormal movement should be tested for only in unconscious patients. Usually it is more important to ask if the patient can move the joints distal to the injury.

Imaging

X-ray examination is mandatory. Remember the rule of twos:

- *Two views*: a fracture or a dislocation may not be seen on a single x-ray film; at least two views (anteroposterior and lateral) must be obtained.
- *Two joints*: the joints above and below the fracture must always be included on the x-ray images; they may be dislocated or fractured.
- *Two limbs*: a pre-existing constitutional abnormality may be mistakenly attributed to the recent injury; and in children, the appearance of immature epiphyses may confuse the diagnosis of a periarticular fracture. X-rays of the uninjured limb are essential for comparison.
- *Two injuries*: severe force often causes injuries at more than one level. Thus, with fractures of the calcaneum or femur it is important also to x-ray the pelvis and spine.
- *Two occasions*: some fractures are notoriously difficult to detect soon after injury, but another x-ray examination a week or two later may show the lesion. Common examples are undisplaced fractures of the distal end of the clavicle, the scaphoid, the femoral neck and the lateral malleolus, and also stress fractures and physeal injuries wherever they occur.

Computed tomography (CT) and *magnetic resonance imaging (MRI)* are useful for displaying fracture patterns in 'difficult' sites such as the vertebral

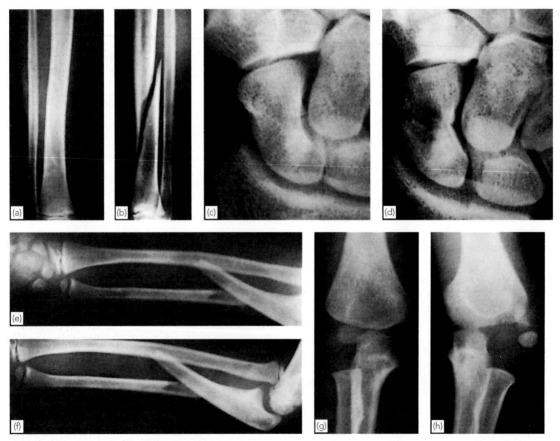

23.5 X-ray examination – the rule of twos X-ray examination must be adequate. (a,b) *Two films* of the same tibia: the fracture may be 'invisible' in one view and perfectly plain in another at right angles to that. (c,d) *Two occasions*: a fractured scaphoid may not be obvious on the day of injury, but clearly seen 2 weeks later. (e,f) *Two joints*: the first x-ray (e) did not include the elbow. This was, in fact, a Monteggia fracture – the head of the radius is dislocated (f). (g,h) *Two limbs*: often the abnormality can be appreciated only by comparison with the normal side; in this case there is a fracture of the lateral condyle of the left humerus (h).

column, the acetabulum and the calcaneum. Three-dimensional reconstructed images are even better. *MRI* may be the only way of showing whether a fractured vertebra is threatening to compress the spinal cord. *Radio-isotope scanning* is helpful in diagnosing a suspected stress fracture or other 'occult' fractures.

Secondary injuries

Certain fractures are apt to cause secondary injuries and *these should always be assumed to have occurred until proved otherwise*.

- *Thoracic injuries*: fractured ribs or sternum may be associated with injury to the lungs or heart. It is essential to check cardiorespiratory function.
- *Spinal cord injury*: with any fracture of the spine, neurological examination is essential: (a) to establish whether the spinal cord or nerve roots have been damaged; and (b) to obtain a baseline for later comparison if neurological signs should change.
- *Pelvic and abdominal injuries*: fractures of the pelvis may be associated with visceral injury. Enquire about urinary function and look for blood at the urethral meatus. Diagnostic urethrograms or cystograms may be necessary.
- *Pectoral girdle injuries*: fractures and dislocations around the pectoral girdle may damage the brachial plexus or the large vessels at the base of the neck. Neurological and vascular examinations are essential.

Testing for fracture union

It is impossible to tell from clinical and x-ray features alone precisely when the bone fragments have joined. What is more important – and what the patient wants to know – is: (a) whether the fracture shows progressive signs of healing; and (b) whether the bone is strong enough to withstand normal loading. Encouraging signs are absence of pain during daily activities, absence of local tenderness, absence of pain on gently stressing the fracture, no hint of mobility at the fracture site and x-ray signs of bone bridging across the fracture site.

Of course, if the fracture has been internally fixed all these criteria may be satisfied and the fracture still not united. Callus formation is usually sparse with internal fixation and one may have to wait for definite x-ray signs of trabecular continuity before declaring the fracture united. Even then it is wise to wait for several more months before removing the fixation implants.

FRACTURES IN CHILDREN

Fractures in growing bones are subject to influences which do not apply to adult bones:

- In very young children the bone ends are largely cartilaginous and therefore do not show up in x-ray images. Fractures at these sites are therefore difficult to diagnose: always x-ray both limbs (for comparison) and an ultrasound scan may be helpful.
- Children's bones are less brittle, and more liable to plastic deformation, than those of adults; hence the frequency of cortical 'buckling' and 'greenstick' fractures.
- In childhood the periosteum is thicker than in adult bones; this may explain why fracture displacement is more controlled. Cellular activity is also more marked, which is why children's fractures heal so much more rapidly than those of adults. The younger the child, the quicker the rate of union. Femoral shaft fractures in infants will heal within 3 weeks, and in young children in 4–6 weeks, compared to 14 weeks or longer in adults.
- Non-union is very unusual in children's fractures.
- Bone growth involves considerable modelling and re-modelling, processes which determine both structure and form. This makes for a great capacity to re-shape fracture deformities (*other than rotational deformities*) over time.
- Injuries of the physis have no equivalent in adults. Damage to the growth plate can have serious consequences however rapidly and securely the fracture might heal.

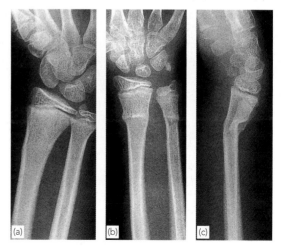

23.6 Fractures in children Childhood fractures are often incomplete: (a) *buckle* or *torus* fracture of the distal third of the radius; (b,c) *greenstick* fractures of the distal ends of the radius and ulna.

INJURIES OF THE PHYSIS

Over 10% of childhood fractures involve injury to the growth plate (or physis). Because this is a relatively weak part of the bone, injuries that cause ligament strains in adults are liable to disrupt the physis in children. The fracture usually runs transversely through the hypertrophic (calcified) layer of the growth plate, often veering off towards the shaft to include a triangular piece of the metaphysis. This has little effect on longitudinal growth, which takes place in the germinal and proliferating layers of the physis. However, if the fracture traverses the cellular 'reproductive' layers of the plate, it may result in premature ossification of the injured part and cessation of growth or deformity of the bone end.

Classification

The most widely used classification of physeal injuries is that of Salter and Harris, which distinguishes five basic types of injury:

- *Type 1*: a transverse fracture through the hypertrophic or calcified zone of the plate. Even if the fracture is quite alarmingly displaced, the growing zone of the physis is usually not injured and growth disturbance is uncommon.
- *Type 2*: this is similar to Type 1, but towards the edge the fracture deviates away from the physis and splits off a triangular piece of metaphyseal bone. Growth is usually not affected.
- *Type 3*: this fracture runs partly along the physis and then veers off through all layers of the physis and the epiphysis into the joint. Inevitably the reproductive zone of the physis is damaged and this may result in growth disturbance.
- *Type 4*: as with Type 3, this fracture splits the epiphysis, but it continues through the physis into the metaphysis. The fracture is particularly liable to displacement and a consequent misfit

between the separated parts of the physis, resulting in asymmetrical growth.
- *Type 5*: a longitudinal compression injury of the physis. There is no visible fracture but the growth plate is crushed and this may result in growth arrest.

Clinical features

Physeal fractures usually result from falls or traction injuries; they occur mostly in road accidents and during sport or playground activities and are more common in boys than in girls. Deformity is usually minimal, but any injury in a child followed by pain and tenderness near the joint should arouse suspicion, and x-ray examination is essential.

X-rays

The physis itself is radiolucent and the epiphysis may be incompletely ossified; this makes it hard to tell whether the bone end is damaged or deformed. The younger the child, the smaller the 'visible' part of the epiphysis and thus the more difficult it is to make the diagnosis; comparison with the normal side is a great help. Telltale features are widening of the physeal 'gap', incongruity of the joint or tilting of the epiphyseal axis. If there is marked displacement the diagnosis is obvious, but even Type 4 fractures may at first be so little displaced that they are hard to see; *if there is the faintest suspicion of a physeal fracture, a second x-ray examination after 4 or 5 days is essential.* Type 5 injuries are usually diagnosed only in retrospect.

Treatment

Undisplaced fractures

These may be treated by splinting the part in a cast or a close-fitting plaster slab for 2–4 weeks (depending on the site of injury and the age of the child). However, *with Type 3 and 4 fractures, a*

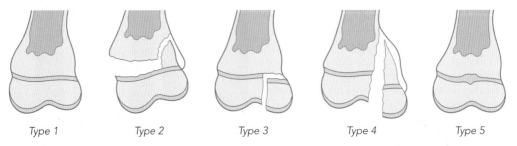

| Type 1 | Type 2 | Type 3 | Type 4 | Type 5 |

23.7 Physeal injuries *Type 1* – separation of the epiphysis. *Type 2* – fracture through the physis and metaphysis (the commonest type). *Type 3* – here the fracture runs along the physis and then veers off into the joint, splitting the epiphysis. *Type 4* – vertical fracture through the epiphysis and the adjacent metaphysis. *Type 5* – crushing of the physis without visible fracture.

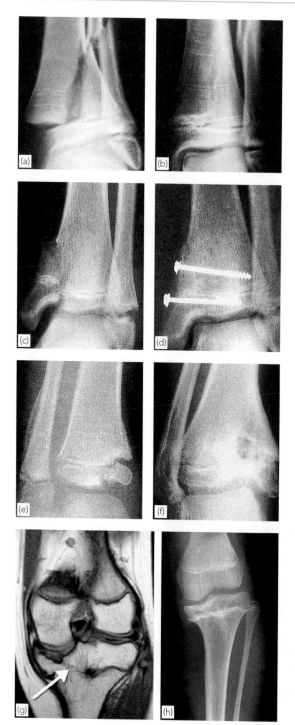

check x-ray after 4 days and again at about 10 days is mandatory in order not to miss late displacement.

Displaced fractures

Displaced fractures must be reduced as soon as possible. With Types 1 and 2 this can usually be done closed; the part is then splinted securely for 3–6 weeks. Type 3 and 4 fractures demand perfect anatomical reduction. An attempt can be made to achieve this by gentle manipulation under general anaesthesia; if this is successful, the limb is held in a cast for 4–8 weeks (the longer periods for Type 4 injuries). Here again, check x-rays at about 4 and 10 days are essential to ensure that the position has been retained. If a Type 3 or 4 fracture cannot be reduced accurately by closed manipulation, immediate open reduction and internal fixation with smooth K-wires is called for. The limb is then splinted for 4–6 weeks, but it takes that long again before the child is ready to resume unrestricted activities.

Complications

Premature fusion

Type 1 and 2 injuries, if properly reduced, usually have an excellent prognosis and bone growth is not adversely affected. Exceptions to this rule are injuries involving the distal femoral and proximal tibial physes; both are undulating in shape, so a transverse fracture may pass through several zones in the physis and result in a focal point of fusion.

Type 3, 4 and 5 injuries are more likely to cause *premature fusion* of part of the growth plate, resulting in *cessation of growth* or *asymmetrical growth and deformity* of the bone end. The size and position of the bony bridge across the physis can be assessed by CT or MRI. If it is relatively small (less than one-third the width of the physis) it can be excised and replaced by a fat graft, with some prospect of preventing or diminishing the growth disturbance. However, if the bone bridge is more extensive, the operation is contraindicated and the remaining part of the physis is closed surgically; the resulting deformity or length discrepancy will have to be dealt with later by osteotomy and/or operative correction of limb length.

23.8 Physeal injuries – x-ray (a) Typical Type 2 injury; after reduction (b) bone growth is normal. (c,d) This Type 4 fracture of the tibial physis was treated immediately by open reduction and internal fixation, giving an excellent result. (e,f) By contrast, in this case accurate reduction was not achieved and the physeal fragment remained displaced; the end result was partial fusion of the physis and severe deformity of the ankle. (g) MRI showing a localized bony bar across the medial part of the proximal tibial physis (arrow). (h) Another case, involving the proximal tibia, in which the plain x-ray shows the deformity caused by lagging growth on the medial side.

Deformity

Established deformity, whether from asymmetrical growth or from malunion of a displaced fracture (e.g. a valgus elbow due to proximal displacement or non-union of a lateral humeral condylar fracture) should be treated by corrective osteotomy. If further growth is abnormal, the osteotomy may have to be repeated.

'SPONTANEOUS' FRACTURES IN CHILDREN

Fractures following minimal trauma may be due to unusual genetic disorders (e.g. osteogenesis imperfecta, which is described in Chapter 8). It is obvious, however, that infants cannot say what happened to them and one should keep in mind the possibility that they may be victims of deliberate injury (the 'battered baby' syndrome). Suspicious features are an unconvincing history, multiple fractures in different stages of healing and bruises elsewhere on the body. X-rays may show florid callus formation, mimicking the appearances of osteomyelitis or scurvy.

STRESS FRACTURES AND INSUFFICIENCY FRACTURES

A *stress or fatigue fracture* is one occurring in the normal bone of a healthy patient. It is caused not by a specific traumatic incident but by unaccustomed or repetitive loading of the bone. This is most likely to occur in new army recruits, athletes in training and ballet dancers. *Insufficiency fractures* are those that occur following minimal trauma to bones that are inherently weaker than normal, typically osteoporotic and osteomalacic bones.

Sites affected

Sites usually affected are the metatarsal bones (the so-called *march fracture*), the distal shaft of fibula (*runner's fracture*), the proximal half of the tibia, the femoral neck, the pubic rami, the pars interarticularis of the fifth lumbar vertebra and the ala of the sacrum.

Clinical features

There may be a history of unaccustomed and repeated activity. A common sequence of events is

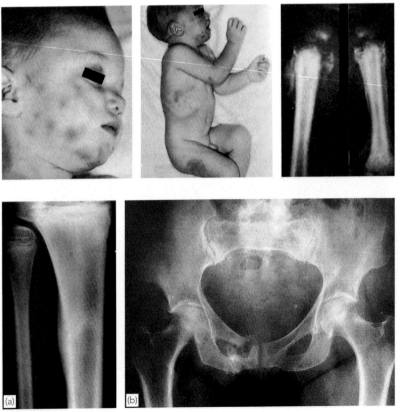

23.9 The battered baby syndrome Note the multiple bruises and bilateral metaphyseal fractures with marked callus formation.

23.10 Stress fractures Stress fractures are often missed or wrongly diagnosed. (a) This tibial fracture was at first thought to be an osteosarcoma; even the biopsy was confusing. (b) Stress fractures and 'insufficiency fractures' in elderly people can be mistaken for metastases (of the pubic rami on the right side in this case).

pain after exercise → pain during exercise → pain without exercise. Occasionally the patient presents only after the fracture has healed, leaving a tender lump on the bone.

Imaging

At first the fracture is difficult to detect, but *radioscintigraphy* will show increased activity at the painful spot. A few weeks later *x-rays* may show a small transverse defect in the cortex and, later still, localized periosteal new-bone formation. These appearances have occasionally been mistaken for those of an osteosarcoma, a horrifying trap for the unwary. *CT* and *MRI* may be helpful in dubious cases.

Diagnosis

Many disorders, including osteomyelitis, scurvy and the battered baby syndrome, can be confused with stress fractures. The great danger, however, is a mistaken diagnosis of osteosarcoma; scanning shows increased uptake in both conditions and even biopsy may be misleading.

Missed diagnosis is even more common than incorrect diagnosis. When dealing with elderly osteoporotic patients, sudden pain in the back, the sacroiliac region or the hip should alert one to the possibility of an insufficiency fracture. Likewise with younger individuals who develop pain in the foot, leg or thigh after stressful activity.

Treatment

Most stress fractures need no treatment other than an elastic bandage and avoidance of the painful activity until the lesion heals; surprisingly, this can take many months and the enforced inactivity is not easily accepted by the hard-driving sportsperson or dancer.

An important exception is a stress or insufficiency fracture of the femoral neck. If the diagnosis is confirmed by bone scan, CT or MRI, the femoral neck should be internally fixed as a prophylactic measure.

PATHOLOGICAL FRACTURES

When abnormal bone gives way this is referred to as a pathological fracture. The causes are numerous and varied (*Table 23.1*). Often the diagnosis is not made until a biopsy is examined.

Table 23.1 Causes of pathological fracture

Local benign conditions	Generalized bone disease
Chronic infection	Osteogenesis imperfecta
Solitary bone cyst	Postmenopausal osteoporosis
Fibrous cortical defect	Metabolic bone disease
Chondromyxoid fibroma	Myelomatosis
Aneurysmal bone cyst	Polyostotic fibrous dysplasia
Chondroma	Paget's disease
Monostotic fibrous dysplasia	Hypercortisonism

Primary malignant tumours	Metastatic tumours
Chondrosarcoma	Carcinoma in breast, lung,
Osteosarcoma	kidney, thyroid, colon,
Ewing's tumour	prostate

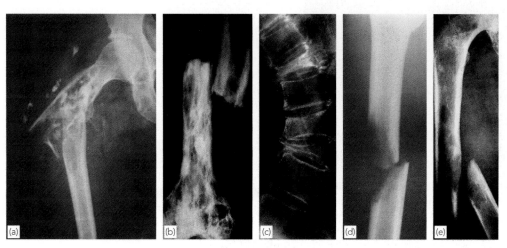

23.11 Pathological fractures Fractures due to: (a) primary chondrosarcoma; (b) Paget's disease; (c) vertebral metastases; (d) metastasis in the midshaft of the femur; and (e) myelomatosis.

Clinical features

Bone that fractures spontaneously or after trivial injury must be regarded as abnormal until proved otherwise. Under the age of 20 years the common causes are benign bone tumours and cysts. Over the age of 40 years the common causes are metabolic bone disease, myelomatosis, secondary carcinoma and Paget's disease. Ask about previous illnesses or operations: a history of gastrointestinal disease, chronic alcoholism or prolonged corticosteroid therapy should suggest a metabolic bone disorder; a malignant tumour, no matter how long ago it occurred, may be the source of a late metastatic lesion.

Local signs of bone disease should not be missed. *General examination* may show features suggestive of hypercortisonism or Paget's disease, or generalized tissue wasting due to malignant disease.

X-rays

Understandably, the fracture itself attracts most attention. But the surrounding bone must also be examined and features such as cyst formation, cortical erosion, abnormal trabeculation and periosteal thickening should be sought. The type of fracture, too, is important: vertebral compression fractures may be due to severe osteoporosis or osteomalacia, but they can also be caused by skeletal metastases or myeloma. Radio-isotope scans may reveal deposits elsewhere in the skeleton, where further imaging studies can be concentrated.

Special investigations

Investigations should include a full blood count, erythrocyte sedimentation rate, protein electrophoresis and tests for metabolic bone disease. Urinalysis may reveal blood from a tumour or Bence–Jones protein.

Biopsy

Some lesions are so typical that a biopsy is unnecessary (solitary cyst, fibrous cortical defect, Paget's disease). Others are more obscure and a biopsy is essential for diagnosis. If open reduction of the fracture is indicated, the biopsy can be done at the same time; otherwise a definitive procedure should be arranged.

Treatment (see also Chapter 9)

The principles are the same as for other fractures, though the choice of method will be influenced by the condition of the bone. The underlying pathological disorder may also need treatment in its own right.

Generalized bone disease

In most of these conditions (including Paget's disease) the bones fracture more easily, but they heal quite well provided the fracture is properly immobilized. Internal fixation is therefore advisable (and for Paget's disease almost essential); this also reduces the risk of re-fracture. Patients with osteomalacia, hyperparathyroidism, renal osteodystrophy and Paget's disease may need systemic treatment as well.

Local benign conditions

Fractures through benign cyst-like lesions usually heal quite well and they should be allowed to do so before tackling the underlying lesion. Treatment is therefore the same as for simple fractures in the same area, although in some cases it will be necessary to take a biopsy before immobilizing the fracture. When the bone has healed, the tumour can be dealt with by curettage or local excision.

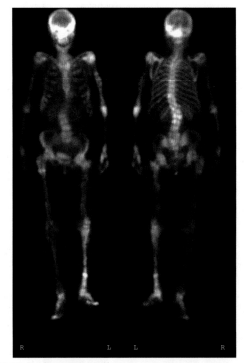

23.12 Radioscintigraphy Isotope bone scans can identify 'hidden' bone lesions. In this patient with polyostotic fibrous dysplasia, multiple sites of involvement ('hot spots') are seen in the skull, spine, pelvis, right proximal femur, left humerus, left distal radius and left tibia.

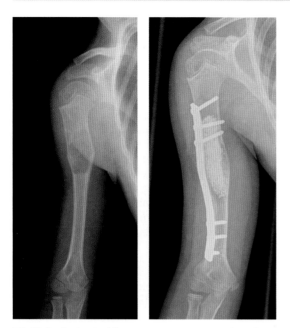

23.13 Pathological fractures – treatment Discrete bone lesions may require local treatment through curettage and bone grafting (here a bone substitute was used) and internal fixation.

Primary malignant tumour

The fracture may need splinting but this is merely a prelude to definitive treatment of the tumour, which by now will have spread to the surrounding soft tissues. The prognosis depends on the type of tumour. Limb-sparing surgery is often possible with modern endoprosthetic replacements.

Metastatic tumours

Metastasis is a frequent cause of pathological fracture in older people. Breast cancer is the commonest source and the femur the commonest site. Nowadays cancer patients (even those with metastases) often live for several years and effective treatment of the fracture will vastly improve their quality of life. Preoperatively, imaging studies should be performed to detect other bone lesions; these may be amenable to 'prophylactic' fixation.

Fracture of a long-bone shaft should be treated by internal fixation; intramedullary nails are more suitable than plates and screws and, if necessary, the site is also packed with acrylic cement. This may be followed by local irradiation.

Fracture near a bone end can often be treated by excision and prosthetic replacement, especially in the case of femoral neck fracture.

Pathological compression fractures of the spine cause severe pain. This is due largely to spinal instability and treatment should include operative stabilization. If there are clinical or imaging features of actual or threatened spinal cord or cauda equina compression, the affected segment should be decompressed; postoperative irradiation may also be needed.

Pre-emptive surgery

Prophylactic fixation of a localized deposit may forestall the difficulties of dealing with a

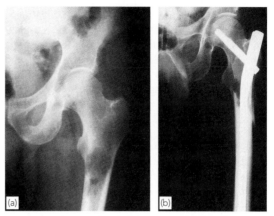

23.14 Pathological fractures – treatment (a) This patient with a secondary deposit below the lesser trochanter was advised to have 'prophylactic' nailing. In the event, the bone actually fractured during the operation (b).

pathological fracture. Once the wound has healed, local irradiation should be applied to reduce the risk of progressive osteolysis.

JOINT INJURIES

Joints are usually injured by twisting or tilting forces that stretch the ligaments and capsule. If the force is great enough the ligament will tear, or the bone to which it is attached may be pulled apart. The articular cartilage, too, may be damaged if the joint surfaces are compressed or if there is a fracture into the joint.

As a general principle, forceful angulation will tear the ligaments rather than crush the bone, but in older people with osteoporotic bone the ligaments may hold and the bone on the opposite side of the joint is crushed instead; in children there may be a fracture–separation of the physis.

SPRAINS AND STRAINS

There is much confusion about the use of the terms 'sprain', 'strain' and 'rupture'. In clinical parlance a *sprain* is any painful wrenching (twisting or pulling) of a joint, short of actual tearing of the ligaments or capsule. *Strain* is more specific: it implies stretching or microscopic tearing of some fibres in the ligament. If the force is great enough, the ligament may be strained to the point of complete *rupture*.

Sprained joint

A twisted joint is painful but there is little or no swelling or bruising. In superficial joints, tenderness can sometimes be localized to a particular ligament. In deep joints, and in the neck and back, it is usually impossible to tell whether it is the ligaments or the muscles which have been injured.

Treatment consists of reassurance and, most importantly, encouragement of movement and exercise from the outset.

Strained ligament

The joint is momentarily twisted or bent into an abnormal position. Some of the fibres in the ligament are torn (perhaps only microscopically) but the joint remains stable. The patient presents with pain, swelling and bruising around one or other aspect of the joint. Tenderness is localized to the injured ligament and stretching the tissues on that side causes a sharp increase in pain.

Treatment

The joint should be firmly strapped and rested until the acute pain subsides. Ice packs and non-steroidal anti-inflammatory medication are helpful if swelling is marked. As soon as pain permits, active movements and muscle-strengthening exercises are encouraged.

Following strains around the knee and ankle there is often a tendency for the joint to give way repeatedly due to unexpected pain rather than true instability. The patient should be warned about this and shown how to protect the ligament during weightbearing.

Ruptured ligament

The ligament is completely torn and the joint is unstable. Hinge joints (the knee, ankle, fingers and thumb) are more vulnerable than others.

As with a strain, the joint is suddenly forced into an abnormal position; sometimes the patient actually hears a snap. Pain is severe and there may be considerable bleeding under the skin; if the joint is swollen, this is probably due to a haemarthrosis. The patient is unlikely to permit a searching examination, but under general anaesthesia instability can be demonstrated by stressing the joint; it is this that distinguishes the lesion from a strain. If the ligament is avulsed rather than torn, x-ray examination may show a detached flake of bone.

Treatment

A torn ligament will heal spontaneously by fibrosis if it is held without tension for 4–6 weeks. However, scarring is diminished and strength improved by early movement. Treatment aims to encourage these natural processes.

Most ligament ruptures can be treated non-operatively. Initially, measures will be needed to control pain and swelling: these are splintage of the joint, ice packs and non-steroidal anti-inflammatory medication. A tense haemarthrosis should be aspirated. After 1 or 2 weeks the splint can usually be exchanged for a functional brace that allows joint movement but at the same time prevents repeated injury to the ligament. Physiotherapy is applied to maintain muscle strength and later proprioceptive exercises are added. If residual instability causes a problem, reconstructive surgery can be undertaken at a later stage.

This non-operative approach has produced better results than were formerly achieved with more aggressive early operative repair, not only in the strength of the healed ligament but in the nature of healing – there is less fibrosis. Exceptions to this rule are: (a) when the ligament is avulsed with an attached

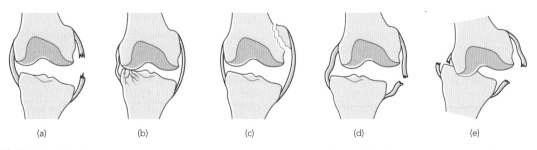

(a)   (b)   (c)   (d)   (e)

23.15 Joint injuries Severe stress and strain may cause various types of injury. (a) A ligament may rupture, leaving the bone intact. If the soft tissues hold, the bone on the opposite side may be crushed (b), or a fragment of bone may be pulled off by the taut ligament (c). (d) Subluxation. (e) Dislocation.

piece of bone: if the fragment is large enough, it should be re-attached; and (b) when dealing with a joint that relies entirely on ligamentous continuity for stability (e.g. the metacarpophalangeal joint of the thumb): this is best treated by early operative repair of the ruptured ligament.

DISLOCATION AND SUBLUXATION

'Dislocation' means that the joint surfaces are completely displaced and are no longer in contact; 'subluxation' implies a lesser degree of displacement, such that the articular surfaces are still partly apposed.

Clinical features

Following an injury the joint is painful and the patient tries at all costs to avoid moving it. The shape of the joint is abnormal and the bony landmarks may be displaced. The limb is often held in a characteristic position; movement is painful and restricted. X-rays will usually clinch the diagnosis; they will also show whether there is an associated bony injury affecting joint stability – i.e. a fracture–dislocation.

If the dislocation is reduced by the time the patient is seen, the diagnosis may be in doubt. This is where the *apprehension test* is useful. The joint is stressed it as if almost to reproduce the suspected dislocation: the patient develops a sense of impending disaster and violently resists further manipulation.

Recurrent dislocation

If the ligaments and joint margins are damaged, repeated dislocation may occur. This is seen especially in the shoulder and the patellofemoral joint.

Habitual (voluntary) dislocation

Some patients acquire the knack of dislocating (or subluxating) the joint by voluntary muscle contraction. Ligamentous laxity may make this easier, but the habit often betrays a manipulative and neurotic personality. It is important to recognize this because such patients are seldom helped by operation.

Treatment

The dislocation must be reduced as soon as possible; usually a general anaesthetic is required, and sometimes a muscle relaxant as well. The joint is rested or immobilized until soft-tissue healing occurs – usually after 2 or 3 weeks – and this is followed by a course of physiotherapy. Occasionally surgical reconstruction is called for if the joint remains unstable.

Complications

Complications such as vascular injury, nerve injury, avascular necrosis of bone, heterotopic ossification, joint stiffness and secondary osteoarthritis are the same as those following fractures and are dealt with in Chapter 25.

CHAPTER 24

FRACTURES – PRINCIPLES OF TREATMENT

Treat the patient, not only the fracture: that is the first injunction. The principles are discussed in Chapter 22.

Treatment of the fracture consists of *manipulation* to improve the position of the fragments, followed by *splintage* to hold them together until they unite; meanwhile, joint *movement* and function must be preserved. Fracture healing is promoted by muscle activity and bone loading, so *exercise* and early *weightbearing* are encouraged. These objectives are covered by three simple rules: REDUCE! HOLD! EXERCISE!

CLOSED FRACTURES

REDUCE

Although general treatment and resuscitation must always take precedence, there should be no undue delay in attending to the fracture; swelling of the soft parts during the first 12 hours makes reduction increasingly difficult. However, there are some situations in which reduction is unnecessary: (1) when there is little or no displacement; (2) when displacement does not initially matter (e.g. in some fractures of the clavicle); and (3) when reduction is unlikely to succeed (e.g. with compression fractures of the vertebrae).

Reduction should aim for *adequate apposition* and *normal alignment* of the bone fragments. The greater the contact surface area between fragments the more likely is healing to occur; a gap between the fragments is a common cause of delayed union or non-union. However, so long as the fragments are in contact and properly aligned, some overlap

at the fracture surfaces is permissible; the exception is a fracture involving an articular surface, which should be reduced as near to perfection as possible.

Reduction may be 'closed' or 'open'.

Closed reduction

Closed manipulation is suitable for all minimally displaced fractures, for most fractures in children and for fractures that are likely to be stable after reduction. Unstable fractures are sometimes reduced 'closed' prior to mechanical fixation.

Under anaesthesia and muscle relaxation, the fracture is reduced by a threefold manoeuvre: (1) the distal part of the limb is pulled in the line of the bone; (2) as the fragments disengage, they are repositioned (by reversing the original direction of force if this can be deduced); and (3) alignment is adjusted in each plane. This is most effective when the periosteum and muscles on one side of the fracture remain intact; the soft-tissue strap prevents over-reduction and stabilizes the fracture after it has been reduced.

Some fractures (e.g. of the femoral shaft) are difficult to reduce by manipulation because of counterforces exerted by powerful muscles. Often, however, they can be reduced by sustained mechanical traction, which then serves also to hold the fracture until it starts to unite. This method was widely employed in the past but with modern technical improvements it has fallen out of favour.

Open reduction

Operative reduction under direct vision is indicated: (1) when closed reduction fails, either because of difficulty in holding the fragments together

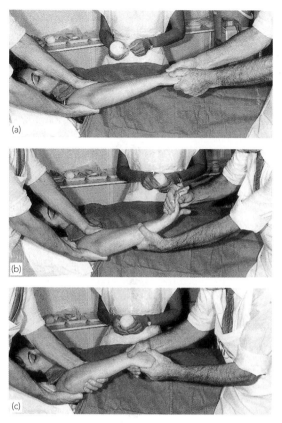

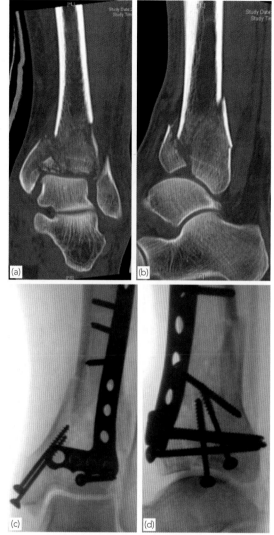

24.1 Closed reduction (a) Traction and countertraction. (b) Manipulation to disimpact the fragments. (c) Pressing the distal fragment into the reduced position.

24.2 Open reduction (a,b) Displaced fractures of a major joint surface need precise reduction.
(c,d) Postoperative x-rays. Fractures stabilized by plates and screws.

or because soft tissues are interposed between them; (2) when there is a large articular fragment that needs accurate positioning; (3) for avulsion fractures in which the fragments are held apart by muscle pull; (4) when an operation is needed for associated injuries (e.g. arterial damage). Generally open reduction is the first step to internal fixation.

HOLD

The word 'immobilization' is avoided because the objective is seldom complete immobility; usually it is the prevention of displacement. Some restriction of movement is also needed to alleviate pain, to promote soft-tissue healing and to allow free movement of the unaffected parts. *The aim is to splint the fracture, not necessarily the entire limb.*

The available methods of holding reduction are: (1) sustained traction; (2) cast splintage; (3) functional bracing; (4) internal fixation; and (5) external fixation.

Closed methods are most suitable for fractures with intact soft tissues (the muscles surrounding a fracture act as a fluid compartment; traction or compression creates a hydraulic effect that is capable of splinting the fracture) and are liable to fail if they are used for fractures with severe soft-tissue damage. Other contraindications to non-operative methods are inherently unstable fractures, multiple fractures and fractures in confused or unco-operative patients.

Sustained traction

Traction is applied to the limb distal to the fracture, so as to exert a continuous pull in the long axis of the bone. In most cases a counterforce will be needed to prevent the patient simply being dragged along the bed. The method is particularly useful for spiral fractures of long-bone shafts, which are easily displaced by muscle contraction. The hold is obviously not perfect, but traction is safe (provided it is not excessive); the bone is gradually pulled out to length and meanwhile the patient can move their joints and exercise their muscles. The problem is *speed* (or rather lack of it): not because the fracture unites slowly (it does not) but because sustained lower limb traction keeps the patient in bed for a long time, thus increasing the likelihood of complications such as thromboembolism, respiratory problems and general weakness. For this reason sustained traction is best avoided in elderly patients, and even in younger patients traction should be replaced by cast splintage or functional bracing as soon as the fracture becomes 'sticky' (deformable but not displaceable). There are several ways of applying traction.

Traction by gravity is suitable only for upper limb injuries. Thus, with a wrist sling the weight of the arm provides continuous traction to the humerus. For comfort and stability, a U-slab of plaster may be bandaged on or, better, a removable plastic sleeve from the axilla to just above the elbow is held on with Velcro (humeral bracing).

Skin traction will sustain a pull of no more than 4 or 5 kg. Holland strapping or one-way stretch Elastoplast is stuck to the shaved skin and held on with a bandage. The malleoli are protected by Gamgee tissue, and cords or tapes are used for traction.

Skeletal traction can withstand much greater force and is therefore used mainly for lower limb injuries. A stiff wire or pin is inserted – usually behind the tibial tubercle for hip, thigh and knee injuries, or through the calcaneum for tibial fractures – and cords are attached to them for applying traction.

Whether by skin or skeletal traction, the fracture is reduced and held in one of three ways: fixed traction, balanced traction or a combination of the two. In *fixed traction* the limb is held in a Thomas's splint, the traction cords are tied to the distal end of the splint while the proximal padded ring of the splint abuts firmly against the pelvis. This method is particularly useful when the patient has to be transported. With *balanced traction* the cords

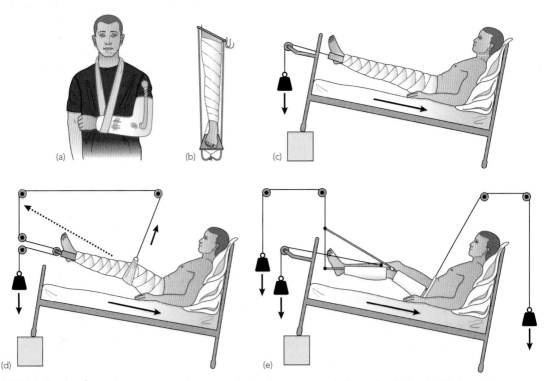

24.3 Methods of traction (a) Traction by gravity. (b–d) Skin traction, which may be (b) fixed, (c) balanced or (d) Russell traction. (e) Skeletal traction with a splint and a knee flexion piece.

are guided over pulleys at the foot of the bed and loaded with weights; counter-traction is provided by the weight of the body when the foot of the bed is raised. The limb is usually supported, both for comfort and to prevent sagging at the fracture site, in a type of cradle – Thomas's splint for the femur or Braun's frame for the tibia. In *combined traction* the tapes are tied to the end of the splint and the entire splint is then suspended, as in balanced traction.

Note: sustained traction does carry certain risks. In children especially, traction tapes and circular bandages may constrict the circulation; for this reason 'gallows traction', in which the baby's legs are suspended from an overhead beam, should never be used for children over 12 kg in weight. In older people, leg traction may predispose to peroneal nerve injury and cause a drop-foot; the limb should be checked repeatedly to see that it does not roll into external rotation during traction. If skeletal traction is used, the pin sites must at all times be kept clean and checked for infection.

Cast splintage

Plaster of Paris (or one of the newer lightweight substitutes) is still widely used as a splint, especially for distal limb fractures and for most children's fractures. It is safe enough, so long as one is alert to the danger of a tight cast and provided pressure sores are prevented. The speed of union is neither greater nor less than with traction, but the patient can go home sooner.

Holding reduction is usually no problem if the correct fracture type is chosen for cast splintage and patients with tibial fractures can bear weight on the cast. However, joints encased in plaster cannot move and are liable to stiffen; this can be minimized by: (a) *delayed splintage* – that is, by using traction until movement has been regained, and only then applying plaster – or (b) using the cast till the limb can be handled without too much discomfort and then replacing it with a functional brace which permits joint movement. The technique of applying a plaster cast is shown in Figure 24.4.

Complications

Tight cast – the cast may be put on too tightly, or it may become tight if the limb swells. The patient complains of diffuse pain; only later – sometimes much later – do the signs of vascular compression appear. The limb should be elevated, but if the pain does not subside during the next hour the only safe course is to split the cast, ease it open throughout its length and cut through all the padding down to skin. Whenever swelling is anticipated the cast should be applied over thick padding and then split before it sets, so as to provide a firm but not absolutely rigid splint.

Pressure sores – even a well-fitting cast may press upon the skin over a bony prominence (the patella, the heel, the elbow or the head of the ulna). The patient complains of localized pain precisely over the pressure spot. Such localized pain demands immediate inspection through a window in the cast.

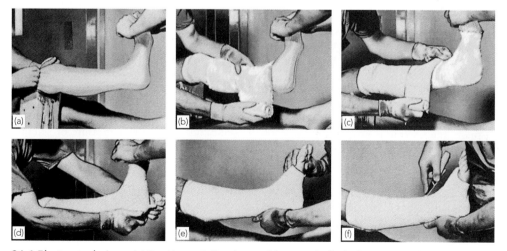

24.4 Plaster technique (a) Stockinette is fitted smoothly on to the limb. (b) For a padded plaster, wool-bandage is rolled on and it must be even. (c) Plaster is next applied smoothly, taking a tuck with each turn, and (d) smoothing each layer firmly on to the one beneath. (e) While still wet, the cast is moulded away from the bony points. (f) With a recent injury, the plaster should then be split to avoid compression by swelling.

Skin abrasion or laceration – this is really a complication of removing the cast, especially if an electric saw is used. Complaints of nipping or pinching during plaster removal should never be ignored.

Loose cast – once the swelling has subsided, the cast may no longer hold the fracture securely. If it is loose the cast should be replaced.

Functional bracing

Functional bracing, using either plaster of Paris or one of the lighter materials, is one way of preventing joint stiffness while still permitting fracture splintage and loading. Segments of a cast are applied only over the shafts of the bones, leaving the joints free; cast segments above and below a joint can be connected by metal or plastic hinges which allow movements in one plane. The splints are 'functional' in that joint movements are less restricted than with conventional casts.

Functional bracing is used most widely for fractures of the femur or tibia but, since the brace is not very rigid, it is usually applied only when the fracture is beginning to unite, i.e. after 3–6 weeks of traction or restrictive splintage. Used in this way, this method comes out well on all of the basic requirements: the fracture can be *held* reasonably well; the joints can be *moved*; the fracture joins at normal *speed* without keeping the patient in hospital and the method is *safe*.

Internal fixation

Bone fragments may be fixed with screws, transfixing pins or nails, a metal plate held by screws, a long intramedullary rod or nail (with or without locking screws), circumferential bands, or a combination of these methods.

Properly applied, internal fixation holds a fracture securely so that movements can begin at once; with early movement the 'fracture disease' (stiffness and oedema) is abolished. *Speed* is not an issue; the patient can leave hospital as soon as the wound is healed, but even though the bone moves in one piece, the fracture is not united – it is merely held by a metal bridge and unprotected weightbearing is, for some time, unsafe.

The greatest *danger*, however, is sepsis; if infection supervenes, all the manifest advantages of internal fixation (precise reduction, immediate stability and early movement) may be lost. The risk of infection depends upon: (1) the patient – devitalized tissues, a dirty wound and an unfit patient are all dangerous; (2) the surgeon – thorough training, a high degree of surgical dexterity and adequate assistance are all essential; and (3) the facilities – a guaranteed aseptic routine, a full range of implants and staff familiar with their use are all indispensable.

Indications for internal fixation

- Fractures that cannot be reduced except by operation.
- Fractures that are inherently unstable and prone to re-displacement after reduction (e.g. midshaft fractures of the forearm and some ankle fractures).
- Fractures that unite poorly and slowly, principally fractures of the femoral neck.
- Pathological fractures, in which bone disease may prevent healing.
- Multiple fractures, where early fixation reduces the risk of general complications.
- Fractures in patients who present severe nursing difficulties.

More controversial is the use of internal fixation as a preferred, rather than a necessary, form of treatment. The introduction of reliable image-guided techniques for 'closed' reduction and nailing of long-bone fractures has gained wide acceptance as an alternative to more difficult and cumbersome non-operative methods.

Types of internal fixation

Screws – interfragmentary screws (lag screws) are useful for fixing small fragments onto the main bone.

Wires – stiff, Kirschner wires (often inserted percutaneously without exposing the fracture) can hold fracture fragments together. They are used in situations where fracture healing is predictably quick; some form of external splintage (usually a cast) is applied as supplementary support.

Plates and screws – this form of fixation is useful for treating both tubular and flat bones. When used on tubular bones, firm coaption of the fragments can be achieved by compression devices before tightening the screws. Recently there has been a move towards using long plates that span the fracture and length of the bone, thus achieving a measure of stability without totally sacrificing the biological (and callus producing) effect of some movement.

Plates can also be shaped; e.g. buttress plates are often used to prop up the overhang of an expanded metaphysis, as in fixing fractures of the proximal tibial plateau.

In tension-band plating the plate is applied on the tensile surface of the bone, thus allowing compression to be applied to the biomechanically more advantageous side of the fracture.

Antiglide plates have also come into use: by

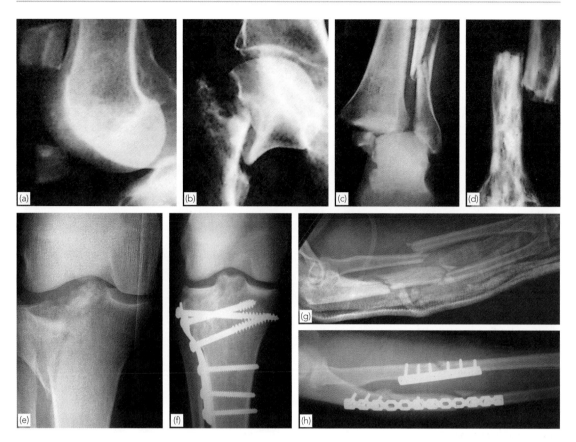

24.5 Indications for open reduction and internal fixation (a) Traction lesions with wide separation of fragments as in this patellar fracture. (b) Fractures that unite poorly, e.g. of the femoral neck. (c) Fractures that are inherently unstable and prone to re-displacement. (d) Pathological fractures. (e,f) Large fragments involving a joint surface. (g,h) Fractures that are very difficult to reduce and likely to re-displace after reduction.

fixing the plate over the tip of a spiral or oblique fracture and then using the plate as a reduction aid, the anatomy can be restored with minimal stripping of soft tissues. The position of the plate acts to prevent shortening and therefore displacement of the fragments.

Intramedullary nails – these are suitable for long bones. A nail (or long rod) is inserted into the medullary canal to splint the fracture; rotational forces are resisted by introducing *locking screws* which transfix the bone cortices and the nail proximal and distal to the fracture. Nails can be used with or without prior reaming of the medullary canal; reaming achieves an interference fit which

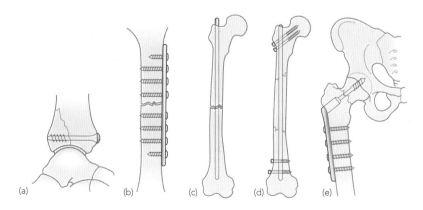

24.6 Types of internal fixation (a) A single interfragmentary screw. (b) Plate and screws. (c) Intramedullary nail. (d) Locked intramedullary nail. (e) Dynamic hip screw.

further improves fracture stability, though at the expense of some damage to the intramedullary blood supply.

Complications of internal fixation

Most of the complications of internal fixation are due to poor technique, poor equipment or poor operating conditions.

Infection: iatrogenic infection is now the most common cause of chronic osteomyelitis; the metal does not predispose to infection but the quality of the patient's tissues and the open operation do. If the infection is not rapidly controlled by intravenous antibiotic treatment, the implants should be replaced with some form of external fixation.

Non-union: causes of non-union are excessive stripping of the soft tissues, unnecessary damage to the blood supply in the course of operative fixation and rigid fixation with a gap between the fragments.

Implant failure: metal is subject to fatigue, and undue stresses should therefore be avoided until the fracture has united. Patients with femoral or tibial fractures should still use crutches until there are signs of fracture healing (6 weeks at least). Pain at the fracture site is a danger signal!

Re-fracture: it is important not to remove metal implants too soon, or the bone may re-fracture; a year is the minimum and 18 or 24 months safer. For several weeks after implant removal the bone is weak, so full weightbearing should be avoided.

External fixation

The principle of external fixation is simple: the bone is transfixed above and below the fracture with screws or pins or tensioned wires and these are then clamped to a frame, or connected to each other by rigid bars. There are numerous variations in fixation devices and techniques of applying them, providing different degrees of rigidity and stability. All of them permit adjustment of length and angulation, and some allow reduction of the fracture in all three planes. This is especially applicable to the long bones and the pelvis, but the method can be used for fractures of almost any part of the skeleton.

Indications

■ Fractures associated with severe soft-tissue damage where internal fixation is risky, or to allow the wound to be left open for inspection, dressing or definitive coverage.

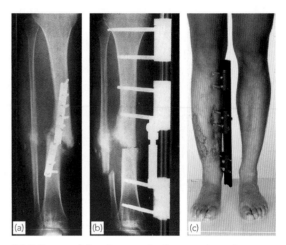

24.8 External fixation (a) The fracture shown here was fixed with a plate and screws but it did not unite. (b) The sclerotic fracture surfaces were excised, leaving a gap, which was dealt with by external fixation and bone transport. (c) The patient was able to walk about while the fracture healed.

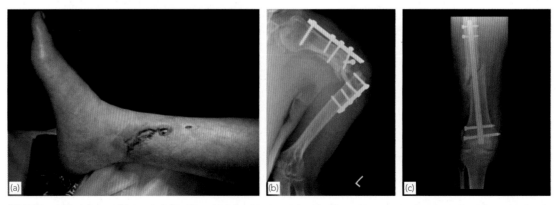

24.7 Complications of internal fixation (a) Infection is a risk with all operations – in this case after plating a distal tibial fracture. (b) If union is long delayed, the implant may develop a fatigue fracture. (c) With rigid internal fixation the fracture may still fail to unite if the fragments are not properly apposed.

- Severely comminuted and unstable fractures, which can be held out to length while healing.
- Patients with multiple severe fractures.
- Fractures of the pelvis, which often cannot be controlled quickly by any other method.
- Fractures associated with major vessel damage.
- Infected fractures, for which internal fixation might not be suitable.
- Ununited fractures which require bone reconstruction.

Complications of external fixation

Damage to soft-tissue structures by transfixing pins or wires. Nerves or vessels may be inadvertently injured, or ligaments may be tethered. The surgeon must be thoroughly familiar with the cross-sectional anatomy before operating.

Over-distraction may prevent contact between the fragments, making union unlikely.

Pin-track infection is unlikely with good operative technique; nevertheless, meticulous pin-site care is essential, and antibiotics should be administered immediately if infection occurs.

EXERCISE

More correctly, 'restore function' – not only to the injured parts but also to the patient as a whole. The objectives are to reduce oedema, preserve joint movement, restore muscle power and guide the patient back to normal activity.

Prevention of oedema

Swelling is almost inevitable after a fracture and may cause tissue tension and blistering. It is also an important cause of joint stiffness, especially in the hand, and should be prevented or treated energetically by a combination of elevation and active exercises. The patient should be encouraged to use the limb (within reason) and to keep moving the joints that are free. The essence of soft-tissue care may be summed up thus: *elevate and exercise; never dangle, never force.*

Active exercise

Active movement, in addition to reducing oedema, stimulates the circulation, prevents soft-tissue adhesion and promotes fracture healing. Even a limb encased in plaster is capable of muscle contraction and the patient should be taught how to do this. When splintage is removed, joint movement is increased and muscle-building exercises encouraged. The unaffected joints also need exercising; it is all too easy to neglect a stiffening shoulder while caring for an injured hand.

Assisted movement

It has long been taught that passive movement can be deleterious, especially with injuries around the elbow where there is a high risk of developing myositis ossificans. Certainly forced movements should never be permitted, but gentle assistance during active exercises helps to retain function or regain movement after fractures involving the articular surfaces. Nowadays this is done with machines that can be set to provide a specified range and rate of movement (*continuous passive motion*).

Functional activity

As the patient's mobility improves, an increasing amount of directed activity is introduced. He or she may need to be taught again how to perform everyday tasks such as walking, getting in and out of bed, bathing, dressing or handling eating utensils. Experience is the best teacher and the patient is encouraged to use the injured limb as much as possible. Those with very severe or extensive injuries may benefit from spending time in a special rehabilitation unit. But the best incentive to full recovery is the promise of re-entry into family life, recreational pursuits and meaningful work.

OPEN FRACTURES

INITIAL MANAGEMENT

Many patients with open fractures have multiple injuries and severe shock; for them, appropriate treatment at the scene of the accident is essential. After splinting the limb, the wound should be covered with a sterile dressing or clean material and left undisturbed until the patient reaches the accident department. This will reduce the risk of further contamination and wound desiccation.

In hospital a rapid general assessment is the first step, and any life-threatening conditions are addressed (see Chapter 22). Tetanus prophylaxis is administered: toxoid for those previously immunized, human antiserum if not. Antibiotics should be given once the diagnosis of an open fracture is confirmed – the sooner the better. This is usually co-amoxiclav or cefuroxime, but clindamycin if the patient is allergic to penicillin.

The wound is carefully inspected; ideally it should be photographed with a Polaroid or digital camera, so that it can again be kept covered until the patient is in the operating theatre. Important

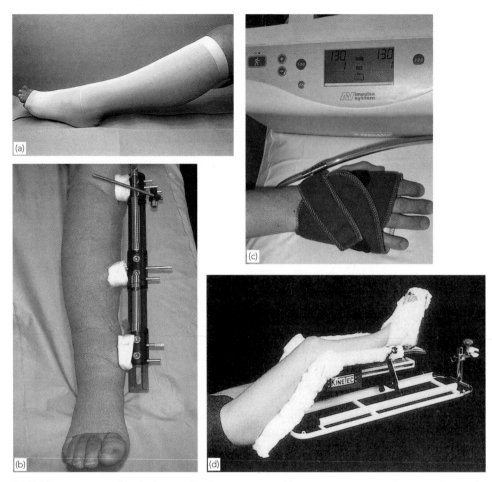

24.9 Management of soft tissues Swelling is minimized by improving venous drainage. This can be accomplished by elevation and firm support. Stiffness is minimized by movement and exercise. (a) A made-to-measure pressure garment helps reduce swelling and scarring. (b) A Coban wrap around a limb to control swelling during treatment. (c) An intermittent venous plexus pump for use on the hand or foot. (d) Continuous passive motion provided by a motorized frame.

features to be noted are the site and size of the wound, whether it is tidy or ragged, clean or dirty, and whether it communicates with the fracture. Other important factors are the condition of the soft tissues and the state of the circulation and nerve supply.

CLASSIFYING THE INJURY

Gustilo's classification of open fractures is widely used:

- *Type 1* is a low-energy fracture with a small, clean wound and little soft-tissue damage.
- *Type II* is a moderate-energy fracture with a clean wound more than 1 cm long, but no skin

flap, not much soft-tissue damage and no more than moderate comminution of the fracture.
- *Type III* is a high-energy fracture with extensive damage to skin, soft tissue and neurovascular structures, and contamination of the wound. In *Type III A* the fractured bone can be adequately covered by muscle or skin, despite the laceration; in *Type III B* there is extensive periosteal stripping and fracture cover is not possible without the use of local or distant flaps; the fracture is classified as *Type III C* if there is an arterial injury which needs to be repaired, regardless of the amount of other soft-tissue damage.

The incidence of wound infection correlates directly with the extent of soft-tissue damage, rising from less than 2% in Type I to over 10% in Type III fractures. The risk of infection also rises with increasing delay in obtaining soft-tissue coverage of the fracture.

TREATMENT OF OPEN FRACTURES

All open fractures, no matter how trivial they may seem, must be assumed to be contaminated; it is important to try to prevent them from becoming infected. The four essentials are:

- Antibiotic prophylaxis.
- Prompt wound debridement.
- Stabilization of the fracture.
- Early definitive wound cover.

Repeated examination of the limb is important; remember that open fractures also can be associated with a compartment syndrome.

Sterility and antibiotic cover

The wound should be kept covered until the patient reaches the operating theatre. At the time of debridement, gentamicin is added to a second dose of the first antibiotic. Both antibiotics provide prophylaxis against the majority of Gram-positive and Gram-negative bacteria that may have entered the wound at the time of injury. Only co-amoxiclav or cefuroxime (or clindamycin) is continued thereafter; the total period of antibiotic use for these fractures should not be longer than 72 hours. This advice is based on evidence that later infections are caused mostly by hospital-acquired bacteria and not seeded at the time of injury. Protracted use of wide-spectrum antibiotics prior to definitive wound closure only serves to select resistant bacteria from the hospital environment to contaminate the wound. Correspondingly, gentamicin and vancomycin (or teicoplanin) are given as a single dose at the time of definitive wound cover as these antibiotics are effective against methicillin-resistant *Staphylococcus aureus* and *Pseudomonas*, both of which are near the top of the league table of bacteria responsible for deep infection after open fractures.

Table 24.1 Antibiotics for open fractures[1]

	Grade I	Grade II	Grade III A	Grade III B/III C
As soon as possible (within 3 hours of injury)	Co-amoxiclav[2]	Co-amoxiclav[2]	Co-amoxiclav[2]	Co-amoxiclav[2]
At debridement	Co-amoxiclav[2] and gentamicin	Co-amoxiclav[2] and gentamicin	Co-amoxiclav[2] and gentamicin	Co-amoxiclav[2] and gentamicin
At definitive fracture cover	Wound cover is usually possible at debridement; delayed closure unnecessary	Wound cover is usually possible at debridement. If delayed, gentamicin and vancomycin (or teicoplanin) at the time of cover	Wound cover is usually possible at debridement. If delayed, gentamicin and vancomycin (or teicoplanin) at the time of cover	Gentamicin and vancomycin (or teicoplanin)
Continued prophylaxis	Only co-amoxiclav[2] continued after surgery	Only co-amoxiclav[2] continued between procedures and after final surgery	Only co-amoxiclav[2] continued between procedures and after final surgery	Only co-amoxiclav[2] continued between procedures and after final surgery
Maximum period	24 hours	72 hours	72 hours	72 hours

[1]Based on the Standards for the Management of Open Fractures of the Lower Limb, British Orthopaedic Association and British Association of Plastic, Reconstructive and Aesthetic Surgeons, 2009.
[2]Or cefuroxime (clindamycin for those with penicillin allergy).

Debridement and wound excision

The operation aims to render the wound free of foreign material and dead tissue, leaving a clean surgical field with a good blood supply throughout. Because open fractures are often associated with severe tissue damage, the operation should be performed by someone skilled in dealing with both skeletal and soft tissues; *ideally this should be a joint effort by orthopaedic and plastic surgeons.* The following principles must be observed:

- *Wound excision* – the wound margins are excised, but only enough to leave healthy skin edges.
- *Wound extension* – thorough cleansing necessitates adequate exposure; poking around in a small wound to remove debris can be dangerous. The safest extensions are to follow the line of fasciotomy incisions; these avoid damaging important perforator vessels that can be used to raise skin flaps for eventual fracture cover.
- *Delivery of the fracture* – examination of the fracture surfaces cannot be adequately performed without extracting the bone from within the wound. The simplest (and gentlest) method is to bend the limb in the manner in which it was forced at the moment of injury; the fracture surfaces will be exposed through the wound without any additional damage to the soft tissues.
- *Removal of devitalized tissue* – devitalized tissue provides a nutrient medium for bacteria. All doubtfully viable tissue, whether soft or bony, should be removed.
- *Wound cleansing* – all foreign material and tissue debris is removed by excision or through a wash with copious quantities of normal saline. A common mistake is to inject syringefuls of fluid through a small aperture – this only serves to push contaminants further in. Adding antibiotics or antiseptics to the solution has no added benefit.

As a general rule it is best to leave cut nerves and tendons alone, though if the wound is absolutely clean and no dissection is required – and provided the necessary expertise is available – they can be sutured.

Wound closure and stabilization

A small, uncontaminated wound in a Grade I or II fracture may (after debridement) be sutured, provided this can be done without tension. In the more severe grades of injury, fracture stabilization and wound cover using split-skin grafts, local or distant flaps is ideal, provided both orthopaedic and plastic surgeons are satisfied that the wound is clean and viable after debridement.

If a combined plastic-and-orthopaedic approach is not available at the time of debridement, the fracture is stabilized by external fixation and then left open and dressed with an impervious dressing.

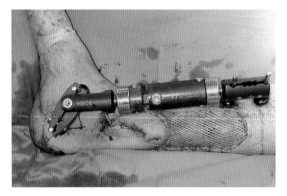

24.11 Stabilizing the limb in open fractures
External fixation is a useful method of holding the fracture while the wound remains accessible. If necessary this can be replaced by internal fixation, provided the wound is clean and covered, and the interval between the two procedures is less than 7 days.

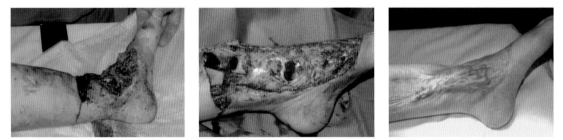

24.10 Debridement Detritus and devitalized tissue is painstakingly removed to leave a healthy soft-tissue bed. Early closure of the wound minimizes infection risk.

Return to surgery for a 'second look' should have definitive fracture cover as an objective. this should ideally be performed within 48–72 hours, and not later than 5–7 days. The external fixator can be replaced by internal fixation at the time of definitive wound closure, should the surgeon deem the fracture pattern appropriate and the degree of contamination at the time of injury mild. Open fractures do not fare well if left exposed for long and repeated debridement can be self-defeating. If wound cover is delayed, then external fixation is the safest means of definitive fracture stabilization.

Skin grafting is most appropriate if the wound cannot be closed without tension and the recipient bed is clean, free of obvious infection and well vascularized; it is not necessary to wait until the bed is covered with granulation tissue. Partial-thickness grafts can, if necessary, be laid on periosteum or paratenon but they should not be applied directly over bare bone or tendons or metal implants.

Extensive skin loss over a fracture, or in an open area where the blood supply is suspect, is better dealt with by transposing a *local* or *regional fasciocutaneous or musculocutaneous flap*, if this can be fashioned without risk to its blood supply. Occasionally the only option is to transfer a *free flap*, with its blood vessels, using microsurgical techniques. Where blood vessels are preserved, they should be sutured outside the zone of injury.

CHAPTER 25

COMPLICATIONS OF FRACTURES

General complications of trauma are dealt with in Chapter 22. *Local complications* can be divided into *early* (those that arise during the first few weeks following injury) and *late*.

Table 25.1 Local complications of fractures

Urgent	Less urgent	Late
Vascular injury	Pressure sores and	Malunion
Local visceral	blisters	Non-union
injury	Nerve entrapment	Avascular necrosis
Compartment	Heterotopic	Muscle contracture
syndrome	ossification	Joint instability
Haemarthrosis	Ligament injury	Regional pain
Nerve injury	Tendon lesions	syndrome
Infection	Joint stiffness	Osteoarthritis
Gas gangrene	Regional pain	
	syndrome	

EARLY COMPLICATIONS

Early complications may present as part of the primary injury or may appear only after a few days or weeks.

VISCERAL INJURY

Fractures around the trunk are often complicated by injuries to underlying viscera, the most important being penetration of the lung with life-threatening pneumothorax following rib fractures and rupture of the bladder or urethra in pelvic fractures. These injuries require emergency treatment, before the fracture is dealt with.

VASCULAR INJURY

Fractures most often associated with damage to a major artery are those around the knee and elbow and those of the humeral and femoral shafts. The artery may be cut, torn, compressed or contused, either by the initial injury or subsequently by jagged bone fragments. Even if its outward appearance is normal, the intima may be detached and the vessel blocked by thrombus, or a segment of artery may be in spasm. The effects vary from transient diminution of blood flow to profound ischaemia, tissue death and peripheral gangrene.

Clinical features

The injured limb is cold and pale, or slightly cyanosed, and the pulse is weak or absent. *X-rays* will probably show that the fracture is at one of the 'high-risk' sites mentioned above.

If a vascular injury is suspected, urgent exploration to establish the diagnosis and restore circulation is mandatory. An angiogram is performed on the operating table if needed, but the damage is usually at the level of the fracture or joint dislocation anyway. Warm ischaemia times greater than 4–6 hours can lead to limb loss.

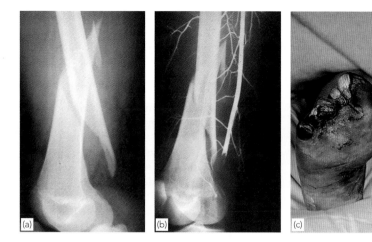

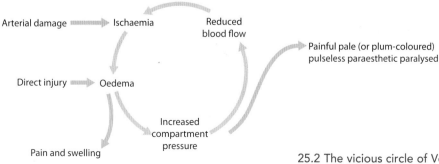

25.1 Vascular injury (a) X-ray of a patient with a fractured femur and early signs of vascular insufficiency. The point of the proximal fragment seems to be dangerously close to the popliteal vessels. Angiography (b) shows that the artery is interrupted at precisely that point. (c) Despite vein grafting, the patient ended up with peripheral gangrene.

Table 25.2 Injuries associated with vascular trauma

Injury	Vessel
First rib fracture	Subclavian artery
Shoulder dislocation	Axillary artery
Humeral supracondylar fracture	Brachial artery
Elbow dislocation	Brachial artery
Pelvic fracture	Presacral and internal iliac vessels
Femoral supracondylar fracture	Femoral artery
Knee dislocation	Popliteal artery
Proximal tibial fracture	Popliteal artery or its branches

Treatment

All bandages and splints should be removed. The fracture is re-x-rayed and, if the position of the bones suggests that the artery is being compressed or kinked, prompt reduction is necessary. The circulation is then reassessed repeatedly over the next 30 minutes. If there is no improvement, the vessels must be explored by operation – preferably with the benefit of perioperative angiography. An early temporary shunt across the damaged zone will restore the circulation promptly. If vessel repair is undertaken, stable fixation is imperative; where it is practicable, the fracture should be fixed internally.

COMPARTMENT SYNDROME

Fractures of the arm or leg can give rise to severe ischaemia even if there is no damage to a major vessel. Bleeding, oedema or inflammation (infection) may increase the pressure within one of the osteofascial compartments; there is reduced capillary flow which results in muscle ischaemia, further oedema, still greater pressure and yet more profound ischaemia – a vicious circle that ends, after 12 hours or less, in necrosis of nerve and muscle within the compartment. Nerve is capable of regeneration but muscle, once infarcted, can never recover and is replaced by inelastic fibrous tissue (*Volkmann's ischaemic contracture*). A similar cascade of events may be caused by swelling of a limb inside a tight plaster cast.

Arterial damage ⟶ Ischaemia ⟶ Reduced blood flow

Direct injury ⟶ Oedema

Increased compartment pressure

Pain and swelling

Painful pale (or plum-coloured) pulseless paraesthetic paralysed

25.2 The vicious circle of Volkmann's ischaemia

353

Clinical features

High-risk injuries are fractures of the elbow, the forearm bones, the proximal one-third of the tibia and multiple fractures of the hand or foot. Other precipitating factors are operation (usually for internal fixation) or infection. Be aware that a compartment syndrome may also arise in a crush injury, a circumferential burn or even in a tight plaster cast.

The classic features of ischaemia are the five Ps: **P**ain, **P**araesthesia, **P**allor, **P**aralysis and **P**ulselessness. However, in a compartment syndrome the ischaemia occurs at the capillary level, so pulses may still be felt and the skin may not be pale! The earliest of the 'classic' features are pain (or a 'bursting' sensation), altered sensibility and paresis (or, more usually, weakness in active muscle contraction). Skin sensation should be carefully and repeatedly checked.

Ischaemic muscle is highly sensitive to stretch, so when the toes or fingers are passively hyperextended, there is increased pain in the calf or forearm.

Confirmation of the diagnosis can be made by measuring the intracompartmental pressures; indeed, so important is the need for early diagnosis that some surgeons advocate the use of continuous compartment pressure monitoring for high-risk injuries and especially for forearm or leg fractures in patients who are unconscious. A split catheter is introduced into the compartment and the pressure is measured close to the level of the fracture. A differential pressure (ΔP) – the difference between the general diastolic pressure and the compartment pressure – of less than 30 mmHg (4.00 kP) is an indication for immediate compartment decompression.

Treatment

The threatened compartment (or compartments) must be promptly decompressed. Casts, bandages and dressings must be completely removed – merely splitting the plaster is utterly useless – and the limb should be nursed flat (elevating the limb causes a further decrease in end-capillary pressure and aggravates the muscle ischaemia). The ΔP should be carefully monitored; if it falls below 30 mmHg, immediate open fasciotomy is performed. *In the case of the leg, 'fasciotomy' means opening all four compartments through medial and lateral incisions.* The wounds should be left open and inspected 2 days later: if there is muscle necrosis, debridement can be done; if the tissues are healthy, the wound can be sutured (without tension), or skin grafted.

If facilities for measuring compartmental pressures are not available, the decision to operate will have to be made on clinical grounds. If three or more of the 'classical' signs are present, the diagnosis is almost certain. If the signs are equivocal, the limb should be examined at 15 minute intervals and if there is no improvement within 2 hours of splitting the dressings, fasciotomy should be performed. Muscle will be dead after 4–6 hours of total ischaemia – there is no time to lose!

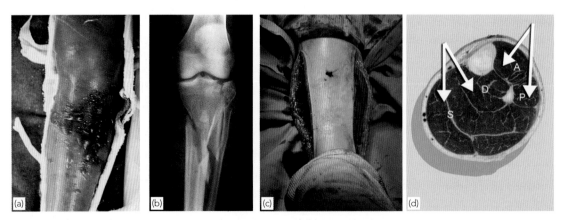

25.3 Compartment syndrome (a,b) A fracture at this level is always dangerous. This man was treated in plaster; pain became intense and when the plaster was split (which should have been done immediately after its application), the leg was swollen and blistered. (c) Tibial compartment decompression is best done through two separate incisions and requires fasciotomies of all compartments (d). (A: anterior, P: peroneal, S: superficial posterior, D: deep posterior.)

Table 25.3 Common nerve injuries

Injury	Nerve
Shoulder dislocation	Axillary
Humeral shaft fracture	Radial
Humeral supracondylar	Radial or median
Elbow medial condyle	Ulnar
Elbow dislocation	Ulnar
Montegia fracture	Posterior interosseous
Hip dislocation	Sciatic
Knee dislocation	Peroneal

NERVE INJURY (see also Chapter 11)

Nerve injury is particularly common with fractures of the humerus or injuries around the elbow or knee. The telltale signs should be looked for (*and documented!*) during the initial examination and again after reduction of the fracture.

In *closed injuries* the nerve is seldom severed, and spontaneous recovery should be awaited – it occurs in 90% of cases within 4 months. If recovery has not occurred by the expected time, and if nerve conduction studies fail to show evidence of recovery, the nerve should be explored.

Early exploration should also be considered if signs of a nerve injury appear *after manipulation of the fracture.*

In *open fractures* any nerve lesion is more likely to be complete; the nerve should be explored during wound debridement and repaired at the time of wound closure.

Nerve compression, as distinct from a direct injury, sometimes occurs with fractures or dislocations around the wrist. Complaints of numbness or paraesthesia in the distribution of the median or ulnar nerves should be taken seriously and the patient monitored closely; if there is no improvement within 48 hours of fracture reduction or splitting of bandages around the splint, the nerve should be explored and decompressed.

HAEMARTHROSIS

Fractures involving a joint may cause acute haemarthrosis. The joint is swollen and tense and the patient resists any attempt at moving it. The blood should be aspirated before dealing with the fracture.

INFECTION (see also Chapter 2)

Open fractures may become infected; closed fractures hardly ever do unless they are opened by operation. Post-traumatic wound infection is now the most common cause of chronic osteomyelitis. This does not necessarily prevent the fracture from uniting, but union will be slow and the chance of re-fracturing is increased.

Clinical features

Following an open fracture or operation, the wound becomes inflamed and starts draining seropurulent fluid. A sample should be submitted immediately for microbiological investigation; while awaiting the result, intravenous antibiotic administration can be started.

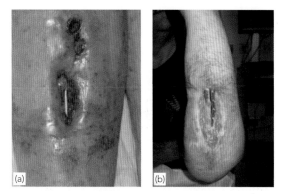

25.4 Infection Wound sinuses and exposed metalwork are sorry sights. X-rays often show that the fracture is ununited

Treatment

All open fractures should be regarded as potentially infected and treated by giving prophylactic antibiotics and meticulously excising all devitalized tissue. If there are signs of acute infection and pus formation, the tissues around the fracture should be opened and drained; the choice of antibiotic is dictated by tests for bacterial sensitivity.

If internal fixation has been used, this does not necessarily have to be removed; even worse than an infected fracture is one that is both infected and unstable. However, if the infection does not respond to antibiotic treatment, it may be necessary to remove the implants and replace them with an external fixation device.

Late signs of infection may appear in the form of a sinus and/or x-ray evidence of a sequestrum. The implants and all avascular pieces of bone should be removed; robust soft-tissue cover (ideally a flap) will be needed. An external fixator can be used to bridge the fracture. If the resulting defect is too large for bone grafting at a later stage, the patient should be referred to a centre with the necessary experience and facilities for limb reconstruction.

GAS GANGRENE

This terrifying condition is produced by clostridial infection (especially *C. welchii*). These are anaerobic organisms that can survive and multiply only in tissues with low oxygen tension; the prime site for infection, therefore, is a dirty wound with dead muscle that has been closed without adequate debridement. Toxins produced by the organisms destroy the cell wall and rapidly lead to tissue necrosis, thus promoting the spread of the disease.

Clinical features appear within 24 hours of the injury: the patient complains of intense pain and swelling around the wound and a brownish discharge may be seen; gas formation is usually not very marked. There is little or no pyrexia but the pulse rate is increased and a characteristic smell becomes evident (once experienced this is never forgotten). Rapidly the patient becomes toxaemic and may lapse into coma and death.

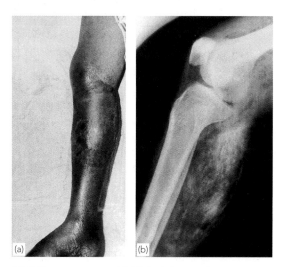

25.5 Gas gangrene (a) Clinical picture of gas gangrene. (b) X-rays show diffuse gas in the muscles of the calf.

It is essential to distinguish gas gangrene, which is characterized by myonecrosis, from anaerobic cellulitis, in which superficial gas formation is abundant but toxaemia usually slight. Failure to recognize the difference may lead to unnecessary amputation for the non-lethal cellulitis.

Prevention

Deep, penetrating wounds in muscular tissue are dangerous; they should be explored, all dead tissue should be completely excised and, if there is the slightest doubt about tissue viability, the wound should be left open. Unhappily there is no effective antitoxin against *C. welchii*.

Treatment

The key to life-saving treatment is early diagnosis. General measures, such as fluid replacement and intravenous antibiotics, are started immediately. Hyperbaric oxygen has been used as a means of limiting the spread of gangrene. However, the mainstay of treatment is prompt decompression of the wound and removal of all dead tissue. In advanced cases, amputation may be essential.

FRACTURE BLISTERS

Two distinct types of blistering are sometimes seen after fractures: clear fluid-filled vesicles and blood-stained ones. Both occur during limb swelling and are due to elevation of the epidermal layer of skin from the dermis. There is no advantage in puncturing the blisters (it may even lead to increased local infection) and surgical incisions through blisters, whilst generally safe, should be undertaken only when limb swelling has decreased.

PLASTER SORES AND PRESSURE SORES

Plaster sores occur where skin is pressed directly onto bone. They should be prevented by padding the bony points and by moulding the wet plaster so that pressure is distributed to the soft tissues around the bony points. While a plaster sore is developing the patient feels localized burning pain. A window must immediately be cut in the plaster, as warning pain quickly abates and skin necrosis proceeds unnoticed.

Pressure sores may be produced by splints and other appliances. These should be checked at frequent intervals to ensure that they fit correctly and comfortably.

Bed sores are liable to occur in elderly or paralysed patients. The skin over the sacrum and heels is especially vulnerable. They can usually be prevented by careful nursing and early activity; once they have developed, treatment is difficult and it may be necessary to excise the necrotic tissue and cover the defect by plastic surgery.

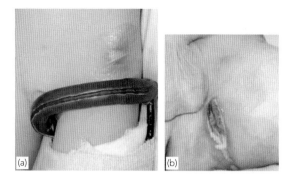

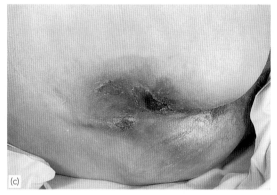

25.6 Pressure sores Pressure sores are a sign of carelessness. (a,b) Sores from poorly supervised treatment in a Thomas' splint. (c) Bed sores in an elderly patient, which kept her in hospital for months.

LATE COMPLICATIONS

DELAYED UNION

Causes

Factors causing delayed union are either biological, biomechanical or patient related.

Poor blood supply

A badly displaced fracture will cause tearing of the periosteum and interruption of the intramedullary blood supply. The fracture surface may become necrotic and the normal healing process will take longer than usual.

Severe soft-tissue damage

Severe soft-tissue damage is the most important cause of delayed union and non-union. It disrupts the blood supply, reduces osteogenesis from mesenchymal stem cells and impairs the effectiveness of muscle splintage.

Periosteal stripping

Over-enthusiastic periosteal stripping during internal fixation is an avoidable cause of non-union.

Imperfect splintage

Excessive traction (creating a fracture gap) or excessive movement at the fracture site will delay ossification in the callus. In forearm or leg fractures, an intact fellow bone may also serve to splint a fracture apart.

Over-rigid fixation

Contrary to popular belief, rigid fixation delays rather than promotes fracture union. It is only because the fixation device holds the fragments securely that the fracture seems to 'unite'. Union by primary bone healing is slow, but provided stability is maintained throughout, the fracture does eventually unite.

Infection

Tissue healing is severely hampered by bone lysis, necrosis and pus formation. In addition, fixation implants tend to loosen and fracture stability is lost.

Implant failure

Implants may loosen or break apart.

Patient related

Patients come in all shapes and forms. They are sometimes immense, immoderate, immovable or impossible. Proper care can overcome most of these problems.

Clinical features

Fracture tenderness persists and if the bone is subjected to stress, pain may be acute. On x-ray the fracture line remains visible and there is very little callus formation or periosteal reaction. However, the bone ends are not sclerosed or atrophic. The appearances suggest that, although the fracture has not united, it eventually will.

Treatment

Conservative

The two important principles are: (1) to eliminate any possible cause of delayed union (see above); and (2) to promote healing by providing the most appropriate biological environment. Immobilization (whether by cast or by internal fixation) should be sufficient to prevent movement at the fracture site; but fracture loading is an important stimulus to union and this can be enhanced by encouraging muscular exercise and weightbearing in the cast or brace. The watchword is patience; however, there comes a point with every fracture where the ill-effects of prolonged immobilization outweigh the advantages of non-operative treatment, or where the risk of implant breakage begins to loom.

Operative

Each case should be treated on its merits; however, if union is delayed for more than 6 months and there is no sign of callus formation, internal fixation and bone grafting are indicated. The operation should be planned in such a way as to cause the least possible damage to the soft tissues.

NON-UNION

In a minority of cases delayed union gradually turns into non-union, i.e. it becomes apparent that the fracture will never unite without intervention. Movement can be elicited at the fracture site and pain diminishes; the fracture gap turns into a pseudarthrosis.

On x-ray the fracture is clearly visible and the bone on either side of it may be either exuberant or rounded off. This contrasting appearance has led to non-unions being divided into hypertrophic and atrophic types. In *hypertrophic non-union* the bone ends are enlarged, suggesting that osteogenesis is still active but not quite capable of bridging the gap. In *atrophic non-union* osteogenesis seems to have ceased; the bone ends are tapered or rounded with no suggestion of new bone formation.

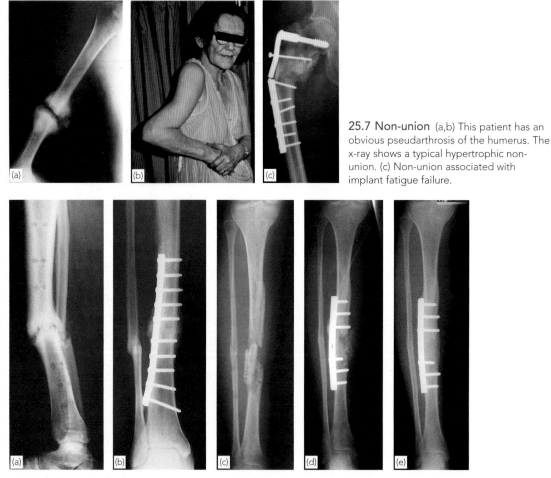

25.7 Non-union (a,b) This patient has an obvious pseudarthrosis of the humerus. The x-ray shows a typical hypertrophic non-union. (c) Non-union associated with implant fatigue failure.

25.8 Non-union – treatment (a) This patient with fractures of the tibia and fibula was initially treated by internal fixation with a plate and screws. The fracture failed to heal and developed the typical features of hypertrophic non-union. (b) After a further operation, using more rigid fixation (and no bone grafts), the fractures healed solidly. (c,d) This patient with atrophic non-union needed both internal fixation and bone grafts to stimulate bone formation and union (e).

Treatment

Conservative

Non-union is occasionally symptomless, needing no treatment or, at most, a removable splint. Even if symptoms are present, operation is not the only answer; with hypertrophic non-union, functional bracing may be sufficient to induce union, but treatment often needs to be prolonged.

Operative

With hypertrophic non-union and in the absence of deformity, rigid fixation alone (internal or external) may lead to union. With atrophic non-union, fixation alone is not enough. Fibrous tissue in the fracture gap, as well as the hard, sclerotic bone ends, should be excised and bone grafts packed around the fracture. If there is significant 'die-back', this will require more extensive excision and the gap is then dealt with by bone advancement using the Ilizarov technique (see Chapter 12).

MALUNION

When the fragments join in an unsatisfactory position (unacceptable angulation, rotation or shortening) the fracture is said to be malunited. Causes are failure to reduce a fracture adequately, failure to hold reduction while healing proceeds or gradual collapse of comminuted or osteoporotic bone.

Clinical features

The deformity is usually obvious, but sometimes the true extent of malunion is apparent only on x-ray. Rotational deformity of the femur, tibia, humerus or forearm may be missed unless the limb is compared with its opposite fellow.

X-rays are essential to check the position of the fracture while it is uniting. This is particularly important during the first 3 weeks when the situation may change without warning (and when deformity can still be easily corrected). At this stage it is sometimes difficult to decide what constitutes 'malunion'; acceptable norms differ from one site to another and these are discussed under the individual fractures.

Treatment

Incipient malunion may call for treatment even before the fracture has fully united; the decision on the need for re-manipulation or correction may be extremely difficult. A few guidelines are offered:

- In adults, fractures should be reduced as near to the anatomical position as possible; apposition is important for healing whereas alignment and rotation are important for function. Angulation of more than 10–15 degrees in a long bone, or a noticeable rotational deformity, may need correction by re-manipulation, or by osteotomy and internal fixation.
- In young children, angular deformities near the bone ends will often re-model with time; rotational deformities will not.
- In the lower limb, shortening of more than 2 cm is seldom acceptable to the patient and a shoe raise may be indicated; in cases of severe discrepancy, limb lengthening should be considered.
- The patient's expectations (often prompted by cosmesis) may be quite different from the surgeon's; they should not be ignored. Early discussion with the patient, and a guided view of the x-rays, will help in deciding on the need for treatment and may prevent later misunderstanding.
- Little is known of the long-term effects of small angular deformities on joint function. However, it seems likely that malalignment of more than 15 degrees in any plane may cause asymmetrical loading of the joint above or below and the late development of secondary osteoarthritis; this applies particularly to the large weightbearing joints.

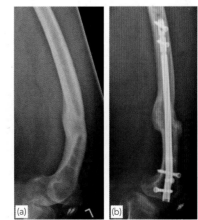

25.9 Malunion (a) This malunited fracture was treated by corrective osteotomy and internal fixation (b).

AVASCULAR NECROSIS (see also Chapter 6)

Certain regions are notorious for their propensity to develop ischaemia and bone necrosis after injury. They are: (1) the head of the femur (after fracture of the femoral neck or dislocation of the hip); (2) the proximal part of the scaphoid (after fracture through its waist); (3) the lunate (following dislocation); and (4) the body of the talus (after fracture of its neck).

Avascular necrosis (AVN) is really an early complication of bone injury, because ischaemia occurs during the first few hours following fracture or dislocation. However, the clinical and radiological effects are not seen until weeks or even months later.

Clinical features

There are no symptoms associated with AVN, but if the fracture fails to unite or if the bone collapses the patient may complain of pain. X-ray shows the characteristic increase in bone density (the consequence of new bone ingrowth in the necrotic segment and disuse osteoporosis in the surrounding parts).

Treatment

Treatment usually becomes necessary when joint function is threatened. In elderly people with necrosis of the femoral head, an arthroplasty is the obvious choice; in younger people, re-alignment osteotomy (or even arthrodesis) may be wiser. AVN in the scaphoid or talus may need no more than symptomatic treatment, but arthrodesis of the wrist or ankle is sometimes needed.

GROWTH DISTURBANCE

In children, damage to the physis may lead to abnormal or arrested growth of the bone. This problem is dealt with on page 332.

JOINT INSTABILITY

Bone loss or malunion close to a joint may lead to instability or recurrent dislocation. The commonest sites are the shoulder, the elbow and the patella.

A more subtle form of instability is seen after fractures around the wrist. Patients complaining of persistent discomfort or weakness after wrist injury should be fully investigated for chronic carpal instability (see page 196).

OSTEOARTHRITIS

A fracture involving a joint may damage the articular cartilage and give rise to post-traumatic osteoarthritis within a period of months. Even if the cartilage heals, irregularity or incongruity of the joint surfaces may cause localized stress and so predispose to secondary osteoarthritis years later. Little can be done to prevent this once the fracture has united.

LATE SOFT-TISSUE COMPLICATIONS

Joint stiffness

Joint stiffness after a fracture commonly occurs in the knee, the elbow, the shoulder and (worst of all) the small joints of the hand. Sometimes the joint itself has been injured; a haemarthrosis forms and leads to synovial adhesions. More often the stiffness is due to oedema and fibrosis of the capsule, the ligaments and the muscles around the joint, or adhesions of the soft tissues to each other or to the underlying bone. All these conditions are made worse by prolonged immobilization; moreover, if the joint has been held in a position where the ligaments are at their shortest, no amount of exercise will afterwards succeed in stretching these tissues and restoring the lost movement completely.

Treatment

The best treatment is prevention: elevation to minimize oedema, functional bracing rather than full cast immobilization, and exercises that keep the joints mobile from the outset. If a joint has to be splinted, make sure that it is held in the 'position of safe immobilization' (see page 397).

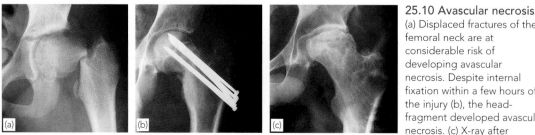

25.10 Avascular necrosis
(a) Displaced fractures of the femoral neck are at considerable risk of developing avascular necrosis. Despite internal fixation within a few hours of the injury (b), the head-fragment developed avascular necrosis. (c) X-ray after removal of the fixation screws.

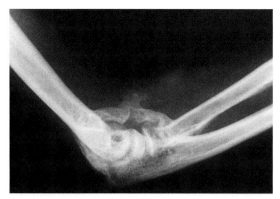

25.11 Myositis ossificans This followed a fractured head of radius.

Joints that are already stiff take time to mobilize, but prolonged and patient physiotherapy can work wonders. However, surgical release of tight structures is sometimes necessary.

Heterotopic ossification

Heterotopic ossification in the muscles sometimes occurs after an injury, particularly around the elbow. The patient (usually a fit young man) complains of pain and local swelling. X-ray is normal at first but a bone scan may show increased activity. Over the next 2–3 weeks the pain gradually subsides, but joint movement is limited and x-ray may show fluffy calcification in the soft tissues. By 8 weeks bony mass is easily palpable and is clearly defined in the x-ray.

Heterotopic ossification sometimes occurs spontaneously in unconscious patients.

Treatment

This condition was much more common in bygone years when joints, after plaster immobilization, were treated by vigorous muscle-stretching exercises. This must be avoided; active movements should be introduced gently and gradually, alternating with rest periods in the position of function. If heterotopic bone has already appeared and is blocking movement, it may be helpful to excise the bony mass. Indomethacin or radiotherapy should be given to help prevent recurrence.

Muscle contracture

Following arterial injury or a compartment syndrome, the patient may develop ischaemic contractures of the affected muscles (*Volkmann's ischaemic contracture*). Nerves injured by ischaemia sometimes recover, at least partially; thus the patient presents with deformity and stiffness, but numbness is inconstant. The sites most commonly

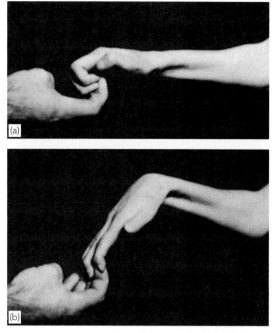

25.12 Muscle contracture (a) Typical claw-finger deformity due to Volkmann's ischaemic contracture of the forearm muscles. With the wrist extended, the fingers are drawn into flexion; (b) when the wrist is allowed to flex, the fingers can be straightened, thus indicating that the deformity is due to muscle shortening.

affected are the forearm and hand, the leg and the foot. In a severe case affecting the forearm, there will be muscle wasting and clawing of the fingers.

Treatment

Detachment of the flexor muscles at their origin and along the interosseous membrane in the forearm may improve the deformity, but function is no better if sensation and active movement are not restored. Nerve grafts may provide protective sensation in the hand, and tendon transfers (wrist extensors to finger and thumb flexors) will allow active grasp. In less severe cases, median nerve sensibility may be quite good and, with appropriate tendon releases and transfers, the patient regains a considerable degree of function.

Tendon rupture

Rupture of the extensor pollicis longus tendon may occur after a fracture of the lower radius. Direct suture is seldom possible and the resulting disability is treated by transferring the extensor indicis proprius tendon to the distal stump of the ruptured thumb tendon. Late rupture of the long head of biceps after a fractured neck of humerus usually requires no treatment.

Nerve compression

Nerve compression may damage the lateral popliteal nerve if an elderly or emaciated patient lies with the leg in full external rotation. Radial palsy may follow the faulty use of crutches. Both conditions are due to lack of supervision.

Nerve entrapment

Bone or joint deformity may result in local nerve entrapment with typical features such as numbness or paraesthesia, loss of power and muscle wasting in the distribution of the affected nerve. Common sites are the *ulnar nerve* (due to a post-traumatic valgus deformity of the elbow), the *median nerve* (following injuries around the wrist), and the *posterior tibial nerve* (following fractures around the ankle). Treatment is by early decompression of the nerve.

Complex regional pain syndrome

Sudeck, in 1900, described a condition characterized by pain, stiffness and osteoporosis of the hand. The same condition sometimes occurs after fractures of the extremities and for many years it was called *Sudeck's atrophy*. More recently it was held to be due to some type of neurovascular

dysfunction and it came to be known variously as *reflex sympathetic dystrophy or algodystrophy*. Because of continuing uncertainty about its nature, these names have been replaced by the term *complex regional pain syndrome*.

The condition is much more common than was previously recognized and it may occur even after relatively trivial injury. The patient complains of continuous pain, often described as 'burning' in character. At first there is local swelling, redness and warmth, as well as tenderness and moderate stiffness of the joints near the site of injury. As the weeks go by the skin becomes pale and atrophic, movements are increasingly restricted and the patient may develop fixed deformities. X-rays characteristically show patchy rarefaction of the bone.

Treatment

The earlier the condition is recognized and treatment begun, the better the prognosis. Elevation and active exercises are important after all injuries, but in this condition they are essential. During the early stage anti-inflammatory drugs and amitriptyline are helpful. Sympathetic block or sympatholytic drugs have been advocated for this condition. They do sometimes appear to help but their effect is unpredictable. Prolonged and dedicated physiotherapy will usually be needed.

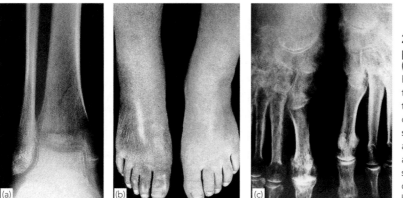

25.13 Complex regional pain syndrome ('algodystrophy') Following a fracture of the tibia, this patient developed the typical features of complex regional pain syndrome affecting the right ankle and foot. The skin is atrophic and shiny; the x-ray shows marked regional osteoporosis above and below the ankle.

CHAPTER 26

INJURIES OF THE SHOULDER, UPPER ARM AND ELBOW

The great bugbear of upper limb injuries is stiffness. In elderly patients especially, it is as important to preserve movement as it is to treat the fracture.

FRACTURES OF THE CLAVICLE

A fall on the shoulder or the outstretched hand may fracture the clavicle; the lateral fragment is pulled down by the weight of the arm, while the medial fragment is held up by the sternomastoid muscle.

Special features

The fracture is almost always displaced, producing a lump along the 'collar-bone'. Fractures of the outer third are easily mistaken for acromioclavicular injuries. Vascular and neurological complications are rare.

Imaging

X-rays show that the fracture is usually in the middle third of the bone and the lateral fragment lies below the medial. Outer-third injuries need special views to define any fracture.

A *computed tomography (CT) scan* is occasionally needed to define the fracture configuration and to exclude a sternoclavicular dislocation.

Treatment

For the usual middle-third fracture, accurate closed reduction is neither possible nor essential. In most cases all that is needed is to support the arm in a sling until the pain subsides (usually 1–3 weeks). Thereafter, active shoulder exercises should be encouraged; this is particularly important in older patients.

By contrast, outer-third fractures are quite troublesome and may need open reduction and internal fixation.

Complications

Malunion is inevitable in displaced fractures; in children the bone is soon re-modelled, but in adults the slight deformity has to be accepted unless there is a very unsightly bump with skin irritation.

Non-union sometimes occurs in middle-third fractures and is treated by bone graft and plating.

FRACTURES OF THE SCAPULA

The *body of the scapula* is fractured by a crushing force, which usually also fractures ribs and may dislocate the sternoclavicular joint. The *neck of the scapula* may be fractured by a blow or by a fall on the shoulder.

Special features

Shoulder movements are painful but possible. If breathing also is painful, thoracic injury must be excluded.

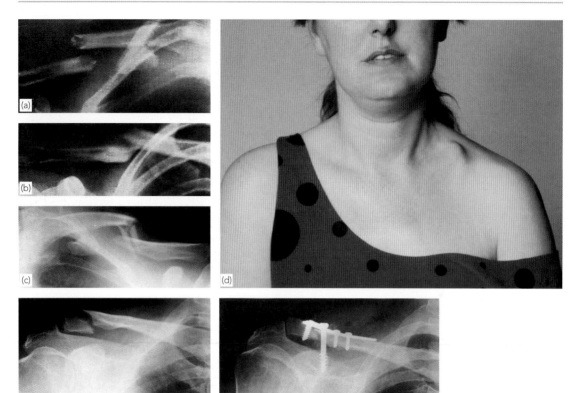

26.1 Fractured clavicle (a) The common site and displacement. Often the fracture unites in a somewhat faulty position (b) but this seldom worries the patient. However, the severely displaced fracture shown in (c), though it united well enough, left an unsightly deformity (d); it would have been better treated by open reduction and internal fixation with a small plate and screws. Fractures of the outer (lateral) third with elevation of the clavicular shaft due to rupture of the coracoclavicular ligament may also require internal fixation (e,f).

Imaging

X-rays may show a comminuted fracture of the *body* of the scapula, or a fractured *scapular neck* with the outer fragment pulled downwards by the weight of the arm. Occasionally a crack is seen in the acromion or the *coracoid process*. CT is useful for demonstrating *glenoid* fractures.

Treatment

Reduction is usually unnecessary. The patient wears a sling for comfort and from the start practises active exercises of the shoulder, elbow and fingers.

Check repeatedly for dislocation of the shoulder; a large glenoid fragment may require open reduction and internal fixation.

SCAPULOTHORACIC DISSOCIATION

This is a high-energy injury in which the shoulder is literally wrenched away from the torso. There is a great chance of death due to the associated vascular

rupture. Treatment requires resuscitation and then reconstruction of the vascular, neurological and muscuoskeletal injuries. The arm rarely recovers.

ACROMIOCLAVICULAR JOINT INJURIES

A fall on the shoulder tears the acromioclavicular ligaments, and upward subluxation of the clavicle may occur; more severe injury also tears the coracoclavicular (conoid and trapezoid) ligaments and results in complete dislocation of the joint.

Special features

The patient can usually point to the site of injury. If there is tenderness but no deformity (or very little deformity), it is probably a strain or a subluxation. With dislocation, the patient is in more pain and a prominent 'step' can be seen and felt.

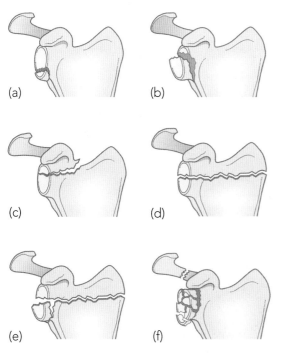

26.2 Fractures of the glenoid socket Diagrams showing the six main types of glenoid fracture.

X-rays

The films show either a subluxation with only slight elevation of the clavicle, or dislocation with considerable separation. A stress view, taken with the patient holding a 5 kg weight in each hand, may reveal the displacement more clearly.

Treatment

Subluxation does not affect function and does not require any special treatment; the arm is rested in a sling until pain subsides (usually no more than 1 week), and shoulder exercises are then begun.

Dislocation is poorly controlled by padding and strapping. Nevertheless, surgery is controversial and it is doubtful whether it improves the outcome except in those whose work or hobbies involve using the arm above shoulder height for long periods.

One of the more reliable techniques is to reduce the dislocation by open operation, then reconstruct the ligament and support it with a graft.

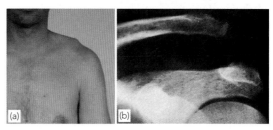

26.4 Acromioclavicular dislocation (a) The clinical picture is unmistakable: a definite step in the contour at the outer end of the clavicle. (b) X-ray showing complete separation of the acromioclavicular joint.

Complications

Long-standing, unreduced dislocation of the acromioclavicular joint, though still compatible with reasonably good function, may leave the patient with an ill-defined feeling of discomfort and weakness of the shoulder, especially when attempting strenuous overhead activities. If the symptoms warrant active treatment, reconstructive surgery can be advised, but the patient must be warned that improvement cannot be guaranteed. One approach is to excise a small segment of the lateral end of the clavicle and then to tether the 'floating' clavicle by transferring the coracoacromial ligament to the lateral end of the clavicle; the structure may be further stabilized by holding the clavicle down with a screw between the clavicle and the coracoid process.

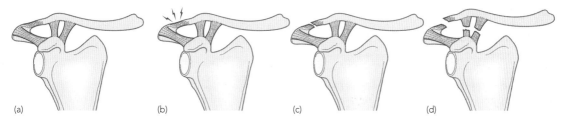

26.3 Acromioclavicular joint injuries (a) Normal joint. (b) Sprained acromioclavicular joint; no displacement. (c) Torn capsule and subluxation but coracoclavicular ligaments intact. (d) Dislocation with torn coracoclavicular ligaments.

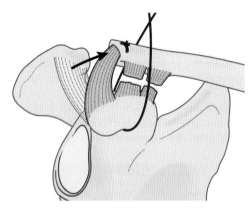

26.5 Modified Weaver Dunn operation The lateral end of the clavicle is excised; the acromial end of the coracoacromial ligament is detached and fastened to the lateral end of the clavicle. Tension on the ligament is lessened by placing a 'sling' around the clavicle and the coracoid process. (Dotted lines show former position of coracoacromial ligament.)

A very late complication is osteoarthritis of the acromioclavicular joint; this can usually be managed conservatively, but if pain is marked, the outer end of the clavicle can be excised.

STERNOCLAVICULAR DISLOCATION

Anterior dislocation

This uncommon injury is caused by a fall on the shoulder. The inner end of the clavicle springs forward, producing a visible and palpable prominence. The joint can usually be reduced quite easily by direct pressure on the prominent clavicle while the shoulders are relaxed. The problem is keeping it there. Splintage is unsatisfactory and internal fixation carries unnecessary risks (great vessels and pericardium are too close for comfort!). The patient should be persuaded to accept the slight residual deformity and mild discomfort during strenuous activity.

Posterior dislocation

This is very rare, but it can cause compression of the large vessels in the neck and should be reduced as a matter of urgency. Closed reduction can sometimes be achieved by lying the patient supine with a sandbag between the shoulder blades and then pulling on the arm with the shoulder abducted and extended; the joint reduces with a snap. The shoulders are braced backwards with

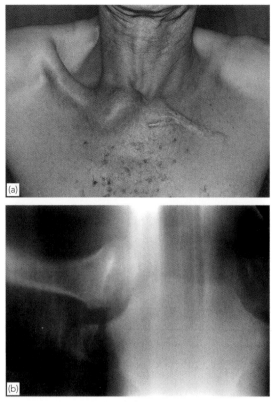

26.6 Sternoclavicular dislocation (a) The bump over the sternoclavicular joint may be obvious, though this is difficult to demonstrate on plain x-ray. (b) Tomography (or better still CT) will show the lesion.

a figure-of-eight bandage, which is kept in place for 3 weeks. If closed reduction fails, operative reduction is called for. The displaced clavicle is pulled forward with a hook.

DISLOCATION OF THE SHOULDER

The glenohumeral joint is very shallow and stability is maintained largely by the glenoid labrum (which slightly deepens the socket) and the surrounding ligaments and muscles. Traumatic dislocation is common; humeral head displacement is usually anterior, less often posterior.

ANTERIOR DISLOCATION

Anterior dislocation is caused either by a fall on the backward-stretching hand or by forced abduction and external rotation of the shoulder. The head of the humerus is driven forward, tearing the capsule or avulsing the glenoid labrum, and usually ends up just below the coracoid process. There may be an associated fracture of the proximal end of the humerus.

Special features

Pain is severe. The patient supports the arm with the opposite hand and is loath to permit any kind of examination. The lateral outline of the shoulder is flattened and a small bulge may be seen and felt just below the clavicle. Looking from above, the usual forward bulge is altered compared with the other side. The arm must always be examined for nerve and vessel injury.

X-rays

This will show the overlapping shadows of the humeral head and glenoid fossa, with the head usually lying below and medial to the socket. A lateral view is essential to show whether or not the head is in the socket.

Treatment

In those with recurrent dislocations, the reduction may be achieved spontaneously by the patient or by the doctor with no sedation. Otherwise, for those with a first dislocation, prompt reduction can be achieved under sedation but if the muscle spasm and pain are overwhelming then a general anaesthetic may be required. X-rays prior to dislocation are mandatory to exclude a fracture–dislocation.

While the patient is waiting, they can be placed in the prone position with the arm hanging over the side of the bed – the dislocation may reduce. Otherwise, the simplest and safest method is to pull on the arm in slight abduction and flexion while the body is steadied by an assistant who has wrapped a towel around the torso for counter-traction.

An x-ray is taken to confirm reduction and exclude a fracture. When the patient is fully awake, active abduction is gently tested to exclude an axillary nerve injury or rotator cuff tear. The arm is then supported in a sling.

For those over 30 years of age, stiffness is more of a risk than recurrent dislocation so movements are begun after 1 week. For those under 30 years, recurrence is more of a risk and so the sling is retained for 3 weeks before mobilizing.

> ⚠ Direct blow to the shoulder: x-ray for associated cervical spine injury.

Complications

Rotator cuff tear

The rotator cuff is often torn, particularly in older people. This is suggested by the patient's inability to initiate abduction of the arm. An ultrasound or magnetic resonance imaging (MRI) will readily confirm the diagnosis. The lesion may later require surgical repair (see page 175).

Nerve injury

The axillary nerve may be injured; the patient is unable to contract the deltoid muscle and there may be a small patch of anaesthesia over the muscle. The lesion is usually a neurapraxia, which recovers spontaneously after a few weeks. This must be distinguished from a rotator cuff tear.

Occasionally the posterior cord of the brachial plexus, the median nerve or the musculocutaneous nerve may be injured. This is alarming, but these injuries usually recover with time.

Vascular injury

The axillary artery may be damaged before or during reduction. The limb should always be examined for signs of ischaemia.

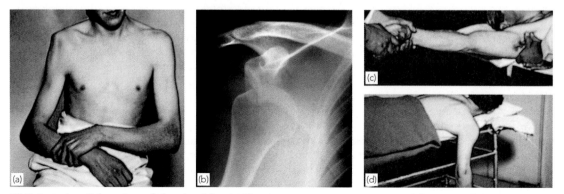

26.7 Anterior dislocation of the shoulder (a) The prominent acromion process and flattening of the contour over the deltoid are typical signs. (b) X-ray confirms the diagnosis of anterior dislocation. (c,d) Two methods of reduction.

Fracture–dislocation

If there is an associated fracture of the proximal humerus, open reduction and internal fixation may be necessary.

Recurrent dislocation

If the glenoid labrum has been damaged or detached, recurrent dislocation is likely (see page 178).

POSTERIOR DISLOCATION

This is much rarer than an anterior dislocation but is commonly missed. It should always be suspected if the patient had suffered an epileptic fit or a severe electric shock. It is otherwise caused by forced internal rotation of the abducted arm or by a direct blow on the front of the shoulder.

Special features

The diagnosis is frequently missed because, in the anteroposterior x-ray, the humeral head may seem to be in contact with the glenoid socket. However, clinically the condition is unmistakable because the arm is held in medial rotation and is locked in that position.

X-rays

In the anteroposterior projection, the humeral head, because it is medially rotated, looks somewhat globular. A lateral film is essential; it shows posterior subluxation and, sometimes, indentation of the humeral head.

Treatment

The arm is pulled and rotated laterally, while the head of the humerus is pushed forwards. After reduction, the management is the same as for anterior dislocation. The management of late-presenting posterior dislocation is complicated.

RECURRENT DISLOCATION

Once a shoulder has been dislocated, this may happen repeatedly – and with increasing ease – over the ensuing months or years. In these cases the capsule and labrum have usually been stripped from the margin of the glenoid and the humeral head may be indented. In the vast majority of cases, recurrence is anterior, but occasionally it is posterior; the distinction is not as easy as it may seem, because often by the time the patient is examined the head is back in the socket and there is only the history to go by.

With recurrent anterior dislocation, the patient complains that the shoulder 'slips out'

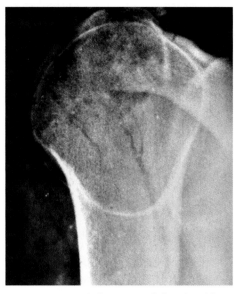

26.8 Posterior dislocation of the shoulder The characteristic x-ray image. Because the head of the humerus is internally rotated, the anteroposterior x-ray shows a head-on projection giving the classic 'electric light-bulb' appearance.

when the arm is lifted into abduction and lateral rotation, as in swimming or dressing or reaching backwards and upwards. At first it has to be 'put back' by someone; as time goes by, reduction becomes easier and often patients learn to do it themselves. The *apprehension test* is positive: if the shoulder is passively manipulated into abduction, extension and lateral rotation, the patient tenses up and anxiously resists further movement.

Imaging

An anteroposterior x-ray with the shoulder in internal rotation will often show a posterolateral defect of the humeral head (Hill–Sachs lesion) where the bone has been damaged by the rim of the glenoid fossa. CT or MRI will show the damaged glenoid labrum (Bankart lesion).

Treatment

If the patient is disabled, an operation will be needed: for anterior dislocation, some form of anterior capsular reconstruction is usually successful; recurrent posterior dislocation is more difficult and may require soft-tissue reconstruction combined with a bone operation to block abnormal movement at the back of the shoulder.

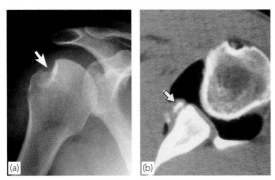

26.9 Recurrent dislocation of the shoulder (a) The classic x-ray sign is a depression in the posterosuperior part of the humeral head (the Hill–Sachs lesion). (b) MRI showing the Bankhart lesion.

FRACTURES OF THE PROXIMAL HUMERUS

Fractures of the proximal humerus usually occur after middle age and are most common in osteoporotic individuals. The patient falls on the outstretched hand, fracturing the surgical neck; one or both tuberosities may also be fractured.

Special features

Pain may not be very severe because the fracture is often firmly impacted. However, the appearance of a large bruise in the upper arm is very suspicious. The patient should be examined for signs of axillary nerve or brachial plexus injury.

Imaging

X-ray examination in elderly patients often appears to show a single, impacted fracture extending across the surgical neck; sometimes a separate fracture of the greater tuberosity is also seen. However, with good definition x-rays several undisplaced fragments may be visible. *In younger patients* the fragments are usually more clearly defined. Axillary and scapular lateral views should always be obtained, to exclude dislocation of the shoulder.

According to Neer's classification, a *one-part fracture* is one in which the fragments are undisplaced or firmly impacted (i.e. the humerus appears to be 'in one piece'); a *two-part fracture* is one in which the neck fracture is displaced (i.e. there are only two fragments, the humeral head and the rest of the bone); *three-part or four-part fractures* are those in which, in addition to the neck fracture, one or both of the tuberosities is also fractured. This sounds systematic and straightforward, but it is not easy to distinguish the radiographic outlines of comminuted fractures.

In common with so many other complex fractures, *a CT scan* will help to diagnose the fracture configuration and plan treatment.

As the fracture heals, the humeral head is sometimes seen to be subluxated downwards (inferiorly); this is due to muscle atony and it usually recovers once exercises are begun.

Treatment

Impacted or minimally displaced fractures need no treatment apart from a short period of rest with

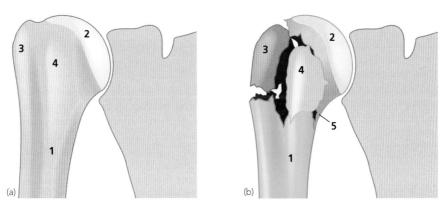

26.10 Fractures of the proximal humerus Diagram of (a) the normal and (b) a fractured proximal humerus, showing the four main fragments, two or more of which are seen in almost all proximal humeral fractures 1, shaft of humerus; 2, head of humerus; 3, greater tuberosity; 4, lesser tuberosity. In this figure there is a sizeable medial calcar spike, 5, suggesting a low risk of avascular necrosis.

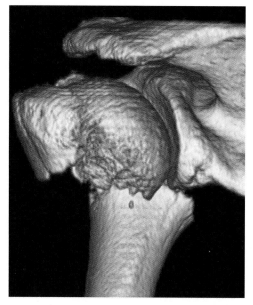

26.11 CT with three-dimensional reconstruction
Advanced imaging provides a much clearer picture of
the injury, allowing better preoperative planning.

the arm in a sling. Active movements are begun as
soon as practicable, but the sling is retained until
the fracture has united (usually after 6 weeks).

Two-part fractures can usually be reduced
closed; the arm is then bandaged to the chest for
3 or 4 weeks, after which shoulder exercises are
commenced (the elbow and hand are, of course,
exercised throughout). If the fragments cannot
be reduced then fixation, particularly in younger
patients, is considered.

Three-part fractures in young, active individuals
usually require open reduction and internal fixation
with a plate and screws. In elderly patients with
osteoporotic bone, the results are less certain and
manipulative reduction followed by physiotherapy
may be equally satisfactory in the long term.
Alternatives for osteoporotic patients include bone
sutures, intramedullary nails or locking plates.

Four-part fractures, which carry additional risks
of incomplete reduction, non-union and avascular
necrosis of the humeral head, are best treated by
prosthetic replacement, particularly in elderly
patients.

Complications

Shoulder dislocation

Combined fracture and dislocation of the shoulder
is difficult to manage. The dislocation should be
reduced (this may require an operation) and the
fracture can then be tackled in the usual way.

Vascular and nerve injuries

These may occur with three-part and four-part
fractures and should be sought at the initial
examination.

Stiffness

Shoulder stiffness is common. It can be minimized
by starting exercises as early as possible.

FRACTURES OF THE PROXIMAL HUMERUS IN CHILDREN

These are often angulated and will re-model well
following simple treatment in a sling for a few
weeks. Occasionally the fracture is through a
benign (or very rarely malignant) bone lesion.

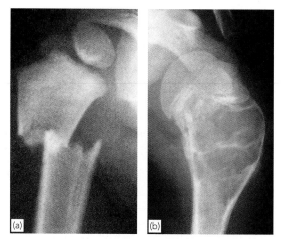

**26.12 Fractures of the proximal humerus in
children** (a) The typical metaphyseal fracture. Reduction
need not be perfect as re-modelling will compensate for
malunion. (b) Fracture through a benign cyst.

FRACTURES OF THE SHAFT OF THE HUMERUS

A fall on the hand may twist the humerus, causing
a spiral fracture. A fall on the elbow with the arm
abducted may hinge the bone, causing an oblique
or transverse fracture. A direct blow to the arm
causes a fracture which is either transverse or
comminuted. A fracture of the shaft in an elderly
patient may be through a metastasis.

Special features

The arm is painful, bruised and swollen. Active
extension of the wrist and fingers should be tested
before and after treatment because the radial nerve
may be damaged.

X-rays

The fracture is usually obvious, but don't forget to look for features suggesting a pathological lesion (e.g. fracture through a bone cyst or metastasis).

Treatment

Fractures of the humerus require neither perfect reduction nor total immobilization; the weight of the arm with an external cast is usually enough to pull the fragments into alignment. The cast is applied from the shoulder to the wrist with the elbow flexed to 90 degrees; after 2–3 weeks, it may be replaced by a shorter cast (shoulder to elbow) or by a removable brace. Exercises of the shoulder can be started within 1 week, but abduction is avoided until the fracture has united. It takes at least 6 weeks for simple spiral fractures to heal. Other fractures may take 3 months or even longer.

If the fracture is very unstable and difficult to control, if it is open, if discomfort is prolonged and a sling is unacceptable or if it is a pathological fracture, internal fixation is preferable. In most cases a plate and screws or a long intramedullary nail with locking screws will suffice. High-energy segmental fractures and some open fractures may be treated with external fixation.

Complications

Nerve injury

Radial nerve palsy (wrist-drop and paralysis of the metacarpophalangeal [MCP] extensors) may occur with oblique fractures of the shaft. In closed injuries the nerve is very seldom divided, so there is no hurry to operate. Passive and active movements of the wrist and hand are encouraged while recovery is awaited.

If there is no sign of recovery by 12 weeks, the nerve should be explored. In complete lesions (neurotmesis), nerve grafting is undertaken but the results are not always satisfactory. If so, function can be largely restored by tendon transfers: pronator teres to extensor carpi radialis brevis for wrist extension; flexor carpi radialis to extensor digitorum for MCP extension; and palmaris longus to abductor pollicis longus for thumb abduction.

Non-union

Midshaft fractures sometimes fail to unite. This is treated by bone grafting and internal fixation.

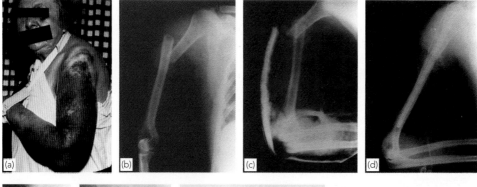

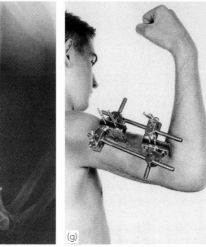

26.13 Fractured shaft of humerus

(a) Bruising is always extensive. Closed transverse fractures with moderate displacement can often be treated by using a sling or a plaster U-slab hanging cast (or ready-made brace). These methods demand careful supervision if excessive angulation and malunion are to be prevented. Beware the upper third fracture (b) which tends to angulate at the proximal border of the splint (c). This particular fracture would have been better managed by (d) intramedullary nailing (and better still with a locking nail). Other methods of fixation – especially for lower-third fractures (e) or open fractures – are compression plating (f) or external fixation (g).

Care must be taken not to injure the radial nerve.

FRACTURES OF THE DISTAL HUMERUS IN CHILDREN

The elbow is second only to the distal forearm for frequency of fractures in children. Most of these injuries are supracondylar fractures, the remainder being divided between condylar, epicondylar and proximal radial and ulnar fractures. Boys are injured more often than girls and more than one-half of the patients are under 10 years old.

The usual accident is a fall directly on the point of the elbow or onto the outstretched hand with the elbow forced into valgus or varus. Pain and swelling are often marked and examination is difficult. X-ray interpretation also has its problems: the bone ends are largely cartilaginous and therefore radiographically incompletely visualized. *A good knowledge of the normal anatomy is essential if fracture displacements are to be recognized.*

Points of anatomy

The elbow is a complex hinge. Its stability is due largely to the shape and fit of the bones that make up the joint and this is liable to be compromised by any break in the articulating structures. The surrounding soft-tissue structures also are important, especially the capsular and collateral ligaments.

With the elbow extended, the forearm is normally in slight valgus in relation to the upper arm, the average carrying angle in children being about 15 degrees. When the elbow is flexed, the forearm comes to lie directly upon the upper arm. Malunion of a supracondylar fracture will inevitably disturb this relationship.

Since the epiphyses are in some part cartilaginous, only the secondary ossific centres can be seen on x-ray; they should not be mistaken for fracture fragments! The average ages at which they appear are easily remembered by the mnemonic CITE: Capitulum – 2 years; Internal (medial) epicondyle – 6 years; Trochlea – 8 years; External (lateral) epicondyle – 12 years. Epiphyseal displacements will not be detectable on x-ray before these ages, but they are inferred from radiographic indices such as *Baumann's angle* (see Figure 26.14).

SUPRACONDYLAR FRACTURES

These are among the commonest fractures in children. The distal fragment may be displaced and/or tilted either posteriorly or anteriorly, medially or laterally; sometimes it is also rotated. *Posterior displacement and tilt* is the commonest (95% of all cases), suggesting a hyperextension injury, usually due to a fall on the outstretched hand. The jagged end of the proximal fragment pokes into the soft tissues anteriorly, sometimes injuring the brachial artery or median nerve. *Anterior displacement* is rare, but may result from over-reduction of the usual posterior displacements.

Special features

Following a fall, the child is in pain and the elbow is swollen; with a posteriorly displaced fracture, the S-deformity of the elbow is usually obvious. It is essential to feel the pulse and check the capillary return.

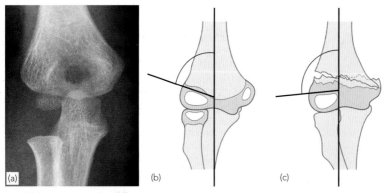

(a) (b) (c)

26.14 Baumann's angle Anteroposterior x-rays are sometimes difficult to make out, especially if the elbow is held flexed after reduction of the supracondylar fracture. Measurement of *Baumann's angle* is helpful. This is the angle subtended by the longitudinal axis of the humeral shaft and a line through the coronal axis of the capitellar physis, as shown in (a) the x-ray of a normal elbow and the accompanying diagram (b). Normally this angle is less than 80 degrees. If the distal fragment is tilted in varus, the increased angle is readily detected (c).

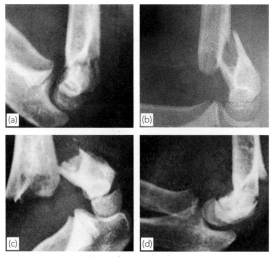

26.15 Supracondylar fractures X-rays showing supracondylar fractures of increasing severity. (a) Undisplaced. (b) Distal fragment posteriorly angulated but in contact. (c) Distal fragment completely separated and displaced posteriorly. (d) A rarer variety with anterior angulation.

X-rays

Undisplaced fractures are easily missed; there may be no more than subtle features of a soft-tissue haematoma. In the common *posteriorly displaced fracture* the distal fragment is tilted backwards and/or shifted backwards. In the rare *anteriorly displaced fracture* the fragment is tilted forwards.

The anteroposterior x-ray is often difficult to interpret because it is taken with the elbow flexed. The degree of sideways tilt (angulation) may therefore not be appreciated. This is where Baumann's angle is most helpful; wherever possible it should be accurately measured and compared with that of the uninjured side (Figure 26.14).

Treatment

If there is even a suspicion of a fracture, the elbow is gently splinted in 30 degrees of flexion to prevent movement and possible neurovascular injury during the x-ray examination.

Undisplaced fractures

The elbow is immobilized at 90 degrees and neutral rotation in a lightweight splint or cast and the arm is supported by a sling. *It is essential to obtain an x-ray 5–7 days later to check that there has been no displacement.* The splint is retained for 3 weeks and supervised movement is then allowed.

Posteriorly minimally angulated fractures

Swelling is usually not severe and the risk of vascular injury is low. If the posterior cortices are in continuity, the fracture can be reduced under general anaesthesia by the following step-wise manoeuvre: (1) traction for 2–3 minutes in the length of the arm with counter-traction above the elbow; (2) correction of any sideways tilt or shift and rotation (in comparison with the other arm); (3) gradual flexion of the elbow to 120 degrees, and pronation of the forearm, while maintaining traction and exerting finger pressure behind the distal fragment to correct posterior tilt. *Then feel the pulse and check the capillary return* – if the distal circulation is suspect, immediately relax the amount of elbow flexion until it improves.

X-rays are taken to confirm reduction, checking carefully to see that there is no varus or valgus angulation and no rotational deformity. If the acutely flexed position cannot be maintained without disturbing the circulation, or if the reduction is unstable, the fracture should be fixed with percutaneous crossed Kirschner wires (K-wires) (take care not to skewer the ulnar nerve!).

Following reduction, the arm is held in a collar and cuff; the circulation should be checked repeatedly during the first 24 hours. An x-ray is obtained after 3–5 days to confirm that the fracture has not slipped. If it has, do not delay – a further attempt at reduction is still possible. If reduction is satisfactory, the splint is retained for 3 weeks, after which movements are begun.

Posteriorly displaced fractures

These are usually associated with *severe swelling*, are difficult to reduce and are often unstable; moreover, there is a considerable risk of neurovascular injury or circulatory compromise due to swelling. The fracture should be reduced under general anaesthesia as soon as possible, by the method described above, and then held with percutaneous crossed K-wires; this obviates the necessity to hold the elbow acutely flexed. Care should be taken not to injure the ulnar and radial nerves. Postoperative management is the same as for simple angulated fractures.

Anteriorly displaced fractures

The fracture is reduced by pulling on the forearm with the elbow semi-flexed, applying thumb pressure over the front of the distal fragment and then extending the elbow fully. A posterior slab is bandaged on and retained for 3 weeks. Thereafter, the child is allowed to regain flexion gradually.

Complications

Vascular injury

The great danger of supracondylar fracture is injury to the brachial artery, which, before the introduction of percutaneous pinning, was reported as occurring in more than 5% of cases. Nowadays the incidence is probably less than 1%. Peripheral ischaemia may be immediate and severe, or the pulse may fail to return after reduction. More commonly, the injury is complicated by forearm oedema and a mounting *compartment syndrome*, which leads to necrosis of the muscle and nerves without causing peripheral gangrene. Undue pain plus one positive sign (pain on passive extension of the fingers, a tense and tender forearm, an absent pulse, blunted sensation or reduced capillary return on pressing the finger pulp) demands urgent action. The flexed elbow must be extended and all dressings removed. If the circulation does not promptly improve, angiography (on the operating table if it saves time) is carried out, the vessel repaired or grafted and a forearm fasciotomy performed. If angiography is not available, or would cause much delay, Doppler assessment should be used. In extreme cases, operative exploration would be justified on clinical criteria alone.

Nerve injury

The median nerve may be injured. Fortunately, loss of function is usually temporary and recovery can be expected in 6–8 weeks.

Malunion

Malunion is common. However, backward or sideways shifts are gradually smoothed out by modelling during growth and they seldom give rise to visible deformity. Forward or backward tilt may limit flexion or extension, but consequent disability is slight.

By contrast, uncorrected sideways tilt (angulation) and rotation may lead to serious deformity of the elbow which will not improve with growth. Cubitus varus is disfiguring and cubitus valgus may cause late ulnar palsy. If deformity is marked, it will need correction by supracondylar osteotomy.

Elbow stiffness

Full movement may take months to return and must not be hurried. Forced movement will only make matters worse and may contribute to the development of heterotopic ossification (see page 379).

> ⚠ Beware of leaving varus angulation of the distal fragment.
> Double check the position and measure Baumann's angle.

FRACTURE–SEPARATION OF THE LATERAL CONDYLE

The distal humeral epiphysis begins to ossify at the age of about 2 years and fuses with the shaft at about 16 years; between these ages, the condylar or epicondylar parts of the epiphysis may be sheared off or avulsed by the sudden pull of the forearm muscles during a fall on the hand. Only two of these injuries are at all common: fracture–separation of the entire condyle on the lateral side, and separation of the epicondyle on the medial side.

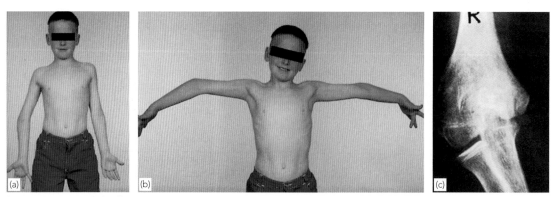

26.16 Supracondylar fractures – complications (a) Varus deformity of the right elbow following incomplete correction of the varus displacement in a supracondylar fracture. (b) The 'gun-stock deformity' becomes more obvious when the arms are raised. (c) X-ray showing the malunion.

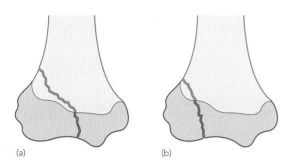

26.17 Physeal fractures of the lateral condyle
(a) The commonest is a fracture starting in the metaphysis and running along the physis of the lateral condyle into the trochlea (Salter–Harris Type II injury). (b) Less common is a fracture running right through the lateral condyle to reach the articular surface in the capitulotrochlear groove (Salter–Harris Type IV): though uncommon, this latter injury is important because of its potential for causing growth defects.

Special features

If the child falls with the elbow stressed in varus, a large fragment including the lateral condyle can be avulsed by the attached wrist extensors. The fracture line usually runs along the physis to enter the joint through the trochlea or (less often) through the capitulatrochlear groove.

The extent of the injury is often not appreciated because the capitellar epiphysis is largely cartilaginous and only the ossific centre in the fragment is visible on x-ray. If the fracture runs through the trochlea, the elbow joint can dislocate. The fragment may be grossly displaced and capsized.

> ⚠ The condylar fragment is always larger than the image shown on x-ray.

Treatment

An *undisplaced fracture* can be treated by splinting the elbow for 2 weeks and then starting exercises. A check x-ray should be obtained after 5 days to make sure that the fracture has not displaced.

A *displaced fracture* may be reduced by manipulation, but if this fails, operative reduction must be carried out and the fragment fixed in position with a screw or K-wires; the arm is immobilized in a cast. The wires are moved after 3–4 weeks and the cast can then be discarded.

Complications

Non-union and malunion

If the condyle is left capsized, *non-union* is inevitable; with growth, the elbow becomes

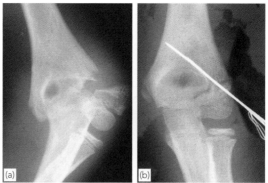

26.18 Fractured lateral condyle – treatment
If displacement is more than 2 mm, open reduction and internal fixation is the treatment of choice.

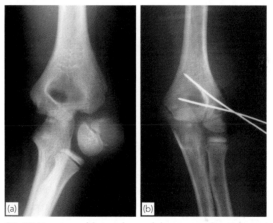

26.19 Fractured lateral condyle – complications
(a) Sometimes the fractured condyle is capsized; it should be reduced and held with a Kirchner wire (b), otherwise it will result in a valgus deformity of the elbow.

increasingly valgus, and ulnar nerve palsy is then likely to develop. *Malunion*, likewise, can result in cubitus valgus. If deformity is marked, it should be corrected by supracondylar osteotomy.

Recurrent dislocation of the elbow

Occasionally condylar displacement results in *recurrent posterolateral dislocation* of the elbow. The only effective treatment is reconstruction of the bony and soft tissues on the lateral side.

SEPARATION OF THE MEDIAL EPICONDYLAR APOPHYSIS

If the wrist is forced into extension, the medial epicondylar apophysis is avulsed by the attached wrist flexors; if the elbow opens up on that side, the epicondylar fragment may be pulled into the joint.

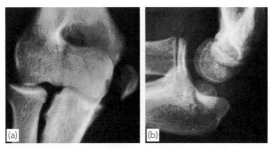

26.20 Fractured medial epicondyle (a) Avulsion of the medial epicondyle following valgus strain. Sometimes the epicondylar fragment is trapped in the joint (b); the serious nature of the injury is liable to be missed unless the surgeon specifically looks for the trapped fragment.

The inner side of the elbow is swollen and acutely tender. The x-ray has to be studied very carefully to detect the tiny ossific centre which marks the epicondylar fragment.

Treatment

Minor displacement may be disregarded; the elbow is splinted for 2–3 weeks to relieve pain, and exercises are then encouraged. However, if the epicondyle is markedly displaced, it should be sutured back in position. If it is trapped in the joint, it must be freed. Manipulation with the elbow in valgus and the wrist hyperextended (to pull on the flexor muscles) may be successful; if this fails, the joint must be opened and the fragment retrieved before being replaced.

FRACTURE OF THE MEDIAL CONDYLE IN CHILDREN

This is much rarer than a lateral condyle fracture. It can be difficult to visualize on a plain x-ray. An arthrogram or MRI scan can be helpful. These are treated in the same way as lateral condyle fractures.

FRACTURE–SEPARATION OF THE ENTIRE DISTAL HUMERAL EPIPHYSIS

Up to the age of 7 years, the distal humeral epiphysis is a solid cartilaginous segment with maturing centres of ossification. With severe injury it may separate en bloc. This is likely to occur with fairly severe violence, such as a birth injury or child abuse.

Special features

The child is distressed and the elbow is markedly swollen. The history may be deceptively uninformative.

X-rays

In a very young child, in whom the bony outlines are still unformed, the x-ray may look normal. Medial displacement of either the capitellar ossification centre or the proximal radius and ulna is very suspicious. In older children the deformity is usually obvious.

Treatment

The injury is treated like a supracondylar fracture. If the diagnosis is uncertain, the elbow is merely splinted in flexion for 2 weeks; any resulting deformity (which is rare) can be dealt with at a later age.

FRACTURES OF THE DISTAL HUMERUS IN ADULTS

There are three types of distal humeral fracture: extra-articular supracondylar fracture, intra-articular unicondylar fracture and bicondylar fractures.

SUPRACONDYLAR FRACTURES

Supracondylar fractures are rare in adults. When they do occur, they are usually displaced and unstable or severely comminuted (high-energy injuries).

Treatment

Closed reduction is unlikely to be stable and K-wire fixation is not strong enough to permit early mobilization. Open reduction and internal fixation is therefore the treatment of choice. The distal humerus is approached through a posterior exposure and reflection of the triceps tendon. A transverse or oblique fracture can usually be reduced and fixed with a single contoured plate and screws. Comminuted fractures may require double plates and transfixing screws.

CONDYLAR FRACTURES

Except in osteoporotic individuals, intra-articular condylar fractures should be regarded as high-energy injuries with soft-tissue damage. A severe blow on the point of the elbow drives the olecranon process upwards, splitting the condyles apart. Swelling is considerable and the bony landmarks are difficult to feel. *The patient should be carefully examined for evidence of vascular or nerve injury;* vascular insufficiency must be addressed as a matter of urgency.

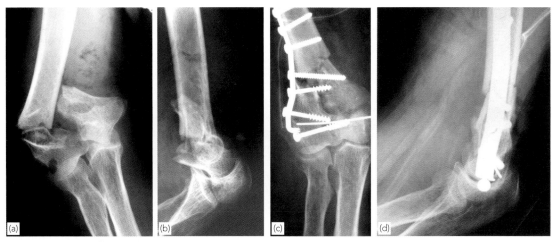

26.21 Bicondylar fractures in adults X-rays taken before (a,b) and after (c,d) open reduction and internal fixation. An excellent reduction was obtained in this case; however, often the elbow ends up with marked loss of movement, even though the general anatomy has been restored.

X-rays

The fracture extends from the lower humerus into the elbow joint; it may be difficult to tell whether one or both condyles are involved, especially with an undisplaced condylar fracture. Sometimes the fracture extends into the metaphysis as a T-shaped or Y-shaped break, and the bone between the condyles may be comminuted.

Treatment

These are usually severe injuries associated with joint damage; prolonged immobilization will certainly result in a stiff elbow. Early movement is therefore a prime objective.

Undisplaced fractures

These can be treated by applying a posterior slab with the elbow flexed almost 90 degrees; gentle movements are commenced after 1 week, but only after obtaining another x-ray to exclude late displacement.

Displaced condylar fractures

Open reduction and internal fixation through a posterior approach is the treatment of choice. The best exposure is obtained by performing an intra-articular olecranon osteotomy. The ulnar nerve should be identified and protected throughout. The fragments are reduced and held temporarily with K-wires. A unicondylar fracture without comminution can then be fixed with screws; if the fragment is large, a contoured plate is added to prevent re-displacement. Bicondylar and comminuted fractures will require double plate and

screw fixation, and sometimes also bone grafts in the gaps. Postoperatively, movement is encouraged but should never be forced.

The fracture heals in about 8 weeks but the elbow often does not regain full movement; in severe injuries, movement may be markedly restricted, however beautiful the postoperative x-ray.

In elderly osteoporotic patients, elbow replacement is often a more reliable option.

Complications

Vascular injury

Always check the circulation (repeatedly!). Vigilance is required to make the diagnosis and institute treatment as early as possible.

Nerve injury

There may be damage to either the median or the ulnar nerve. It is important to examine the hand and record the findings before treatment is commenced and again after treatment. The ulnar nerve may shut down following surgery but it usually recovers in time.

Stiffness

Comminuted fractures of the elbow always result in some degree of stiffness. However, the disability may be reduced by encouraging an energetic exercise programme. Late operations to improve elbow movement are difficult but can be rewarding.

Heterotopic ossification

Severe soft-tissue damage may lead to heterotopic ossification. Forced movement should be avoided.

FRACTURED CAPITULUM

This is an articular fracture which occurs only in adults. The patient falls on the hand, usually with the elbow straight. The anterior part of the capitulum is sheared off and displaced.

Fullness in front of the elbow is the most notable feature. The lateral side of the elbow is tender and flexion is grossly restricted.

Imaging

In the lateral x-ray view the capitulum (or part of it) is seen in front of the lower humerus, and the radial head is not opposed to it. The images can be difficult to interpret and a CT scan is invaluable in planning treatment.

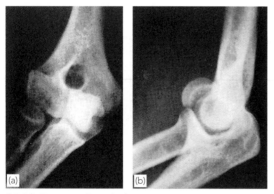

26.22 Fractured capitulum Anteroposterior and lateral x-rays showing proximal displacement and tilting of the capitular fragment.

Treatment

Undisplaced fractures can be treated by resting the arm in a sling for 4–5 days and then starting movement.

Displaced fractures should be treated by operative reduction and fixation with small buried screws.

If this proves too difficult, the fragment is best excised. Movements are commenced as soon as discomfort permits.

DISLOCATION OF THE ELBOW

A fall on the outstretched hand may dislocate the elbow. In 90% of cases the forearm bones are pushed backwards and dislocate posteriorly or posterolaterally. Provided there is no associated fracture, reduction will usually be stable and recurrent dislocation unlikely.

Special features

Deformity is usually obvious and the bony landmarks are displaced. In very severe injuries, pain and swelling are so marked that examination of the elbow is impossible; however, the hand should be examined for signs of vascular or nerve damage.

X-ray examination is essential: (a) to confirm the presence of a dislocation and (b) to identify any associated fractures.

Treatment

Uncomplicated dislocation

The patient should be fully relaxed under anaesthesia. The surgeon pulls on the forearm while the elbow is slightly flexed. With one hand, sideways displacement is corrected, then the elbow is further flexed while the olecranon process is pushed forward. Unless almost full flexion can be obtained, the olecranon is not in the trochlear groove.

After reduction, the elbow should be put through a full range of movement to see whether it is stable. Nerve function and circulation are checked again and the x-ray is repeated to confirm that the joint is reduced and that there are no associated fractures.

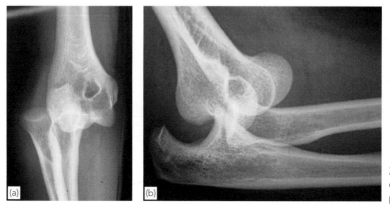

26.23 Dislocation of the elbow X-rays showing lateral and posterior displacement.

The arm is held in a light cast with the elbow flexed to just above 90 degrees and the wrist supported in a collar and cuff. After 1 week the cast can be removed and gentle exercises begun; at 3 weeks the collar and cuff are discarded. Elbow movements are allowed to return spontaneously and should never be forced.

Fracture–dislocation

The combination of radial head fracture, coronoid fracture and medial collateral ligament injury is known as the *'terrible triad'* – a fitting acknowledgement of the severe instability and poor outcome in these cases. Associated fractures of the radial head, coronoid process or the olecranon process, will need internal fixation. In cases where the elbow remains unstable after the bone and joint anatomy has been restored, the ligaments may need repair and a hinged external fixator can be applied in order to maintain mobility while the tissues heal.

Complications

Vascular injury

The brachial artery may be damaged. Absence of the radial pulse is a warning. If there are other signs of ischaemia, this should be treated as an emergency. Splints must be removed and the elbow should be straightened somewhat. If there is no improvement, an arteriogram is performed; the brachial artery may have to be explored.

Nerve injury

The median or ulnar nerve is sometimes injured. Spontaneous recovery usually occurs after 6–8 weeks.

Stiffness

Loss of 20–30 degrees of extension is not uncommon after elbow dislocation. Physiotherapy may help, but forceful manipulation must be avoided.

Heterotopic ossification

Heterotopic bone formation may occur in the damaged soft tissues in front of the joint. In former years 'myositis officans' was a fairly common complication, usually associated with forceful reduction and over-enthusiastic passive movement of the elbow. Nowadays it is rarely seen, but one should be alert for signs such as excessive pain, tenderness, and slow recovery of active movements. X-rays may show soft-tissue ossification as early as 4–6 weeks after injury. If the condition is suspected, exercises are stopped and the elbow is splinted in comfortable flexion

until pain subsides; gentle active movements and continuous passive motion are then resumed. Anti-inflammatory drugs may help to reduce stiffness; they are also used prophylactically to reduce the risk of heterotopic bone formation.

A bone mass which markedly restricts movement and elbow function should be excised once the bone is 'mature', i.e. has well-defined cortical margins and trabeculae. This is followed by anti-inflammatory medication, bisphosphonates or radiotherapy to prevent recurrence.

Osteoarthritis

Secondary osteoarthritis is a late complication. Symptoms can usually be treated conservatively, but if pain and stiffness are intolerable, total elbow replacement can be considered.

ISOLATED DISLOCATION OF THE RADIAL HEAD

Isolated dislocation of the radial head is very rare; if it is seen, search carefully for an associated fracture of the ulna (the Monteggia injury), which may be difficult to detect in a child because the fracture is often incomplete. Even a minor deformity of the ulna may prevent full reduction of the radial head dislocation.

'PULLED ELBOW'

In young children the elbow is sometimes injured by a sharp tug on the wrist. The child is in pain; the elbow is held in extension and he or she will not allow it to be moved. There are no x-ray changes. What has happened is that the radius has been pulled distally and the annular ligament has slipped up over the head of the radius. A dramatic cure is achieved by forcefully supinating and then flexing the elbow; the ligament slips back with a snap.

FRACTURES OF THE PROXIMAL END OF THE RADIUS

Fractures of the proximal end of the radius are fairly common in young adults and children. A fall on the outstretched hand with the elbow extended and the forearm pronated causes impaction of the radial head against the capitulum. In adults this may fracture the *head of the radius*; in children, it is more likely to fracture the *neck of the radius* (possibly because the head is largely cartilaginous). In addition, the articular cartilage of the capitulum may be bruised or chipped; this cannot be seen on x-ray but is an important complication.

Special features

Following a fall on the oustretched arm, the patient complains of pain and local tenderness posterolaterally over the proximal end of the radius. A further clue is a marked increase in pain on pronation and supination of the forearm.

X-rays

In children the fracture is through the neck; the proximal fragment may be tilted forwards and outwards.

The *typical adult fracture* is a vertical split or marginal fracture through the radial head; less often there is a transverse neck fracture. Sometimes the head is crushed or comminuted. Impacted fractures are easily missed unless several views are obtained. The wrist also should be very carefully examined to exclude a concomitant injury of the distal radioulnar joint – the Essex Lopresti lesion – which if not recognized early can be almost impossible to treat.

Treatment

Children

In fractures of the radial neck, up to 30 degrees of radial head tilt and up to 3 mm of transverse displacement are acceptable. The arm is rested in a collar and cuff, and exercises are commenced after 1 week.

Displacement of more than 30 degrees should be corrected. With the patient's elbow extended, traction and varus force are applied; the surgeon then pushes the displaced radial fragment into position with his or her thumb. If this fails, open reduction is performed; there is no need for internal fixation. Following operation, the elbow is splinted in 90 degrees of flexion for 1–2 weeks and then movements are encouraged. *The head of the radius must never be excised in children because this will interfere with the synchronous growth of radius and ulna.*

Fractures that are seen 1 week or longer after injury should be left untreated (except for light splintage).

Adults

Undisplaced fractures of the radial head can be treated by supporting the elbow in a collar and cuff for 2 weeks; active flexion, extension and rotation are encouraged.

Displaced fractures are treated by open reduction and fixation with small screws.

Comminuted fractures have in the past been treated by excising the radial head. However, if there are associated forearm injuries or disruption of the distal radioulnar joint, the risk of proximal migration of the radius is considerable and the patient may develop intractable symptoms of pain and instability in the forearm. In such cases, every effort should be made to reconstruct the radial head or, if it has to be excised, it should be replaced by a metal prosthesis.

Complications

- *Joint stiffness* is common and may involve both the elbow and the radioulnar joints.
- *Recurrent instability of the elbow* can occur if the medial collateral ligament was injured and the radial head then excised.

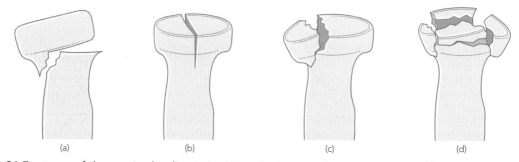

26.24 Fractures of the proximal radius (a) In children the injury usually causes a fracture of the neck of the radius. (b–d) In adults the injury is usually a vertical split (b), a marginal fragment (c) or a comminuted fracture of the head of the radius (d).

■ *Osteoarthritis of the radiocapitellar joint* is a late complication of adult injuries. This may call for excision of the radial head.

FRACTURES OF THE OLECRANON PROCESS

Two types of injury are seen: (1) a *comminuted fracture*, which is due to a direct blow or a fall on the elbow; and (2) a *clean transverse fracture*, due to traction when the patient falls onto the hand while the triceps muscle is contracted.

Special features

A graze or bruise over the elbow suggests a comminuted fracture: the triceps is intact and the elbow can be extended against gravity. With a transverse fracture there may be a palpable gap and the patient is unable to extend the elbow against resistance.

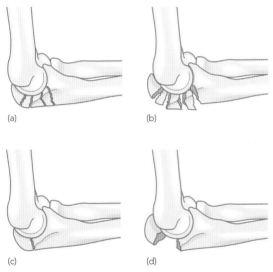

26.25 Fractured olecranon (a,b) Comminuted fractures, undisplaced and displaced. (c,d) Transverse fractures, undisplaced and displaced.

X-rays

A properly orientated lateral view is essential to show details of the fracture, as well as the associated joint damage. The position of the radial head should be checked: it may be dislocated.

Treatment

An *undisplaced comminuted fracture* with the triceps intact can occasionally be treated conservatively if the patient is old and osteoporotic; internal fixation is challenging and immobilizing the elbow will lead to stiffness. The arm is rested in a sling until the pain subsides; a further x-ray is obtained to ensure that there is no displacement, and the patient is then encouraged to start active movements. Comminuted fractures in others should be treated by operation, using meticulous technique to preserve the soft-tissue attachments. Modern metal plates are specially contoured for these fractures and can 'bridge' across the fragments.

An *undisplaced transverse fracture* that does not separate when the elbow is flexed can be treated by immobilizing the elbow in a cast in about 60 degrees of flexion for 1 week; then exercises are begun. The fracture must be examined carefully with repeat x-rays to make sure it does not distract.

Displaced transverse fractures can, theoretically, be held by splinting the arm absolutely straight – but stiffness in that position would be disastrous. Operative treatment is therefore preferred. The fracture is reduced under vision and held by one of three methods: (a) fixation with a long cancellous screw inserted from the tip of the olecranon; or (b) tension-band wiring – two stiff wires driven across the fracture, leaving their ends protruding proximally and distally to anchor a tight loop of wire which will pull the fragments together; or (c) a contoured low-profile plate and screws. Early mobilization should be encouraged.

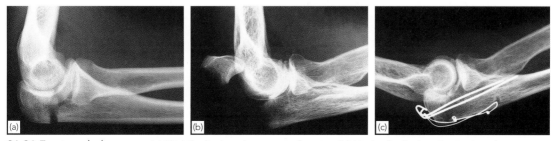

26.26 Fractured olecranon (a) Slightly displaced transverse fracture. (b) Markedly displaced transverse fracture – the extensor mechanism is no longer intact. Treatment in this case was by open reduction and tension-band wiring (c).

Complications

Stiffness used to be common, but with secure internal fixation and early mobilization the residual loss of movement should be minimal.

Non-union sometimes occurs after inadequate reduction and fixation of a transverse fracture. If elbow function is good, it can be ignored; if not, rigid internal fixation and bone grafting will be needed.

Osteoarthritis is a late complication, especially if the articular surface in the trochlear notch is poorly reduced. This can usually be treated with modification of activities and occasional cortisone injections. Joint replacement is considered for severe symptoms but heavy work and sport would not be permissible afterwards.

CHAPTER 27

INJURIES OF THE FOREARM AND WRIST

FRACTURES OF THE RADIUS AND ULNA

A twisting force (usually a fall on the hand) produces spiral fractures with the bones broken at different levels. A direct blow or an angulating force causes transverse fractures of one or both bones at the same level. The bone fragments are easily displaced by contraction of strong muscles attached to the radius. Bleeding and swelling in the muscle compartments of the forearm may cause circulatory impairment.

Special features

The diagnosis is usually quite obvious, but the wrist and hand must be carefully examined for signs of nerve damage or circulatory impairment.

X-rays

In adults the fractures are easy to see; in children they are often incomplete and the bones may appear bent rather than broken.

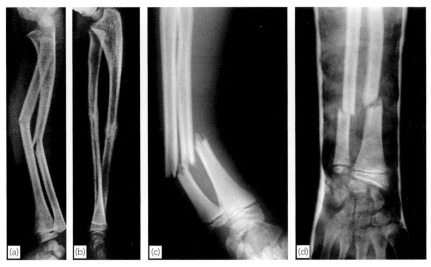

27.1 Fractured radius and ulna in children Greenstick fractures (a) need only correction of angulation (b) and plaster splintage. Complete fractures (c) are harder to reduce; however, provided alignment is corrected and held in plaster (d), re-modelling will restore the anatomy.

Treatment

Children

In children, closed reduction is usually successful and the fragments can be held in a well-moulded, full-length cast extending from the axilla to the metacarpal shafts (to control rotation). The cast is applied with the elbow at 90 degrees. If the radial fracture is proximal to pronator teres, the forearm is supinated; if it is distal to pronator teres, the forearm is held in neutral. The position is checked by x-ray after 1 week and, if it is satisfactory, splintage is retained until both fractures are united (usually 6–8 weeks).

Throughout this period, hand and shoulder exercises are encouraged. If reduction is impossible or unstable, then fixation with small plates or intramedullary pins is needed. The pins are inserted with great care taken to avoid the growth plates.

Adults

Unless the fragments are in close apposition, reduction is difficult and re-displacement in the cast almost inevitable. Consequently, most surgeons opt for open reduction and internal fixation from the outset. The fragments are held by plates and screws. The deep fascia is left open to prevent a build-up of pressure in the muscle compartments, and only the skin and subcutaneous tissues are sutured.

After the operation, the arm is kept elevated until the swelling subsides, and during this period active exercises of the hand are encouraged. If the fracture is not comminuted and the patient is reliable, early range-of-movement exercises are commenced, but lifting and sports are avoided. It takes 8–12 weeks for the bones to unite.

Complications

Nerve injury

Nerve injuries are rarely caused by the fracture, but they may be caused by the surgeon! Exposure of the radius in its proximal third risks damage to the posterior interosseous nerve where it is covered by the superficial part of the supinator muscle. Surgical technique is particularly important here; the anterior Henry approach is safest to protect the nerve.

Compartment syndrome

Fractures (and operations) of the forearm bones are always associated with swelling of the soft tissues, with the attendant risk of a compartment syndrome. The threat is even greater, and the diagnosis more difficult, if the forearm is wrapped up in plaster. The byword is 'watchfulness'; if there are any signs of circulatory embarrassment, treatment must be prompt and uncompromising (see page 353).

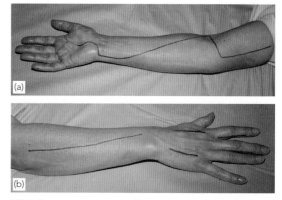

27.3 Compartment syndrome Incisions to relieve a compartment syndrome in the forearm.

Delayed union and non-union

Most fractures of the radius and ulna heal within 8–12 weeks. However, one of the bones may take longer than usual, and immobilization may have to be continued beyond the usual time. High-energy and open fractures are at risk of developing non-union, which will require bone grafting and internal fixation.

Malunion

With closed reduction there is always a risk of malunion, resulting in angulation or rotational

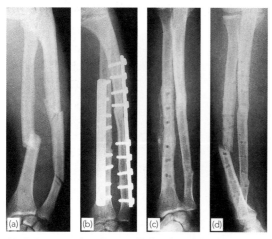

27.2 Fractured radius and ulna in adults
(a,b) Forearm fractures in adults have a strong tendency to re-displace after closed reduction and are therefore usually treated by internal fixation with sturdy plates and screws. Removal of the implants is not without risk. In this case (c,d) the radius fractured through one of the screw holes.

deformity of the forearm, cross-union of the fragments, or shortening of one of the bones and disruption of the distal radioulnar joint. If pronation or supination is severely restricted, and there is no cross-union, mobility may be improved by a corrective osteotomy.

Complications of plate removal

Removal of plates and screws is often regarded as a fairly innocuous procedure. Beware! Complications are common, and they include damage to vessels and nerves, infection, and fractures through screw holes.

FRACTURE OF A SINGLE FOREARM BONE

Fracture of either the radius or the ulna alone is uncommon. Its importance lies in the fact that deformity or shortening of one bone (while the partner bone remains intact) usually involves a concomitant disruption of either the proximal or distal radioulnar joint. This associated injury must always be looked for by obtaining a full-length x-ray of the forearm, including the elbow and wrist.

Special features

Ulnar fractures are easily missed – even on x-ray. If there is local tenderness, a further x-ray 1–2 weeks later is wise. Always examine the elbow and wrist.

X-rays

The fracture may be anywhere in the radius or ulna. It usually follows a direct blow – the so-called 'nightstick fracture' when the victim's arm is raised to protect the face and the assailant's weapon strikes the ulna. The fracture line is transverse and displacement is slight. In children, the intact bone sometimes bends without actually breaking ('*plastic deformation*').

Treatment

Isolated fracture of the ulna

The fracture must be perfectly reduced. Even a slight angulation will affect rotation at the distal radioulnar joint. Surgical fixation will ensure an anatomical reduction and obviate the need for a cast.

Isolated fracture of the radius

Radial fractures are prone to rotary displacement; to achieve reduction, the forearm needs to be supinated for upper-third fractures, neutral for middle-third fractures and pronated for lower-third fractures. The position is usually difficult to hold, so for almost all of these fractures, rigid internal fixation with a compression plate and screws is preferred. Following the operation early movement is encouraged.

MONTEGGIA FRACTURE – DISLOCATION OF THE ULNA

The injury originally described by Monteggia was a fracture of the shaft of the ulna associated with disruption of the proximal radioulnar joint and dislocation of the radiocapitellar joint. Nowadays, the term includes also fractures of the olecranon combined with radial head dislocation.

Special features

Usually the cause is a fall on the hand and forced pronation of the forearm. The radial head usually dislocates forwards and the upper third of the ulna fractures and bows forwards. The forearm deformity is obvious but the radial head dislocation may be missed.

X-rays

Any apparently isolated fracture of the ulna should raise the suspicion of a proximal radial dislocation.

27.4 Monteggia fracture–dislocation of the radius and ulna (a–c) The Monteggia injury is a fracture of the ulna and dislocation of the proximal end of the radius. X-rays that include the elbow joint will show that the head of the radius no longer points to the capitulum. In a child, closed reduction and plaster is usually satisfactory; in the adult (b,c), the crucial step is to restore the ulna to its full length by reducing the fracture and holding it with internal fixation; in most cases the radial head will then reduce by itself but if it does not then open reduction is required.

A good lateral view of the elbow will confirm the diagnosis: normally the head of the radius points directly to the capitulum; if it is dislocated, it lies in a plane anterior to the capitulum.

Treatment

The secret of successful treatment is to restore the length of the fractured ulna; only then can the dislocated proximal radioulnar joint be fully reduced and remain stable. In adults, this means an operation. The ulnar fracture must be accurately reduced, with the bone restored to full length, and then fixed with a plate and screws. The radial head usually reduces once the ulna has been fixed. Stability must be tested through a full range of movement. If the radial head does not reduce, or is not stable after reduction, open reduction should be performed.

If the elbow is completely stable, flexion/extension and rotation can be started after 10 days. If there is doubt, the arm should be immobilized in plaster with the elbow flexed for 6 weeks.

Complications

Unreduced dislocation

If the diagnosis has been missed or the dislocation imperfectly reduced, the radial head remains dislocated and limits both elbow flexion and forearm rotation. In children no treatment is advised until the end of growth, and then only if function is significantly impaired. In adults operative reduction or excision of the radial head may be needed.

GALEAZZI FRACTURE – DISLOCATION OF THE RADIUS

The counterpart of the Monteggia injury is a fracture of the distal third of the radius and dislocation or subluxation of the distal radioulnar joint.

Special features

The Galeazzi fracture is much more common than the Monteggia. Prominence or tenderness over the lower end of the ulna is the striking feature. It is important also to test for an ulnar nerve lesion, which is common.

X-rays

The displaced fracture in the lower third of the radius is obvious; check the inferior radioulnar joint for subluxation or dislocation.

Treatment

As with the Monteggia fracture, the important step is to restore the length of the fractured bone. In

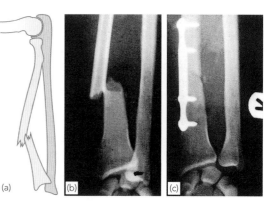

27.5 Galeazzi fracture–dislocation (a) In the Galeazzi fracture–dislocation it is the radius that is fractured and thereby 'shortened', causing the head of the ulna to dislocate. (b,c) X-rays before and after reduction and plating.

children, closed reduction is often successful; in adults, reduction is best achieved by open operation and compression plating of the radius. An x-ray is taken to ensure that the distal radioulnar joint is reduced and stable. If it is, no further action is needed; the arm is rested for a few days, after which gentle active movements are encouraged. If it is reduced but unstable, the radioulnar joint should be fixed with a Kirschner wire (K-wire) and the forearm splinted in an above-elbow cast for 6 weeks. If there is a large ulnar styloid fragment, it should be reduced and fixed.

FRACTURES OF THE DISTAL RADIUS IN ADULTS

COLLES' FRACTURE

The injury which Abraham Colles described in 1814 is a transverse fracture of the radius just above the wrist, with dorsal displacement of the distal fragment. It is the most common of all fractures in older people, the high incidence being related to the onset of postmenopausal osteoporosis. Thus the patient is usually an older woman who gives a history of falling on her outstretched hand.

Special features

With undisplaced fractures, there may be pain and swelling but little or no deformity. Displaced fractures produce a distinctive dorsal tilt just above the wrist – the so-called 'dinner-fork deformity'.

X-rays

The radius is fractured at the corticocancellous junction, about 2 cm from the wrist; often the ulnar styloid is also fractured. Characteristically, the distal fragment is shifted and tilted both dorsally and towards the radial side; in some cases the fracture is impacted, in others it may be severely comminuted.

Treatment

Undisplaced fractures

If the fracture is undisplaced a dorsal splint is applied for 1–2 days until the swelling has resolved, then the cast is completed. The fracture is stable and the cast can usually be removed after 4 weeks to allow mobilization.

Displaced fractures

Displaced fractures must be reduced under anaesthesia (haematoma block, Bier's block or axillary block). The hand is grasped and traction is applied in the length of the bone to disimpact the fragments; the distal fragment is then pushed into place by pressing on the dorsum while manipulating the wrist into moderate flexion, ulnar deviation and pronation. The position is then checked by x-ray. If it is satisfactory, a dorsal plaster slab is applied, extending from just below the elbow to the metacarpal necks and two-thirds of the way round the circumference of the wrist. It is held in position by a crepe bandage. *Extreme positions of flexion and ulnar deviation must be avoided*: 20 degrees in each direction is adequate.

The arm is kept elevated for the next day or two; shoulder and finger exercises are started as soon possible. If the fingers become swollen, cyanosed or painful, there should be no hesitation in splitting the bandage.

It is essential to check the position again by x-ray 10 days later. Often the fracture re-displaces in the cast; if re-manipulation is needed, this should be done within the first 2 weeks.

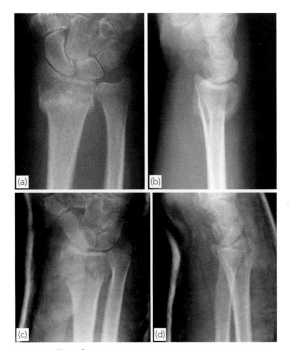

27.6 Colles' fracture (a,b) The typical Colles' fracture is both displaced and angulated towards the dorsum and towards the radial side of the wrist. (c,d) Note how, after successful reduction, the radial articular surface faces correctly both distally and slightly volarwards.

The fracture usually unites in about 5 weeks and, even in the absence of radiological proof of union, the slab may then be discarded and exercises begun.

Comminuted and unstable Colles' fractures

If plaster immobilization alone cannot hold the fracture, then surgery is considered. Options include percutaneous K-wire fixation; the plaster

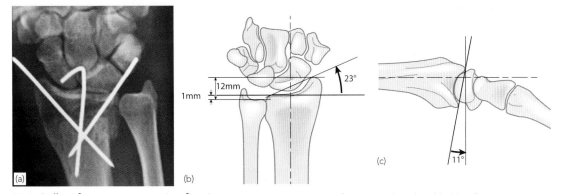

27.7 Colles' fracture – operative fixation (a) Comminuted Colles' fracture reduced and held with percutaneous wires. Make sure that the articular surface angles are correctly restored (b,c).

and wires are removed after 5 weeks and exercises begun. For very unstable fractures and osteoporotic bone, external fixation may be added to prevent collapse around the wires. Proximal pins are placed through the radius and distal pins through the shaft of the second metacarpal. Bone grafts may be added if the radius has markedly collapsed.

Internal fixation with metal plates applied to the front of the distal radius is becoming increasingly popular. The plates have a special design such that the screws lock into the plate which holds the plate–bone combination very firmly even in relatively osteoporotic and comminuted bone, allowing early functional movement.

Complications

Circulatory impairment

Circulation in the fingers must be checked; the bandage holding the slab may need to be split or loosened.

Nerve injury

The median nerve may be compressed by swelling in the carpal tunnel. If the symptoms are mild, they may resolve with release of the dressings and elevation of the arm. If symptoms are severe or persistent, the transverse carpal ligament should be divided.

Malunion

Malunion is common, either because reduction was not complete or because displacement within the plaster was overlooked. In most cases, treatment is not necessary. However, if disability is marked, the radial deformity can be corrected by osteotomy.

Associated radioulnar and carpal injuries

Compression fractures in osteoporotic bone may result in shortening of the radius relative to the ulna (positive ulnar variance) and displacement of the radioulnar joint, which can be painful.

Ligament strains around the wrist are more common than generally recognized and may be a source of pain and weakness long after the fracture has healed.

Tendon rupture

Rupture of the extensor pollicis longus tendon occasionally occurs several weeks after the fracture. The frayed fibres cannot easily be sutured; a tendon transfer, using one of the extensor tendons of the index finger, will restore lost function.

Joint stiffness

Stiffness of the shoulder, elbow and fingers can be avoided by encouraging active movement.

Complex regional pain syndrome

This troublesome condition (formerly called Sudeck's atrophy or reflex sympathetic dystrophy) may appear after a Colles' fracture. Early signs are swelling and tenderness of the finger joints – a warning not to neglect the daily exercises. By the time the plaster is removed, the hand is stiff and painful and there are signs of vasomotor instability. X-rays show osteoporosis and there is increased activity on the bone scan. Treatment is discussed on page 362.

SMITH'S FRACTURE

Smith (a Dubliner, like Colles) described a similar fracture about 20 years later. However, in this injury the distal fragment is displaced and tilted anteriorly (which is why it is sometimes called a 'reversed Colles'). It is caused by a fall on the back of the hand.

Treatment

The fracture is reduced by traction and extension of the wrist. The forearm can be immobilized in a cast for 6 weeks. If the fracture is unstable (and they usually are), percutaneous wires will add support. However, rigid fixation with a volar locking plate allows earlier return of function.

FRACTURE OF THE RADIAL STYLOID PROCESS

This injury is caused by forced radial deviation of the wrist, usually the result of a fall. The fracture line is transverse, just proximal to the radial styloid process.

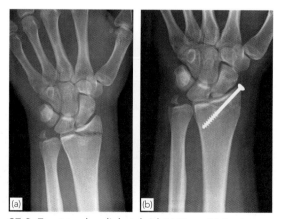

27.8 Fractured radial styloid (a) X-ray; (b) fixation with cannulated percutaneous screw.

Treatment

If the styloid fragment is displaced, it should be reduced and held with screws or K-wires.

FRACTURE–SUBLUXATION OF THE WRIST (BARTON'S FRACTURE)

Barton's injury is an oblique fracture which runs from the volar surface of the distal end of the radius into the wrist joints. The fragment is often displaced anteriorly, carrying the carpus with it as a fracture–dislocation. The significance of recognizing this fracture is that it can be expected to be unstable.

Treatment

The fracture may be easily reduced, but it is just as easily re-displaced. Internal fixation, using a small anterior buttress plate, is recommended.

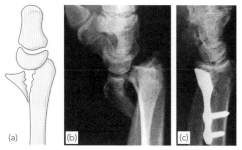

27.9 Fracture–subluxation (Barton's fracture) (a,b) The true Barton's fracture is a split of the volar edge of the distal radius with anterior (volar) subluxation of the wrist. This has been reduced and held (c) with a small anterior plate.

COMMINUTED INTRA-ARTICULAR FRACTURES IN YOUNG ADULTS

In the young adult, a comminuted intra-articular fracture is a high-energy injury. A poor outcome

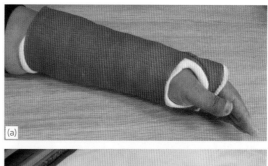

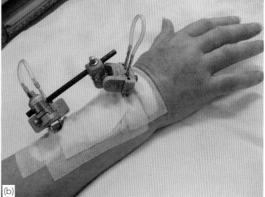

27.10 Distal radius fracture Options include a simple cast (a) or external fixation (b) depending on the amount of comminution, stability of the fracture and patient demands.

will result unless intra-articular congruity, fracture alignment and length are restored and movements started as soon as possible.

Treatment

The simplest option is a manipulation and cast immobilization but only if a perfect reduction is achieved. If highly comminuted then open reduction can disrupt the soft-tissue envelope; distraction with an external fixator and percutaneous wires may

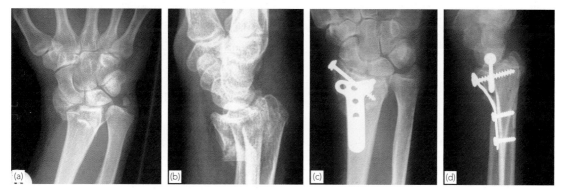

27.11 High-energy injuries in younger patients Perfect reduction is required.

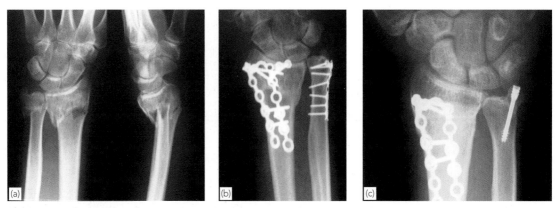

27.12 Don't forget the ulna (a) Fracture of radius and ulna, both unstable. (b) Both bones fixed. (c) Ulnar styloid fracture fixed to prevent instability of distal radioulnar joint.

be the most suitable option. In fractures where the anatomy is not restored, and there are identifiable fragments (computed tomography [CT] scanning can help to decide) open reduction and volar plate fixation may be necessary. Sometimes a separate dorsal approach is required as well.

COMPLICATIONS OF DISTAL RADIUS FRACTURES

Carpal instability

Any serious injury of the distal radius and ulna, and especially those involving the wrist joint, may be associated with unsuspected injuries of the carpus. These can be excluded only by careful clinical and x-ray examination. If they are overlooked, the patient may return months or years later with symptoms and signs of carpal instability (see page 196).

Secondary osteoarthritis

Injuries around the wrist joint may eventually lead to secondary osteoarthritis. It is difficult to predict when (or even whether) this is likely to occur: symptoms develop slowly and disability is often not severe. If pain and weakness interfere significantly with function, then partial arthrodesis, total arthrodesis or even joint replacement of the wrist may be needed.

DISTAL FOREARM FRACTURES IN CHILDREN

The distal radius and ulna are among the commonest sites of childhood fractures. The break may occur through the distal radial physis or in the metaphysis of one or both bones. Metaphyseal fractures are often incomplete or greenstick.

The usual injury is a fall on the outstretched hand with the wrist in extension; the distal fragment is usually forced posteriorly (this is often called a 'juvenile Colles' fracture'). Lesser force may do no more than buckle the metaphyseal cortex (a type of compression fracture, or torus fracture).

Special features

The wrist is painful, and often quite swollen; sometimes there is an obvious 'dinner-fork deformity'.

X-rays

Physeal fractures are almost invariably Salter–Harris Type 1 or 2, with the epiphysis shifted and tilted backwards and radially. Metaphyseal injuries may appear as mere buckling of the cortex, as angulated greenstick fractures, or as complete fractures with displacement and shortening. If only the radius is fractured, the ulna may be bent though not fractured.

Treatment

Physeal fractures are reduced, under anaesthesia, by pressure on the distal fragment. The arm is immobilized in a full-length cast with the wrist slightly flexed and ulnar deviated, and the elbow at 90 degrees. The cast is retained for 4 weeks. These fractures do not interfere with growth. Even if reduction is not absolutely perfect, further growth and modelling will obliterate any deformity within a year or two.

Buckle fractures require no more than 2 weeks in plaster, followed by another 2 weeks of restricted activity.

Greenstick fractures are usually easy to reduce – but apt to re-displace in the cast! Some degree of angulation can be accepted: in children under the

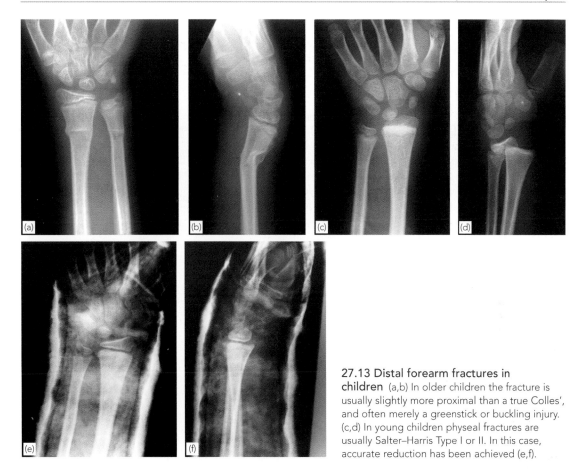

27.13 Distal forearm fractures in children (a,b) In older children the fracture is usually slightly more proximal than a true Colles', and often merely a greenstick or buckling injury. (c,d) In young children physeal fractures are usually Salter–Harris Type I or II. In this case, accurate reduction has been achieved (e,f).

age of 10 years, up to 30 degrees, and in children over 10 years, up to 15 degrees. If the deformity is greater, the fracture is reduced by thumb pressure and the arm is immobilized in a full-length cast with the wrist and forearm in neutral and the elbow flexed 90 degrees. The cast is changed and the fracture re-x-rayed at 1 week; if it has re-displaced, a further gentle manipulation can be carried out. The cast is finally discarded after 6 weeks. Occasionally surgical stabilization, preferably with intramedullary pins, is required.

Complete fractures can be difficult to reduce – especially if the ulna is intact. The fracture is manipulated in much the same way as a Colles' fracture; the reduction is checked by x-ray and a full-length cast is applied with the wrist neutral and the forearm supinated. After 1 week, a check x-ray is obtained; the cast is kept on for 6 weeks. If the fracture slips, especially if the ulna is intact, it should be stabilized with a percutaneous K-wire.

Complications

Forearm swelling and a threatened compartment syndrome are prevented by avoiding over-forceful or repeated manipulations, splitting the plaster, elevating the arm for the first 24–48 hours and encouraging exercises.

Malunion as a late sequel is uncommon in children under 10 years of age. Deformity of as much as 30 degrees will straighten out with further growth and re-modelling over the next 5 years. This should be carefully explained to the worried parents.

INJURIES OF THE CARPUS

Injuries of the wrist comprise soft-tissue strains and fractures or dislocations of individual carpal bones. However, they should never be regarded as isolated injuries: the entire carpus suffers, and sometimes, long after the fracture has healed, the patient still complains of pain and weakness in the wrist.

Clinical assessment

Following a fall, the patient complains of pain in the wrist, perhaps accompanied by swelling. Tenderness can often be localized to a particular spot, providing a clue to the diagnosis. Movements are likely to be restricted and painful.

X-rays

Fractures are often quite obvious, but sometimes multiple views – and examination on multiple occasions – are needed to detect an undisplaced crack.

Study the shape of the carpus and the relationship of the bones to each other. Familiarity with the normal anatomy is essential. Unusual gaps (e.g. between the scaphoid and the lunate) suggest disruption of ligaments; more subtle changes appear in the alignment of the bones. In the lateral x-ray, the axes of the radius, lunate, capitate and third metacarpal are co-linear, and the scaphoid projects at an angle of about 45 degrees to this line. With traumatic instability, the linked carpal segments collapse (like the buckled carriages of a derailed train). Two patterns are recognized: dorsal intercalated segment instability (DISI), in which the lunate is torn from the scaphoid and tilts backwards; and volar intercalated segment

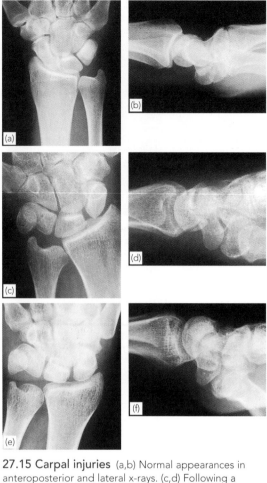

27.15 Carpal injuries (a,b) Normal appearances in anteroposterior and lateral x-rays. (c,d) Following a 'sprained wrist' this patient developed persistent pain and weakness. X-rays showed (c) scapholunate dissociation and (d) dorsal rotation of the lunate (the typical dorsal intercalated segmental instability pattern). (e,f) This patient, too, had a sprained wrist. The anteroposterior and lateral x-rays show foreshortening of the scaphoid and volar rotation of the lunate (volar intercalated segmental instability).

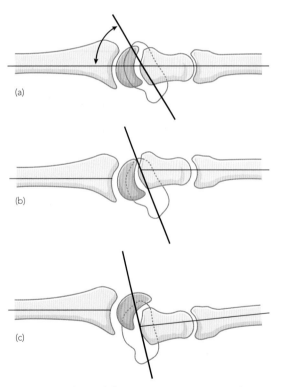

27.14 Carpal instability – x-ray patterns (a) Normal lateral view. The radius, capitate and middle metacarpal lie in a straight line and the scaphoid axis is angled at 45 degrees to the line of the radius. (b) Dorsal intercalated segmental instability. The lunate is tilted dorsally and the scaphoid is tilted somewhat volarwards; the axes of the capitate and metacarpals now lie behind (dorsal to) that of the radius. (c) Volar intercalated segmental instability. The lunate and scaphoid are tilted somewhat volarwards and the capitate and metacarpals lie anterior (volar) to the radius.

instability (VISI), in which the lunate is torn from the triquetrum and tilts forwards.

Principles of management

A diagnosis of 'wrist sprain' should not be accepted until a more serious injury has been excluded with certainty. Even with apparently trivial injuries, ligaments are sometimes torn and the patient may later develop carpal instability.

If the initial x-rays seem to be normal but the clinical signs suggest a carpal injury, a splint or plaster should be applied and the x-ray examination repeated 2 weeks later; a fracture or dislocation may then be more obvious. A magnetic resonance imaging (MRI) scan is very helpful to settle uncertainty and allow either earlier definitive treatment or reassurance that there is not a serious injury after all.

If splintage is needed, the fingers should be left free so that movements are not unnecessarily impeded.

FRACTURE OF THE SCAPHOID

Scaphoid fractures account for almost 75% of all carpal fractures. The usual mechanism is a fall on the hand with wrist extended. The critical movement is probably a combination of dorsiflexion and radial deviation, with the force passing between the two rows of carpal bones; the scaphoid, lying partly in each row, fractures across its waist. The injury is rare in children and in the elderly.

The blood supply of the scaphoid diminishes proximally. This accounts for the fact that 1% of distal-third fractures, 20% of middle-third fractures and 40% of proximal fractures result in non-union or avascular necrosis of the proximal fragment.

Special features

There may be slight fullness in the anatomical snuffbox; precisely localized tenderness in the same place is an important diagnostic sign. However, examination must also include pressure backwards over the scaphoid tubercle, palpation over the proximal pole and telescoping of the thumb base. If any of these are positive then the suspicion for a scaphoid fracture should be high.

Imaging

X-rays should offer anteroposterior, lateral and two oblique views; even then, the fracture may not be seen in the first few days after the injury. Two weeks later, the break is usually much clearer, due to bone resorption at the fracture site and slight displacement of fragments. The crack is usually transverse through the narrowest part of the bone (the waist), but it may be more proximal or more distal. Always look for signs of associated carpal displacement.

A *CT scan* is more sensitive for diagnosing a scaphoid fracture; it is particularly useful in confirming the alignment of the bone fragments if surgery is planned, or to confirm whether the fracture has united or not.

MRI is the definitive way to confirm or exclude a diagnosis of scaphoid fracture if the technique is available.

Treatment

If the x-ray looks normal but the clinical features are suggestive of a fracture, the patient must not be discharged. The diagnosis has to be confirmed one way or another. The usual advice is to return for a second x-ray 2 weeks later. Meanwhile, the wrist is immobilized in a cast extending from the upper forearm to just short of the metacarpophalangeal joints of the fingers, but incorporating the proximal phalanx of the thumb; the wrist is held dorsiflexed and the thumb forwards in the 'glass-holding' position (the so-called scaphoid plaster). An alternative is to arrange an MRI scan (or, if not available, a CT scan) which will definitely detect the fracture even if it was not visible on the x-ray.

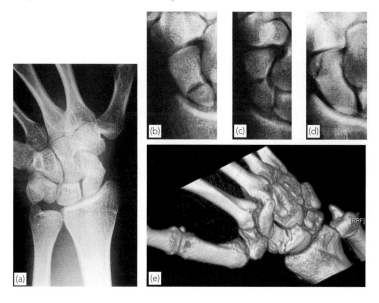

27.16 Fractures of the scaphoid – diagnosis

(a) The initial anteroposterior view often fails to show the fracture. The fracture may be (b) through the proximal pole, (c) the waist, or (d) the scaphoid tubercle. (e) A CT scan is useful for showing the fracture configuration.

If a fracture is confirmed, treatment will depend on the type of fracture and the degree of displacement.

Fracture of the scaphoid tubercle usually needs no splintage and should be treated as a wrist sprain; a crepe bandage is applied and movement is encouraged.

Undisplaced fractures of the waist need no reduction and can be treated in plaster; 90% should heal. After 8 weeks, the plaster is removed and the wrist examined clinically and radiologically. If there is no tenderness and the x-ray shows that the fracture has fully healed, the wrist is left free; if there is doubt a CT scan should be used to confirm whether it has indeed healed. For those who do not wish, or cannot afford, to have so long in plaster with a potentially uncertain outcome, the alternative is to treat the fracture with surgery as soon as it is diagnosed, passing a compression screw percutaneously through the fracture. This allows earlier functional movement and may also increase the chance of union.

If the scaphoid is tender, or the fracture still visible on x-ray, when non-operative treatment is chosen, the cast is re-applied and retained for a further 6 weeks. If, at that stage, there are signs of *delayed union* (bone resorption and cavitation around the fracture), healing can be hastened by bone grafting and internal fixation.

Displaced fractures can be manipulated and treated in plaster, but the outcome is less predictable. It is better to reduce the fracture and to fix it with a compression screw.

Proximal pole fractures have such a poor rate of healing that unless the patient is prepared to spend a long time in plaster (and even then sometimes the fracture does not heal), or unless the techniques are not available, then there is a tendency to fix these with a percutaneous screw.

Complications

Non-union

By 2–3 months it may be obvious that the fracture will not unite. If so, bone grafting should be considered. The aim is to reduce the pain from the non-union and to reduce the chance of secondary osteoarthritis. Bone graft on a vascular pedicle can be taken from the back of the distal radius. Once a fracture of the waist fails to heal, it starts to collapse into a 'hump back' deformity. A wedge of bone taken from the iliac crest can be carved into shape and placed into the non-union to restore the proper shape and encourage healing.

Avascular necrosis

X-ray examination at 2–3 months may show increased density of the proximal fragment, a pathognomonic sign of avascular necrosis. Although spontaneous re-vascularization and union are possible, they take years and meanwhile the wrist collapses and arthritis develops. Vascularized bone grafting may be successful. If the wrist becomes painful, the dead fragment can be excised but the wrist tends to collapse after this procedure; a better option is to remove the entire proximal row of carpal bones, or else to remove the scaphoid and fuse the proximal to the distal row.

Osteoarthritis

Non-union or avascular necrosis may lead to secondary osteoarthritis of the wrist. If the arthritis is confined to the distal pole, excising the radial styloid may help. As the arthritis progresses, changes appear in the scaphocapitate joint. Salvage procedures include proximal row carpectomy, partial wrist fusion and radiocarpal fusion.

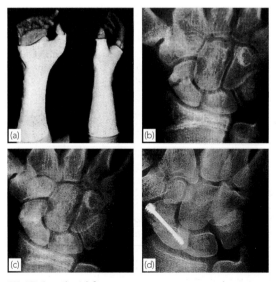

27.17 Scaphoid fractures – treatment and complications (a) Scaphoid plaster. (b) Fracture going on to (c) union at 10 weeks. (d) Delayed union treated by inserting a Herbert screw.

FRACTURES OF OTHER CARPAL BONES

Carpal fractures, other than those of the scaphoid, can be difficult to diagnose on the usual x-ray views. However, the diagnosis, if suspected, can usually be confirmed by special carpal tunnel views, CT or MRI.

Undisplaced fractures are usually treated by splinting until healed. Displaced fractures will need open reduction and internal fixation.

ULNAR-SIDE WRIST INJURIES

The distal radioulnar joint is often injured with fractures of the radius; less often as an isolated event. Injuries comprise tears of the triangular fibrocartilage complex (TFCC), avulsion of the ulnar styloid process and articular fractures of the head of the ulna.

Special features

There is tenderness over the distal radioulnar joint and pain on rotation of the forearm. The distal ulna may be unstable; the *piano-key sign* is elicited by holding the patient's forearm pronated and pushing sharply on the prominent head of the ulna.

X-rays

X-ray examination may show a fracture or signs of incongruity of the distal radioulnar joint. Arthrography, MRI and arthroscopy help to confirm the diagnosis.

Treatment

Dislocation of the distal radioulnar joint can usually be reduced by closed manipulation; the arm and wrist are then immobilized in an above-elbow cast (to prevent rotation) for 4 weeks. If the joint cannot be reduced or is still unstable, operative reduction, repair of the injured structures and pinning may be needed.

SCAPHOLUNATE DISSOCIATION

What is thought to be a sprain giving rise to persistent tenderness over the dorsum of the wrist may be shown by x-ray or arthrography to be a much more significant injury due to disruption of the ligaments between scaphoid and lunate. The pathognomonic features are foreshortening of the scaphoid and the appearance of a large gap between scaphoid and lunate.

Treatment

If the condition is diagnosed fewer than 4 weeks after injury, the bones should be repositioned by open operation and held in place with K-wires; it may be possible at the same time to repair the ligaments with interosseous sutures. The wrist is immobilized in a cast for 8 weeks.

If the diagnosis is missed, the patient may develop carpal instability (see page 196).

LUNATE AND PERILUNATE DISLOCATIONS

A fall with the hand forced into dorsiflexion may tear the tough ligaments that normally bind the carpal bones. The lunate usually remains attached to the radius, and the rest of the carpus is displaced backwards (*perilunate dislocation*). Usually the hand immediately snaps forwards again but, as it does so, the lunate may be levered out of position to be displaced anteriorly (*lunate dislocation*). Sometimes the scaphoid remains attached to the radius and the force of the perilunar dislocation causes it to fracture through the waist (*trans-scaphoid perilunate dislocation*).

Special features

The wrist is painful and swollen and is held immobile. If the carpal tunnel is compressed, there may be paraesthesia or blunting of sensation in the territory of the median nerve, and weakness of palmar abduction of the thumb.

X-rays

Most dislocations are *perilunate*. In the anteroposterior view, the carpus is diminished in height and the bone shadows overlap abnormally. One or more of the carpal bones may be fractured (usually the scaphoid). *Lunate* dislocation can be recognized by the abnormal shape of the lunate anteroposterior x-ray image – triangular instead of quadrilateral.

In the lateral view, it is easy to distinguish a lunate from a perilunate dislocation. The dislocated lunate is tilted forwards and is displaced in front of the radius, while the capitate and metacarpal bones are in line with the radius. With a perilunate dislocation, the lunate is not displaced forwards.

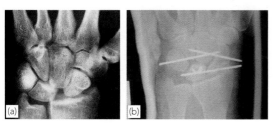

27.18 Scapholunate dissociation (a) After a fall, this patient complained of pain and tenderness in the anatomical snuff box. X-ray (a) shows that the scaphoid is intact but the image is markedly foreshortened and there is a wide gap between the scaphoid and the lunate. (b) After open reduction and repair of the dorsal ligaments, the scaphoid was held in position with Kirschner wires.

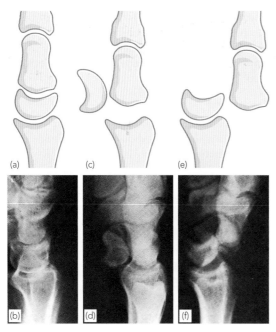

27.19 Lunate and perilunate dislocations
(a,b) Lateral x-ray of normal wrist; (c,d) lunate dislocation; (e,f) perilunate dislocation.

Treatment

Closed reduction

Pulling on the hand with the wrist in extension and applying thumb pressure to the displaced bones may succeed. A plaster slab is applied, holding the wrist neutral. Percutaneous K-wires may be needed to hold the reduction.

Open reduction

If closed reduction fails, open reduction is imperative. The carpus is exposed by an anterior approach, which has the advantage of decompressing the carpal tunnel. While an assistant pulls on the hand, the lunate is levered into place and kept there by a K-wire which is inserted through the lunate into the capitate. If the scaphoid is fractured, this too can be reduced and fixed with a screw or K-wires. Torn ligaments should be repaired through palmar and dorsal approaches. At the end of the procedure, the wrist is splinted. Fingers, elbow and shoulder are exercised throughout this period. The splint and K-wires are removed at 8 weeks.

Complications

Avascular necrosis of the lunate may follow disruption of its blood supply. The x-ray shows progressive increase in bone density. Treatment is required only if symptoms demand it. If the wrist is stiff and painful, removal of the lunate and partial arthrodesis may be preferable.

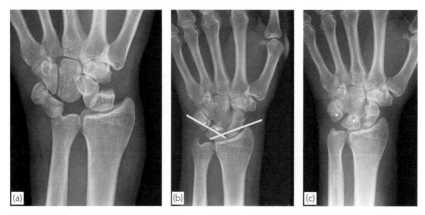

27.20 Perilunate dislocation (a) Lunate still in its original position while the rest of the carpus is dislocated around it. (b) The dislocation has been reduced and held with K-wires. (c) The lunotriquetral ligament is re-attached with ligament anchors.

CHAPTER 28

INJURIES OF THE HAND

Hand injuries are important out of all proportion to their apparent severity, because of the need for perfect function. Local oedema and stiffness of the joints – common accompaniments of all injuries – are more threatening in the hand than anywhere else. Fractures may heal and joints re-stabilize, and yet the patient may still be left with a useless hand because of insufficient attention to splintage, the prevention of swelling, the preservation of movement and rehabilitation.

The patient should be examined in a clean environment with the hand displayed on sterile drapes. The history should include details of the accident, as well as the patient's age, occupation, leisure activities and 'handedness'. Examination should establish: (1) the degree of mutilation; (2) the presence of any deformity; (3) the state of the circulation; (4) nerve function; and (5) tendon function.

Closed injuries and small wounds can often be treated under regional block anaesthesia. Large wounds and multiple fractures are better dealt with under general anaesthesia.

Definitive treatment is dictated by the nature of the injury, but common to all injuries are three important requirements:

■ Safe splintage.
■ Prevention of swelling.
■ Dedicated rehabilitation.

Splintage must be kept to a minimum. If only one finger is injured, it alone should be splinted – either by strapping it to its neighbour so that both move as one ('buddy-strapping'), or by fashioning a splint that does not impede movement in the uninjured fingers. If the whole hand is splinted or bandaged, this must always be in the '*position of safe immobilization*' – with the knuckle joints flexed at least 70 degrees, the finger joints straight and the thumb abducted. That way the ligaments are at full stretch, so if they do become adherent it is still possible to regain movement with physiotherapy.

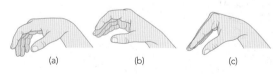

28.1 Splintage of the hand Three positions of the hand: (a) the position of relaxation; (b) the position of function (ready for action); and (c) the position of safe immobilization, with the ligaments taut.

Prevention of swelling means keeping the hand elevated and performing early and repeated active exercises.

Physiotherapy and rehabilitation are best undertaken by a dedicated and experienced hand therapist.

CARPOMETACARPAL INJURIES

DISLOCATION OF THE FINGER CARPOMETACARPAL JOINTS

Dislocation of the finger carpometacarpal (CMC) joints is caused by forceful dorsiflexion of the wrist combined with a longitudinal impact. Thus it is seen typically in boxers and in motorcyclists. There may be an associated intra-articular fracture at the base of the metacarpals. The x-rays must be carefully inspected and if there is any doubt about the nature of the injury a CT scan will usually help.

Treatment

The dislocation is reduced by traction, manipulation and thumb pressure. A protective slab is worn for 6 weeks, during which time the fingers are kept moving. If reduction is unstable, especially if there are associated fractures, then holding with percutaneous wires is necessary.

If the thumb alone is dislocated it should be reduced and then carefully re-examined. If it is stable a plaster cast for 6 weeks will suffice; if it is unstable (and it usually is) then it should be held with a Kirschner wire (K-wire) until the soft tissues heal.

BENNETT'S FRACTURE–SUBLUXATION OF THE FIRST METACARPAL

This is a fracture at the base of the thumb metacarpal with extension into the CMC joint. It is an unstable injury: the smaller fragment remains in contact with the trapezium while the metacarpal shaft is pulled proximally by the powerful abductor pollicis longus. The fracture–dislocation is easy to reduce by traction but difficult to keep in position. It can be held in a plaster cast but it usually slips so it is best to fix the fracture with a simple percutaneous wire or screw.

Complications

If the CMC joint is seriously damaged or subluxated, osteoarthritis may ensue. Treatment is usually conservative, but if pain becomes intolerable an operation may be needed – either arthrodesis of the joint or excision of the trapezium.

FRACTURED METACARPALS

The metacarpal bones are vulnerable to blows and falls upon the hand, or the force of a boxer's punch. The bones may fracture at their base, in the shaft or through the neck.

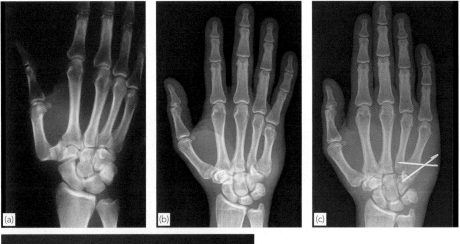

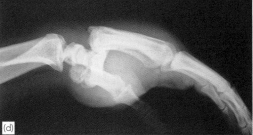

28.2 Carpometacarpal (CMC) dislocation
(a) Thumb dislocation. (b) Dislocation of the fourth and fifth CMC joints treated by closed reduction and Kirschner wires (c). Complete CMC dislocation (d).

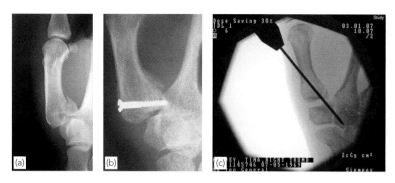

28.3 Bennett's fracture–subluxation
(a) This fracture at the base of the thumb metacarpal with extension into the carpometacarpal joint is inherently unstable. It is therefore best treated by reduction and internal fixation with a small screw (b) or a percutaneous K-wire (c).

In the midshaft, angular deformity is usually not marked, and even if it persists it does not interfere much with function. Rotational deformity, however, is serious and may result in malposition of the entire ray when the hand is closed in a fist.

In fractures of the neck – and particularly the neck of the fifth metacarpal – the small distal fragment may be tilted markedly towards the palm.

Special features

If the fragments are displaced, there may be a bump on the back of the hand, or one of the knuckles may be flattened. The metacarpal head can be prominent in the palm, a particular problem with grip if the index finger is involved. There is considerable swelling and local tenderness.

Fractures of the metacarpal head are associated with a punching injury. If an opponent's tooth has punctured the skin over the metacarpal head – a 'fight-bite' – then the joint will surely be infected. Immediate exploration and thorough washout of the wound, however small, is essential to avoid destruction of the joint.

X-rays

Fractures of the base of the metacarpal are usually impacted. Fractures of the shaft are either transverse or oblique; there may be shortening or angulation of the fragments. Fractures of the metacarpal neck may result in forward tilting of the distal fragment.

Treatment

Undisplaced fractures

Fractures that are undisplaced (or only slightly displaced) require only a firm crepe-bandage (for comfort), which is worn for 2 or 3 weeks. This should not be allowed to interfere with active movements of the fingers, which must be practised assiduously.

Displaced fracture of the shaft

If there is marked displacement or shortening of the bone, open reduction and internal fixation with small plates and screws is the best option. Careful attention should be given to correcting rotation, otherwise the finger will go awry during flexion. A

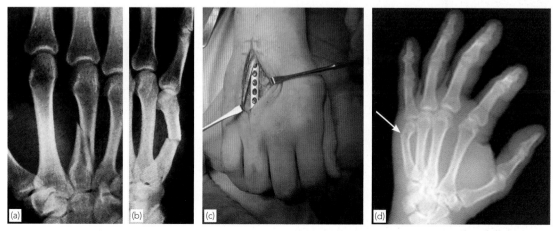

28.4 Metacarpal fractures (a) A spiral fracture of a single metacarpal is usually held adequately by neighbouring bones and muscles. (b) A displaced transverse fracture will often require internal fixation with rigid wires or a small plate (c). Fractures of the metacarpal neck (d) can usually be managed by early mobilization.

useful guide is to remember that in flexion every finger should point towards the thenar crease (compare with the other side). After operation, movements are started as soon as possible.

Displaced fracture of the neck

With fractures of the metacarpal neck, angulation of up to 50 degrees in the fourth and fifth metacarpals and 20 degrees in the second and third can be accepted. All other displaced metacarpal fractures should be reduced by traction and pressure. Reduction can be held by a plaster slab extending from the forearm over the fingers (only the damaged ones); however, displacement is likely and also there is a risk of stiffness in the splinted finger. Therefore, fixation with percutaneous intramedullary wires passed from the base is usually preferred.

Fractures of the head

Closed fractures can be treated non-operatively if the fragments are undisplaced. Displaced fragments, like any intra-articular fracture, must be perfectly reduced. Tiny buried screws are used. A fight-bite needs immediate washout (Figure 28.5).

Complications

Malunion

Angulation may result in a visible bump or a flattened knuckle, but function is usually good.

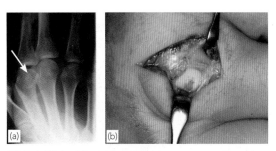

28.5 A 'fight-bite' The underlying metacarpal head was damaged by the attacker's tooth.

Rotational deformity is much more serious because the patient cannot properly close the fist. This may need correction by osteotomy.

Stiffness

Metacarpal fractures invariably unite and, even if angulation persists, malunion is less disabling than stiffness of the hand. Early movement and the avoidance of swelling is essential (see page 397).

METACARPOPHALANGEAL DISLOCATION

Usually the thumb is affected, sometimes the fifth finger and rarely the other fingers. A hyperextension force may dislocate the phalanx backwards, and the volar capsule may be torn. If the metacarpal head has been forced like a button through the hole, closed reduction may be impossible. Sometimes one or other collateral ligaments are avulsed, pulling a triangular fragment of bone.

For a dislocation, closed reduction is attempted by pulling on the thumb and levering the phalanx forwards. If this fails, the joint is exposed from the dorsum and, while strong traction is applied, the metacarpal head is levered into place. The joint is then strapped in the flexed position for 1 week before mobilizing.

A collateral ligament avulsion is usually treated by strapping the finger to its neighbour for 3 or 4 weeks. A markedly displaced or unstable fracture can be fixed with a small screw or bone suture.

TORN ULNAR COLLATERAL LIGAMENT OF THE THUMB METACARPOPHALANGEAL JOINT

In former years, gamekeepers who twisted the necks of little animals ran the risk of tearing the ulnar collateral ligament of the thumb metacarpophalangeal (MCP) joint. The injury came to be known as *gamekeeper's thumb*. Nowadays, it is seen in skiers who fall onto the extended thumb,

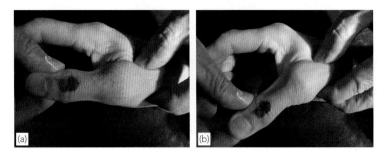

28.6 'Skier's thumb' A fall onto the extended thumb may force the metacarpophalangeal joint into hyperabduction. (a,b) Gentle examination shows that the ulnar collateral ligament has ruptured. Urgent repair is indicated.

forcing it into hyperabduction. A small flake of bone may be pulled off at the same time.

Special features

The ulnar side of the joint is swollen and very tender, yet the condition is often under-diagnosed as a simple 'sprain'. Before testing the ligament, an x-ray must be obtained to exclude any fracture. A local anaesthetic is then injected into the tissues along the inner (adductor) aspect of the joint, and the thumb is stressed in abduction with the MCP joint flexed 30 degrees; if there is no undue laxity (compared with the normal side), a serious injury can be excluded. If there is significant laxity, this is at least a partial rupture. The test is then repeated with the thumb fully extended: if there is still significant laxity, it is probably a complete rupture. The ligament can become jammed proximally under the adductor pollicis tendon (the so-called Stener lesion) and requires operative repair. An ultrasound scan can be helpful in clarifying the degree of injury.

Treatment

Partial tears can be treated by immobilization of the thumb in a cast or splint for 4 weeks. This is followed by increasing movement and pinching and gripping exercises.

Complete tears need operative repair. Care should be taken during the exposure not to injure the superficial radial nerve branches. Postoperatively, the joint is immobilized in a removable thumb splint (leaving the interphalangeal joint free) for 6 weeks. Gentle flexion–extension movements out of the splint are allowed early to prevent stiffness, but no pinch against the repair is permissible for 6 weeks.

FRACTURED PHALANGES

Phalangeal fractures usually result from direct trauma and therefore any part of the bone may be broken.

Treatment

Open wounds should always be treated first. Skin must be preserved and carefully sutured, and wound healing must not be jeopardized by the treatment of the fractures.

Undisplaced fractures

These need the minimum of splintage. The type of splint depends on the fracture and the direction of potential instability. This may necessitate strapping the finger to its uninjured neighbour ('buddy-strapping') or a splint on the digit alone. Early movement, without compromising stability, is encouraged.

Displaced fracture of the proximal or middle phalanx

The bone should be straightened under local anaesthesia, carefully avoiding malrotation; the

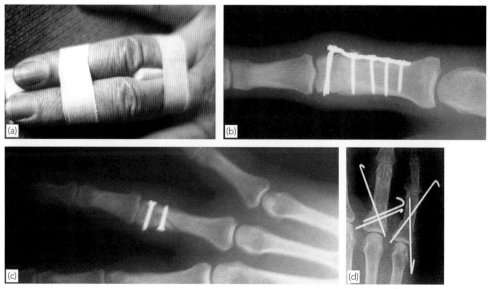

28.7 Phalangeal fractures Depending on the 'personality' of the fracture, the equipment available and the experience of the surgeon, these injuries can be treated by neighbour strapping (a), plate fixation (b), percutaneous screw fixation (c) or percutaneous wire fixation (d).

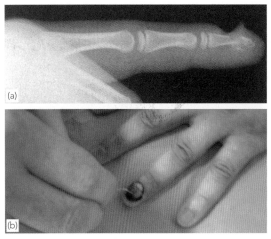

(a)

(b)

> ⚠️ As in all hand injuries, the danger of stiffness is ever present, and a stiff finger can be worse than no finger. The principles of soft-tissue care should never be neglected: elevate, keep splintage to a minimum, move, exercise.

28.8 Distal phalangeal injury (a) A fracture of the tuft, caused by a hammer blow, is treated by a protective dressing. The subungual haematoma should be evacuated using a red-hot paper clip tip (b) or a small drill.

injured finger is then splinted, leaving the other fingers free. The splint can be discarded after 3 weeks. If reduction cannot be held in this way, fixation with K-wires, a small plate or screws is indicated depending on the type of fracture. Surgery is challenging and invites stiffness. Meticulous attention to surgical technique and postoperative rehabilitation is needed.

Fractures of the distal phalanx
Distal phalangeal fractures are usually due to crushing injuries or a blow from a hammer. The soft-tissue damage must be treated; the fracture can be ignored.

FINGER JOINT INJURIES

SPRAINS OF THE FINGER JOINTS

Partial or complete tears of the ligaments are common and usually due to forced angulation at the joint. Milder injuries require no treatment; with more severe strains, the finger should be splinted for 1–2 weeks. However, the patient should be warned that the joint is likely to remain swollen and slightly painful for 6–12 months.

INTERPHALANGEAL DISLOCATION

Dislocation at the proximal joint is common and is easily reduced by pulling on the finger. If there is no associated fracture, then minimal splintage is needed. However, the patient should be warned that swelling and slight loss of movement may persist for months.

If there is a fracture, the joint may be unstable, requiring surgery under local anaesthesia with wires or even a spring-loaded external fixator.

MALLET FINGER

If the fingertip is forcibly bent during active extension, the extensor tendon may rupture or a flake of bone may be avulsed from the base of the distal phalanx. This sometimes occurs when the finger is stubbed when making a bed or catching a ball.

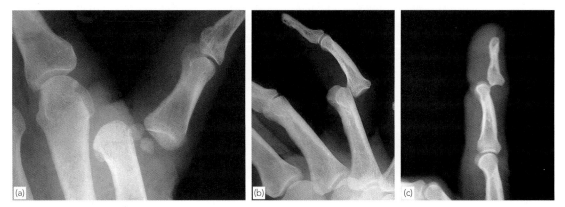

(a)

(b)

(c)

28.9 Finger dislocation (a) Metacarpophalangeal dislocation in the thumb occasionally buttonholes and needs open reduction; (b,c) interphalangeal dislocations are easily reduced (and easily missed if not x-rayed!).

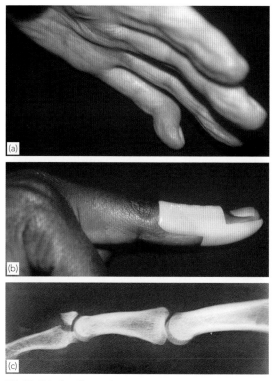

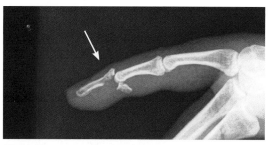

28.11 Flexor tendon avulsion Avulsion at the distal interphalangeal joint.

28.10 'Mallet finger' (a,b) The typical deformity in the little finger. This is best treated with a splint for 6 weeks. (c) Sometimes a small fragment is avulsed from the base of the distal phalanx; this also can be treated with a splint – surgery may well make the outcome worse.

A pure soft-tissue injury can be treated by splinting the distal joint continuously in extension for 8 weeks and then at night only for another 4 weeks. If there is a large flake of bone, a shorter term of splintage will usually suffice. Operative fixation is rarely needed; it is unlikely to improve outcome in any but the most markedly displaced fractures. The risk of stiffness and wound problems is rather high.

FLEXOR TENDON AVULSION

Avulsion of the flexor tendon from the base of the distal phalanx is a rare injury, but it should not be missed. It usually affects the left ring finger; it is sometimes known as a 'rugby jersey finger', reflecting the fact that it is often caused when the finger is caught in an opponent's shirt. The patient cannot actively flex the tip of the finger.

X-rays sometimes show a fragment of avulsed bone either at the tip or further down the finger (Figure 28.11).

Treatment is urgent and requires operative reattachment of the tendon.

OPEN INJURIES OF THE HAND

Open injuries range from clean cuts to ragged lacerations, crushing, injection of foreign material, pulp defects and amputations. Knowing the mechanism of injury helps immensely in assessing the type and degree of damage.

Clinical assessment

Examination must be gentle and painstaking. It should be carried out in a clean (and preferably a sterile) environment, and may have to be repeated in the operating theatre when the patient is anaesthetized. *X-rays* are obligatory: they may show fractures or foreign bodies.

Skin damage is important, but remember that even a tiny, clean cut may conceal nerve or tendon injury. The *circulation* to the hand and fingers must be assessed; *sensation* and *motor activity* are tested in the territory of each nerve.

Tendons are examined with similar care. Note the posture of the hand and fingers; comparison with the opposite hand may show that the normal postural tension in one or other finger is absent, suggesting a tendon injury. If the patient will allow it, active wrist and finger movements are then assessed. *Flexor digitorum profundus* is tested by holding the proximal finger joint straight and instructing the patient to bend the distal joint. *Flexor digitorum superficialis* is tested by asking the patient to flex one finger at a time while the examiner holds the other fingers in full extension; this immobilizes all the deep flexors because they have a common muscle belly, so any active flexion of the injured finger must be performed by the superficial flexor (see Figure 28.12).

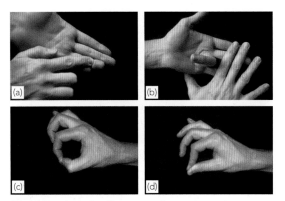

28.12 Testing the flexor tendons Testing for (a) flexor digitorum profundus (FDP) lesser fingers, (b) flexor digitorum superficialis (FDS) lesser fingers, (c) FDP index, (d) FDS index.

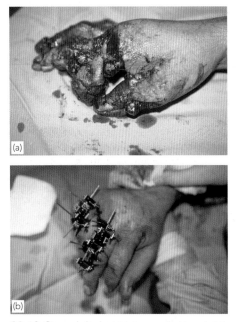

28.13 Open injuries (a) A mangled hand; (b) open fractures treated with external fixation.

Severe lacerations and fractures can produce a daunting picture. Yet even a 'mangled hand' deserves painstaking examination to see what is salvageable.

Treatment

Preoperative care

The patient will need painkillers. If the wound is contaminated, it should be rinsed with sterile saline, and antibiotics should be given as soon as possible. Prophylaxis against tetanus may also be needed. The wound is covered with a sterile dressing and the hand is lightly splinted.

Wound exploration

Under general or regional anaesthesia, the wound is cleaned and explored. A pneumatic tourniquet is essential unless there is a crush injury and muscle viability is in doubt. Skin is too precious to waste, and only obviously dead skin should be excised. For adequate exposure, the wound may need enlarging, but *incisions must never cross a skin crease or an interdigital web* because healing will result in a soft-tissue contracture across the crease. Through the enlarged wound, loose debris is picked out, dead tissues are excised and the wound is thoroughly irrigated with isotonic crystalloid solution. A more thorough assessment of the extent of the injury is then undertaken.

Tissue repair

Fractures are reduced and held with K-wires or plates or an external fixator depending on the configuration. Bone defects can be treated with bone graft or may be simply bridged with a metal device for later expert attention. The *joint capsule and ligaments* are repaired with fine sutures.

Artery and vein repair (or grafting) may be needed if the hand or finger is ischaemic. *Severed nerves* are

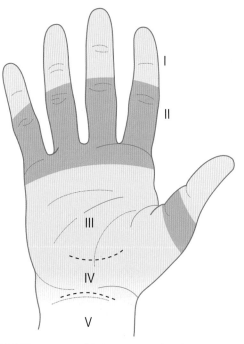

28.14 The zones of injury (I) Distal to the insertion of flexor digitorum superficialis. (II) Between the opening of the flexor sheath (the distal palmar crease) and the insertion of flexor superficialis. (III) Between the end of the carpal tunnel and the beginning of the flexor sheath. (IV) Within the carpal tunnel. (V) Proximal to the carpal tunnel.

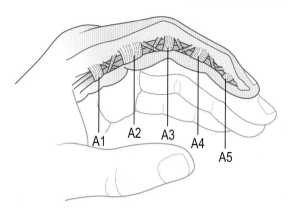

28.15 The flexor tendon sheath and pulleys
Fibrous pulleys – designated A1 to A5 – hold the flexor
tendons to the phalanges and prevent bowstringing
during movement. *A2 and A4 have a crucial tethering
effect and must always be preserved or reconstructed.*

sutured with the finest, non-reactive material. If the
repair cannot be achieved without tension, a nerve
graft (e.g. from the posterior interosseous nerve at
the wrist) should be performed. These procedures
are carried out under high magnification (loupes or
an operating microscope).

Extensor tendon repair is usually quite straightforward.

Flexor tendon repair is more challenging,
particularly in the region between the distal
palmar crease and the flexor crease of the proximal
interphalangeal joint (Zone II), where both the
superficial and deep tendons run together in a
common sheath. This area has been called – rather
portentously – 'no man's land'. Primary repair with
at least four sutures across the cut and fastidious
postoperative supervision gives the best outcome,
but calls for a high level of expertise and specialized
physiotherapy. If the necessary facilities are not
available, the wound should be washed out and
loosely closed, and the patient transferred to a
special centre. A delay of several days, with a clean

wound, is unlikely to affect the outcome. Tendon
grafting, sometimes with a temporary silicone
'spacer', may be needed (see below).

Division of the *superficialis tendon alone*
should also be repaired. Even though the loss of
superficialis action does not altogether prevent
finger flexion, it noticeably weakens the hand and
may lead to a swan-neck deformity of the finger.

*Cuts above the wrist, in the palm or distal to the
superficialis insertion* have a better outcome than
injuries in 'no man's land'.

Amputation of a finger as a primary procedure
should be avoided unless the damage involves
many tissues and is clearly irreparable.

Closure

The tourniquet is deflated and bipolar diathermy is
used to stop bleeding; haematoma formation leads
to poor healing and tendon adhesions. Unless the
wound is contaminated, the skin is closed – either
by direct suture without tension or, if there is skin
loss, by skin grafting (skin grafts are conveniently
taken from the inner aspect of the upper arm).
If tendon or bare bone is exposed, this must
be covered by a rotation skin flap or a pedicled
flap. If the wound is very large, a free flap with
a microvascular attachment may be needed. If a
severely mutilated finger has to be sacrificed, its
skin can be used as a rotation flap or a source of
graft to cover an adjacent area of loss.

Dressing and splintage

The wound is covered with a single layer of
paraffin gauze and ample wool roll. A light plaster
slab holds the wrist and hand in the position of
safe immobilization (wrist extended, MCP joints
flexed to 70 degrees, interphalangeal joints straight,
thumb abducted – see Figure 28.17). This is the
position in which the MCP and interphalangeal
ligaments are fully stretched and fibrosis is
therefore least likely to cause contractures. *Failure
to appreciate this point is the commonest cause of*

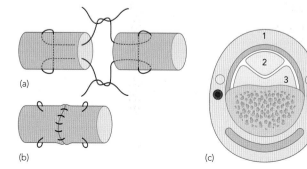

28.16 Flexor tendon repair A core suture
(a) is supplemented by circumferential sutures
(b). The relationships of the important
structures in 'no man's land' are shown in (c):
1, the tendon sheath; 2, flexor digitorum
profundus; 3, flexor digitorum superficialis;
4, digital nerves; 5, artery; 6, extensor tendon.

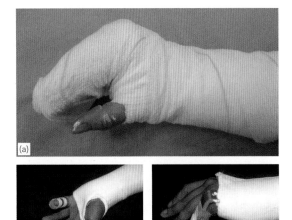

28.17 Splintage (a) The 'position of safe immobilization'. (b,c) For a single metacarpal or phalangeal injury immobilize only the affected ray.

persistent stiffness after injury. The rule is slightly modified in two circumstances: (a) after primary flexor tendon suture, the wrist is held in about 20 degrees of flexion to take tension off the repair; and (b) after extensor tendon repair, the MCP joints are flexed to only about 30 degrees so that there is less tension on the repair.

Postoperative management

The hand is kept elevated in a roller towel or high sling, which can be removed several times a day to exercise the elbow and shoulder. As soon as possible the sling is discarded but dependency of the limb must be avoided.

Rehabilitation

Movements of the hand must be commenced within a few days at most. Splintage should allow as many joints as possible to be exercised, consistent with protecting the repair. Extensor tendon injuries are splinted for about 4 weeks. Various protocols are followed for flexor tendon injuries, including passive, active or elastic-band-assisted flexion. Early movement promotes tendon healing and excursion. In all cases, the risk of rupture is balanced against the need for early mobilization. Close supervision and attention to detail are essential.

Once the tissues have healed, the hand is increasingly used for more and more complex tasks, especially those that resemble the patient's normal work activities. The importance of an experienced hand therapist cannot be over-estimated.

Delayed tendon repair

Primary suture may have been contraindicated by wound contamination, undue delay between injury and repair, massive skin loss or inadequate operating facilities. In these circumstances, secondary repair or tendon grafting may be necessary.

Injury of the profundus tendon with an intact superficialis

Unless the patient's work or hobby demands active flexion of the fingertip, fusion or tenodesis of the distal interphalangeal joint is the most reliable option.

Injury of both the superficialis and profundus tendons

If both tendons have been divided and have retracted, a tendon graft is needed. Full passive joint movement is a prerequisite. If the pulley system is in good condition and there are no adhesions, the tendons are excised from the flexor sheath and replaced with a tendon graft (palmaris longus, duplicated extensor digiti minimi, plantaris or a toe extensor). Rehabilitation is the same as for a primary repair. If the pulleys are damaged, the skin cover poor, the passive range of movement limited or the sheath scarred, a two-stage procedure is preferred. The tendons are excised and the pulleys reconstructed with extensor retinaculum or excised tendon. A Silastic rod is sutured to the distal stump of the profundus tendon and is left free in the palm or distal forearm. Rehabilitation is planned to maintain a good passive range of movement. A smooth gliding surface forms around the rod. No less than 3 months later, the rod is removed through two smaller incisions and a tendon graft (palmaris longus, plantaris or a lesser toe extensor) is sutured to the proximal and distal stumps of flexor digitorum profundus at exactly the right tension. Rehabilitation is as for a primary repair.

Pulp and fingertip injuries

In full-thickness wounds without bone exposure, the best results come with simple non-adherent dressings. These are changed every few days until the wound has re-epithelialized. This might take a few weeks but the alternatives of skin grafts or skin flaps invite cold intolerance and poor sensory recovery. If bone is exposed and length of the digit is important for the individual patient, then an advancement flap or neurovascular island flap should be considered. If not, primary cover can be achieved by shortening the bone and tailoring the skin flaps ('terminalization').

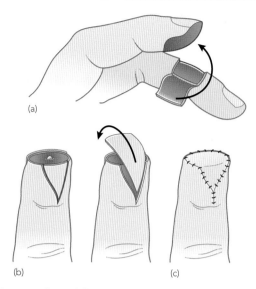

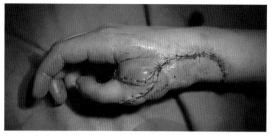

28.19 Late reconstruction The second toe has been transferred to replace the thumb, which was severed in an accident.

28.18 Pulp and fingertip injuries (a) Cross-finger graft for a palmar oblique fingertip injury with exposed bone. (b) V-to-Y advancement for a transverse fingertip injury with exposed bone. Thumb tip loss (c) must always be reconstructed – never amputate.

In young children, the fingertips recover extraordinarily well from injury and they should almost always be treated with dressings rather than grafts or terminalization.

Thumb length should never be sacrificed lightly. Sophisticated techniques such as a free microsurgical toe transfer or metacarpal lengthening may be suitable when the injury leaves the thumb too short for proper function.

Nail-bed injuries

These are often seen in association with fractures of the terminal phalanx. If appearance is important, meticulous repair and split-thickness grafting under magnification will give the best cosmetic result.

The severely mutilated hand

This should be dealt with by a team with special skills in hand surgery. In exceptional cases a new finger or thumb can be constructed by neurovascular microsurgical transfer of a toe, or a lost thumb can be replaced by rotating a surviving finger (pollicization) to restore oppositional movement.

BURNS

These should be, in general, managed in a specialized burns unit because of the devastating loss of function that can follow burns to the hand.

Superficial burns are covered with a moist dressing and the hand is elevated. Early movement is encouraged. *Partial-thickness burns* are dressed in an antimicrobial cream and splinted in the position of safety. *Full-thickness burns* do not heal and require skin grafting.

Constricting burns may need urgent release to preserve the circulation (escharotomy).

Electric burns can cause very widespread damage that may only become apparent a few days later.

Chemical burns require copious irrigation; particular neutralizing agents are suitable for certain chemical burns.

Frostbite needs special attention, with slow re-warming and management of blisters and tissue loss. Amputation is often required, once the area of dead and viable tissue has been demarcated.

CHAPTER 29

INJURIES OF THE SPINE AND THORAX

Spinal injuries are due either to direct force (e.g. penetrating wounds from firearms or knives) or, much more commonly, indirect force – usually following a fall from a height when the spinal column collapses in its vertical axis, or during violent free movements of the neck or trunk. A variety of mechanisms come into play, often simultaneously: axial compression, flexion, extension, rotation, shear and distraction.

The injury carries a double threat: damage to the vertebral column and damage to the neural tissues. Neurological injury is not always immediate and may occur (or be aggravated) only if and when there is movement and displacement of the vertebral fracture or dislocation. Hence the importance of establishing whether the injury is stable or unstable.

A *stable injury* is one in which the vertebral components will not be displaced by normal movements; *an unstable injury* is one in which there is a significant risk of displacement and consequent damage – or further damage – to the neural tissues. Stability depends on the integrity of the vertebral bodies and the posterior arches as well as the ligaments that link adjacent vertebrae.

In assessing spinal stability, three structural elements must be considered: the *posterior column* consisting of the pedicles, facet joints, posterior bony arches, interspinous and supraspinous ligaments; the *middle column* comprising the posterior half of the vertebral body, the posterior part of the intervertebral disc and the posterior longitudinal ligament; and the *anterior column* composed of the anterior half of the vertebral body, the anterior part of the intervertebral disc and the anterior longitudinal ligament. *All fractures involving the middle column and at least one other column should be regarded as unstable.*

Fortunately, only 10% of spinal fractures are unstable and less than 5% are associated with cord damage.

Spinal injuries heal slowly. Non-union is rare but malunion is common and may lead to progressive deformity of the spine.

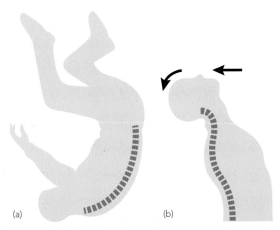

29.1 Mechanism of injury The spine is usually injured in one of two ways: (a) a fall onto the head or the back of the neck; and (b) a blow on the forehead which forces the neck into hyperextension. Sudden acceleration, as in a severe rear-end collision, will also result in the head and neck falling into hyperextension.

PRINCIPLES OF DIAGNOSIS AND MANAGEMENT

Diagnosis and management go hand in hand; inappropriate movement during examination can irretrievably change the outcome for the worse. *If there is the slightest possibility of spinal trauma in an injured patient, the spine must be immobilized until the patient has been resuscitated and other life-threatening injuries have been identified and treated.* Immobilization is abandoned only when a serious spinal injury has been excluded by clinical and radiological assessment.

HISTORY

A high index of suspicion is essential; symptoms and signs may be minimal – the history is crucial. Every patient with a blunt injury above the clavicle, a head injury or loss of consciousness should be considered to have a cervical spine injury until proven otherwise. Every patient who is involved in a fall from a height, a crushing accident or a high-speed deceleration accident should similarly be considered to have a thoracolumbar injury. However, lesser injuries also should arouse suspicion if they are followed by pain in the neck or back or neurological symptoms in the limbs.

EXAMINATION

Neck

Look, Feel but do not Move! If there is an unstable injury movement may imperil the cord. The head and face are thoroughly inspected for bruises or grazes which could indicate indirect trauma to the cervical spine. The neck itself is examined for deformity, bruising or a penetrating injury. The patient may be supporting his or her head with their hands. The bones and soft tissues of the neck are palpated; tenderness, bogginess or an abnormal space between adjacent spinous processes suggests an unstable injury of the posterior part of the cervical spine.

Back

The patient is 'log-rolled' to avoid movement of the thoracolumbar spine. The spine is inspected and palpated as before.

Neurological examination

A full neurological examination should be carried out in every case; this may have to be repeated several times during the first few days. Each dermatome, myotome and reflex is tested.

The unconscious patient is difficult to examine; a spinal injury must be assumed until proven otherwise. Features suggesting a spinal cord lesion

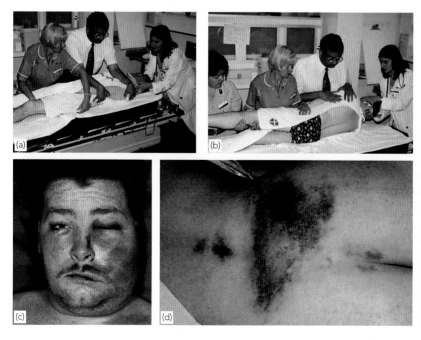

29.2 Examination The neck must be supported throughout the examination, using a semi-rigid collar, sandbags on either side of the head and a tape across the forehead. (a,b) The 'log-rolling technique' is used when turning the patient for examination of the back. Suspicious signs may be noticed immediately: (c) severe facial bruising; (d) bruising over the lower back.

are a history of a fall or rapid deceleration, a head injury, diaphragmatic breathing, a flaccid anal sphincter, hypotension with bradycardia and a pain response above, but not below, the clavicle.

> ⚠ For tests for nerve root function:
> See *Table 29.1*.

Table 29.1 Tests for nerve root motor function

Nerve root	Test	Tendon reflex
C5	Elbow flexion	Biceps
C6	Wrist extension	Brachioradialis
C7	Wrist flexion	Triceps
	Finger extension	
C8	Finger flexion	
T1	Finger abduction	
L1,2	Thigh abduction	
L3,4	Knee extension	Quadriceps
L5, S1	Knee flexion	Tendo Achillis
L5	Great toe extension	
S1	Great toe flexion	

IMAGING

X-ray examination is mandatory for all accident victims complaining of pain or stiffness in the neck or back, all patients with head injuries or severe facial injuries (cervical spine), patients with rib fractures or severe seat-belt bruising (thoracic spine), and those with severe pelvic or abdominal injuries (thoracolumbar spine). Accident victims who are unconscious should have spine x-rays as part of the routine work-up.

Movement should be kept to a minimum. In the cervical spine, anteroposterior and lateral views (with coverage from C1 to T1) and open-mouth views are needed. 'Difficult' areas, such as the lower cervical and upper thoracic segments which are often obscured by shoulder and rib images, may require computed tomography (CT). CT is also ideal for showing structural damage to individual vertebrae and displacement of bone fragments into the vertebral canal. However, for displaying the intervertebral discs, ligamentum flavum and neural structures, *magnetic resonance imaging (MRI)* is the method of choice.

TREATMENT

The objectives of treatment are:

- To preserve neurological function.
- To relieve any reversible neural compression.
- To restore alignment of the spine.
- To stabilize the spine.
- To rehabilitate the patient.

The indications for urgent surgical stabilization are: (a) an unstable fracture with progressive neurological deficit; and (b) an unstable fracture in a patient with multiple injuries.

Patients with no neurological injury

If the spinal injury is stable, the patient is treated by supporting the spine in a position that will cause no further strain; a firm collar or lumbar brace will usually suffice, but the patient may need to rest in bed until pain and muscle spasm subside.

If the spinal injury is unstable it should be held secure until the tissues heal and the spine becomes stable. In the cervical spine this should be done as soon as possible by traction in bed through tongs or a halo device attached to the skull. If the halo is attached to a body cast or a rigid vest, the patient

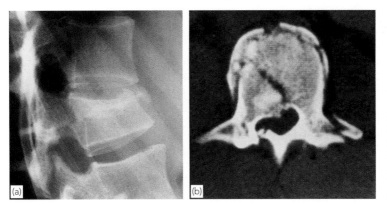

29.3 X-ray diagnosis Plain x-ray alone may be insufficient to show the true state of affairs. (a) This x-ray showed the fracture, but it needed a CT scan (b) to reveal the large fragment encroaching on the spinal canal.

can be got up early and mobilized. Unstable thoracolumbar injuries are more often treated by internal fixation.

Patients with neurological injury

The injury is usually unstable. Conservative treatment is highly demanding and best carried out in a special unit equipped for round-the-clock nursing, 2-hourly turning routines, skin toilet, bladder care and specialized physiotherapy and occupational therapy. After a few weeks the injury stabilizes spontaneously and the patient can be got out of bed for intensive rehabilitation. The benefit of early surgery to neurological recovery is uncertain. However, if neurological loss is incomplete, and especially if progressive, early operative reduction or decompression and stabilization is indicated.

Methods of treatment

Cervical spine

Soft collars can be used for minor sprains during the first few days after injury. *More rigid collars* are better for limiting movements in acute injuries, but they are not adequate for potentially unstable injuries.

Skull tongs with traction is the usual way of reducing cervical fractures and fracture–dislocations. The spine is then held in position until it is considered to be stable. A *halo ring* (a ring attached to the skull by at least four pins) is also suitable; after reduction of the fracture or dislocation the ring can then be fixed to a plaster 'vest' and the patient can be moved about more easily. Halo ring fixation is also used from the outset for lesser injuries where there is a risk of vertebral displacement. However, bear in mind that there can be complications such as pin loosening, pin-site infection and (in elderly patients) respiratory distress.

Operative fixation is necessary in some cases. Various procedures are available, depending on the level and pattern of injury. Odontoid fractures can be fixed with lag screws, burst fractures can be decompressed through an anterior approach and facet dislocations can be reduced through a posterior approach. The spine can be stabilized anteriorly with plates between the vertebral bodies, posteriorly with wires between the spinous processes or with small plates between the lateral masses.

Thoracolumbar spine

Special beds and mattresses are ideally used in the management of all spinal injuries. They are designed to avoid pressure sores and to facilitate turning the patient frequently.

A *thoracolumbar brace* prevents flexion by three-point fixation. It is suitable for some burst fractures, seat-belt injuries and compression fractures.

Operative decompression and stabilization: the aim of surgery is to reduce the fracture, hold the reduction and decompress the neural elements. The anterior (transthoracic, transdiaphragmatic or transperitoneal) approach is suitable for burst fractures with significant canal impingement or as a supplement to posterior fixation in those compression fractures with considerable loss of anterior bone stock. The vertebral body is removed so that the spinal canal is decompressed; a bone graft (rib, fibula or iliac crest) is then inserted and special plates are applied between the intact vertebral bodies above and below the injured level.

The posterior approach is more suitable for flexion–compression injuries. Hook and rod systems provide fixation between intact vertebrae several segments above and below the injury. Bone grafts are added to provide biological fusion.

CERVICAL SPINE INJURIES

Clinical features

The patient usually gives a history of a fall from a height, a diving accident or a vehicle accident in which the neck is forcibly moved. In a patient unconscious from a head injury, a fractured cervical spine should be assumed (and acted upon) until proved otherwise.

An abnormal position of the neck is suggestive, and careful palpation may elicit tenderness. Movement is best postponed until the neck has been x-rayed. Pain or paraesthesia in the limbs is significant, and the patient should be examined for evidence of spinal cord or nerve root damage.

Imaging

Plain x-rays must be of high quality and should be examined methodically. In the anteroposterior view the lateral outlines should be intact, and the spinous processes and tracheal shadow in the midline. An open-mouth view is necessary to show C1 and C2 (for odontoid and lateral mass fractures).

The lateral view must include all seven cervical vertebrae and the upper half of T1, otherwise a serious injury at the cervicothoracic junction will be missed. Four parallel curves should be identified, one running down the front of the vertebral bodies, one down the back of the bodies, one through the bases and one along the tips of the spinous processes (see Figure 29.4). Any deviation from this pattern is suggestive of a vertebral fracture or displacement. Do not forget to look at the soft-tissue outlines: the prevertebral soft-tissue shadow should be less than 5 mm in width above the level of the trachea and less than one vertebral body's width below that level; any increase in this space suggests a prevertebral haematoma.

Children's x-rays can be particularly difficult to interpret. Moderate atlantoaxial displacement in the lateral view may be due to normal ligamentous laxity in childhood; unfused growth plates in the odontoid process or spinous processes can be mistaken for undisplaced fractures; and even a normal looking spine does not exclude the possibility of a cord injury.

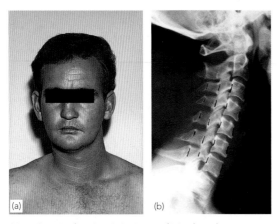

29.4 Cervical spine injuries – clinical and x-ray
(a) Look at the position of the neck. This patient complained of neck pain and stiffness after a fall. X-ray showed an odontoid fracture. (b) The lateral x-ray must include all seven cervical vertebrae – nothing less will suffice. Four parallel lines can be traced unbroken from C1 to C7. They are bounded by the anterior surfaces of the vertebral bodies, the posterior surfaces of the bodies, the posterior borders of the lateral masses and the bases of the spinous processes. A segment that is shifted out of line is abnormal.

FRACTURE OF C1

Sudden severe load on the top of the head may cause a 'bursting' force which fractures the ring of the atlas (Jefferson's fracture). There is no encroachment on the neural canal and, usually, no neurological damage. The fracture is seen on the open-mouth view; the lateral masses are spread away from the odontoid peg. A CT scan is particularly helpful in defining the fracture.

If the fracture is undisplaced, the injury is stable and the patient needs only a rigid collar until the fracture unites. If there is much sideways spreading of the lateral masses, the injury is unstable and should be treated either by skull traction or by the application of a halo–body orthosis for 6 weeks, followed by another 6 weeks in a semi-rigid collar.

Fractures of the atlas are associated with injury elsewhere in the cervical spine in up to 50% of cases; odontoid fractures and 'hangman's fractures' in particular should be excluded.

C2 PARS INTERARTICULARIS FRACTURES (HANGMAN'S FRACTURE)

In the true judicial hangman's fracture, the intervertebral disc at C2/3 is torn and there are bilateral fractures of the pars interarticularis of C2; the mechanism is extension with distraction. In civilian injuries, the mechanism is more complex, with varying degrees of extension, compression and flexion. This is one cause of death in motor vehicle accidents when the forehead strikes the dashboard. Neurological damage, however, is unusual because the fracture of the posterior arch tends to decompress the spinal cord. Nevertheless, the fracture is potentially unstable.

Stable undisplaced fractures are treated in a semi-rigid collar or halo–vest until united (6–12 weeks). Displaced fractures may need reduction before immobilization in a halo–vest for 12 weeks.

FRACTURE OF THE ODONTOID PROCESS

Odontoid fractures are uncommon. They usually occur as flexion injuries in young adults due to high-velocity accidents or severe falls; less often they occur in elderly, osteoporotic people as a result of low-energy trauma in which the neck is forced into hyperextension, e.g. a fall onto the face or forehead. Neurological injury occurs in about one-quarter of cases.

Plain x-rays usually show the fracture. Three types are recognized: avulsion of the tip (Type 1); fracture through the junction of the odontoid peg and body of C2 (Type 2); and a fracture through the body of C2 only (Type 3).

Type 1 fractures need no more than immobilization in a rigid collar until discomfort subsides.

Type 2 fractures are often unstable and prone to non-union. Undisplaced fractures can be held by fitting a halo–vest. Displaced fractures need to be reduced by traction and then held either by operative posterior C1/2 fusion or by anterior screw

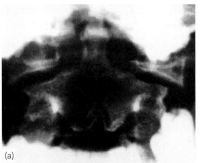

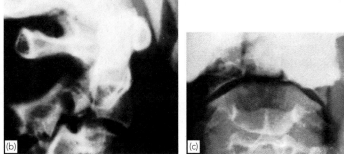

29.5 Fractures of C1 and C2 (a) Jefferson's fracture – bursting apart of the lateral masses of C1. (b) Hangman's fracture – fracture of the pedicle or lateral pillar of C2. (c) Fracture of the base of the odontoid peg of C2. All three fractures can be treated by immobilization of the neck in a 'halo–vest' cast (d).

fixation (provided the fracture is not comminuted, the transverse ligament is not ruptured, the fracture is fully reduced and the bone is solid enough to hold a screw). If full operative facilities are not available, immobilization can be applied by using a halo–vest with repeated x-ray monitoring to check for stability.

Type 3 fractures, if undisplaced, are treated in a halo–vest for 8–12 weeks. If displaced, the fracture must first be reduced by traction before immobilization in a halo–vest for 8–12 weeks; a drawback is that neck rotation will be restricted. Anterior screw fixation is suitable for Type 2 fractures that run from anterior-superior to posterior-inferior; in that way neck rotation is retained.

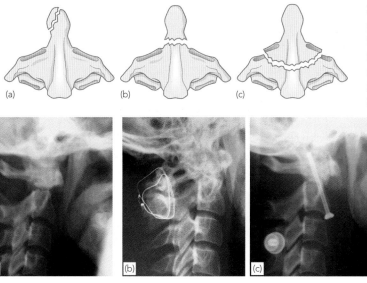

29.6 Fractures of the odontoid process (a) Type I – fracture through the tip. (b) Type II – fracture at the junction of the odontoid process and the body. (c) Type III – fracture through the body of the axis.

29.7 Odontoid fractures that need fusion (a) Severely displaced fracture which was treated by skull traction and (b) posterior fusion. (c) Unstable Type II fracture treated by screw fixation.

POSTERIOR LIGAMENT INJURY

Sudden flexion of the midcervical spine can result in damage to the posterior ligament complex. The upper vertebra tilts forward on the one below, opening up the interspinous space posteriorly.

The patient complains of pain and there is localized tenderness posteriorly. X-ray may reveal a slightly increased gap between the adjacent spines; however, if the neck is held in extension this sign can be missed. A flexion view would, of course, show the widened interspinous space more clearly, but flexion should not be permitted in the early postinjury period. This is why the diagnosis is often made only some weeks after the injury, when the patient goes on complaining of pain.

The assessment of stability is essential in these cases. If the angulation of the vertebral body with its neighbour exceeds 11 degrees, if there is anterior displacement of one vertebral body upon the other of more than 3.5 mm or if the facets are fractured, then the injury is unstable and it should be treated as a subluxation. If it is certain that the injury is stable, a semi-rigid collar for 6 weeks is adequate; if the injury is unstable then posterior fixation and fusion is advisable.

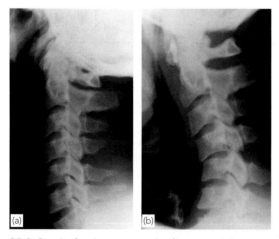

29.8 Cervical spine – posterior ligament injury
(a) The x-ray taken in extension shows no displacement of the vertebral bodies. (b) On carefully controlled flexion there is an unusually wide gap between the spinous processes of C4 and C5.

WEDGE COMPRESSION FRACTURE

This usually occurs in the middle and lower cervical segments. A pure flexion injury causes compression of the anterior part of the vertebral body (wedge compression). The middle and posterior columns remain intact and the injury is stable. All that is needed is a comfortable collar for 6–8 weeks.

BURST AND COMPRESSION–FLEXION FRACTURES

These severe injuries result from axial compression of the cervical spine, usually in diving or athletic accidents. Persistent neurological injury is common.

Plain x-rays show either a crushed vertebral body (a burst fracture) or a flexion deformity with a small triangular fragment separated from the anteroinferior edge of the fractured vertebra (the innocent-looking image which has given the name 'tear-drop fracture' to this injury). *The x-ray should be carefully examined for evidence of middle column damage and posterior displacement (even very slight displacement) of the main body fragment.* Traction must be applied immediately and CT or MRI should be performed to look for retropulsion of bone fragments into the spinal canal.

If there is no neurological deficit, the patient can be treated by confinement to bed and traction for 2–4 weeks, followed by a further period in a halo–vest for 6–8 weeks. (The halo–vest alone is unsuitable for initial treatment because it does not provide axial traction.)

If there is any sign of neurological deterioration and the MRI shows that there is a threat of cord compression, then urgent anterior decompression, bone grafting and plate fixation is considered – and sometimes also posterior stabilization.

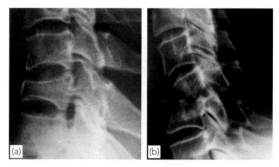

29.9 Cervical compression fractures (a) A simple wedge compression of a single vertebral body is a stable fracture because the middle and posterior elements remain intact. (b) In this case the middle column is broken and the posterior part of the vertebral body is driven backwards. CT or MRI will show the true state of affairs. The fracture is unstable and the cord is threatened.

FRACTURE–DISLOCATIONS BETWEEN C3 AND T1

The displacement must be reduced as a matter of urgency. Skull traction is used, starting with 5 kg and increasing the weight step-wise up to about 30 kg; intravenous muscle relaxants and a bolster beneath the shoulders may help. The entire procedure should be done without anaesthesia (or under mild sedation only) and neurological examination should be repeated after each incremental step. If neurological symptoms or signs develop, or increase, further attempts at closed reduction must be stopped.

When x-rays show that the dislocation has been reduced, traction is diminished and then maintained at 5 kg for 6 weeks; the patient should then wear a collar for another 6 weeks. Alternatively, it may be more convenient simply to immobilize the neck in a halo–vest for 12 weeks. Some surgeons may prefer to perform a posterior fusion as soon as reduction has been achieved; the patient is then allowed up in a cervical brace which is worn for 6–8 weeks. Posterior open reduction and fusion is also indicated if closed reduction fails.

Unilateral facet dislocation

This is a flexion–rotation injury in which only one apophyseal joint is dislocated. There may be an associated fracture of the facet. On the lateral x-ray the vertebral body appears to be partially displaced (less than one-half of its width); on the anteroposterior x-ray the alignment of the spinous processes is distorted. Cord damage is unusual and the injury is stable.

Management is the same as for bilateral dislocation. Sometimes complete reduction is prevented by the upper facet becoming perched upon the lower. When no further progress occurs, it is tempting to assist by gently manipulating the patient's head in extension and rotation; this should be attempted only by an experienced operator. As a general rule, if closed reduction fails, open reduction and posterior fixation are advisable.

After reduction, if the patient is neurologically intact the neck is immobilized in a halo–vest for 6–8 weeks. However, in about 50% of the patients surgery may still have to be considered at the end of this period. If there is an associated facet fracture or recurrent dislocation in the external fixator, then posterior fusion again becomes necessary. Patients left with an unreduced unilateral facet dislocation may develop neck pain and nerve root symptoms long term, if poorly managed.

AVULSION INJURY OF C7 SPINOUS PROCESS

Fracture of the C7 spinous process may occur with severe voluntary contraction of the muscles at the back of the neck; it has earned the name 'clay-shoveller's fracture'. The injury is painful but harmless. No treatment is required; as soon as symptoms permit, neck exercises are encouraged.

SPRAINED NECK (WHIPLASH INJURY)

Soft-tissue sprains (or wrenching injuries) of the neck are so common after car accidents that they now constitute a veritable epidemic; and the imaginative term 'whiplash injury' has served effectively to enhance public apprehension at its occurrence. It usually follows a rear-end collision in which the occupant's body is thrown forwards and

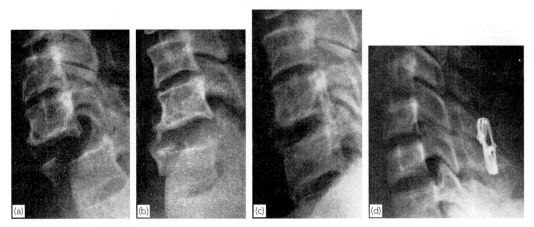

29.10 Cervical fracture–dislocation (a) Fracture–dislocation in the lower cervical spine. (b,c) Stages in the reduction of this fracture–dislocation by skull traction; (d) subsequent posterior wiring to ensure stability.

the head jerked backwards with hyperextension of the lower cervical spine; however, it can also occur with flexion and rotation injuries. Women are affected more often than men. There is disagreement about the exact pathology and there is no correlation between the amount of damage to the vehicle and the severity of complaints.

Pain and stiffness of the neck usually appear during the next 12–48 hours, or occasionally only several days later. Some patients complain of more ill-defined symptoms such as headache, dizziness, blurring of vision, paraesthesiae in the arms, temporomandibular discomfort and tinnitus. Neck muscles are tender and movements often restricted. X-ray examination may show straightening out of the normal cervical lordosis, a sign of muscle spasm; in other respects the appearances are usually normal though in some cases there are features of long-standing intervertebral disc degeneration.

Simple pain-relieving measures, including analgesic medication, may be needed during the first few weeks. However, the emphasis should be on graded exercises for return of neck movement.

The long-term prognosis is variable and a small group of patients appear never to be free of symptoms. Negative prognostic indicators are increasing age, severity of symptoms at the outset, prolonged duration of symptoms and the presence of pre-existing intervertebral disc degeneration.

THORACIC SPINE INJURIES

Most thoracic spine injuries result from hyperflexion. Wedge compressions are relatively common in osteoporotic people; they are usually mechanically stable but may lead to progressive kyphosis, especially if more than one vertebra is involved.

Severe injuries in younger people carry a high risk of cord damage, particularly those involving T11 and T12 which are not 'splinted' by the rib-cage. If there is any doubt about the presence of fragmentation or displacement of the posterior part of the vertebral body, CT or MRI will be needed to demonstrate the real risk to the spinal cord.

Plain x-rays, whilst showing the lower thoracic spine quite clearly, may be difficult to interpret for the upper thoracic spine because the scapula and shoulders get in the way. Here again CT or MRI will be helpful.

Treatment

Stable fracture patterns with less than about 30 degrees of kyphosis and without neurological

injury are managed symptomatically. If angulation is more marked, bracing or posterior fusion is indicated to avoid an increasing kyphosis.

If there is complete paraplegia and no improvement after 48 hours, conservative management is adequate; the patient can be rested in bed for 5–6 weeks, then gradually mobilized in a brace. However, if there is severe bony injury, with the risk of increasing kyphosis, internal fixation should be considered.

THORACOLUMBAR INJURIES

Most injuries of the thoracolumbar spine occur in the transitional area (T11–L2) between the somewhat fixed thoracic spine and the more mobile lumbar spine. The upper thoracic vertebrae are also protected by the rib-cage and fractures in this region tend to be mechanically stable. However, the spinal canal in that area is relatively narrow, so cord damage is not uncommon; when it does occur it is usually complete.

The spinal cord ends at L1 and below that level it is the lower nerve roots that are at risk.

Types of fracture

Low-energy fractures comprise those that occur in osteoporotic bone and minor fractures of the vertebral processes. *High-energy fractures and fracture–dislocations* are due to major injuries sustained in vehicle collisions, falls or diving from heights, horse-riding and collapsed buildings. It is mainly in the second group that one encounters neurological complications.

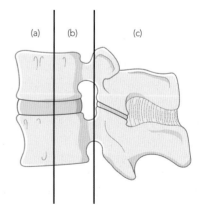

29.11 Structural elements of the lumbar spine The three important structural elements are: (a) the anterior column; (b) the middle column; and (c) the osseoligamentous complex forming the posterior column.

It is most important to establish whether the injury is *stable* or *unstable*. As mentioned at the beginning of the present chapter, this hinges on the integrity of the three structural elements: the *posterior osseoligamentous complex (or posterior column)*, the *middle column*, which includes the posterior half of the vertebral body and the posterior longitudinal ligament, and the *anterior column* composed of the anterior half of the vertebral body, the anterior part of the intervertebral disc and the anterior longitudinal ligament. Fractures involving the middle column and at least one of the other columns should be regarded as unstable.

Examination

Patients complaining of back pain following an injury or showing signs of bruising and tenderness over the spine, as well as those suffering head or neck injuries, chest injuries and pelvic fractures should undergo a careful examination of the spine and a full neurological examination, including rectal examination to assess sphincter tone.

Imaging

X-rays should be carefully examined for loss of vertebral height or splaying of the vertebral body. Widening of the distance between the pedicles or an increased distance between successive spinous processes suggests posterior column damage. The lateral view is examined for vertebral alignment and structural integrity. Look particularly for evidence of fragment retropulsion towards the spinal canal. *Rapid screening CT scans* are more reliable than x-rays in showing bone injuries. MRI also may be needed to evaluate neurological or other soft-tissue injuries.

Treatment

Treatment depends on: (a) the type of anatomical disruption; (b) whether the injury is stable or unstable; (c) whether there is neurological involvement; and (d) the presence or absence of concomitant injuries.

FRACTURES OF THE TRANSVERSE PROCESSES

The transverse processes can be avulsed with sudden muscular activity. Isolated injuries need no more than symptomatic treatment. More ominous than usual is a fracture of the transverse process of L5, which should alert one to the possibility of a vertical shear injury of the pelvis.

FLEXION–COMPRESSION INJURY

This is by far the most common vertebral fracture and is due to severe spinal flexion with the posterior ligaments remaining intact. In osteoporotic individuals fracture may occur with minimal trauma. Pain may be quite severe but the fracture is usually stable (only the anterior column is damaged) and neurological injury is extremely rare.

Patients with minimal wedging and a stable fracture pattern are kept in bed for 1–2 weeks until pain subsides and are then mobilized; no support is needed.

Those with moderate wedging (loss of 20–40% of anterior vertebral height) and a stable injury can be allowed up after 1 week, wearing a thoracolumbar brace or a body cast applied with the back in extension. At 3 months, flexion–extension x-rays

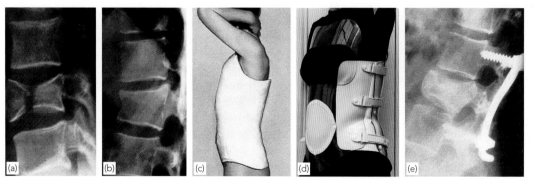

29.12 Wedge-compression fractures (a) Central compression fracture of the vertebral body and (b) anterior wedge-compression fracture with less than 20% loss of vertebral body height. In both cases the middle and posterior columns are intact; further collapse can be prevented by immobilization for 8–12 weeks in (c) a plaster 'jacket' or (d) a lightweight removable orthosis. (e) More severe and potentially unstable compression fractures may need posterior internal fixation.

are obtained with the patient out of the orthosis; if there is no instability, the brace is gradually discarded. If the deformity increases, posterior fixation and spinal fusion should be considered.

AXIAL COMPRESSION OR BURST INJURY

Severe axial compression may 'explode' the vertebral body, shattering the posterior part of the vertebral body and extruding fragments of bone into the spinal canal. The injury is usually unstable.

The x-ray appearance may superficially resemble the wedge compression fracture (see above) but the posterior border of the vertebral body is damaged; this is seen most clearly on CT scans.

If there is minimal anterior wedging, little or no retropulsion of bone and no neurological damage, the patient is kept in bed until the acute symptoms settle and is then mobilized in a thoracolumbar brace or body cast which is worn for about 12 weeks.

Even if CT shows that there is considerable compromise of the spinal canal, provided there are no neurological symptoms or signs non-operative treatment is still appropriate; the fragments usually re-model. However, any new symptoms such as tingling, weakness or alteration of bladder or bowel function must be reported immediately and should call for further imaging by MRI; anterior decompression and stabilization may then be needed if there are signs of present or impending neurological compromise.

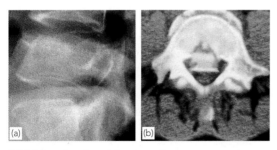

29.13 Lumbar burst fracture Severe compression may cause retropulsion of the vertebral body (a). The extent of spinal canal encroachment is best shown by CT (b).

JACK-KNIFE INJURY (THE CHANCE FRACTURE)

This unusual injury was described by Chance in 1948. Combined flexion and posterior distraction (seen typically in severe seat-belt injuries) may cause the midlumbar spine to jack-knife around an axis anterior to the vertebral column. There is little or no crushing of the vertebral body; the tear passes transversely through the bones or the ligament structures, or both. Because the posterior and middle columns fail, the injury is by definition unstable but neurological damage is uncommon.

The injury usually heals quite rapidly. Three months in a body cast or well-fitting brace will usually suffice.

FRACTURE–DISLOCATION

Segmental displacement may occur with various combinations of flexion, compression, rotation and shear. The spine is grossly unstable. These are the most dangerous injuries and are often associated with neurological damage to the lowermost part of the cord or the cauda equina.

X-rays may show fractures through the vertebral body, pedicles, articular processes and laminae; there may be varying degrees of subluxation or even bilateral facet dislocation. CT helps to demonstrate the degree of spinal canal occlusion.

If there is no neurological injury, most patients will benefit from early surgery. Operative stabilization will prevent later neurological damage, facilitate nursing, shorten the hospital stay, make rehabilitation easier and reduce the chance of painful deformity. If specialized surgery cannot be performed, these injuries can be managed non-operatively with postural reduction, bed rest and bracing.

For patients with paraplegia, if they can be treated in a specialized spinal injuries unit, there is no convincing evidence that surgery will shorten the hospital stay or reduce the chance of painful deformity.

For patients with a partial neurological deficit, there is likewise no evidence that surgical decompression and stabilization provide a better neurological outcome than high-level conservative treatment. Our advice, therefore, is that these patients too should be treated non-operatively – provided the appropriate levels of nursing and rehabilitative care can be assured.

TRAUMATIC PARAPLEGIA

Injuries of the spine may be complicated by damage to the spinal cord or cauda equina. The injuries most likely to do this are 'burst' fractures and fracture–dislocations of the thoracolumbar region or the lower cervical spine.

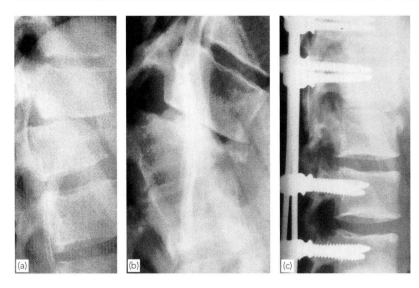

29.14 Thoracolumbar fracture–dislocation
(a) Fracture–dislocation at T11/12 in a 32-year-old woman who was a passenger in a truck that overturned. She was completely paraplegic and operation was not thought worthwhile. (b) Four weeks later the deformity had increased, leaving her with a marked gibbus. (c) Treatment by open reduction and internal fixation.

Complete transection of the cord results in either paraplegia (thoracic and lumbar lesions) or quadriplegia (cervical lesions). Initially there is complete flaccid paralysis and anaesthesia, with loss of the anal reflex (spinal shock). At this stage, and for the first 24 hours, the diagnosis cannot be absolutely certain. However, if the anal reflex returns during the first 48 hours and the neural deficit persists, the cord lesion must be assumed to be complete. Gradually the features of an upper motor neuron lesion appear, with spastic paralysis and exaggerated reflexes.

Incomplete cord transection results in partial sensory and motor loss below the level of the lesion. Signs vary according to which part of the cord is damaged.

Nerve root transection causes motor paralysis, sensory loss and visceral paralysis in the distribution of the damaged roots. Root transection differs from cord transection in two ways: recovery may occur and residual motor paralysis remains permanently flaccid.

ANATOMICAL LEVEL

With cervical spine injuries the segmental level of cord transection nearly corresponds to the level of bony damage. High cervical cord transection is fatal because all the respiratory muscles are paralysed.

At the C5 vertebra, cord transection isolates the lower cord with paralysis of the upper and lower limbs, the trunk and the viscera.

Cord transection at the T10 vertebra causes paralysis of the lower limbs and viscera. *Between T10 and L1* the cord forms a bulge, the conus medullaris; it then tapers to an end at the interspace between the L1 and L2 vertebrae.

The L2–S4 nerve roots from the conus medullaris stream downwards in a bunch (the *cauda equina*) to emerge at successive levels of the lumbosacral spine. These roots supply the muscles of the ankles and feet, the anal and penile reflexes, as well as bladder and bowel continence.

Therefore, spinal injuries above the T10 vertebra cause cord transection, those between the T10 and L1 vertebrae cause cord and nerve root lesions, and those below the L1 vertebra only nerve root lesions.

PROGNOSIS

Complete paralysis and anaesthesia below the level of injury suggest cord transection. Complete lesions lasting more than 72 hours have only a small chance of neurological recovery.

Persistence of any sensation distal to the injury (perianal pinprick is most important) suggests an incomplete lesion. Cord hemisection causes the *Brown–Séquard syndrome* (loss of motor power on the side of the lesion and loss of pain and temperature sensation on the opposite side); this is usually caused by penetrating thoracic injuries. Most of these patients improve and regain bowel and bladder function and some walking ability.

A well-established method of recording the functional deficit after an incomplete spinal cord injury was that described by Frankel (*Table 29.2*).

Most patients with Grades B, C or D improve by one grade regardless of the type of treatment, though only 5% reach Grade D or E.

419

Table 29.2 Frankel grading

Grade A	Absent motor and sensory function
Grade B	Sensation present, motor power absent
Grade C	Sensation present, motor power present but not useful
Grade D	Sensation present, motor power present and useful (MRC Grade 4 or 5)
Grade E	Normal motor and sensory function

MANAGEMENT

Whether management is by decompression and stabilization (favoured by some surgeons for partial paralysis) or by conservative treatment, it is the overall care of the patient that is the most important. The patient must be transported with great care to prevent further damage, and preferably taken directly to a spinal centre. The principles of treatment are outlined below.

Skin

Within a few hours anaesthetic skin may develop large pressure sores; this can be prevented by meticulous nursing. Creases in the sheets and crumbs in the bed are not permitted. Every 2 hours the patient is gently rolled onto his or her side and the back is carefully washed (without rubbing), dried and powdered. After a few weeks the skin becomes a little more tolerant and the patient can turn in bed without assistance. Later the patient should be taught how to relieve skin pressure intermittently during periods of sitting. If sores have been allowed to develop, they may never heal without excision and skin grafting.

Bladder and bowel

For the first 24 hours the bladder distends only slowly, but, if the distension is allowed to progress, overflow incontinence occurs and infection is probable. In special centres it is usual to manage the patient from the outset by intermittent catheterization under sterile conditions. If early transfer to a paraplegia centre is not possible, continuous closed drainage through a fine Silastic catheter is advised. The disposable bag should be changed twice weekly to prevent blockage. If infection supervenes, antibiotics are given.

As the local reflexes gradually return, automatic emptying of the bladder may occur whenever it becomes distended. If the cauda equina is damaged, this reflex is lost and bladder emptying has to be initiated by manual suprapubic pressure. Bladder training is begun as early as possible and patients learn to manage this function themselves.

The bowel is more easily trained, with the help of enemas, aperients and abdominal exercises.

Muscles and joints

The paralysed muscles, if not treated, may develop severe flexion contractures. These are usually preventable by moving the joints passively through their full range twice daily.

With lesions below the cervical cord, the patient should be up within 6 weeks; standing and walking are valuable in preventing contractures. Calipers are usually necessary to keep the knees straight and the feet plantigrade. The calipers are removed at intervals during the day while the patient lies prone, and while he or she is having physiotherapy. The upper limbs must be trained until they develop sufficient power to enable the patient to use crutches and a wheelchair.

If flexion contractures have been allowed to develop, tenotomies may be necessary. Painful flexor spasms are rare unless skin or bladder infection occurs. They can sometimes be relieved by tenotomies, neurectomies, rhizotomies or the intrathecal injection of alcohol.

Heterotopic ossification is a common and disturbing complication; it is more likely to occur with high lesions and complete lesions. It may restrict or abolish movement, especially at the hip. Once the new bone is mature it can safely be excised.

Tendon transfer operations in the upper limbs may be feasible for some patients with low cervical cord injuries.

Morale

The morale of a paraplegic patient is liable to reach a low ebb, and the restoration of self-confidence is an important part of treatment. Constant enthusiasm and encouragement by doctors, physiotherapists and nurses are essential. Their scrupulous attention to the patient's comfort and toilet are of primary importance; the unpleasant smells associated with skin or urinary infection must be prevented. The earlier the patient gets up the better, and he or she must be trained for a new job as quickly as possible.

FRACTURES OF THE THORACIC CAGE

FRACTURES OF THE STERNUM

The sternum may be fractured by a direct blow to the chest, or indirectly during a flexion injury of the spine.

The patient complains of severe pain directly over the sternum. X-ray signs are sometimes difficult to discern, particularly if the fracture is undisplaced. *Unless it is certain that the only injury was a direct blow to the front of the chest, it is important to x-ray the spine to exclude an associated vertebral compression fracture.*

If displacement is minimal, treatment is needed only to control pain and encourage breathing exercises. If the fracture is severely displaced, it will require operative treatment: the sternum can be lifted forwards (under general anaesthesia) with the aid of a bone-hook. The patient should be kept under observation to make sure that there are no pulmonary complications.

RIB FRACTURES

Rib fractures are almost always due to direct injury. However, in osteoporotic patients ribs may fracture with minor stresses such as coughing or sneezing.

The patient complains of a sharp pain in the chest. This is markedly aggravated by deep breathing or coughing, or by anteroposterior compression of the chest wall. X-ray shows one or more fractures, usually near the rib angle. Because the bones are often osteoporotic, it may be difficult to obtain clear images of these fractures, especially if the fragments are undisplaced. A radionuclide scan 10 days later will show localized activity at the fracture sites.

In most cases treatment is needed only for pain; an injection of local anaesthetic will bring immediate relief. Breathing exercises are encouraged.

A note of warning: even a benign looking rib fracture occasionally penetrates the pleura and during the next few days the patient may complain of respiratory difficulty due to a tension pneumothorax. Always enquire about any recent chest injury.

COMPLEX THORACIC INJURIES

Complex fractures of the thorax include secondary injuries to mediastinal structures. These conditions require emergency treatment. They are dealt with in Chapter 22.

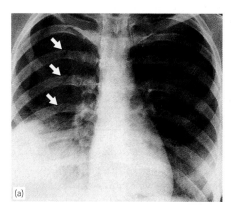

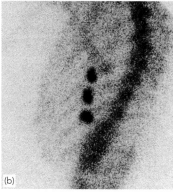

29.15 Fractures of ribs
(a) Rib fractures are usually obvious on plain x-ray (arrows). (b) Undisplaced fractures are difficult to see; a week later they show up clearly on the radionuclide scan.

CHAPTER 30

FRACTURES OF THE PELVIS

Fractures of the pelvis are particularly serious because they are often complicated by damage to the pelvic soft tissues (bowel, bladder, urethra, reproductive organs, nerve plexuses, and a network of supporting ligaments), causing massive blood loss which can be fatal. The overall mortality in pelvic trauma is 9%, although this is significantly increased (up to 50%) if the patient is haemodynamically unstable at presentation.

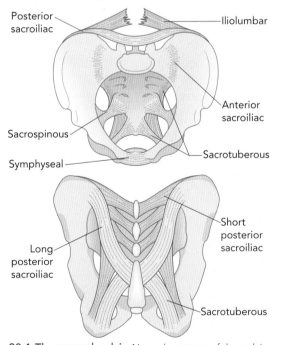

30.1 The normal pelvis Normal anatomy of the pelvis and its stabilizing ligaments.

Clinical assessment

A fracture of the pelvis should be suspected in every patient with serious abdominal or lower limb injuries. The patient may be severely shocked due to blood loss and visceral damage. Resuscitation should be started even before the examination is complete (the ATLS approach is described in Chapter 22).

Local bruising or abrasions may be obvious; ecchymoses often extend into the thigh and perineum, and there may be gross swelling of the labia or scrotum. Bleeding from the urethra or genitalia suggests serious visceral damage. Abdominal tenderness and guarding suggest intraperitoneal bleeding, possibly due to rupture of the spleen or liver.

Pain may be elicited if the pelvic ring is sprung by gentle but firm pressure – first from side to side on the iliac crests, then outwards on the anterior superior iliac spines, and then directly on the symphysis pubis. If the patient is haemodynamically unstable this manoeuvre should be performed only once, as repeated examinations may disturb a pelvic haematoma and cause further bleeding.

During rectal examination (which is mandatory), the coccyx and sacrum can be felt; more importantly, the position of the prostate can be gauged: if it is abnormally high, it suggests a urethral injury. A ruptured bladder should be suspected in patients who do not void or in whom a bladder is not palpable after adequate intravenous fluid replacement.

Neurological examination is essential. There may be damage to the lumbosacral plexus; a

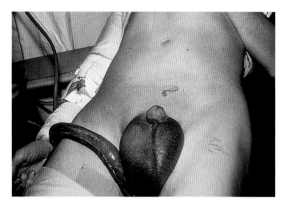

30.2 Fractures of the pelvis – clinical examination This young man crashed on his motorcycle and was brought into the Accident and Emergency Department with a fractured femur. His perineum and scrotum were swollen and bruised; he was unable to pass urine and a streak of blood appeared at the external meatus. X-rays confirmed that he had a fractured pelvis.

common presenting sign is a foot-drop as a result of damage to the L5 nerve root.

Imaging

A good anteroposterior view of the pelvis is mandatory; ideally inlet and outlet views and oblique views of each half of the pelvis should also be obtained.

Nowadays all patients with suspected major trauma undergo a 'trauma computed tomography (CT) scan', comprising the head, neck, chest, abdomen and pelvis. Axial CT scans provide the best images to reveal and diagnose pelvic injuries, particularly those around the sacroiliac joints and sacrum (e.g. sacroiliac disruption). Three-dimensional CT reconstructions can be formatted from the 'trauma CT'. An intravenous contrast preparation can also be given, providing a CT cystogram.

TYPES OF FRACTURE

Pelvic fractures fall into four groups: (1) isolated fractures with an intact pelvic ring; (2) fractures with a broken ring – these may be stable or unstable; (3) fractures of the acetabulum: although these are ring fractures, involvement of the joint raises special problems and therefore they are considered separately; and (4) sacrococcygeal fractures.

ISOLATED FRACTURES

Avulsion fractures

A piece of bone is pulled off by violent muscle contraction; this is usually seen in sports participants and athletes. The sartorius may pull off the anterior superior iliac spine, the rectus femoris the anterior

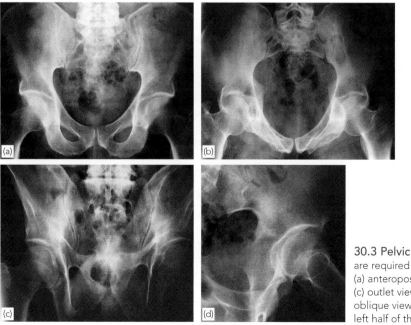

30.3 Pelvic x-rays At least five views are required for diagnosis: (a) anteroposterior; (b) inlet view; (c) outlet view; and (d) right and left oblique views, similar to this view of the left half of the pelvis.

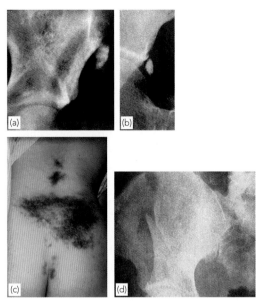

30.4 Isolated injuries (a,b) Avulsion fractures. Powerful muscle contraction may tear off a piece of bone at its attachment. Two examples are shown here: (a) avulsion of sartorius attachment and (b) avulsion of rectus femoris origin. (c,d) Fractured iliac blade. The bruise suggests the site of the injury. The fracture looks alarming and is certainly painful but, if the remainder of the bony pelvis is intact, it poses no threat to the patient.

inferior iliac spine, the adductor longus a piece of the pubis, and the hamstrings part of the ischium. All are essentially muscle injuries, needing only rest for a few days and reassurance.

Direct fractures

A direct blow to the pelvis, usually after a fall from a height, may fracture the ischium or the iliac blade. Bed rest until pain subsides is usually all that is needed.

Stress fractures

Fractures of the pubic rami are fairly common (and often quite painless) in severely osteoporotic or osteomalacic patients.

FRACTURES OF THE PELVIC RING

The innominate bones and the sacrum form a ring which is held together by the weak symphyseal joint anteriorly and the strong sacroiliac and iliolumbar ligaments posteriorly. Because of the rigidity of the adult pelvis, a break at one point in the ring must be accompanied by disruption at a second point. (Try breaking a ring-shaped biscuit at one point only!) Exceptions are comminuted fractures due to direct blows (including fractures of the acetabular floor), or ring fractures in children, whose symphyses and sacroiliac joints are springy.

Mechanisms of injury

The basic mechanisms of pelvic ring injury are anteroposterior compression (APC), lateral compression (LC), vertical shear (VS) and combinations of these. The degree of stability can usually be judged from the fracture pattern; fractures are either stable, partially stable or unstable (Tile classification).

Anteroposterior compression

APC injury is usually seen in motorcyclists where the patient straddles the petrol tank of the motorcycle at the point of impact with sudden deceleration. Initially the pubic symphysis is disrupted; as the force of energy increases, the sacroiliac joints posteriorly are disrupted – the so-called 'open-book' injury. The sacroiliac ligaments may be torn; there may be a fracture of the posterior part of the ilium or a vertical sacral fracture. This fracture pattern increases the pelvic volume and is associated with the largest amount of blood loss.

Lateral compression

Side-to-side compression of the pelvis causes the ring to buckle and break. This is usually due to a side-on impact in a pedestrian accident or a side-on collision in a car accident. Anteriorly the pubic rami on one or both sides are fractured, and posteriorly there is a severe sacroiliac strain or a fracture of the ilium or sacrum. If the sacroiliac injury is much displaced, the pelvis is unstable.

Vertical shear

The innominate bone on one side is displaced vertically, fracturing the pubic rami and disrupting the sacroiliac region on the same side. This occurs typically when someone falls from a height onto one leg. These are usually severe, unstable injuries with gross tearing of the soft tissues and retroperitoneal haemorrhage.

Combination injuries

In severe pelvic injuries there may be a combination of the above, e.g. a pedestrian hit by a car and thrown into the air or a motorcyclist ejected from the bike at impact.

Clinical features

With *isolated fractures and stable injuries* the patient is not severely shocked but has pain on attempting

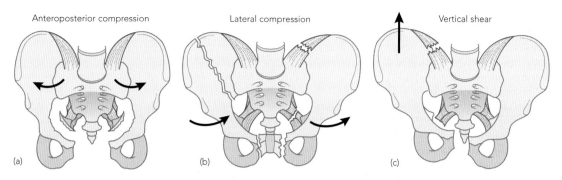

Anteroposterior compression   Lateral compression   Vertical shear

(a)   (b)   (c)

30.5 Fractures of the pelvic ring (a) Anteroposterior compression with lateral rotation causes disruption of the anterior part of the ring – the 'open book' injury. (b) Lateral compression causes the ring to buckle and break, fracturing the pubic rami on one or both sides; posteriorly the iliac blade may break or the sacrum is crushed. (c) Vertical shear injury, causing disruption of both the sacroiliac and symphyseal regions on one side.

to walk. There is localized tenderness but seldom any damage to pelvic viscera.

With *unstable injuries* the patient is severely shocked, in great pain and unable to stand; he or she may also be unable to pass urine. There may be blood at the external meatus. Tenderness is widespread and attempting to move the ilium is very painful. There may be a foot-drop due to a L5 nerve root injury, or one leg may be partly anaesthetic because of sciatic nerve injury. These are extremely serious injuries, carrying a high risk of associated visceral damage.

As a rule, it is only the mechanically unstable displaced fractures that lead to haemodynamic instability; if a patient has a stable pelvic fracture but is haemodynamically unstable, one must look for another source of bleeding, e.g. chest or abdomen.

Open pelvic fractures are also associated with major blood loss, so it is always important to 'log-roll' patients and ensure there is no external blood loss posteriorly.

Early management

Treatment should not await full and detailed diagnosis. It is vital in treating any severely injured patient to follow the priorities set out in Chapter 22.

Any patient with a suspected pelvic fracture should have a pelvic compression binder applied by the ambulance crew or paramedics attending the accident; this provides immediate stability to any pelvic ring disruption and is potentially life-saving.

The diagnosis of persistent blood loss is straightforward but it is not always easy to determine the source of the bleeding. In the rare case of a patient in extremis due to haemodynamic

instability, it is not safe to perform a 'trauma CT' to locate the precise source of bleeding. A routine chest x-ray will show any evidence of a haemothorax (which should be treated with a chest drain) and pelvic x-ray will show if the pelvis is unstable. In addition a 'FAST scan' (Focussed Assessment with Sonography for Trauma) is obtained to exclude intraperitoneal haemorrhage. If there is fluid in the abdomen, it should be explored via a laparotomy in an attempt to find and deal with the source of bleeding.

If the 'FAST scan' is negative, the likely bleeding source is the pelvis: this is 80% low-pressure venous plexus bleeding, 10% arterial, and 10% cancellous bone. Although most hospital protocols call for binder application and transfer for angiography and embolization of the bleeding vessels, this does not stop the venous bleeding and the mortality rate in patients treated by that routine is up to 50%.

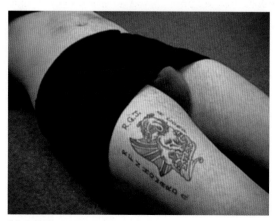

30.6 Early management A pelvic binder is applied at the level of the greater trochanters, to provide pelvic stability.

More recent studies have shown a better outcome and lower mortality rate following immediate transfer to the operating theatre for emergency preperitoneal pelvic packing and application of an external fixator.

Urological injury occurs in about 10% of patients with pelvic ring fractures. One attempt at urethral catheterization may be attempted; this usually results in successful bladder drainage. If unsuccessful (due to a presumed urethral injury) a suprapubic cystostomy is performed.

Treatment of the fracture

Traditional treatments of prolonged bed rest and traction are avoided due to the incidence of pressure sores, venous thromboembolism and chest sepsis. Stable fractures are treated with early mobilization, and the principles of operative treatment are to convert an unstable pelvis to a stable pelvic ring to allow mobilization.

Undisplaced ring fractures

These commonly include LC injuries involving a pubic ramus fracture anteriorly and an undisplaced sacral fracture posteriorly. Pain usually subsides after a few days, and patients can be mobilized partially weightbearing on the affected side for 6 weeks.

Anteroposterior compression injuries

'*Open-book*' *injuries* involve anterior symphysis pubis widening and posterior sacroiliac joint (SIJ) disruption. Anteriorly, a wide symphysis is treated by open reduction and internal fixation, and posteriorly the SIJ injury is fixed with iliosacral screws.

Even minimal disruptions are treated because of the increased incidence of long-term pain with non-operative treatment. Where patients have suffered bilateral rami fractures anteriorly and posterior sacral fractures, treatment is by using iliosacral screws posteriorly and an external fixator to stabilize the pelvic ring anteriorly. Patients can be mobilized following this treatment.

Vertical shear fractures and displaced lateral compression fractures

Severe VS and LC injuries can be challenging. The fracture or dislocation must be reduced and then stabilized. Posteriorly, reduction is achieved with the use of either traction and percutaneous

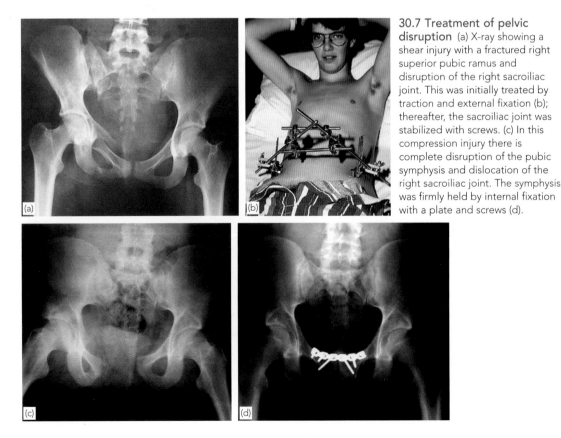

30.7 Treatment of pelvic disruption (a) X-ray showing a shear injury with a fractured right superior pubic ramus and disruption of the right sacroiliac joint. This was initially treated by traction and external fixation (b); thereafter, the sacroiliac joint was stabilized with screws. (c) In this compression injury there is complete disruption of the pubic symphysis and dislocation of the right sacroiliac joint. The symphysis was firmly held by internal fixation with a plate and screws (d).

iliosacral screw fixation, or open reduction and internal fixation. Anteriorly, stabilization is achieved either by open reduction and internal fixation of the symphysis or the application of an external fixator.

Complications

Urogenital damage

APC fractures are the usual cause of urogenital tract damage; symphyseal widening is associated with urethral injury, and displaced rami fractures may cause bladder injury. All that needs to be provided urgently in a seriously ill patient is adequate urinary drainage, which is accomplished by suprapubic cystostomy. Definitive repair can be delayed while the patient's general condition improves and expert urological advice is sought. Late complications include urethral stricture, incontinence and impotence.

Bowel injury

If there is a bowel injury at presentation, a defunctioning colostomy is performed so as not to contaminate the pelvis. A re-anastomosis is performed at 6–12 months once healing has occurred.

Vaginal injury

Displaced pubic ramus fractures can tear the lateral wall of the vagina, in which case there is an open injury. Tears should be washed out and repaired.

Nerve injury

Displacement of the sacroiliac joint or fracture of the sacrum may injure the lumbosacral plexus, commonly the L5 nerve root. Recovery is usually rare.

Persistent sacroiliac pain

This usually occurs if a SIJ injury has been left untreated. Late treatment involves fusion if symptoms are severe.

Venous thromboembolic disease

Patients with pelvic fractures are prone to the development of venous thromboembolism (VTE), especially if they undergo operative fixation. VTE prophylaxis is initiated at diagnosis, and continued for 6–12 weeks if surgery has been performed.

FRACTURES OF THE ACETABULUM

Fractures of the acetabulum occur when the head of the femur is driven into the pelvis. This is caused either by a blow on the side (as in a fall from a height) or by a blow on the front of the knee, usually in a dashboard injury when the femur also may be fractured.

Patterns of fracture (see Figure 30.8)

It is the position of the leg (i.e. rotation and abduction/adduction) that determines the fracture pattern. The Letournel classification, although complex, allows accurate description of the fracture pattern and guides the surgical approach if operative treatment is indicated. Fractures are divided into five 'elements', and five 'associated fractures'.

The five 'elements' are as follows:

Posterior wall fractures

This is the commonest fracture. It usually occurs with the leg flexed and the knee hitting the dashboard in a motor vehicle accident. On impact the femoral head is thrust against the posterior wall of the acetabulum. The hip is dislocated and either remains so, or is spontaneously reduced.

Anterior wall fractures

Here the fracture produces a trapezoid fragment with anterior subluxation of the femoral head. This is the rarest fracture pattern.

Posterior column fractures

This fracture runs upwards from the obturator foramen into the sciatic notch, separating the posterior ischiopubic column of bone and breaking the weightbearing part of the acetabulum. It is usually associated with medial migration of the femoral head.

Anterior column fractures

The fracture runs through the anterior part of the acetabulum, separating a segment between the anterior inferior iliac spine and the obturator foramen.

Transverse fracture

This is an uncomminuted fracture running transversely through the acetabulum and separating the iliac portion above from the pubic and ischial portions below; the femoral head usually follows the ischiopubic segment. The fracture is often associated with a SIJ injury.

The five 'associated fractures' are combinations of the elemental fractures. In these cases the articular surface is more severely disrupted, and the fractures usually need operative reduction and internal fixation.

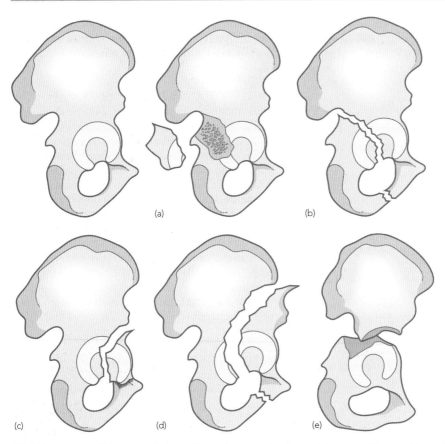

30.8 Fractures of the acetabulum Shown here are drawings of the normal hemipelvis and the five main elements in Letournel's classification. (a) Posterior wall fracture. (b) Posterior column fracture. (c) Anterior wall fracture. (d) Anterior column fracture. (e) Transverse fracture.

The five types are:

A T-shaped fracture

This is a transverse fracture with an additional vertical split into the obturator foramen.

Posterior column plus posterior wall

This is a posterior column fracture with an associated posterior wall fracture. The femoral head is dislocated and the level of the fracture is through the sciatic notch.

Transverse plus posterior wall

This is a transverse fracture with an additional posterior wall fracture due to dislocation of the femoral head. There is a high incidence of sciatic nerve injury (up to 70%).

Anterior column plus posterior hemitransverse

This is a fracture of the anterior column with an additional posterior column fracture at the posterior half of a transverse fracture.

Combined posterior and anterior columns

All articular segments are separate from the ilium – a 'floating acetabulum'. This is the most severe form of injury.

Clinical features

There has usually been a severe injury, either a traffic accident or a fall from a height. Associated fractures are not uncommon and, because they may be more obvious, they are liable to divert attention from a more urgent pelvic ring injury. Whenever a fractured femur, a severe knee injury or a fractured calcaneum is diagnosed, the hips also should be x-rayed.

The patient may be severely shocked, and the complications associated with all pelvic fractures should be sought. There may be bruising around the hip and the limb may lie in internal rotation (if the hip is dislocated). Test for sciatic nerve palsy.

X-rays

An anteroposterior view of the pelvis is mandatory. Oblique views are also important: they allow an accurate classification to be made and guide any surgical approach. CT scanning excludes any other pelvic fracture and shows evidence of marginal impaction of the articular surface. Three-dimensional CT reconstructions allow excellent visualization of fracture fragments.

Treatment

Initial management

Emergency treatment consists of treating associated injuries and reducing a dislocation. Traction is then applied to the limb (10 lb [4.5 kg] will suffice). Definitive treatment of the fracture is ideally performed at 2–5 days post injury. The delay should not exceed 7 days, as it becomes increasingly difficult to reduce the fragments accurately.

Conservative treatment

Undisplaced fractures or stable fractures may be treated conservatively with minimal weightbearing and early mobilization. The joint must be congruent with minimal articular displacement. Close monitoring over the first 6 weeks is necessary to ensure the position is maintained.

Operative treatment

Operative treatment is indicated for all unstable hips and fractures resulting in significant distortion of joint congruence, as well as for associated fractures of the femoral head and/or retained bone fragments in the joint. The aim should be a perfect anatomical reduction, and the operation is best undertaken in a centre specializing in this form of treatment.

Associated fractures are difficult to reduce, and require a combination of surgical expertise, specialized reduction clamps and a special orthopaedic table allowing traction to be applied and appropriate imaging.

Complications

Nerve injury

With posterior fractures involving a hip dislocation, the sciatic nerve may be injured. The nerve is usually not severed, but recovery is seldom complete.

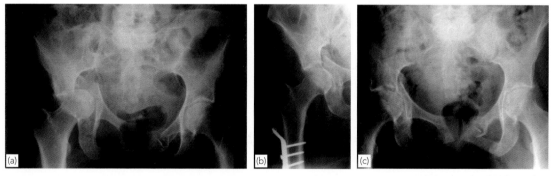

30.9 Fractured acetabulum – conservative treatment This severely displaced acetabular fracture (a) was almost completely reduced by (b) longitudinal and lateral traction. (c) The fracture healed and the patient regained a congruent joint with a fairly good range of movement.

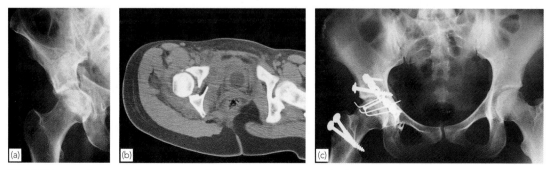

30.10 Fractured acetabulum – internal fixation (a) X-ray shows the fracture, but the degree of displacement is better demonstrated by CT (b). This was treated by open reduction and internal fixation (c).

Avascular necrosis

As in all severe injuries of the hip, femoral head necrosis may occur. The changes take months or even years to develop. If this progresses to fragmentation and collapse of the femoral head, arthroplasty may be indicated.

Heterotopic bone formation

Heterotopic bone formation is common after severe soft-tissue injury and extended surgical dissections (particularly any posterior approach involving elevation of the abductor muscles). In cases where this is anticipated, prophylactic indomethacin is useful.

Osteoarthritis

The principle reason for surgical treatment is to prevent osteoarthritis and disability. Secondary osteoarthritis of the hip is a common (late) complication, especially if the fracture involves the weightbearing surface. If the joint is not congruent, the patient will develop osteoarthritis within months. The progression to osteoarthritis is directly related to the quality of the fracture reduction. Osteoarthritis is also more common in patients over 55 years of age.

INJURIES OF THE SACRUM AND COCCYX

A blow from behind, or a fall onto the 'tail', may fracture the sacrum or coccyx, or sprain the joint between them.

If the fracture is markedly displaced, reduction is worth attempting. The lower fragment may be pushed backwards by a finger in the rectum. The reduction is stable, which is fortunate. The patient is allowed to resume normal activity, but is advised to use a rubber-ring cushion when sitting.

Vertical fractures of the sacrum are associated with pelvic ring injuries. The fractures are classified according to their relation to the sacral foramina: Type 1 fractures lie lateral to the sacral foramina; Type 2 through the foramina; and Type 3 medial to the foramina.

Below the level of S2 the sacrum does not articulate with the pelvis so mechanical instability is less of a concern.

Low transverse fractures below the level of S2 are caused by a fall onto the 'tail'. The only indication for operative treatment is if there is significant displacement in the sagittal plane leading to nerve dysfunction in the bowel and bladder. In this situation the sacral canal may need urgent decompression and reduction.

Persistent pain, especially on sitting, is common after coccygeal injuries. If the pain is not relieved by the use of a cushion or by the injection of local anaesthetic into the tender area, excision of the coccyx may be considered.

CHAPTER 31

INJURIES OF THE HIP AND FEMUR

DISLOCATION OF THE HIP

The incidence of hip dislocation has paralleled the rise in the number of road accidents. The injuries are classified according to the direction of dislocation: posterior occurs most frequently, followed by anterior and central.

POSTERIOR DISLOCATION

Usually this occurs in a road accident when someone seated in a truck or car is thrown forwards, striking the knee against the dashboard. The femur is thrust in a posterior direction and the femoral head is forced out of its socket; often a piece of bone at the back of the acetabulum is sheared off (fracture–dislocation).

Special features

In a straightforward case the diagnosis is easy: the leg is short and lies adducted, internally rotated and slightly flexed. However, if one of the long bones is fractured – usually the femur – the injury can be missed. *The golden rule (whenever the facilities exist) is to obtain a 'trauma computed tomography (CT)' scan which includes the pelvis, the entire femur and the knee in every case of severe injury*; and, even with isolated femoral fractures, to insist on x-rays that include the hip and the knee. The lower limb should be examined for signs of sciatic nerve injury.

X-rays

In the anteroposterior film the femoral head is seen out of its socket and above the acetabulum.

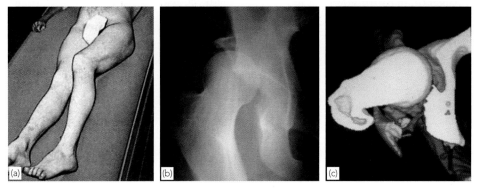

31.1 Posterior dislocation of the hip (a) Typical posture in a patient with posterior dislocation: the left hip slightly flexed and internally rotated. (b) The x-ray in this case showed a dislocated hip with an associated acetabular rim fracture. (c) Three-dimensional CT image revealing the full extent of the associated acetabular injury.

Multiple views (and better still CT scans) may be needed to exclude a fracture of the acetabular rim or the femoral head.

Treatment

The dislocation is usually reduced under general anaesthesia. An assistant steadies the pelvis; the surgeon flexes the patient's hip and knee to 90 degrees and pulls the thigh vertically upwards. X-rays are essential to confirm reduction and to exclude a fracture. Once closed reduction has been performed, CT is needed to make sure that bone fragments are not trapped in the joint.

After reduction the hip is usually stable, but it has been injured and needs to be rested. The simplest way is to apply traction and maintain it for 3 weeks. Movement and exercises are begun as soon as pain allows. At the end of 3 weeks the patient is allowed to walk with crutches.

Complications

Sciatic nerve injury

The sciatic nerve is damaged in 10–20% of cases, but fortunately it usually recovers. If, after reducing the dislocation, a sciatic nerve lesion and an unreduced acetabular fracture are diagnosed, the nerve should be explored and the fracture reduced and stabilized. Recovery often takes months and in the meantime the limb must be protected from injury and the ankle splinted to overcome the foot-drop.

Avascular necrosis

The blood supply of the femoral head is seriously impaired in at least 10% of traumatic hip dislocations; if reduction is delayed by more than a few hours, the figure rises to 40%. If there is a necrotic segment, operative treatment should be considered (see Chapter 6). In patients over the age of 50 years a total hip replacement is better.

Osteoarthritis

Secondary osteoarthritis is not uncommon and is due to: (1) cartilage damage at the time of the dislocation; (2) the presence of retained fragments in the joint; or (3) ischaemic necrosis of the femoral head. The options are discussed in Chapter 5.

ANTERIOR DISLOCATION

This is rare compared with posterior dislocation. The leg lies externally rotated, abducted and slightly flexed. Seen from the side, the anterior bulge of the dislocated head is unmistakable.

X-rays

In the anteroposterior view the dislocation is usually obvious, but occasionally the head is almost directly in front of its normal position; any doubt is resolved by a lateral film.

Treatment

The manoeuvres employed are almost identical to those used to reduce a posterior dislocation, except that while the flexed thigh is being pulled upwards, it should be adducted; an assistant then helps by applying lateral traction to the thigh. The subsequent treatment is similar to that employed for posterior dislocation. Avascular necrosis is a recognized complication.

CENTRAL DISLOCATION

A fall on the side, or a blow over the greater trochanter, may force the femoral head medially through the floor of the acetabulum. Although this is called 'central dislocation', it is really a complex fracture of the acetabulum. The condition is dealt with in Chapter 30.

FRACTURE OF THE FEMORAL NECK

The fracture usually results from a fall directly onto the greater trochanter. In younger individuals, the usual cause is a fall from a height or a blow sustained in a road accident; these patients often have multiple injuries and in 20% there is an associated fracture of the femoral shaft. However, this injury is most commonly seen in elderly osteoporotic people; here less force is required – perhaps no more than catching a toe in the carpet and twisting the hip into external rotation.

In Garden's classification, Stage I is an incomplete impacted fracture, Stage II is a complete but undisplaced fracture, Stage III is a complete fracture with moderate displacement and Stage IV is a severely displaced fracture. Left untreated, a comparatively benign-looking Stage I fracture may rapidly disintegrate to Stage IV.

With displaced fractures there is an increased risk of damage to the femoral head blood supply and thus a significant incidence of avascular necrosis.

Special features

There is usually a history of a fall, followed by pain in the hip. If the fracture is displaced, the patient lies with the limb in lateral rotation and the leg looks short.

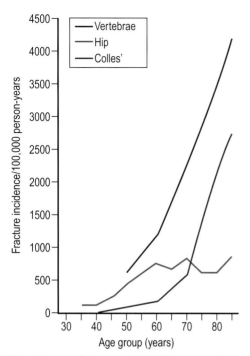

31.2 **Incidence of 'osteoporotic' fractures** The incidence of brittle fractures in women rises sharply from the menopause onwards.

X-rays

Two questions must be answered: is there a fracture, and is it displaced? Usually the break is obvious, but an impacted fracture can be missed by the unwary. Displacement is judged by the abnormal shape of the bone images and the degree of mismatch of the trabecular lines in the femoral head and neck and the innominate (supraacetabular) bone. This assessment is important because impacted or undisplaced fractures do well after internal fixation, whereas displaced fractures have a high rate of non-union and avascular necrosis.

Treatment

Operative treatment is almost mandatory. Displaced fractures will not unite without internal fixation, and in any case elderly people should be got up and kept active without delay if pulmonary complications and bed sores are to be prevented. Impacted fractures can be left to unite, but there is always a risk that they may become displaced, even while lying in bed, so fixation is safer.

When should the operation be performed? In young patients operation is urgent: interruption of the blood supply will produce irreversible cellular changes after 12 hours and the way to prevent this is to obtain accurate reduction and internal fixation as soon as possible. In older patients also the longer the delay the greater is the likelihood of

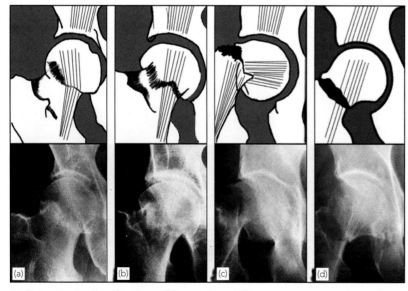

31.3 **Garden's classification of femoral neck fractures** (a) *Stage I*: Impacted fracture, which in some cases may be an incomplete fracture. (b) *Stage II*: Complete but only slightly displaced fracture. The innominate trabeculae are still directly in line with the femoral neck trabeculae. (c) *Stage III*: Partially displaced fracture. The femoral head trabeculae are no longer in line with those of the innominate bone. (d) *Stage IV*: Complete fracture with full displacement; the proximal fragment appears to be normally aligned with the innominate trabeculae, but that is because the completely detached femoral head has resumed its normal position in the acetabulum.

433

complications; however, here speed is tempered by the need for adequate preparation, especially in the very elderly, who are often ill and debilitated.

What if operation is considered too dangerous? Lying in bed on traction may be even more dangerous! And leaving the fracture untreated too painful. The patient least fit for operation may need it most. Prophylaxis against thromboembolism is very important (see page 162).

The principles are accurate reduction, secure fixation and early activity. Under anaesthesia the fracture is manipulated and reduction is checked by x-ray. If it is satisfactory, the fracture is securely fixed with cannulated screws, or with a sliding ('dynamic') compression screw which attaches to the femoral shaft. Impacted fractures can be fixed as they lie.

What if the fracture cannot be accurately reduced? In patients over 60 years old partial or total hip replacement should be seriously considered. In patients under 60 years it is worth trying open reduction rather than sacrificing the joint.

From the first day the patient should sit up in bed or in a chair. Walking with crutches is encouraged as soon as possible.

Fractures in children

If the fracture is undisplaced it can be held in a plaster cast (a hip spica) until it unites. If it is displaced it should be reduced and fixed with screws.

Complications

General complications

There is a high incidence of general complications in these elderly and often frail patients. Thromboembolism, pneumonia and bed sores are constant dangers, not to mention the disorders that might have been present before the fracture.

Avascular necrosis

Necrosis of the femoral head occurs in about 30% of patients with displaced fractures and 10% of those with undisplaced fractures. The reason is simple. The femoral head derives its blood supply from three sources: the nutrient artery, vessels reflected from the capsule, and vessels in the ligamentum teres. When the femoral neck is fractured and severely displaced, the branches from the nutrient artery are severed, the retinacular vessels from the capsule are torn, and the remaining blood supply via the ligamentum teres may be insufficient to prevent ischaemia of the femoral head. The bone dies and eventually collapses. The fracture may still unite but the femoral head becomes distorted and the joint irreversibly damaged.

In patients over 45 years of age, treatment is by total joint replacement. In younger patients re-alignment osteotomy may be suitable for small superomedial necrotic segments. Arthrodesis is still favoured by some surgeons, particularly for patients

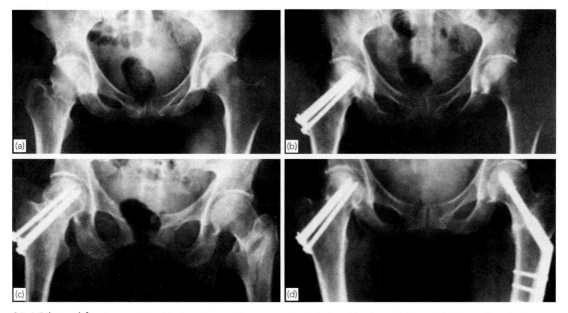

31.4 Bilateral fractures This elderly osteoporotic woman stumbled and fractured (a) her right femoral neck. The fracture was fixed with 3 long screws (b) and it united soundly. Then, a year later, she tripped and sustained an intertrochanteric fracture on the left side (c). This needed more secure fixation – a compression screw and plate fixed to the femoral shaft (d).

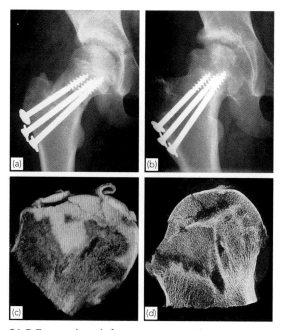

31.5 Femoral neck fracture – avascular necrosis (a) The postreduction x-ray may look splendid but the blood supply is compromised and 6 months later (b) there is obvious necrosis of the femoral head. (c) Section across the excised femoral head, showing the large necrotic segment and splitting of the articular cartilage. (d) Fine detail x-ray of the same.

under 30 years; however, the functional outcome is at best unpredictable and at worst unacceptable.

Non-union

More than one-third of all femoral neck fractures fail to unite, and the risk is particularly high in those that are severely displaced. There are many causes: poor blood supply, imperfect reduction, inadequate fixation, and the tardy healing that is characteristic of intra-articular fractures. The bone at the fracture site is ground away, the fragments fall apart and the nail or screw cuts out of the bone or is extruded laterally. The patient complains of pain, shortening of the limb and difficulty with walking. The x-ray shows the sorry outcome.

Treatment of non-union depends on the age of the patient. In those under 50 years an attempt may be made to secure union by placing a bone graft across the fracture and reinserting a fixation device. In older patients, prosthetic replacement of the femoral head, or total replacement of the joint, must be considered.

Osteoarthritis

Subarticular bone necrosis or femoral head collapse may lead, after several years, to secondary osteoarthritis. If the symptoms warrant it, the joint should be replaced.

INTERTROCHANTERIC FRACTURES

As with femoral neck fractures, these injuries are common in elderly, osteoporotic women. However, in sharp contrast to the intracapsular neck fractures, the extracapsular intertrochanteric fractures usually unite quite easily and seldom cause avascular necrosis.

Intertrochanteric fractures can be classified according to the degree of comminution, and thus the degree of instability (Figure 31.6).

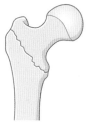
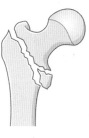
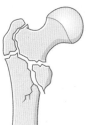
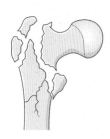

TYPE 1	TYPE 2	TYPE 3	TYPE 4
Undisplaced	Displaced	Displaced	Severely comminuted
Uncomminuted	Slightly comminuted	Greater trochanter fracture	Subtrochanteric extension
	Lesser trochanter fracture	Comminuted	(Also reverse oblique)
	Varus	Varus	

31.6 Intertrochanteric fractures – classification Types 1 to 4 are arranged in increasing degrees of instability and complexity. Types 1 and 2 account for the majority (nearly 60%). Included in Type 4 are the 'reverse oblique' type of intertrochanteric fracture, which is particularly difficult to fix securely.

Clinical features

Following a fall the patient is in pain and unable to stand. The limb is shortened and lies in external rotation.

X-rays

The fracture usually runs diagonally from the greater to the lesser trochanter; it may be comminuted and severely displaced, but in some cases the crack can hardly be seen.

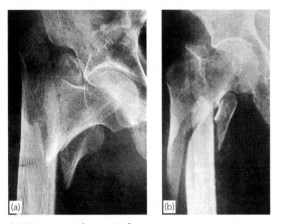

31.7 Intertrochanteric features – x-rays
(a) A typical Type 2 fracture, running obliquely downwards from the lateral to medial cortex; in this case associated with a lesser trochanter fracture and resulting in a varus deformity. (b) Type 4 'reverse oblique' fracture: here the fracture line runs downwards from medial to lateral cortex, to produce an unstable geometry.

Treatment

These fractures are almost always treated by early internal fixation – not because they fail to unite with conservative treatment (they unite quite readily), but (1) to obtain the best possible position and (2) to get the patient up and walking as soon as possible.

The common type of intertrochanteric fracture can be reduced under x-ray control and then fixed with a compression screw and plate. The patient is allowed to weightbear early, using crutches until the fracture has united (8–12 weeks). Severely comminuted and 'reverse' fractures are inherently unstable and require more complex fixation, similar to the devices used for subtrochanteric fractures (see Figure 31.8).

Complications

General

Early complications are the same as with femoral neck fractures, reflecting the fact that most of these patients are in poor health.

Failure of fixation

Screws may cut out of the osteoporotic bone if reduction is poor or if the fixation device is incorrectly positioned; reduction and fixation may have to be re-done.

Malunion

Varus and external rotation deformities are common. Fortunately they are seldom severe and rarely interfere with function.

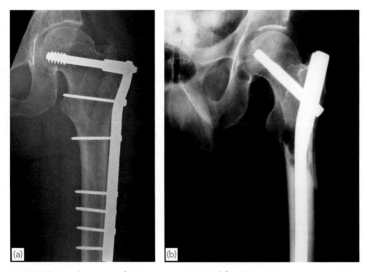

31.8 Subtrochanteric fractures – internal fixation Two methods of fixation are shown here: (a) a 95-degree screw and plate device; and (b) an intramedullary nail with a proximal interlocking screw into the femoral head – in this case for a pathological fracture through a metastatic deposit.

SUBTROCHANTERIC FRACTURES

Subtrochanteric fractures may occur at any age if the injury is severe enough; but most occur with relatively trivial injury, in elderly patients with osteoporosis, osteomalacia, Paget's disease or a secondary deposit. Blood loss is greater than with femoral neck or trochanteric fractures.

The leg lies externally rotated and short, and the thigh is markedly swollen. Movement is excruciatingly painful.

X-ray examination shows that the fracture is through or below the lesser trochanter and is frequently comminuted.

Treatment

Open reduction and internal fixation is the treatment of choice. Intramedullary nails with locking screws into the femoral head or else a compression (dynamic) hip screw and long plate will provide satisfactory fixation.

Postoperatively the patient is allowed partial weightbearing (with crutches) until union is secure.

Complications

Malunion is fairly common and, if marked, may need operative correction.

HIP FRACTURES IN CHILDREN

These comparatively rare injuries are usually due to high-velocity trauma; for example, falling from a height or a car accident. In children under 2 years, the possibility of non-accidental injury should be considered.

In infants the area between the capital epiphysis and greater trochanter is incompletely ossified and unusually vulnerable to trauma. Fractures through the middle and basal parts of the femoral neck are the most common. Between the ages of 4 and 8 years the ligamentum teres contributes very little to the blood supply of the epiphysis; hence its susceptibility to post-traumatic ischaemia and avascular necrosis.

Clinical features

Diagnosis can be difficult, especially in infants where the epiphysis is not easily defined on x-ray. Ultrasonography, magnetic resonance imaging (MRI) and arthrography may help. In older children the diagnosis is usually obvious on plain x-ray examination.

It is important to establish whether the fracture is displaced or undisplaced; the former carries a much higher risk of complications.

Treatment

These fractures should be treated as a matter of urgency, and certainly within 24 hours of injury. Initially the hip is supported or splinted while investigations are carried out. Early aspiration of the intracapsular haematoma is advocated by some authors as a means of reducing the risk of epiphyseal ischaemia.

Undisplaced fractures may be treated by immobilization in a plaster spica for 6–8 weeks. However, fracture position is not always maintained and there is a considerable risk of late displacement and malunion or non-union.

Displaced intertrochanteric fractures also can be treated non-operatively: closed reduction, traction and spica immobilization. Careful follow-up is essential; if position is lost, operative fixation will be needed.

Fractures through the physis or femoral neck are treated by closed reduction (one gentle manipulation) and then internal fixation with smooth pins or cannulated screws. If this fails, open reduction is performed. In small children, operative fixation is supplemented by a spica cast for 6–12 weeks.

Complications

Avascular necrosis of the femoral head

This is the most common (and most feared) complication. It occurs in about 30% of all cases; important risk factors are: (1) an age of more than 10 years; (2) high-velocity injury; (3) a fracture through the proximal part of the femoral neck; and (4) fracture displacement.

The child complains of pain and loss of movement; x-ray changes usually appear within 3 months of injury.

Treatment is problematic; most end up with pain and restriction of movement, sometimes calling for reconstructive surgery. Arthrodesis may be considered as a late salvage procedure.

Coxa vara

Femoral neck deformity may result from malunion, avascular necrosis or premature physeal closure. If the deformity is mild, re-modelling may occur. If the neck–shaft angle is less than 110 degrees, subtrochanteric valgus osteotomy will probably be needed.

Diminished growth

Physeal damage may result in retarded femoral growth. Limb length equalization may be needed.

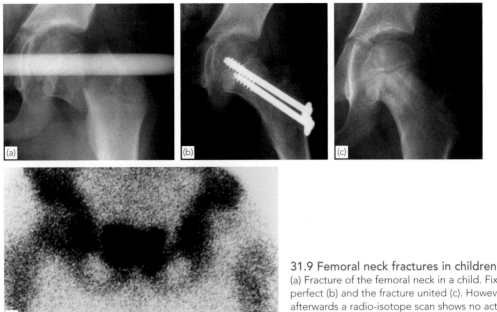

31.9 Femoral neck fractures in children
(a) Fracture of the femoral neck in a child. Fixation was perfect (b) and the fracture united (c). However, soon afterwards a radio-isotope scan shows no activity in the left femoral head (d), i.e. ischaemic necrosis.

FEMORAL SHAFT FRACTURES

The femoral shaft is well padded with muscles – an advantage in protecting the bone from all but the most powerful forces, but a disadvantage in that fractures are often severely displaced by muscle pull, making reduction difficult.

Special features

This is essentially a fracture of young adults and usually results from a high-energy injury. Diaphyseal fractures in elderly patients should be considered 'pathological' until proved otherwise. In children under 4 years of age the possibility of physical abuse must be kept in mind.

X-rays

Most fractures of the femoral shaft have some degree of comminution, although it is not always apparent on x-ray; it is a reflection of the amount of force involved in these injuries. Displacement may be in any direction. Sometimes there are two fracture lines separated by an unbroken length of bone – the 'segmental fracture'. *The pelvis and knee must always be x-rayed to avoid missing an associated injury.*

Treatment

The risk of systemic complications in these high-energy injuries can be significantly reduced by early stabilization of the fracture. Traction can reduce and

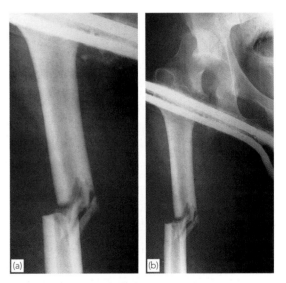

31.10 Femoral shaft fractures – a diagnostic trap (a) Note that the upper fragment is adducted, suggesting that the hip also may be affected. (b) Always x-ray the pelvis; in this case the hip was dislocated.

hold most fractures in reasonable alignment and certainly the patient should be transported from the scene of the accident with the limb splinted – many emergency splints incorporate a facility to apply traction as well. Definitive treatment will depend on the type of fracture and patient.

Traction and bracing

The main indications for traction are: (1) fractures in children; (2) contraindications to anaesthesia; and (3) lack of suitable skill or facilities for internal fixation. It is a poor choice for elderly patients, for pathological fractures and for those with multiple injuries. The chief drawback is the length of time spent in bed (10–14 weeks for adults) with its attendant problems. Some of these difficulties are overcome by reducing the time in traction and then changing to a plaster spica or – in the case of lower-third fractures – functional bracing; this is applicable once the fracture is 'sticky', usually around 6–8 weeks.

While the patient is in traction, joint mobility must be preserved by encouraging movement and exercises. The position of the fragments should be checked repeatedly by x-ray and the system adjusted if necessary.

Open reduction and plating

Fixation with plates and screws was popular at one time but it went out of favour because of the high complication rate, including implant failure. The main indications today are (1) the combination of shaft and femoral neck fractures and (2) a shaft fracture with an associated vascular injury.

Intramedullary nailing

Intramedullary nailing is the method of choice for most femoral shaft fractures. The basic implant system consists of an intramedullary nail (in a range of sizes) which is perforated near each end so that locking screws can be inserted transversely at the proximal and distal ends; this controls rotation and ensures stability even for subtrochanteric and distal-third fractures.

External fixation

The main indications for external fixation are: (1) the treatment of severe open injuries; (2) management of patients with multiple injuries (damage control orthopaedics); and (3) dealing with severe bone loss by the technique of 'bone transport' (see Chapter 12). External fixation is also useful for (4) treating femoral fractures in adolescents.

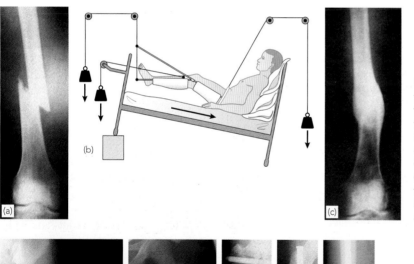

31.11 Femoral shaft fracture – conservative treatment Conservative treatment is sometimes the best option, though it does call for a long period in bed. (a) Fracture of the femur. (b) Balanced skeletal traction. (c) The fracture has healed in excellent alignment.

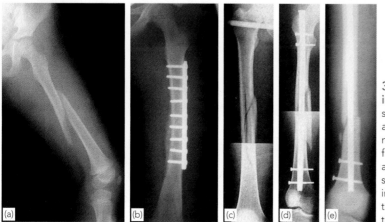

31.12 Femoral shaft fractures – internal fixation (a) Unstable shaft fractures in children and adolescents, especially those with multiple injuries, can be securely fixed (b) with a plate and screws. In adults, shaft fractures are usually stabilized with a locked intramedullary nail (c,d); this treatment is suitable even for distal-third fractures (e).

Complications

General

Complications such as blood loss, shock, fat embolism and acute respiratory distress are common in high-energy injuries such as this. These conditions are dealt with in Chapter 22.

Vascular injury

The vascular lesion takes priority and the vessel must be repaired or grafted without delay. At the same operation the fracture is secured by internal fixation.

Thromboembolism

Prolonged traction in bed predisposes to thrombosis. Movement and exercise are important in preventing this; they can be supplemented by foot compression devices or prophylactic doses of anticoagulants. Constant vigilance is needed and full anticoagulant treatment is started immediately if thigh vein or pelvic vein thrombosis is diagnosed.

Infection

In open injuries, and following internal fixation, there is always a risk of infection. Prophylactic antibiotics, and careful attention to the principles of fracture surgery, should keep the incidence below 2%.

Delayed union and non-union

A fractured femur may take 3–6 months to unite. If union is delayed beyond this time, an exchange nailing is performed using a slightly larger nail; in addition the fracture may need bone grafting.

Malunion

Fractures treated by traction and bracing often develop some deformity; no more than 15 degrees of angulation should be accepted.

Until the x-ray shows solid union, the fracture is too insecure to permit weightbearing; the bone will bend and what previously seemed a satisfactory reduction may end up with lateral or anterior bowing. Shortening is seldom a major problem; if it occurs, and is not too marked, the shoe can be built up.

Joint stiffness

It is surprising how often the knee is affected after a femoral shaft fracture. The joint may be injured at the same time, or it stiffens due to soft-tissue adhesions during treatment; hence the importance of exercise and knee movements.

OPEN FRACTURES

Open femoral fractures should be carefully assessed for: (1) skin loss; (2) wound contamination; (3) muscle ischaemia; and (4) injury to vessels and nerves.

The immediate treatment is similar to that of closed fractures. Antibiotics are started and wound cleansing and debridement are carried out with as little delay as possible. The major decision then is how to stabilize the fracture. With small, clean wounds and little delay from the time of injury, the fracture can be treated as for a closed injury, with the addition of prophylactic antibiotics. With large wounds, contaminated wounds, skin loss or tissue destruction, internal fixation should be avoided initially; after debridement the wound should be left open and the fracture stabilized by applying an external fixator.

FEMORAL FRACTURES IN CHILDREN

Infants need no more than 1 or 2 weeks in balanced traction followed by a spica for another 3 or 4 weeks.

Children up to 6 years can be treated in a similar manner.

Teenagers may require even longer in traction before changing to a spica. However, if satisfactory reduction cannot be obtained or held, internal fixation with a plate and screws or intramedullary nails is justified – especially in those with multiple injuries.

SUPRACONDYLAR FRACTURES OF THE FEMUR

Supracondylar fractures of the femur are seen (a) in young adults, usually as a result of high-energy trauma, and (b) in elderly, osteoporotic individuals. Direct trauma is the usual cause. The fracture line is just above the condyles, but it may branch off distally between them. The pull of the gastrocnemius attachments may tilt the distal fragment backwards.

Special features

The knee is swollen and deformed; movement is too painful to be attempted. The tibial pulses should always be palpated.

X-rays

The fracture is just above the femoral condyles and is transverse or comminuted. The distal fragment is often tilted backwards. The entire femur must be x-rayed so as not to miss a proximal fracture or dislocated hip.

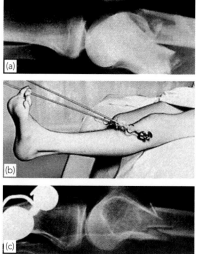

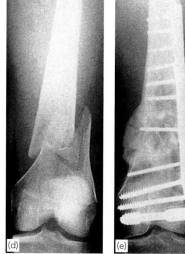

31.13 Supracondylar fractures (a,b,c) These fractures were, for many years, treated successfully by traction through the upper tibia. (d,e) If the bone is not too osteoporotic, internal fixation with a dynamic condylar screw and plate is a good alternative.

Treatment

If the fracture is only slightly displaced and extra-articular, or if it reduces easily with the knee in flexion, it can be treated quite satisfactorily by skeletal traction through the proximal tibia; the limb is cradled on a Thomas' splint with a knee flexion piece, and movements are encouraged. If the distal fragment is displaced by gastrocnemius pull, a second pin above the knee, and vertical traction, will correct this. At 4–6 weeks, when the fracture is beginning to unite, traction can be replaced by a cast-brace and the patient allowed up and partially weightbearing with crutches. Non-operative treatment is most likely to be considered if the patient is young and has not suffered multiple injuries.

If closed reduction fails, open reduction and internal fixation with fixed angle and locked plates, though difficult, may be successful. This does not necessarily lead to earlier mobilization because the bone is often osteoporotic and the patient may be old and frail, but nursing in bed is easier and knee movements can be started sooner. Unprotected weightbearing is not permitted until the fracture has consolidated (usually around 12 weeks).

Locked intramedullary nails which are introduced retrograde through the intercondylar notch are also used for these fractures. They provide adequate stability, even in the presence of osteoporotic bone, but unprotected weightbearing is best avoided until union is assured.

Complications

Joint stiffness

Knee stiffness is almost inevitable. A long period of exercise is necessary but full movement is rarely regained.

Non-union

Knee stiffness increases the likelihood of non-union. This combination is difficult to treat and, unless great care is exercised, the ultimate range of movement at the knee may be less than that at the fracture.

Osteoarthritis

Supracondylar fractures often extend into the joint surface; anatomical restoration by accurate reduction is necessary to reduce the risk of this late complication.

CONDYLAR FRACTURES

One or both femoral condyles may be fractured. The knee is swollen and has the doughy feel of a haemarthrosis.

X-rays

One condyle may be fractured and shifted upwards; occasionally the condyles are split apart and there may be a supracondylar fracture, too.

Treatment

The haemarthrosis must be aspirated as soon as possible. Because the articular surface is involved, accurate reduction is important. Open reduction and internal fixation are therefore often employed (Figure 31.14).

An intra-articular multifragmentary condylar fracture in osteoporotic bone poses the most difficult challenge; there may be no alternative to performing a hinged joint replacement.

441

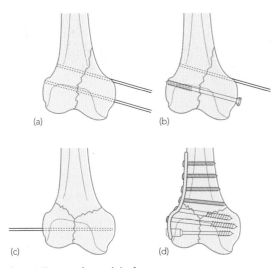

(a)   (b)

(c)   (d)

31.14 Femoral condyle fractures (a) A single condylar fracture can be reduced open and held with Kirschner wires preparatory to (b) inserting compression screws. (c,d) More complex fractures are best fixed with a dynamic condylar screw and plate.

Complications

Stiffness of the knee

This is a common complication. It usually responds to prolonged physiotherapy, although movement may not be fully restored.

Osteoarthritis

As with other intra-articular fractures, secondary osteoarthritis is a late complication.

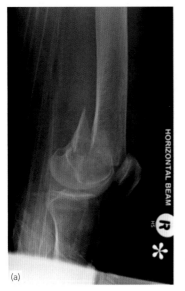

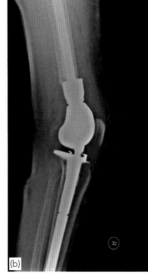

(a)   (b)

31.15 Fragmented condylar fractures (a) A displaced, multifragmentary, intra-articular fracture in an elderly patient may be difficult to stabilize surgically. (b) These fractures can be treated by a segmental knee replacement, allowing early, full weightbearing mobilization.

CHAPTER 32

INJURIES OF THE KNEE AND LEG

TIBIAL PLATEAU FRACTURES

Fractures of the tibial plateau are caused by strong bending forces combined with axial loads, e.g. a car striking a pedestrian on the side of the knee (hence the term 'bumper fracture') or a fall from a height in which the knee is forced into valgus or varus. One or both tibial condyles are crushed or split by the opposing femoral condyle.

Special features

The patient is nearly always an adult. The joint is swollen and has the doughy feel of a haemarthrosis. There is diffuse tenderness on the side of the fracture, and also on the opposite side if a ligament is injured. Severe fractures can be associated with major vascular injury and in fact may represent a knee dislocation that has reduced.

X-rays

Multiple views (and often computed tomography [CT] scans) are needed to show the true extent of the fracture. Several classifications have been proposed. The one used here is based on Schatzker's classification.

Treatment

These fractures all involve the articular surface of the tibia. The guiding principle in their management is straightforward: function is more important than an anatomical reduction. Traction alone often produces a well-functioning knee, though there may be some residual deformity.

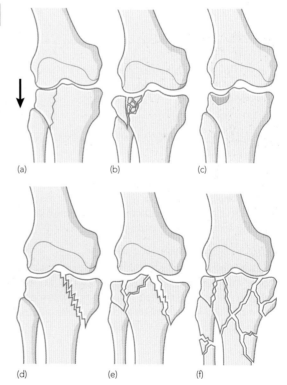

32.1 Tibial plateau fractures (a) Type 1 – simple split of the lateral condyle. (b) Type 2 – a split of the lateral condyle with a more central area of depression. (c) Type 3 – depression of the lateral condyle with an intact rim. (d) Type 4 – a fracture of the medial condyle. (e) Type 5 – fractures of both condyles, but with the central portion of the metaphysis still connected to the tibial shaft. (f) Type 6 – combined condylar and subcondylar fractures.

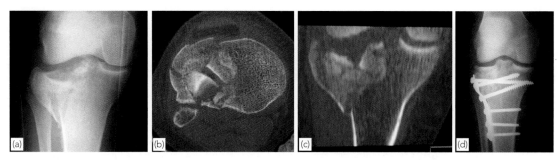

32.2 Tibial plateau fractures – imaging (a) X-rays provide information about the position of the main fracture lines and areas of articular surface depression. (b,c) CT reconstructions reveal the extent and direction of displacements. (d) Postoperative x-ray showing perfect fixation with a buttress plate and screws.

On the other hand, obsessional surgery to restore a shattered surface can produce a good x-ray appearance – and a stiff knee.

Undisplaced and minimally displaced fractures of the lateral condyle

These can be treated conservatively. The haemarthrosis is aspirated if the skin is threatened and a compression bandage is applied. Knee movements are begun and, as soon as the acute pain and swelling have subsided (usually within 1 week), a hinged cast-brace is fitted; however, weightbearing is not allowed for another 3 weeks. The fracture usually heals by 8–9 weeks. If there is any doubt about the degree of displacement, open reduction and internal fixation with a lag screw would be safer.

Markedly displaced and/or comminuted fractures of the lateral condyle

These should be treated by open reduction and internal fixation. The condylar surface is examined and depressed areas elevated; bone grafts may be needed to support the reduction. Fixation is usually with lag screws and a buttress plate.

Fractures of the medial condyle

Fractures of the medial tibial condyle are usually more complex than they appear to be at first sight. They are best treated by open reduction and fixation with a buttress plate and screws. Associated lateral ligament damage will need repair.

Bicondylar fractures

These fractures are usually high-energy injuries and do best if reduced and stabilized surgically. Internal fixation with plates and screws is possible, but operative technique needs to be meticulous if wound breakdown problems are to be avoided. A combination of screw fixation and circular external fixation offers satisfactory stabilization with a lower risk of wound complications. *Beware the development of a compartment syndrome.*

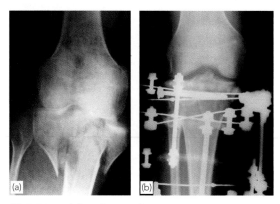

32.3 Bicondylar plateau fractures (a) These injuries are difficult to manage and carry a high risk of soft-tissue complications. If the facilities and expertise are available, they can be treated by a combination of internal and external fixation (b); otherwise non-operative treatment by traction and mobilization may be the better choice.

Osteoporotic condylar fractures

Elderly individuals with osteoporotic fractures can be treated along the same lines as above. However, if the fracture pattern permits, a total knee replacement (using revision surgery components) may offer a more appropriate solution.

Complications

Compartment syndrome

With severe condylar fractures there is a significant risk of developing a compartment syndrome. The leg and foot should be examined repeatedly for suggestive signs (see page 353).

Joint stiffness

Failure to regain full knee bend is an important cause of disability, and is minimized by starting movements early.

Deformity

Some residual valgus or varus deformity is quite common but can be compatible with good function, although constant overloading of one compartment may predispose to osteoarthritis in later life.

Osteoarthritis

If, at the end of treatment, there is marked depression of the plateau, deformity of the knee or ligamentous instability, secondary osteoarthritis is likely to develop after 5–10 years. This may eventually require reconstructive surgery.

FRACTURED PATELLA

Three types of fracture are seen: (1) an undisplaced fracture across the patella, which is probably due to a direct blow; (2) a comminuted or 'stellate' fracture, due to a fall or a direct blow on the front of the knee; and (3) a transverse fracture with a gap between the fragments – this is an indirect traction injury due to forced, passive flexion of the knee while the quadriceps muscle is contracted; the entire extensor mechanism is torn across and active knee extension is impossible.

Special features

The knee is painful and swollen; sometimes the gap can be felt. Usually there is blood in the joint. It is helpful to establish whether the patient can actively extend the knee, as this will influence the choice of treatment.

X-rays

The three types of fracture are usually clearly distinguishable, but it is important not to confuse a fracture with a congenital bipartite patella in which a smooth line extends obliquely across the superolateral angle of the bone.

Treatment

The key to the management of patellar fractures is the state of the extensor mechanism.

Undisplaced or minimally displaced crack

If there is a haemarthrosis threatening the skin, it is aspirated. The extensor mechanism is intact and treatment is mainly protective. A plaster cylinder holding the knee straight is worn for 4–6 weeks and during this time quadriceps exercises are practised every day.

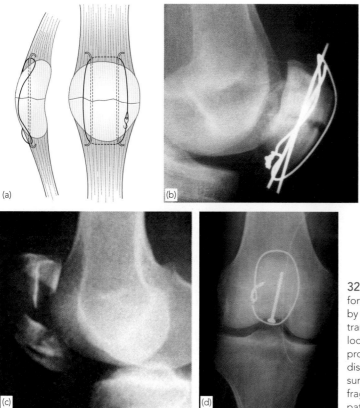

32.4 Fractured patella (a,b) Straight-forward transverse fractures can be treated by *tension-band wiring*: the fragments are transfixed with K-wires and tightened by looping a malleable wire around the protruding ends of the K-wires. (c) For displaced comminuted fractures some surgeons would preserve as many useful fragments as possible (d), but often total patellectomy is preferable.

445

Comminuted (stellate) fracture

The extensor expansions are intact and the patient may be able to lift the leg. However, the undersurface of the patella is irregular and there is a serious risk of damage to the patellofemoral joint. All attempts should be made to preserve the patella. A partial patellectomy might be required, with the fragments held by a circlage wire. After an initial period in a back-slab, a hinged brace can be applied in order to mould the fragments into position and to preserve mobility. Once healed and if symptomatic, in an otherwise well-preserved knee the patella may be resurfaced.

Displaced transverse fracture

The lateral expansions are torn and the entire extensor mechanism is disrupted. Operation is essential; the fragments are held apposed by internal fixation (using the tension band principle) and the extensor expansions are repaired. A brace is worn until active extension of the knee is regained, but flexion and extension exercises are practised each day.

DISLOCATION OF THE PATELLA

Because the knee is normally angled in slight valgus, there is a natural tendency for the patella to pull towards the lateral side when the quadriceps muscle contracts. Traumatic dislocation is due to sudden, severe contraction of the quadriceps muscle while the knee is stretched in valgus and external rotation. Typically this occurs in field sports when a runner dodges to one side. The patella dislocates laterally and the medial retinacular fibres (part of the quadriceps expansion) may be torn along with the medial patellofemoral ligament (MPFL).

Clinical features

In a 'first-time' dislocation, the patient may experience a tearing sensation and a feeling that the knee has gone 'out of joint'; when running, he or she may collapse and fall to the ground. Often the

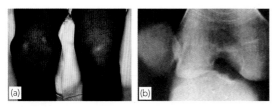

32.5 Dislocation of the patella (a) The right patella has dislocated laterally, giving a broad, flattened appearance to the knee. (b) X-ray showing the patella displaced to the lateral side.

patella springs back into position spontaneously; however, if it remains unreduced, there is an obvious (if somewhat misleading) deformity: the displaced patella, seated on the lateral side of the knee, is not easily noticed but the uncovered medial femoral condyle is unduly prominent and may be mistaken for the patella; neither active nor passive movement is possible.

X-rays

In an unreduced dislocation, the patella is seen to be laterally displaced and tilted or rotated. In 5% of cases there is an associated osteochondral fracture.

Treatment

The patella is easily pushed back into place, and anaesthesia is not always necessary. Early repair of the MPFL has not conclusively been shown to be an advantage.

With the knee straight, a plaster back-slab is applied. It is worn for 2 weeks. When the back-slab has been removed, flexion is easily regained with physiotherapy. A patella-holding brace may be of use for a further 4 weeks after the plaster has been removed.

Recurrent dislocation

Patients treated non-operatively for a first-time dislocation have a 15–20% chance of suffering further dislocations. Predisposing factors are generalized joint laxity, marked genu valgum and an unduly high patella (see page 282).

ACUTE KNEE LIGAMENT INJURIES

The bony structure of the knee joint is inherently unstable; were it not for the strong capsule, intra-articular and extra-articular ligaments and controlling muscles, the knee would not be able to function effectively as a mechanism for support, balance and thrust.

Valgus stresses are resisted by the fascia lata, pes anserinus, superficial and deep layers of the medial collateral ligament (MCL) and the tough posteromedial part of the capsule. The main checks to varus angulation are the iliotibial tract and the lateral collateral ligament (LCL). The anterior and posterior cruciate ligaments (ACL and PCL) provide both anteroposterior and rotary stability; they also help to resist excessive valgus and varus angulation.

Injuries of the knee ligaments are common, particularly in sporting pursuits but also in road accidents, where they may be associated with fractures or dislocations. They vary in severity from a simple sprain to complete rupture. It is important to recognize that these injuries are seldom 'unidirectional'; they often involve more than one structure and it is therefore useful to refer to them in functional terms (e.g. anteromedial instability) as well as anatomical terms (e.g. torn MCL and ACL).

Clinical features

The patient gives a history of a twisting or wrenching injury and may even claim to have heard a 'pop' as the tissues snapped. The knee is painful and, in contrast to the story in meniscal injury, swelling appears almost immediately. Tenderness is most acute over the torn ligament, and stressing one or other side of the joint may produce excruciating pain.

Tests for ligamentous stability can be performed if pain allows (see Chapter 20). Partial tears permit no abnormal movement, but the attempt always causes pain. Complete tears permit abnormal movement, which sometimes causes surprisingly little pain.

Sideways tilting (varus/valgus) is examined, first with the knee at 30 degrees of flexion and then with the knee straight. Movement is compared with the normal side. If the knee angulates only in slight flexion, there is probably an isolated tear of the collateral ligaments; if it angulates in full extension, there is almost certainly rupture of the capsule and cruciate ligaments as well as the collateral ligament.

Anteroposterior stability is assessed first by placing the knees at 90 degrees with the feet resting on the couch and looking from the side for posterior sag of the proximal tibia; when present, this is a reliable sign of PCL instability. The *Lachman test* is a reliable way of showing up ACL instability; anteroposterior glide is tested with the knee flexed 15–20 degrees.

X-rays

Stress x-rays of the knee may provide visual evidence of instability. Plain x-rays may show that the ligament has avulsed a small piece of bone – the MCL usually from the femur, the LCL from the fibula, the ACL from the tibial spine and the PCL from the back of the upper tibia. Another sign is an avulsion fracture off the edge of the lateral tibial condyle (the so-called Segond fracture), indicating an ACL injury.

A magnetic resonance imaging (MRI) scan is usually requested. This is especially good at identifying ligament injuries. It can also highlight areas of bone bruising.

Treatment

Sprains and partial tears

The intact fibres splint the torn ones and spontaneous healing will occur. The hazard is adhesions, so active exercise is prescribed from the start. Aspirating the haemarthrosis may help ease the pain and is necessary if the skin is threatened. However, strict aseptic conditions must be ensured. Applying ice-packs intermittently also helps relieves pain. Weightbearing is allowed, but the knee is protected from rotation or angulation strains by a heavily padded bandage or a functional brace. A complete plaster cast is unnecessary and disadvantageous, as it inhibits movement.

Complete tears

Isolated tears of the MCL or the LCL can be treated as above.

Isolated tears of the ACL may be treated by early operative reconstruction if the individual is a professional sportsman, though there is still debate around this issue. Importantly, the knee must be able to go through a full range of motion prior to reconstruction of the ACL. In all other cases, it is more prudent to follow the conservative regimen described above; the cast-brace is worn only until symptoms subside, and thereafter movement and muscle-strengthening exercises are encouraged. A significant proportion of patients regain sufficiently good function not to need further treatment. The remainder complain of varying degrees of instability; late assessment will identify those who are likely to benefit from ligament reconstruction. The menisci

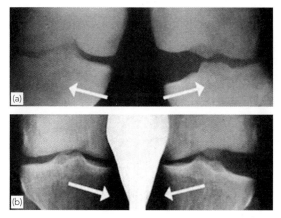

32.6 Ligament injuries Stress x-rays of two different patients showing (a) complete tear of the medial ligament of the left knee and (b) complete tear of the lateral ligament.

remain at risk of damage with an ACL deficient knee.

Isolated tears of the PCL are usually treated conservatively.

Avulsion fractures of the tibial intercondylar eminence

Sometimes a severe strain in the younger patient, instead of rupturing a cruciate ligament, results in an avulsion fracture at the insertion of the ligament. The fragment may be only partially displaced and difficult to detect on x-ray. If the fragment can be manipulated back into position *and allows full extension of the knee*, immobilization in a plaster cylinder for 6 weeks will suffice. If the fragment cannot be reduced, or if there is a block to full extension, operative reduction and fixation with strong sutures (or with small screws if the physis has closed) will be needed. Full movement is usually regained within 3 months.

Combined injuries

With combined ACL and collateral ligament injury, it is wiser to start treatment with joint bracing and physiotherapy in order to restore a good range of movement before following on with ACL reconstruction. The collateral ligament does not usually need reconstruction. A similar approach is adopted for combined injuries involving the PCL, but here all damaged structures will need to be repaired.

Complications

Adhesions

If the knee with a partial ligament tear is not actively exercised, torn fibres stick to intact fibres and to bone. The knee 'gives way' with catches of pain; localized tenderness is present, and pain occurs on medial or lateral rotation. The obvious confusion with a torn meniscus can be resolved by repeating an MRI.

Instability

The knee may continue to give way. The instability tends to get worse and ultimately predisposes to osteoarthritis (OA). Reconstruction before the onset of cartilage degeneration is wise. If OA is already present, ACL reconstruction may mean that the patient will have to accept more pain from their degenerative disease in return for gaining stability. This has to be discussed with the patient before deciding on the best form of treatment.

DISLOCATION OF THE KNEE

The knee can be dislocated only by considerable violence, as in a road accident. The cruciate ligaments and one or both collateral ligaments are torn.

Clinical features

There is severe bruising, swelling and gross deformity. The circulation in the foot must be examined because the popliteal artery may be torn or obstructed. Distal sensation and movement should be tested to exclude nerve injury.

X-rays

In addition to the dislocation, the films occasionally reveal a fracture of the tibial spine due to ligament avulsion. If there is any doubt about the circulation, an arteriogram should be obtained.

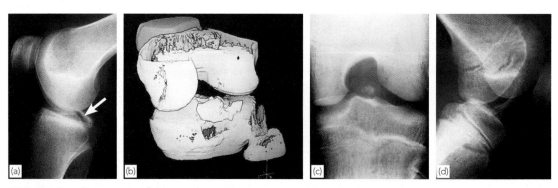

32.7 Cruciate ligament avulsion (a) X-ray showing an avulsion fracture at the insertion of the posterior cruciate ligament. (b) Three-dimensional CT reconstruction, demonstrating the avulsed fragment and its bed. (c,d) Avulsion of the anterior cruciate ligament. In adolescence the avulsed tibial spine seems smaller on x-ray than is actually the case because it is covered by thick articular cartilage.

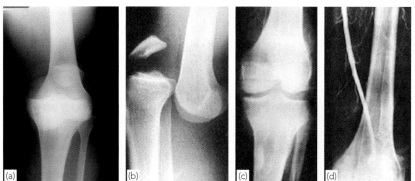

32.8 Dislocation of the knee (a,b) This patient was admitted with a dislocated knee. After reduction (c) the x-ray looked satisfactory, but the circulation did not. (d) An arteriogram showed vascular cut-off just above the knee.

Treatment

Reduction under anaesthesia is urgent. If reduction is achieved, the limb is rested on a back-slab with the knee in 15 degrees of flexion; the circulation is checked repeatedly during the next week. Because of swelling, a plaster cylinder is dangerous. If the joint is unstable, an anterior external fixator can be applied. If there is an open wound, or vascular damage which needs operation, the opportunity is taken to repair the ligaments and capsule. Otherwise, these structures are left undisturbed.

When swelling has subsided, a cast is applied. Quadriceps muscle exercises are practised from the start. Weightbearing in the plaster is permitted as soon as the patient can lift the leg. Knee movements are regained when the plaster is removed.

FRACTURES OF THE TIBIA AND FIBULA

A twisting force causes a spiral fracture of both leg bones at different levels; an angulatory force produces short oblique fractures, usually with a separate triangular 'butterfly' fragment.

Because of its subcutaneous position, the tibia is more commonly fractured, and more commonly sustains an open fracture, than any other long bone. A direct injury may crush or split the skin over the fracture; this is a high-energy fracture and is often from a motorcycle accident. Indirect injuries are low energy; with a spiral or oblique fracture, one of the bone fragments may pierce the skin from within.

Clinical features

The limb should be carefully examined for bruising, severe swelling, crushing or tenting of the skin, an open wound, weak or absent pulses, diminution or loss of sensation and inability to move the toes.

Always be on the alert for signs of an impending compartment syndrome.

X-rays

The entire length of the tibia and fibula, as well as the knee and ankle joints, must be seen.

Management

The main objectives are:

- To limit soft-tissue damage and preserve skin cover.
- To obtain and hold fracture alignment.
- To recognize a compartment syndrome.
- To start early weightbearing (loading promotes healing).
- To start joint movements as soon as possible.

Treatment of low-energy fractures

If the fracture is undisplaced or minimally displaced, a full-length cast from upper thigh to metatarsal necks is applied with the knee slightly flexed and the ankle at a right angle. The pattern of fracture must be such as to permit weightbearing through the cast; i.e. the fracture must be axially stable.

A displaced fracture needs reduction under general anaesthesia with x-ray control before cast application. The limb is elevated and the patient is kept under observation for 48–72 hours. If there is excessive swelling, the cast is split. Patients are usually allowed up (and home) on the second or third day, bearing minimal weight with the aid of crutches. After 2 weeks, the position is checked by x-ray. With stable fractures, the full-length cast may be changed after 4–6 weeks to a functional below-knee cast or brace which is carefully moulded to bear upon the upper tibia and patellar tendon. This liberates the knee and allows full weightbearing. The cast (or brace) is retained until the fracture

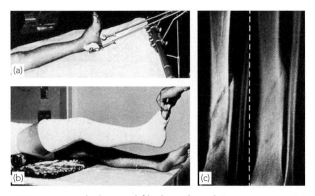

32.9 Fractured tibia and fibula – closed treatment (a) Skeletal traction is used to reduce any overlap, and also as a provisional treatment when skin viability is doubtful. (b) After 10–14 days, a long-leg plaster cast is applied. This method is generally more suited to low-energy fractures where the initial displacement is slight and the soft tissues are well preserved. (c) X-rays showing the position before and after fracture union.

unites, which is around 8 weeks in children but seldom under 16 weeks in adults.

Indications for skeletal fixation

In hospitals where experience and facilities for operative skeletal fixation are lacking, non-operative treatment is not only feasible but positively desirable. It allows for a shorter period of hospitalization, but follow-up is more frequent and prolonged. Where appropriate skills and facilities are available, tibial shaft fractures can be surgically fixed. Indeed, many surgeons would hold that unstable fractures, even of low-energy type, are better treated by skeletal fixation from the outset.

- *Locked intramedullary nailing*: this is the method of choice for diaphyseal (shaft) fractures. Union can be expected in more than 95% of cases. However, the method is less suitable for fractures near the bone ends.
- *Plate fixation*: plating is best for metaphyseal fractures that are unsuitable for nailing. It is also sometimes used for unstable low-energy shaft fractures in children.
- *External fixation*: this is an alternative to closed nailing, but postoperative monitoring is demanding. It can be applied for metaphyseal and shaft fractures.

Treatment of high-energy fractures

Initially, the most important consideration is the viability of the damaged soft tissues and underlying bone. Tissues around the fracture should be disturbed as little as possible, and open operations should be avoided unless there is already an open wound. The risk of compartment syndrome prevails in the first 48 hours.

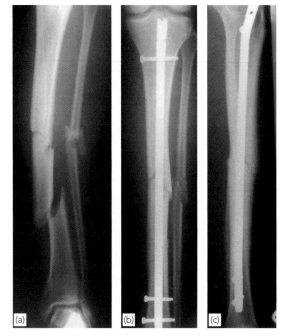

32.10 Fractured tibia and fibula – internal fixation Closed intramedullary nailing for unstable tibial fractures. (a) Position on admission to hospital. (b,c) Anteroposterior and lateral views after intramedullary nailing. Active movements and partial weightbearing were started soon after operation.

In keeping with the principle of inflicting as little surgical damage as possible to a limb that is already badly injured, external fixation offers several advantages as the method of choice for stabilization. Intramedullary nailing is an alternative, but may be difficult.

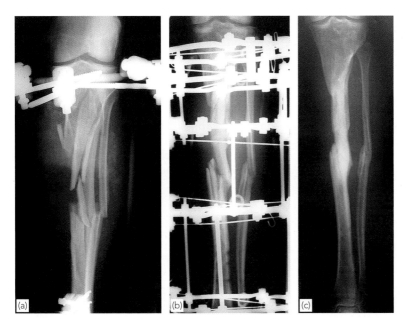

32.11 Fixation (a,b) Severely comminuted fractures treated by external fixation. This offers the benefit of multi-level stability and can be carried out with little additional damage to the soft tissues around the injury. (c) X-ray 6 months later, showing fracture union in a satisfactory position.

Treatment of open fractures

There is a risk of deep infection and chronic osteomyelitis. Gustilo and Anderson's method is popular for classifying these injuries (see page 348).

A suitable regimen for the treatment of open tibial fractures comprises:

- Antibiotics.
- Debridement.
- Stabilization.
- Soft-tissue cover.
- Rehabilitation.

Antibiotics are started immediately and are continued for a full therapeutic course, which is 3 days. A broad-spectrum cephalosporin with an aminoglycoside, such as gentamicin, are used together to cover Gram-positive and Gram-negative bacteria as these are the most likely causes of infection after open fractures. Metronidazole should be added if soil contamination has occurred.

Full wound assessment is done in the operating theatre and not the emergency department. Ideally, the debridement should be carried out with a plastic surgeon so that wound extensions do not compromise the raising of skin flaps for bone cover. Repeat debridement may be necessary, but exposed bone should preferably be covered within 5 days of the injury. Fracture stabilization may be achieved by several methods depending on the energy of injury; external fixation is favoured for the more severe ones.

Complications

Vascular injury

Fractures of the proximal half of the tibia may damage the popliteal artery. This is an emergency of the first order, requiring angiograms, exploration and repair.

Compartment syndrome

Tibial fractures – both open and closed – and intramedullary nailing are the commonest causes of compartment syndrome in the leg. Heightened awareness is all! Early warning symptoms are increasing pain and a feeling of tightness or 'bursting' in the leg. Numbness in the leg or foot, and absent pulses are worrying late signs. The diagnosis can be confirmed by measuring the compartment pressures in the leg and may be the only means of assessment in patients with reduced consciousness or those who are intubated. However, strong clinical suspicion must over-ride any numerical figure obtained by the pressure monitoring. Once the diagnosis is made, decompression by open fasciotomy should be carried out with the minimum delay (see page 354).

Infection

Open fractures are always at risk; even a small perforation should be treated with respect, and debridement carried out before the wound is closed.

451

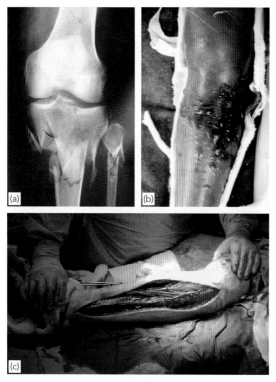

32.12 Compartment syndrome (a) Fractures at this level carry a high risk of causing a compartment syndrome. This patient was initially treated in plaster but he developed intense pain, swelling and blistering (b). Tibial compartment decompression (c) requires two incisions, one medial and one lateral, to reach all compartments in the leg.

With established infection, skeletal fixation should not be abandoned if the system is stable; infection control and fracture union are more likely if fixation is secure. However, if there is a loose implant, it should be removed and replaced by external fixation. Intractable infections also are unlikely to subside unless the implant is replaced by external fixation.

Malunion

Slight shortening (up to 1.5 cm) is usually of little consequence, but angulation should be prevented at all stages. The normal ankle compensates more readily for a valgus deformity than for a varus one; however, anything more than 7 degrees in either plane is unacceptable. Malunion nearer the ends of the tibia is more likely to lead to early osteoarthritis. Deformity, if marked, should be corrected by tibial osteotomy.

Delayed union and non-union

High-energy fractures and fractures associated with bone loss or deep infection are slow to unite and liable to non-union. Bone grafting may solve some 'slow' unions; in others, a different mode of fixation may be needed.

Joint stiffness

Prolonged cast immobilization is liable to cause stiffness of the ankle and foot, which may persist for 12 months or longer in spite of active exercises. This can be avoided by changing to a functional brace as soon as it is safe to do so, usually by 4–6 weeks.

Complex regional pain syndrome (algodystrophy)

With distal-third fractures, algodystrophy is not uncommon. Exercises should be encouraged throughout the period of treatment. The management of established algodystrophy is discussed on page 362.

CHAPTER 33

INJURIES OF THE ANKLE AND FOOT

ANKLE LIGAMENT INJURIES

A sudden twist of the ankle momentarily tenses the structures around the joint. This may amount to no more than a painful wrenching of the soft tissues – a sprained ankle. If more severe force is applied, the ligaments may be strained to the point of rupture. If the tear is partial, healing is likely to restore full function to the joint; however, with complete tears, joint instability may persist.

More than 90% of ankle ligament injuries involve the lateral side – usually the anterior talofibular, or both this and the calcaneofibular ligament; only in the most severe injuries is the posterior talofibular ligament torn.

Special features

A history of a twisting injury followed by pain, bruising and swelling is typical. Tenderness is maximal just distal and slightly anterior to the lateral malleolus, and the slightest attempt at passive inversion of the ankle is extremely painful. *It is essential to examine the entire leg and foot: undisplaced fractures of the ankle, the more proximal fibula or the tarsal bones are easily missed.*

Imaging

About 15% of ankle sprains reaching the Emergency Department are associated with an ankle fracture. X-ray examination is called for if there is:

- Pain around the malleolus.
- Inability to take weight on the ankle immediately after the injury.
- Inability to take four steps in the Emergency Department.
- Bone tenderness at the posterior edge or tip of either of the malleoli or the base of the fifth metatarsal bone.

Treatment

Initial treatment consists of rest, ice, compression and elevation (RICE), which is continued for 1–3 weeks depending on the severity of the injury and the response to treatment. Cold compresses should be applied for about 20 minutes every 2 hours, and after any activity that exacerbates the symptoms.

The ankle may need to be protected (crutches, splint or brace) during a phased approach to mobilization and a supported return to function. An advice leaflet for patients is useful.

The use of non-steroidal anti-inflammatory drugs (NSAIDs) during the acute phase can be helpful; there is evidence that topical non-steroidal anti-inflammatory gels or creams might be as beneficial as oral preparations, probably carrying a better risk profile.

Functional treatment – i.e. protected mobilization without jeopardizing stability – provides earlier recovery of all grades of injury than either rigid immobilization or early operative treatment.

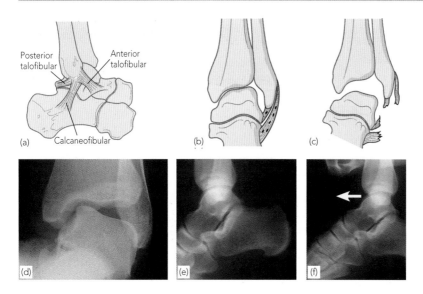

33.1 Ankle ligament injuries (a) The three components of the lateral collateral ligament of the ankle. (b) The commonest injury is a partial tear of one or other component of the lateral ligament. (c) Following a complete tear of the lateral ligament, the talus may be displaced in the ankle mortise. (d) Stress x-ray showing talar tilt. (e,f) X-rays demonstrating anteroposterior instability. Pulling the foot forward under the tibia causes the talus to shift appreciably at the ankle joint; this is usually seen after recurrent sprains.

Operative treatment may be needed if, despite physiotherapy, intrusive symptoms persist for more than 6 weeks. Residual complaints of ankle pain and stiffness, a sensation of instability or giving way and intermittent swelling are suggestive of cartilage damage or impinging scar tissue within the ankle. Arthroscopic repair or ligament substitution is effective in many cases, often allowing a return to full function and sports.

FRACTURES OF THE ANKLE

Fractures and fracture dislocations of the ankle are common. Most are low-energy fractures of one or both malleoli, usually caused by a twisting mechanism. Less common are the more severe fractures involving the tibial plafond – pilon fractures – which are high-energy injuries, often caused by a fall from a height.

The patient usually presents with a history of a 'twisted ankle', the joint typically turned into inversion, followed by immediate pain, swelling and difficulty weightbearing. Bruising often appears soon after injury.

The most obvious feature is a fracture of one or both malleoli; often, though, the 'invisible' part of the injury – rupture of one or more ligaments – is just as serious.

The management of all significant ankle injuries must take account of seven important elements: the fibula, the tibial malleolus, the tibiofibular syndesmosis, the medial collateral (deltoid) ligament, the lateral collateral ligaments, the tibial articular surface and the position of the talus.

As with most fractures, it is the extent of injury to the soft tissue envelope (skin, ligaments, capsule and tendons) that determines the early course of treatment and the eventual outcome.

Clinical features

Ankle fractures are typically seen in skiers, footballers and climbers. They also occur, as a result of much lesser force, in osteoporotic bone.

Following a twisting injury the patient complains of intense pain and inability to stand on the leg – symptoms suggesting something more serious than a simple 'sprain'. The ankle is swollen and deformity may be obvious, especially in a fracture–dislocation.

X-rays

The indications for x-ray examination in ankle injuries are discussed under ankle sprains above. The most obvious finding is a fracture of one or both malleoli; however, the 'invisible' part of the injury is just as important – rupture of the collateral and/or distal tibiofibular ligaments. Three views are advisable: anteroposterior, lateral and a 30-degree oblique projection facing the plane of the inferior tibiofibular joint (the 'mortise' view). Fracture lines should be looked for in both the anteroposterior and the lateral x-rays; separation (diastasis) of the tibiofibular joint is best displayed in the mortise view. Collateral ligament damage is suggested by displacement or tilting of the talus.

Two different but complementary classifications are employed in assessing these injuries. The *Lauge–Hansen classification* is based on the adduced mechanism of injury, which is useful in planning how to reduce the displaced fragments by reversing

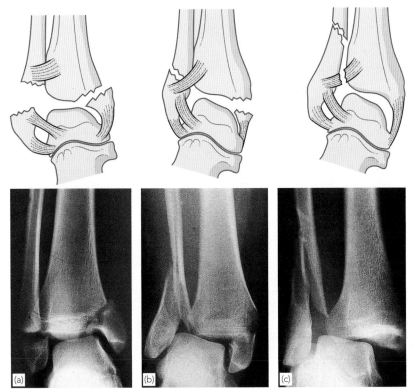

33.2 Ankle fractures – classification (a) The Danis–Weber classification is based on the level of the fibular fracture. (a) *Type A* – a fibular fracture below the tibiofibular syndesmosis and an oblique fracture of the medial malleolus. (b) *Type B* – a fracture at the syndesmosis, often associated with disruption of the anterior fibres of the tibiofibular ligament and fracture of the medial malleolus, or disruption of the medial ligament. (c) *Type C* – a fibular fracture above the syndesmosis; the tibiofibular ligament must be torn, producing an unstable fracture–subluxation of the ankle. Using the Lauge–Hansen classification, (a) would probably have been caused by forced supination and adduction of the foot; (b) by abduction of the ankle; and (c) by severe abduction and external rotation.

the injurious forces during manipulation of the ankle. The *Danis–Weber classification* focuses on the level of the fibular fracture: fractures distal to the tibiofibular joint generally leave the syndesmosis intact, whereas indirect fractures above that level must necessarily have damaged the syndesmotic ligaments. If the mortise becomes unstable, the talus can be displaced. Thus, careful interpretation of the x-rays is important for both diagnosis and treatment.

Principles of treatment

- Swelling is usually rapid and severe. If the injury is not dealt with within a few hours, definitive treatment may have to be deferred for several days while the leg is elevated so that the swelling can subside.
- As with all fractures involving a joint, the anatomy must be accurately restored and held until healing is complete. Residual displacement or incongruity of the joint will lead to focal stress on the articular surface and the gradual emergence of osteoarthritis.
- The key to congruity and stability of the joint is found in the level of the fibular fracture. If the fracture is below (distal to) the tibiofibular joint, the ankle will be stable once the malleolar

fractures are reduced and immobilized; non-operative treatment will often suffice.
- If the fibular fracture is above the level of the tibiofibular joint – even if the fracture appears on x-ray to be undisplaced – one must carefully assess for associated damage to the inferior tibiofibular ligaments and the medial components of the ankle joint. If there is no medial malleolar fracture, check carefully for signs of deltoid ligament disruption and displacement of the talus, as well as x-ray features of tibiofibular diastasis. When there is medial injury or significant fibular displacement then the fibular fracture is best stabilized by internal fixation. Diastasis should be reduced (if necessary under vision) and secured with a screw which transfixes the two bones, a 'diastasis screw'. Immediate postoperative x-ray examination is essential to ensure that the talus is correctly placed in the mortise; if it is laterally displaced (even slightly), the medial collateral ligament must be explored and any obstructing tissue removed.
- Isolated medial malleolar fractures, if undisplaced, can be managed by plaster immobilization for about 6 weeks. Displaced

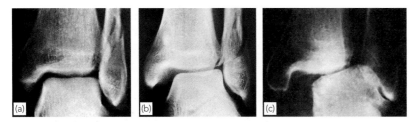

33.3 Stable and unstable ankle fractures It is very important to assess whether the fracture is stable or unstable. (a) This is a stable Type B fracture; after reduction, the ankle joint is symmetrically restored and the width of the joint space is regular both superiorly and medially. (b) In this case, although the fracture of the fibula appears to have been reduced, the medial joint space is abnormally widened, the talus is shifted slightly towards the lateral side and is also slightly tilted. The medial ligament must have been torn and may even be trapped in the medial side of the joint, so it is important to explore the medial side, release any obstructing tissue and position the talus correctly before accepting the reduction and immobilizing the ankle. (c) This is an obvious fracture–dislocation with rupture of the tibiofibular syndesmosis and severe damage to the medial collateral ligament. The fibula must be fixed to full length and the tibiofibular joint secured before the ankle can be stabilized.

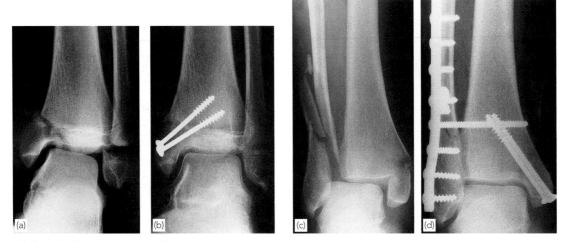

33.4 Ankle fractures – operative treatment (a,b) If the medial malleolar fragment involves a large segment of the articular surface, it is best treated by accurate open reduction and internal fixation with one or two screws. (c,d) An unstable fracture–dislocation almost always needs open reduction and internal fixation. The fibula must be restored to full length and fixed securely; in this case the medial malleolus also needed internal fixation. Because it is assumed that there was a partial disruption of the distal tibiofibular syndesmosis, a tibiofibular screw has been used to secure the diastasis until the ligaments heal (usually 12 weeks).

fractures should be accurately reduced and fixed with one or two screws. If the talus is shifted laterally, look for an associated fibular fracture; it may even be at the proximal end of the fibula, out of range of the ankle x-ray! Also check for tibiofibular diastasis, which may require open reduction and transverse screw fixation.

■ The same principles apply to bi-malleolar fractures and fracture–dislocations. Displaced fractures and fracture–dislocations require accurate reduction and internal fixation.

Postoperative management

The ankle and foot will be immobilized in a below-knee cast or supported in a special boot. The patient is often allowed to walk about, partial weightbearing with the aid of crutches. For stable, low-level fractures, the support can usually be discarded after 4–6 weeks and exercises are then encouraged. For unstable and operatively treated fractures, the cast may need to be retained for somewhat longer.

Complications

Joint stiffness

Swelling and stiffness of the ankle are usually the result of neglect in treatment of the soft tissues. The patient must walk correctly in plaster or support and, when the plaster is removed, he or she must, until circulatory control is regained, use a compression stocking and elevate the leg whenever it is not being used actively. Physiotherapy is key to recovery.

Complex regional pain syndrome

Long-lasting aching, recurrent swelling and regional osteoporosis are fairly common after ankle fractures. There is a spectrum from mild ache and swelling to intrusive or disabling pain, the established complex regional pain syndrome. The management of this condition is discussed on page 362.

Osteoarthritis

Malunion from incomplete reduction will eventually lead to secondary osteoarthritis of the ankle. Symptoms may not become intrusive for 10 or 15 years; however, in some cases (for reasons that are not clear), degenerative changes appear with alarming rapidity and patients may seek treatment within a year or two of the ankle injury.

COMMINUTED FRACTURES OF THE TIBIAL PLAFOND (PILON FRACTURES)

Severe axial compression of the ankle joint (e.g. in a fall from a height) may shatter the tibial plafond. There is considerable damage to the articular cartilage, and the subchondral bone may be broken into several pieces; in severe cases, the comminution extends some way up the shaft of the tibia.

Special features

Swelling is usually severe and fracture blisters are common.

X-rays

This appears as a comminuted fracture of the distal end of the tibia, extending into the ankle

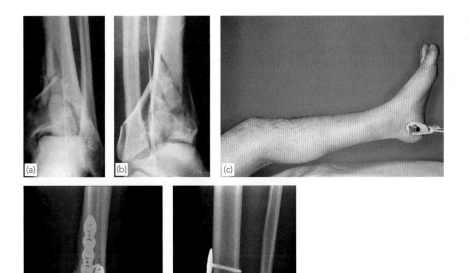

33.5 Pilon fracture of the ankle High-energy pilon fractures (a,b) carry a risk of wound breakdown and infection if treated by wide open reduction and plating. Conservative treatment (c) – traction and movement – is sometimes the best option. (d,e) Another case, treated by minimal approach reduction and internal fixation; 3 months after operation the fractures have healed and the joint is normally aligned.

457

joint. Sometimes the fibula also is fractured. The extent of the injury is usually not obvious in the plain x-rays; accurate definition of the fragments demands a computed tomography (CT) scan.

Treatment

The three points of early management are: *span, scan, plan*. Staged treatment has reduced the complication rate in these injuries.

Control of swelling is a priority; this is best achieved either by elevation or applying an external fixator across the ankle joint. It can take 3 weeks before the soft tissues improve and during this time blisters can be treated rather than hidden under a cast.

Once the skin has recovered, open reduction and fixation with plates and screws (usually with bone grafting) may be possible. However, the more severe injuries do not tolerate large surgical exposures for plating and significant wound breakdown and infection rates have been reported. Better results have followed indirect reduction techniques (applying a bone distractor or using the spanning fixator across the joint to obtain as much reduction as possible) and then plating through a limited exposure or using small screws to hold the articular fragments. Circular frame fixation has also been successful.

After fixation, elevation and early movement help to reduce the oedema; arteriovenous impulse devices applied to the sole of the foot are also helpful.

Outcome

Pilon fractures usually take several months to heal. Postoperatively, physiotherapy is focused on joint movement and reduction of swelling. Function is often impaired following these complex injuries. Although bony union may be achieved, the fate of the joint is decided by the degree of cartilage injury – the 'invisible' factor on x-rays. Secondary osteoarthritis, stiffness and pain are still frequent late complications.

ANKLE FRACTURES IN CHILDREN

Physeal injuries are quite common in children and almost one-third of these occur around the ankle (see page 331).

The foot is fixed to the ground or trapped in a crevice and the leg twists to one or other side. The tibial (or fibular) physis is wrenched apart, usually resulting in a Salter–Harris Type 1 or 2 fracture. Types 3 and 4 fractures are uncommon

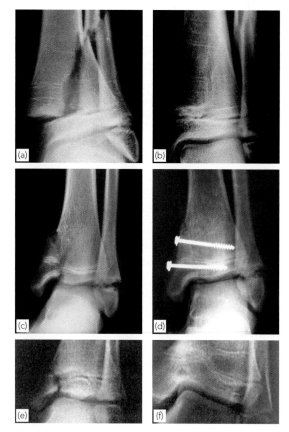

33.6 Physeal injuries (a) Fractures which do not break through the physis can be treated conservatively; after reduction (b) bone growth is normal. (c,d) This Type 4 fracture of the tibial physis was treated immediately by open reduction and internal fixation, giving an excellent result. (e,f) By contrast, in this case accurate reduction was not achieved and the physeal fragment remained displaced; the medial side of the physis fused prematurely, resulting in distorted growth.

but dangerous. The epiphysis is split vertically and one piece of the epiphysis may be displaced; if it is not accurately reduced, it will inevitably result in abnormal growth and deformity of the ankle.

Special features

Following a fracture, the ankle is painful, swollen, bruised and acutely tender.

X-rays

Undisplaced physeal fractures are easily missed. Even a hint of physeal widening should be regarded with great suspicion, and the x-ray examination must be repeated after 1 week.

Treatment

Salter–Harris Types 1 and 2 injuries are treated closed. If it is displaced, the fracture is gently reduced under general anaesthesia. The limb is immobilized in a full-length cast for 3 weeks and then in a below-knee walking cast for a further 3 weeks. Occasionally, surgery is needed to extract a periosteal flap which prevents adequate reduction.

Type 3 or 4 fractures, if undisplaced, can be treated in the same manner, but the ankle must be x-rayed again after 5 days to ensure that the fragments have not slipped. Displaced fractures should be reduced open and fixed with interfragmentary screws which are inserted parallel to the physis. Postoperatively, the leg is immobilized in a below-knee cast for 6 weeks.

Complications

Malunion

Imperfect reduction may result in angular deformity of the ankle – usually valgus. In children under 10 years old, mild deformities may be accommodated by further growth and modelling. In older children the deformity should be corrected by osteotomy.

Asymmetrical growth

Fractures through the epiphysis may result in fusion of the physis. The bony bridge is usually in the medial half of the growth plate; the lateral half goes on growing and the distal tibia gradually veers into varus. CT is helpful in showing where it is. If the bridge is small, it can be excised and replaced by a pad of fat in the hope that physeal growth may be restored. If more than half of the physis is involved, or the child is near the end of the growth period, supramalleolar osteotomy is indicated.

Shortening

Early physeal closure occurs in about 20% of children with distal tibial injuries. Fortunately, the resulting limb length discrepancy is usually mild. If it promises to be more than 2 cm and the child is young enough, proximal tibial epiphysiodesis in the opposite limb may restore equality.

INJURIES OF THE HINDFOOT

Injuries of the foot are apt to be followed by residual symptoms and loss of function which seem out of proportion to the initial trauma. Severe injuries affect the foot as a whole, whatever the particular bone that is fractured. In practice, the entire foot should be examined systematically, no matter that the injury may appear to be localized to one spot.

Multiple fractures, or combinations of fractures and dislocations, are easily missed. The circulation and nerve supply must be carefully assessed: a well-reduced fracture is a useless achievement if the foot becomes ischaemic or insensitive.

FRACTURE OF THE TALUS

Talar injuries are rare and due to considerable violence – car accidents or falls from a height. The injuries include fractures of the head, the neck, the body or the bony processes of the talus, dislocations of the talus or the joints around the talus, osteochondral fractures of the superior articular surface and a variety of chip or avulsion fractures.

Clinical features

The foot and ankle are painful and swollen; if the fracture is displaced, there may be an obvious deformity, or the skin may be tented or split. Tenting is a dangerous sign; if the fracture or dislocation is not promptly reduced, the skin may slough and become infected.

X-rays

Undisplaced fractures are not always easy to see, and sometimes even severely displaced fractures are missed because of unfamiliarity with the normal appearance in various x-ray projections. CT scanning is essential.

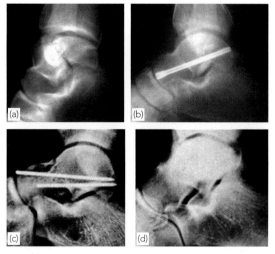

33.7 Fractures of the talus (a) This displaced fracture of the body of the talus was reduced and fixed with a counter-sunk screw (b) giving a perfect result. Fractures of the neck, even if well-reduced (c), are still at risk of developing avascular necrosis (d).

Treatment

When displacement is no more than trivial, reduction is not needed. A split plaster is applied and, when the swelling has subsided, is replaced by a complete plaster in the plantigrade position. This is retained for 6–8 weeks.

Displaced fractures and fracture–dislocations require urgent reduction. Closed manipulation is tried first, but should this fail, there must be no hesitation in performing open reduction. The reduced fracture can be stabilized with screws. A below-knee plaster is needed for 6–12 weeks. Weightbearing must be protected until the state of healing and the vascularity of the talus have been determined.

Complications

Avascular necrosis

Fractures of the neck of the talus often result in avascular necrosis (AVN) of the body (the posterior fragment). The risk of AVN depends on the degree of displacement of the fracture and the related joints. The fracture may fail to unite and the posterior half of the bone eventually collapses. The ankle may need to be arthrodesed.

FRACTURES OF THE CALCANEUM

The patient falls from a height, often from a ladder, onto one or both heels. The calcaneum is driven up against the talus and is split or crushed. More than 20% of these patients suffer associated injuries of the spine, pelvis or hip.

Extra-articular fractures involve the calcaneal processes or the posterior part of the bone. They are easy to manage and have a good prognosis. Treatment is 'closed' unless the fragment is large and badly displaced, in which case it will need to be fixed back in position.

Intra-articular fractures cleave the bone obliquely and run into the superior articular surface; secondary cracks cause further disruption of the bone. The articular facet is split apart and may be displaced into the body of the calcaneum; there may be severe comminution.

Special features

The foot is painful, swollen and bruised; the heel may look broad and squat. The tissues are thick and tender, and the normal concavity below the lateral malleolus is lacking. The subtalar joint cannot be moved but ankle movement is possible. Always check for signs of a compartment syndrome of the foot (intense pain, very extensive swelling and bruising and diminished sensation).

X-rays

Extra-articular fractures are usually fairly obvious. Intra-articular fractures, also, can often be identified in the plain films and, if there is displacement of the fragments, the lateral view may show flattening of Böhler's angle. However, for accurate definition of intra-articular fractures, CT is essential.

With severe injuries – and especially with bilateral fractures – *it is essential to assess the knees, the spine and the pelvis as well.*

Treatment

For all except the most minor injuries, the patient is admitted to hospital so that the leg and foot can be elevated and treated with ice-packs until the swelling subsides. This also gives time to obtain the necessary x-rays and CT scans.

Undisplaced fractures can be treated closed.

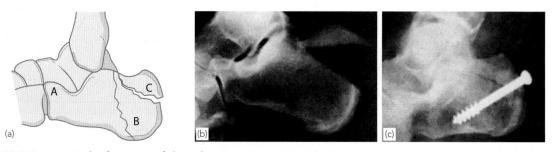

33.8 Extra-articular fractures of the calcaneum (a) Most extra-articular fractures occur through **A**, the anterior process, **B**, the body of calcaneum or **C**, the tuberosity. Sometimes the sustentaculum or the medial tubercle may fracture. (b) Avulsion fracture of the posterosuperior corner, which can be easily fixed by a screw (c).

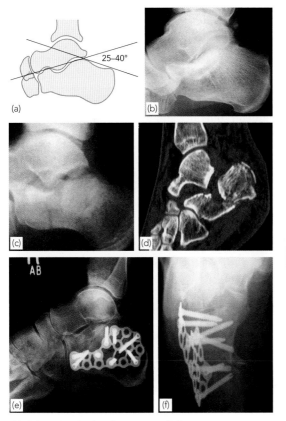

Complications

Broadening of the heel

This is quite common and may cause problems with shoe fitting as well as impingement affecting the peroneal tendons or the sural nerve.

Talocalcaneal stiffness and osteoarthritis

Displaced intra-articular fractures may lead to joint stiffness and, eventually, osteoarthritis. This can usually be managed conservatively, but persistent or severe pain may necessitate subtalar arthrodesis. If the calcaneocuboid joint is also involved, a triple arthrodesis (fusing the subtalar, calcaneocuboid and talonavicular joints) might be indicated.

MIDTARSAL INJURIES

Injuries in this area vary from minor sprains, often incorrectly labelled as 'ankle' sprains, to severe fracture–dislocations which can threaten the survival of the foot. Isolated injuries of the navicular, cuneiform or cuboid bones are rare. Fractures in this region should be assumed to be 'combination' fractures or fracture–subluxations until proved otherwise.

Clinical features

The foot is bruised and swollen. Tenderness is usually diffuse across the midfoot. A medial midtarsal dislocation looks like an 'acute club-foot' and a lateral dislocation produces a valgus deformity. It is important to exclude distal ischaemia or a compartment syndrome.

The extent of the bony injury is best determined by CT scans.

33.9 Intra-articular fractures of the calcaneum Fractures involving the talocalcaneal articular surface are serious injuries. (a,b) Normally the lateral x-ray of the calcaneum shows the superior surface raised at an angle (25–40 degrees) under the talus – *Böhler's angle*. Fracture of the articular surface may result in flattening of Böhler's angle (c). More information is derived from the CT scans (d). With accurate knowledge of the pathological anatomy, open reduction and internal fixation can be undertaken (e,f).

Exercises are encouraged from the outset. When the swelling subsides, a firm bandage is applied and the patient is allowed up, non-weightbearing on crutches for 6 weeks.

Displaced intra-articular fractures are best treated by open reduction and internal fixation with plates and screws. This is difficult surgery, which calls for complete familiarity with the local anatomy. Postoperatively, the foot is lightly splinted and elevated. Exercises are begun as soon as pain subsides and, after 2–3 weeks, the patient can be allowed up, non-weightbearing on crutches. Partial weightbearing is permitted only when the fracture has healed (seldom before 8 weeks), and full weightbearing about 4 weeks after that.

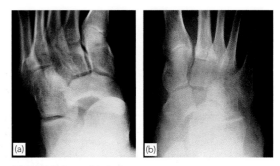

33.10 Midtarsal injuries (a) X-ray showing dislocation of the talonavicular joint. (b) X-ray of another patient showing longitudinal compression fracture of the navicular bone and subluxation of the head of the talus. This injury is often difficult to demonstrate accurately on plain x-ray.

Treatment

Ligamentous strains

The foot may be bandaged until acute pain subsides; thereafter, movement is encouraged. If symptoms do not settle, suspect (and investigate for) a missed fracture!

Undisplaced fractures

The foot is elevated to counteract swelling. After 3 or 4 days, a below-knee cast or similar support is applied and the patient is allowed up on crutches with limited weightbearing. The support is retained for 6 weeks.

Fracture–dislocations

These are severe injuries. Under general anaesthesia, the dislocation can usually be reduced by closed manipulation, but holding it is a problem. If there is the least tendency to re-displacement, Kirschner wires (K-wires) or screws are run across the joints to fix them in position. The foot is immobilized in a below-knee cast for 6–12 weeks. Exercises are then begun and should be practised assiduously; it may be 6–8 months before function is regained.

TARSOMETATARSAL INJURIES

Sprains are quite common but dislocation is rare; twisting and crushing injuries are the usual causes. *A fracture–dislocation should always be suspected if the patient has pain, swelling and bruising of the foot after an accident, even if there is no obvious deformity.*

X-rays

A fracture–dislocation is unlikely to be missed on x-ray examination, but the full extent of the injury is seldom clear on the plain x-ray. CT is the investigation of choice for bony and articular injury, although subtle ligamentous injury will be better seen on a magnetic resonance imaging (MRI) scan. Whether or not the talonavicular joint is dislocated, always look carefully for fractures of the navicular or cuneiform bones, which are more difficult to reduce and hold.

Treatment

Undisplaced sprains require cast immobilization for 4–6 weeks. Subluxation or dislocation calls for accurate reduction. Traction and manipulation under anaesthesia achieves reduction (open reduction is rarely needed); the position is then held with K-wires or screws and cast immobilization. A new cast is applied after the swelling has subsided and the patient is instructed to remain non-weightbearing for 6–12 weeks.

METATARSAL FRACTURES

Metatarsal fracture may be caused by a direct blow, by a severe twisting injury or by repetitive stress. In the usual case there is a history of injury and the foot is painful and somewhat swollen. X-ray examination will show the fracture.

Treatment

A walking plaster may be applied, mainly for comfort, and is retained for 3 weeks. The fracture unites readily.

In the unlikely event of severe displacement, reduction and fixation, possibly just temporary, may be justified. In that case, weightbearing is avoided for 3 weeks and this is followed by a further 3 weeks in a weightbearing cast.

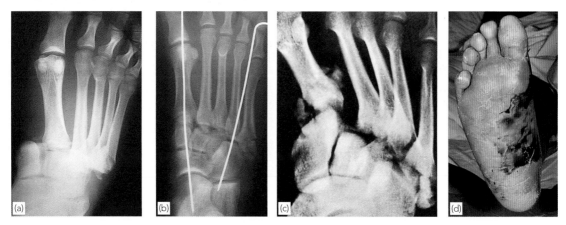

33.11 Tarsometatarsal injuries (a) Dislocation of the tarsometatarsal joints. (b) X-ray after reduction and stabilization with Kirschner wires. (c) X-ray showing a high-energy fracture–dislocation involving the tarsometatarsal joints. These are serious injuries which may be complicated by (d) compartment syndrome of the foot.

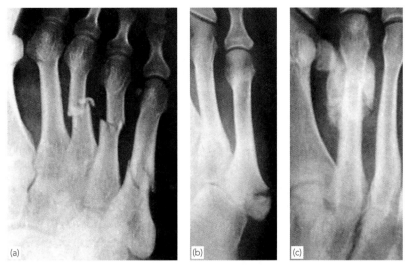

33.12 Metatarsal injuries
(a) Transverse and oblique fractures of three metatarsal shafts. (b) Avulsion fracture of the base of the fifth metatarsal. (c) Florid callus and periosteal new bone formation around the second metatarsal shaft – the classic sign of a stress fracture.

(a) (b) (c)

STRESS INJURY (MARCH FRACTURE)

In a young adult (particularly a new army recruit or a sportsperson) the foot may become painful after over-use. A tender lump is palpable just distal to the mid-shaft of a metatarsal bone, usually the second. The x-ray appearance may at first be normal, but a radio-isotope scan will show an area of intense activity in the bone. MRI also may show stress changes in the bone. Later a hairline crack may be visible, and later still a mass of callus or periosteal new bone is seen, usually 3 weeks or more after the onset of symptoms.

No displacement occurs and neither reduction nor splintage is necessary. The forefoot may be supported and normal walking is encouraged.

FRACTURED TOES

A heavy object falling on the toes may fracture phalanges. If the skin is broken, it must be covered with a sterile dressing. The fracture is disregarded and the patient encouraged to walk in a suitably adapted boot. However, if pain is marked, the toe can be splinted by strapping it to its neighbour for 2–3 weeks.

FRACTURED SESAMOIDS

One of the sesamoids (usually the medial) may fracture from either a direct injury (landing from a height on the ball of the foot) or sudden traction; chronic, repetitive stress is more often seen in dancers and runners.

The patient complains of pain directly over the sesamoid. There is a tender spot in the same area and sometimes pain can be exacerbated by passively hyperextending the big toe. X-rays will usually show the fracture (which must be distinguished from a smooth-edged bi-partite sesamoid).

Treatment is often unnecessary, though a local injection of lignocaine helps for pain. If discomfort is marked, the foot can be immobilized in a short-leg walking cast for 2–3 weeks. Occasionally, intractable symptoms call for excision of the offending ossicle.

INDEX